Exotic Animal Medicine
for the
Veterinary Technician

Exotic Animal Medicine
for the
Veterinary Technician

Edited by
Bonnie Ballard, D.V.M.
and Ryan Cheek, R.V.T.

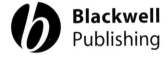

Blackwell Publishing

Dr. Bonnie Ballard has worked in veterinary medicine since 1974, starting as a veterinary assistant, becoming a technician in 1979, and earning a DVM in 1994. In 1997, she began to develop the veterinary technology program at Gwinnett Technical College. The program received full AVMA program accreditation in 2000. Dr. Ballard currently is the program's director and one of two full time faculty members. She also practices small animal and exotic medicine at Winder Animal Hospital in Winder, Georgia.

Ryan Cheek graduated from Gwinnett Technical College in 1999 with an AAT in veterinary technology. After completing an internship at the ZooAtlanta Veterinary Hospital, he went to work at Avalon Animal Hospital in Lawrenceville, Georgia. He also holds a part-time faculty position at Gwinnett Technical College, where he is a lab assistant and teaches exotic animal medicine. Mr. Cheek enjoys keeping reptiles and teaching children about them.

©2003 Iowa State Press
A Blackwell Publishing Company
All rights reserved

Blackwell Publishing Professional
2121 State Avenue, Ames, Iowa 50014

Orders: 1-800-862-6657
Office: 1-515-292-0140
Fax: 1-515-292-3348
Web site: www.blackwellprofessional.com

Printed on acid-free paper in India

First edition, 2003

Library of Congress Cataloging-in-Publication Data

Ballard, Bonnie M.
  Exotic animal medicine for the veterinary technician / Bonnie M. Ballard, Ryan Cheek.—1st ed.
      p. cm.
Includes bibliographical references and index.
  ISBN-13: 978-0-8138-1928-0
  ISBN-10: 0-8138-1928-8 (alk. paper)
  1. Exotic animals—Diseases. 2. Wildlife diseases. 3. Pet medicine. 4. Veterinary nursing.
  [DNLM: 1. Animal Diseases. 2. Animal Technicians. 3. Animals, Wild. 4. Veterinary Medicine. SF 774.5 B189e 2003]
I. Cheek, Ryan. II. Title.
  SF997.5.E95B35 2003
  636.089′073—dc21003004794

The last digit is the print number: 9 8 7 6 5 4 3

Contents

Contributors

Bonnie Ballard has worked in veterinary medicine since 1974, starting as a veterinary assistant, becoming a technician in 1979, and earning a DVM in 1994. In 1997, she began to develop the veterinary technology program at Gwinnett Technical College. The program received full AVMA program accreditation in 2000. Dr. Ballard currently is the program's director and one of two full time faculty members. She also practices small animal and exotic medicine at Winder Animal Hospital in Winder, Georgia.

Denise I. Bounous, DVM, PhD, Diplomate ACVP, was a professor of clinical pathology at the University of Georgia College of Veterinary Medicine before her move into the pharmaceutical industry. Her academic interests included avian and reptilian clinical pathology, and her research was in avian immunomodulation.

Ryan Cheek graduated from Gwinnett Technical College in 1999 with an AAT in veterinary technology. After completing an internship at the ZooAtlanta Veterinary Hospital, he went to work at Avalon Animal Hospital in Lawrenceville, Georgia. He also holds a part-time faculty position at Gwinnett Technical College, where he is a lab assistant and teaches exotic animal medicine. Mr. Cheek enjoys keeping reptiles and teaching children about them.

Cheryl B. Greenacre, DVM, Diplomate ABVP–Avian, graduated from the University of Georgia in 1991 and taught there before moving to the University of Tennessee in July 2001. Besides helping clients with their pets and teaching veterinary students, interns, and residents, she has also codeveloped a "high sensitivity" total T_4 test for use in birds and snakes and is currently studying the use of synthetic TSH on birds.

Melanie Haire, VMT, received an AS degree in veterinary technology from Wilson College and worked in an Atlanta small animal clinic following graduation. She has spent the last decade on the staff of ZooAtlanta where she is the senior veterinary technician and serves as the hospital manager. She is federally licensed to rehabilitate migratory bird species and raptors and has a state DNR permit to rehabilitate rabies vector species. She is on the board of directors of the Rockdale County Animal Control and the Atlanta Wild Animal Rescue Effort (AWARE), a wildlife rehabilitation organization in metro Atlanta.

Anne E. Hudson, LVT, LAT, graduated from Blue Ridge Community College with an AAS in veterinary technology and received AALAS certification. She has worked as a biological laboratory technician for the Department of Defense's Clinical Investigation and Research Department. She teaches veterinary assisting to high school students interested in pursuing careers in the veterinary field.

Michael J. Huerkamp, DVM, Diplomate ACLAM, earned his DVM from the Ohio State University and did postdoctoral training in the specialty of laboratory animal medicine at the University of Michigan. He is a diplomate of the American College of Laboratory Animal Medicine (ACLAM). He is an associate professor of laboratory animal medicine and pathology in the Emory University School of Medicine where he also serves as director of the Division of Animal Resources. Dr. Huerkamp has eighteen years of experience in the medical care and management of laboratory animals including rabbits.

Michael Duffy Jones, DVM, received a BS from Notre Dame and his DVM from Tufts University. He completed an internship at Georgia Veterinary Specialists. He is on the staff at Bells Ferry Veterinary Hospital and has a particular interest in the use of ultrasound as a diagnostic tool, which he uses regularly in his practice and which he teaches other veterinarians.

Trevor Lyon, RVT, graduated from Maple Woods Community College with an AA in veterinary technology. Focusing on internal medicine, he has lectured at several veterinary conferences around the country. He is a technician supervisor at Bells Ferry Veterinary Hospital. He has worked with wildlife rehabilitation programs and participated in programs to educate the public about wildlife.

Julie Mays, LVT, graduated from Snead State Community College with an AA in veterinary technology. She is on the staff of Bells Ferry Veterinary Hospital where she has concentrated on exotic animal medicine and surgery.

James R. McClearen, DVM, graduated from the University of Georgia with a BS in agriculture. He received his DVM from the University of Georgia College of Veterinary Medicine, where he worked for several years in raptor rehabilitation. He is the owner and a practicing veterinarian at Bells Ferry Veterinary Hospital, which opened in 1984. He was one of only two veterinarians in the Atlanta area who routinely saw exotic species at that time. His practice today provides services for small animals, wildlife, and exotic animals.

Shannon Richards, CAT, is a licensed veterinary technician at ZooAtlanta. She operates a reptile and amphibian rescue and is also active in the community, providing educational programs related to these wonderful creatures.

Samuel Rivera, DVM, graduated from Kansas State University College of Veterinary Medicine. He later received a master of science in veterinary pathobiology. He has been practicing in an avian and exotic practice for the past six years and is also a contract veterinarian for ZooAtlanta.

Brad Wilson, DVM, is a veterinarian and partner in two private practice veterinary clinics in north Atlanta. He received his BS in zoology and his DVM from the University of Georgia. He is the consulting veterinarian for the largest wholesale importer and distributor of fish, reptiles, amphibians, pocket pets, ferrets, and birds in north Georgia as well as for the Atlanta Botanical Garden, which has an extensive collection of dendrobatid and Central and South American hylid frogs. He has personally maintained and captively bred many species of snakes and frogs.

Preface

This book was written to provide the veterinary technician with important information about a variety of species commonly seen in exotic practice. This text would be beneficial to the technician who would like to work with these animals but may have graduated years ago before this area of medicine was popular. This text would also be helpful to the technician who works for a veterinarian who would like to add exotic species to his or her practice. While it was not written for veterinarians, they may find it beneficial as well.

With the help of this book, the technician will know what questions to ask to obtain an adequate history, be able to educate the client about husbandry and nutrition, be able to safely handle and restrain common species, and be able to perform necessary procedures when needed. Because the field of exotic animal medicine is a dynamic one, new knowledge is constantly emerging about many of the species kept as pets and new information can in some cases contradict what was thought to be true before. For many species, exotic animal medicine could be said to be in its infancy. For this reason it is essential that those interested in exotics keep up with the latest information. This is best accomplished by attending national conferences where the leaders in this field speak. We realize that for some of the species featured in this book, the information presented may need to be modified in the future.

While some of the contributors provided drug dosages and formularies, we do not take responsibility for what is provided. We also realize that while technicians do not make decisions about what drugs to use in any animal, they are required to be familiar with different pharmaceuticals, know where to find a dosage, and know how to calculate it.

This book was written with the assumption that the technician already is educated in anatomy, physiology, medical terminology, pathology, and pharmacology. Only what is unique to the species featured is presented.

Because what we know about exotic animal medicine is forever changing and much has not been scientifically proven, it is common to find contradicting information from one reputable source to the next. This can create frustration but also provide the challenge of working in a cutting edge area of medicine.

Dedication

In memory of Dr. Stephen M. Soloway—
teacher, mentor, clinician, friend

Acknowledgments

Thank you to all of our contributors, who had the same vision as we did about this book. All wanted it to be the best of its kind and I believe it is. Thank you to Paige Tharpe, RVT, for proofreading the manuscript. I also want to thank my husband, David, who has the patience of a saint, for helping with proofreading and frustrating computer problems.

I appreciate the patience and understanding of my friends and family who heard "I have to work on the book" for way too long! Finally, I would like to thank Ryan for coming up with the idea for this book, born back in the fall of 1999, and keeping me calm through the whole process.

Bonnie Ballard

This book would not have been possible without the help and support of my friends Melissa, Jenny, Lee, Trish, and Desiree, and my family. They motivated me to start on this long and tiresome project and then stood by me with the much-needed support to finish. Also, a big thank you to all of my fellow coworkers at Avalon Animal Hospital and Georgia Veterinary Specialists for allowing me the time off needed to finish this book.

Ryan Cheek

Disclaimer

As exotic animal dosages are based largely on empirical data and not researched facts, the editors and contributors make no guarantee regarding the results obtained from dosages used in this textbook.

Exotic Animal Medicine
for the
Veterinary Technician

CHAPTER ONE

The Role of Veterinary Technicians in Exotic Animal Medicine

Bonnie M. Ballard

Welcome to the world of exotic animal medicine! For those who practice it, it is the variety that provides the spice to veterinary life. In a practice that sees exotics, it would not be uncommon to see a dog for vaccines, a diabetic cat, an iguana with metabolic bone disease, a ferret for a physical examination, a rabbit with hair loss, and a feather-picking cockatoo all in one day. The challenge for those in this field lies in the vast differences in the species seen (fig. 1.1).

In the world of veterinary medicine, an exotic animal is any animal that isn't the dog, cat, horse, or cow. Exotic animals include wildlife species, animals commonly used in research that are kept as pets, and animals native to various regions of the world, such as South America, Australia, and Africa.

There are several scenarios in which a technician faced with exotics may find this book helpful. A technician might take a job in a practice where exotics are seen but knows little about them because graduation happened before exotics became as popular as they are now. This book will help that person get up to speed with what he or she needs to know about popular exotic species. A technician may work for a veterinarian who wants to add exotics to the practice but

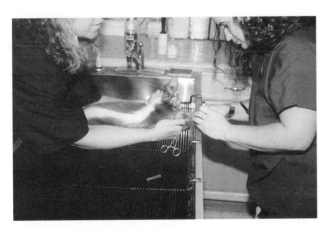

Fig. 1.1. *A technician drawing blood from a skunk. (Photo courtesy of Ryan Cheek)*

doesn't have hands-on experience with them. Alternatively, a technician may find employment at a zoological park or work with a wildlife rehabilitator and wants to brush up on current ideas about exotics. While this book does not cover zoo species specifically, knowledge of exotic animals, their treatment, and their care is desirable in the zoo environment.

For a technician who works for a veterinarian who would like to add exotics to the practice, it is essential that the technician help the veterinarian understand how the practice will need to change to accommodate these species. One must accept the fact that a fifteen or twenty minute appointment will not suffice. In many cases appointments of thirty minutes or longer will be required. Because husbandry and nutrition are typically the two most common causes of illness in exotics, a thorough history in these areas is essential. Also, because of the delicate nature of some of the species seen, more time may be required to perform a physical examination. In many cases the owner will require client education to keep his or her pet healthy, so adequate time to do so will be required.

While the average animal hospital will have most of the necessary equipment needed to treat exotics, there are some items that a clinic will need to purchase. For example, a gram scale will be required to weigh many of the very small patients. Microtainer blood collection tubes are also essential. Appendix 12 provides a list of equipment useful in exotic practices.

The role of the technician in exotic animal medicine is the same as the technician's role in small or large animal medicine. One of the most important roles is that of a meticulous history taker. As each chapter illustrates, a simple history will not do. Detailed questions must be asked about how and where the pet was acquired. Wild-caught species can have different health problems than captive-raised ones. How the pet is housed is vitally important, and this means not only asking what it is housed in but the cage size, construction, substrate used, and where it is kept in the house. If the animal is not brought in the cage it is

3

housed in, the technician, after gathering the history, should be able to create a mental picture of what the cage at home looks like.

The same is true for gathering adequate information about the pet's diet. It is not good enough to ask what is fed as what is fed may not be what is consumed. For example, an owner may report that his or her Amazon parrot's daily diet is made up of fruits, vegetables, and seeds. When asked how much of each is consumed each day, the answer may be mostly seeds, which is an inadequate diet.

In many cases, owners of exotics may have been misinformed about their pet's care from the pet shop where it was purchased. While some may, many pet shop employees simply do not know the correct information about the species they sell. Also an owner may have read information from a less than reputable source. The veterinary technician should be able to give owners the correct information about husbandry and nutrition without chastising them for their mistakes. Many honestly may not know that what they were doing was wrong. Owners may have obtained books that are not written by reputable sources or found information on the Internet that is inaccurate. Clients value information on how to keep their pets healthy and their veterinary clinic should be the source of that information.

The technician can also be of value when helping a client make a decision about what type of exotic pet to buy. For example, an iguana is considered to be a difficult reptile to keep as its housing and nutrition requirements are demanding. A bearded dragon may be a better choice. A parakeet may be a better choice for a first-time bird owner than a macaw, which can be noisy and messy. The topic of conservation of species is important here as well. New exotic pet owners should be encouraged to acquire captive-raised species rather than wild-caught if possible. With many exotic species, numbers in the wild are diminishing. This is especially true of many of the avian species. Most exotic species desired as pets can be obtained from captive-raised sources.

One should never underestimate the strength of the human-animal bond that exists between owners and their exotic pets. An owner can be as bonded to a mouse or a snake as another owner would be to a dog or horse. Just as one should never assume what an owner is willing to spend for medical care on dogs,

cats, and horses, one should never assume what exotic pet owners would be willing to spend for their pets. It is not uncommon to see a devoted owner spend hundreds of dollars for a surgical procedure for a pet rat.

Some veterinary practices that see exotic pets will see primates and venomous species. Because of the dangers to humans from these animals, veterinarians will typically set the "rules of engagement" regarding the care and treatment of these animals. For example the veterinarian may only see a primate or a venomous snake after hours when all employees and clients are gone. Likewise a veterinarian may require that an owner of a venomous snake provide in date antivenin along with the snake.

Some veterinarians will not see large exotic cats in practice due to safety concerns. And yes, there are people who have permits to keep them! Others will see these animals on the owner's premises as long as handling equipment, such as squeeze cages, is provided. It will be important that all employees know the clinic's protocol for seeing primates, venomous species, and large cats.

Every state has different laws regarding which species are legal to keep as pets and which are not. It is up to the veterinarian to decide whether he or she will see pets that may in fact be illegal pets, and to communicate this information to the technicians and other staff.

Continuing education is an important part of a graduate technician's professional enhancement, and its importance in exotic medicine cannot be overemphasized. What is known about the care and treatment of exotic animals is forever changing as more and more is learned. What one may have heard is the proper diet for a particular lizard one year may be something different the next year. More and more drugs are being tried in exotics. This type of cutting-edge information is often presented at conferences and in professional publications. This presents an added challenge to practices that see exotic animals as information is forever changing.

In response to this challenge, we have assembled here for the veterinary technician a survey of the most recent practices in the area of exotic animal care. Exotic animal medicine provides a veterinary technician with the opportunity to utilize all of his or her skills and knowledge in a way that has a direct benefit to the practice and to the patients. Enjoy!

CHAPTER TWO

The Avian Patient

Cheryl B. Greenacre

TAXONOMY AND COMMON SPECIES SEEN IN PRACTICE

The class Aves consists of over 8,500 different species of birds. Among the 27 orders of birds, 2 are commonly kept as pets in the United States: the Psittaciformes (parrots) and the Passeriformes (canaries and finches) (Forshaw & Cooper 1989). (See table 2.1.) Other orders such as Columbiformes (pigeons), Anseriformes (ducks), Galliformes (chickens), Falconiformes (hawks), and Strigiformes (owls) may also be encountered in a clinical practice (King & McLelland 1984).

BEHAVIOR OF SELECTED SPECIES

General Information

All statements regarding behavior of the selected species are generalizations and consideration should be given for individual behavioral differences that may have been molded by environment and experiences. For example, African grey parrots are good talkers and can mimic sounds extremely well, but not all African grey parrots will talk. Also, an aggressive individual bird might be encountered in a species generally known for its nice disposition, and vice versa.

Psittacines

African Grey Parrots

African grey parrots are considered to be very intelligent and subsequently become bored easily. They may feather pick (a behavioral problem, not unlike nail biting and hair twirling/pulling in humans). They are known for their talking and mimicking abilities and playfulness, but can be high strung, require attention and tend to form individual bonds (Perry 1994).

Amazon Parrots

Amazon parrots are very playful, boisterous, independent birds. They are generally extroverts, many with excellent talking abilities. Also, they tend to form individual bonds (Perry 1994).

Budgerigars

Budgerigars (also known as budgies, parakeets) are an excellent choice for a first-time bird owner since a bite from them is relatively harmless, and they are playful, intelligent, and inexpensive to purchase. Also they are nondestructive, gentle, and relatively quiet (Perry 1994). They do have the ability to talk.

Cockatiels

Cockatiels are an excellent choice for a first-time bird owner since a bite from them is relatively harmless, and they are playful and intelligent. Also they are nondestructive, gentle, and relatively quiet (Perry 1994).

Cockatoos

In general, cockatoos are very cuddly, gentle, intelligent birds, but are needy, requiring a great deal of attention. Cockatoos, being dependent on their human family for reassurance, are thought to feather pick primarily due to separation anxiety, but further studies are needed to elucidate the many causes of feather picking in birds (Perry 1994). See color plate 2.1.

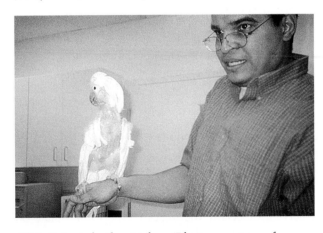

Plate 2.1. *A feather picker. (Photo courtesy of Dr. Sam Rivera) (See also color plates)*

Table 2.1. *Examples of Common Species of Birds Encountered in Practice*

Common name	Scientific name	Color plate number
Cockatoo		
Moluccan	*Cacutua moluccensis*	
Umbrella*	*Cacatua alba*	2.9
Sulfur-crested	*Cacatua sulphurea*	
Macaw		
Blue and gold*	*Ara ararauna*	2.10
Scarlet	*Ara macao*	2.11
Hyacinth	*Anodorhynchus hyacinthinus*	2.12
Military	*Ara militaris*	2.13
Green-winged	*Ara chloroptera*	
Amazon parrot		
Yellow-naped*	*Amazona ochrocephala*	2.14
Red-lored	*Amazona autumnalis*	
Orange-winged	*Amazona amazonica*	
Double yellow-headed	*Amazona ochrocephala*	
Blue-fronted	*Amazona aestiva*	2.15
Mexican red-headed	*Amazona viridigenalis*	
Lory, Rainbow	*Trichoglossus haematodus*	
Conure		
Blue-crowned	*Aratinga acuticaudata*	
Sun	*Aratinga solstitialis*	
Half-moon	*Aratinga canicularis*	
Maroon (Red)-bellied	*Pyrrhura frontalis*	
Nanday	*Nandayus nenday*	
Green-cheeked	*Pyrrhura molinae*	
Mitred	*Aratinga mitrata*	
Lovebird, Peach-faced	*Agapornis rosicollis*	
Cockatiel*	*Nymphicus hollandicus*	
Parakeet		
Standard budgie*	*Melopsittacus undulates*	
Grey-cheeked	*Brotogeris pyrrhopterus*	
Quaker (Monk)	*Myiopsitta monachus*	
Finch		
Zebra	*Poephila castanotis*	
Lady Gouldian	*Poephila gouldiae*	
Parrot		
African grey*	*Psittacus erithacus*	2.16
Eclectus	*Eclectus roratus*	

Source: Forshaw & Cooper (1989).
*Most commonly encountered species.

Conures
Conures are known for their playfulness but can be quite noisy (Perry 1994).

Eclectus Parrots
Eclectus parrots are not playful and are generally reserved, especially the males (Perry 1994). They do have the ability to talk.

Lories
Lories are playful and noisy, but messy due to a fruit diet, which causes their stool to be liquid and projectile (Perry 1994).

Lovebirds
Lovebirds are usually playful and nondestructive, but they can be aggressive (Perry 1994).

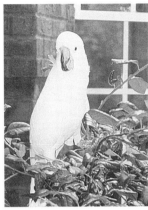

Plate 2.9

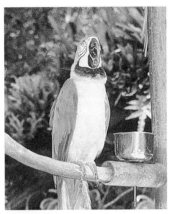

Plate 2.10

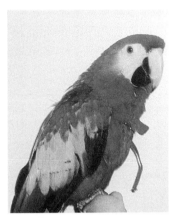

Plate 2.11

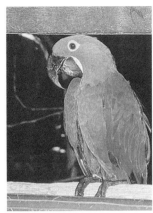

Plate 2.12

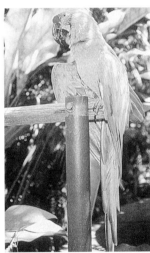

Plate 2.13

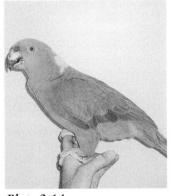

Plate 2.14

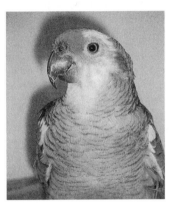

Plate 2.15

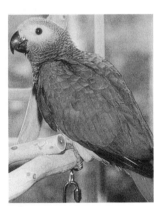

Plate 2.16

Plate 2.9. Umbrella cockatoo. (Photo courtesy of Cherie Fox) (See also color plates)

Plate 2.10. Blue and gold macaw. (Photo courtesy of Cherie Fox) (See also color plates)

Plate 2.11. Scarlet macaw. (Photo courtesy of Dr. Sam Rivera) (See also color plates)

Plate 2.12. Hyacinth macaw. (Photo courtesy of Cherie Fox) (See also color plates)

Plate 2.13. Military macaw. (Photo courtesy of Cherie Fox) (See also color plates)

Plate 2.14. Yellow-naped amazon. (Photo courtesy of Dr. Sam Rivera) (See also color plates

Plate 2.15. Blue-fronted amazon. (Photo courtesy of Dr. Sam Rivera) (See also color plates)

Plate 2.16. Congo African grey. (Photo courtesy of Cherie Fox) (See also color plates)

Macaws

Macaws are intelligent and require a great amount of attention. Being the largest of the parrots, they can be quite destructive and noisy (Perry 1994).

Passerines

Canaries and Finches

Canaries and finches are flighty and easily stressed. They are therefore not usually handled, but are admired from afar (Perry 1994).

ANATOMY AND PHYSIOLOGY

Birds are anatomically and physiologically different from mammals in many respects, and usually these differences are related to an adaptation that enables flight or hatching from an egg.

Integumentary System

Birds have skin that is thinner than mammals requiring smaller suture (4-0 to 5-0). They have feathers for flight and insulation. They usually have only one gland, the uropygial (preen) gland at the base of the tail.

Musculoskeletal System

Birds have 8–25 cervical vertebrae (rather than the usual 7 of mammals) and a very flexible neck.

There is fusing of bones in the spine to form the notarium and synsacrum for greater stability, and fusing of bones of the wing and leg to decrease weight. In addition, there is fusing of the caudal vertebrae to form the pygostyle to support the tail. A keel along the sternum provides for attachment of the large pectoral (flight) muscles. Birds have pneumatic (air-filled) bones to decrease weight. A coracoid bone between the sternum and thoracic girdle helps enable flight. The avian skeletal system is shown in figure 2.1.

Cardiovascular/Lymphatic System

Birds have a relatively large heart when compared to mammals. Lymph tissue and vessels exist, but lymph nodes are absent. The renal-portal system (that system in which blood from caudal half of body can go to the kidney before going to the heart) exists in these patients. It is important to note not to administer injectable medications, especially those that are toxic to the kidneys, in the caudal part of the body such as the leg, since the kidney could eliminate the medication before it could benefit the bird or the kidney

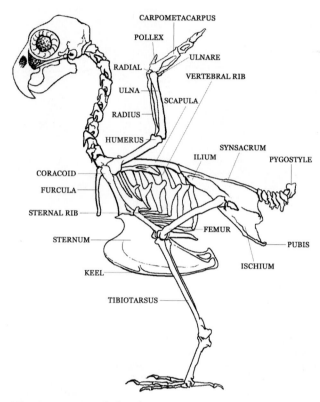

Fig. 2.1. *Avian skeletal anatomy. (Drawing by Scott Stark)*

could sustain damage from being exposed to concentrated medication.

The right jugular vein is larger than the left jugular vein. A phlebotomy is generally performed on the right jugular vein in parrots for this reason.

Renal System

Mammalian and reptilian type nephrons are present, therefore birds produce liquid urine and pasty white urates. Note that kidney function in birds is not measured by BUN and creatinine levels, but by levels of uric acid.

Respiratory System

Birds have a relatively large trachea compared to mammals, therefore they are easy to intubate (fig. 2.2). Their "voice box" is called a syrinx and is located at the bifurcation of the trachea, near the heart. Birds lack a diaphragm, therefore the sternum must be able to move up and down or suffocation can occur.

Air sacs store and warm air, and act as a bellows for moving air through the lungs. They are approximately ten times more efficient at oxygen exchange than mammals. Like mammals, gas exchange occurs in the

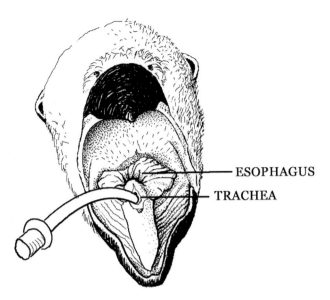

Fig. 2.2. *Oral cavity/intubation. (Drawing by Scott Stark)*

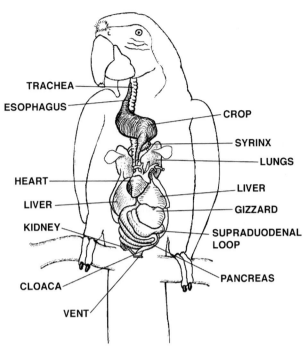

Fig. 2.3. *Avian viscera. (Drawing by Scott Stark)*

lungs, but unlike mammals, oxygen exchange occurs on both expiration and inspiration.

Digestive System

Birds have a beak and no teeth. An out-pouching of esophagus called the crop is used to store food. The esophagus is on the right side of the bird's neck with the crop also located on the right side of the bird's neck at the level of the thoracic inlet.

The proventriculus is the true glandular stomach of the bird. The ventriculus (gizzard) is used for grinding food.

The cloaca is where the reproductive, gastrointestinal, and urinary tracts meet and end before exiting the bird. Avian viscera are shown in figure 2.3.

Reproductive System

Most female birds have one functional ovary (on the left). Male have two testis and a rudimentary fold of tissue called a phallus instead of a penis.

Biologic and Reproductive Data

There is no such thing as a "generic" bird, meaning that different species of birds can have very different biological values. Therefore, it is important to identify the species of bird being evaluated and make comparisons using reference ranges of the same species whenever possible.

Heart Rate and Respiratory Rate

Typically, the smaller the bird the faster the heart rate and respiratory rate. See table 2.2.

Longevity

The average inbred budgie or cockatiel on an all-seed diet lives approximately 5 to 7 years, however some individuals have lived to as old as 18 years. Cockatoos, African grey parrots, macaws, and

Table 2.2. *Representative Heart and Respiratory Rates for Various Species of Birds*

Species	Weight (grams)	HR (rest)	HR (restraint)	RR (rest)	RR (restraint)
Cockatiel	100	200	500–600	40–52	60–80
Amazon	400	150	200–350	25–30	40–60
Macaw	1000	125	150–350	15–20	25–40

Source: Ritchie, Harrison, & Harrison (1994).
Note: HR = heart rate, RR = respiratory rate.

Amazon parrots can live much longer: 40, 50, 50, and 80 years, respectively. On an all-seed diet, these larger parrots do not live much past 15 years of age, due to chronic malnutrition.

Reproductive Activity

The smaller species, such as cockatiels, can be reproductively active as early as 6 months of age, whereas larger species, such as macaws, may not be reproductively active until over 3 years of age (Joyner 1994). Cockatiels are prolific breeders, and females can lay many eggs even in the absence of a male bird. Commonly, egg-laying female cockatiels on a seed diet become egg bound, requiring emergency medical assistance.

Egg Incubation

Many aviaries are present in the United States and are now sustaining the population of parrots for the pet market since the ban on importation of parrots into this country began in the early 1990s. Some aviculturists allow the parent birds to incubate the eggs and then remove the neonates (young birds) from the nest at 10 days of age to be hand-fed, as is commonly practiced with African grey parrots. Other aviculturists remove the eggs immediately after being laid and place them in an incubator, then a hatcher, and then hand-feed the neonates. Typically, an egg is formed in the uterus over 24 hours. The incubation period (from laying to hatching) for budgie and cockatiel eggs is 18 and 21 days, respectively, whereas for the African grey parrots, Amazon parrots, and macaws it is approximately 26 days (Joyner 1994).

HUSBANDRY AND NUTRITION

It is estimated that the majority of health problems observed in pet birds is due to improper husbandry and diet.

Substrate

Although many variations of substrate are available, the best is paper, such as newspaper or paper towels. It is inexpensive, easy to observe droppings, easy to clean (just throw it away), and nontoxic. Other choices for substrate include newspaper pellets or walnut shells, but the droppings are difficult to observe. Avoid use of substrate material that readily grows fungus, such as corncob and wheat straw, as these have been associated with fungal pneumonia. Also avoid use of substrate material that is irritating to the mucous membranes of the eyes and respiratory tract (sinus), such as cedar shavings.

Room Temperature

If a person is comfortable in a T-shirt then the room temperature is probably comfortable for an adult bird. The exception is neonates, which require higher temperatures depending on their age. If a neonate needs to visit the hospital, the owner should be advised to bring supplemental heat and a covered (with air holes) container to keep the neonate warm. Newly hatched chicks can require up to 94°F and greater than 50% humidity (Harrison & Ritchie 1994). The body temperature of different species of birds can vary between 104°F and 112°F (Flammer & Clubb 1994).

Humidity

Tropical parrots prefer 50–60% humidity. Some birds, such as budgies and zebra finches, are from arid regions and may require less. Gas heaters used in homes during the winter months can create dry air within the house and a humidifier may be needed in the bird's room to maintain adequate humidity.

Light Cycle

In general, birds should be exposed to the natural light cycle occurring outside or be kept at 10 hours of light and 14 hours of dark. To avoid stimulating reproductive activity in some birds (i.e., a chronically egg laying cockatiel), the amount of "light time" may need to be decreased even more.

Bathing

Bathing helps maintain healthy feathers and most birds appear to enjoy it, especially those from South America, such as macaws and Amazon parrots. Birds can be placed in the shower or sink, or offered a shallow bowl for bathing. Allow enough time for the bird to completely dry before their usual "dark time." Some owners blow dry their birds, but care must be taken not to burn or overheat the bird. Heated air blowing under the protective feathers easily burns the thin skin of birds.

Perches

Most hardwoods (from trees that lose their leaves in the winter), such as oak, aspen, manzanita, and ribbon wood, make excellent perches. It is best to avoid the soft woods, such as pine, that are high in resin and sap. Also avoid wood from trees that have been sprayed with fungicides, herbicides, or insecticides. The bird should be offered perches of varying diameter in order to exercise the toes and help prevent arthritis. The diameter should allow most of the bird's foot to be in contact with the wood. Plantar erosions can develop on the bottom of the bird's feet if perches are too small in diameter. Sandpaper-covered perches are irritating to the feet and should not be used. If concrete perches are used, they should be offered in conjunction with wooden perches. Perches should be positioned so that when the bird defecates, the food and water bowls are not contaminated.

If a bird is severely ill or incapacitated in some way, it is best to place the perches low right in front of the (preferably elevated) food and water for easy access. Also, since birds prefer to sit on the highest perch available, remove the high perches from the cage of a debilitated bird, or it will waste precious energy climbing to the top perch.

Cage Size
Ideally, the bigger the cage, the better it is for the bird. The bird should at least be able to fully extend their wings in all directions. Birds are commonly allowed out of their cage for supervised play on a play gym or additional perch. The bird should not be able to put its head between the bars.

Cage Construction
Ideally, stainless steel is the best, most inert substance for a cage, but it is also very expensive and difficult to obtain in a form for caging. So the next best, most commonly used substance is plain steel, which can rust. Because of this it is painted, powder coated (a form of powder paint put on the metal via electrolysis), or galvanized (meaning the steel has been coated with zinc). All these coverings can contain toxic levels of lead and/or zinc. Some commercially available cages have been documented to have toxic levels of lead and/or zinc (Van Sant 1998) but most commercially available cages are "safe." Do not use hardware cloth (it has a square mesh and is a dull gray color) as it is welded together with a compound containing lead and is also galvanized (coated in zinc), both of which are highly toxic to birds. Parrots have a high propensity to chew and are more likely to be exposed to lead or zinc. Good alternatives are the silver (chrome-plated) or gold-toned (brass) metal cages that are not painted. It is best to provide a grate on the bottom of the cage so the bird cannot access its own feces or dropped, old food.

Toys
Toys are usually safe if made from hardwoods (either untreated or vegetable dyed), untreated leather, ropes, uncoated steel, stainless steel, or hard plastics. One study in humans showed that some soft plastics contain toxic levels of lead, so these should be avoided for birds. Also, avoid long ropes or chains that can wrap about a bird's neck, foot, or toe. Avoid materials that are galvanized (coated in zinc to prevent rust) or those that contain lead or zinc (see also below, "Noninfectious Diseases—Lead; Zinc").

Nutrition
Fresh, plain water with no additives should be provided at all times. If bottled water is used, spring or drinking water, not distilled water, which lacks necessary salts and minerals, should be chosen.

Seeds are most notably low in vitamin A and protein, and high in fat. Consequently, birds such as an Amazon parrot, which can live past 50 years of age, are dying of malnutrition at 15 years of age on an all-seed diet.

There are three concepts to understand regarding the ideal diet in pet birds: (1) there is no "generic" parrot and each species has its own, different requirements; (2) the requirements are not well known for any species of parrot; and (3) the pelleted diets available today are based on dietary requirements of chickens and cockatiels.

With that said, no one knows the specific dietary requirements of each pet bird, but some are known. The best current recommendation is to feed parrots naturally colored (not artificially colored) pelleted diets made for parrots. As a supplement to the pellets, approximately 10–20% of their daily intake can be fresh dark-green leafy and dark-yellow vegetables, such as carrots, sweet potato, greens, and green beans. Fruits and seeds can be offered as a treat (Brue 1994). Currently, it is recommended to offer small birds (budgies, cockatiels, finches) a diet that is as much as 50% seeds, such as millet, to lower the overall protein intake in these species of birds.

Do not offer a bird chocolate (toxic theobromine), sugar, salt, caffeine, avocados (can cause death), or peanuts (high in aflatoxins, which over time severely affect the liver).

COMMON AND ZOONOTIC DISEASES (INFECTIOUS AND NONINFECTIOUS)

There are over 20 diseases in birds that are zoonotic. One of those that is quite common and serious is listed below (chlamydiosis; Ritchie & Dreesen 1998).

Bacterial

Gram-negative Bacteria and Gram-positive Bacteria
The causative agent is any bacteria, even those categorized as "normal flora," which can cause an infection or disease in certain situations. In general, bacterial infections in parrots are associated with gram-negative bacteria.

Clinical signs vary according to the affected anatomical part. Examples include diarrhea from an enteritis; nasal discharge from a sinusitis; dyspnea from pneumonia; inflamed tissue or abscess from an infection in the skin, joint, or tissue; bumblefoot (ulcerative pododermatitis) from infection in the bottom of the foot; anorexia from hepatitis; regurgitation from infection in the crop (ingluvitis). See color plates 2.2 through 2.6.

A diagnosis is made by a biopsy or cytology of the affected area showing bacteria engulfed within white blood cells. Aerobic and anaerobic cultures of the affected area showing medium to heavy growth consistent with the clinical signs the bird is exhibiting would also be diagnostic. Ancillary diagnostics include a complete blood count (CBC).

Treatment includes broad-spectrum, bactericidal antibiotics based on the sensitivity of the culture.

Chlamydiosis

The causative agent is *Chlamydophila psittaci*. Clinical signs are variable, but can include dyspnea, green urates (biliverdinuria), anorexia, and lethargy.

A diagnosis is made in various ways. Many tests are available including fecal antigen (DNA probe, ELISA), blood antigen (DNA probe), and serum antibody (IFA, EBA) tests. Positive fecal antigen tests suggest the bird is shedding the organism in the feces and is contagious. Positive blood antigen tests suggest the organism is in the blood stream and the bird has an active infection. Positive serum antibody tests suggest the bird has been exposed to the organism sometime during its life, but is not necessarily infected at this time. Ancillary diagnostics include a CBC and radiographs. Ideally, a complete workup includes a *Chlamydophila* panel (fecal and blood DNA probe test, and serum IFA antibody) and ancillary diagnostics such as CBC, chemistry profile (including AST, LDH, and bile acids), and a radiograph in order to evaluate the potential diagnosis of chlamydiosis.

The treatment is doxycycline for 45 days (by law).

Since it is a zoonotic disease, birds can transmit it to people. A positive test needs to be immediately reported to the state veterinarian (in most states), and it should be documented in the record that the owners were informed of the positive results and instructed to consult their physician. It is a treatable disease in people, but if left untreated, it can eventually be fatal.

Clostridiosis

The causative agent is *Clostridium* spp. (i.e., *C. perfringens*), an anaerobic bacteria.

Clinical signs include a fetid, septic-tank-type smell to the diarrhea, which may be accompanied by gas.

To diagnosis this disease, a fecal gram stain should be performed. It will show relatively large (3 microns wide), gram-positive bacteria, oftentimes with clear spores in the center (safety-pin shape) or on the end (racquet shaped). An anaerobic culture can also be performed.

The treatment is clindamycin or other drugs based on the anaerobic culture.

Fungal/Yeast (Mycotic)

Aspergillosis

The causative agent is *Aspergillus flavus* or *fumigatus*. Clinical signs include none to dyspnea or loss of voice. This disease can be diagnosed with *Aspergillus* antigen and antibody serology, plasma electrophoresis, radiographs, rigid endoscopy to visualize a mass in the air sacs or tracheal bifurcation, and fungal culture. Ancillary diagnostics include a CBC. Treatment involves antifungal medications such as itraconazole, ketaconazole, or amphotericin-B. (Note: Itraconazole causes severe depression in African grey parrots, therefore an alternative antifungal should be utilized in these birds.)

Candidiasis

The causative agent is *Candida albicans*. Clinical signs include regurgitation or diarrhea, anorexia, delayed crop emptying, and sweet/sour smell to crop contents.

A diagnosis is made with a crop and/or fecal gram stain showing the egg-shaped purple-stained organism with more than three budding yeast per 40X field.

Treatment includes nystatin (acts topically throughout the GI tract), or ketaconazole if the infection is severe and invading the mucosa.

Note that usually this infection is diagnosed in neonates or immunosuppressed birds of any age.

Viral

Psittacine Beak and Feather Disease (PBFD)

The causative agent is a circovirus, Psittacine Beak and Feather Disease Virus. Clinical signs include none to feather dystrophy and loss, sometimes beak necrosis. Old World species (cockatoo, cockatiel, budgie, lovebird, African grey parrot, etc.) are most susceptible. PBFD can have a very long incubation period. Birds can be infected and spreading the virus to other birds while looking clinically normal for years. See color plate 2.7.

A diagnosis is made with a blood test using a DNA probe test, and/or DNA in situ hybridization on a feather follicle biopsy.

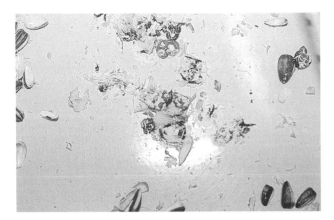

Plate 2.2. *Normal feces. (Photo courtesy of Ryan Cheek) (See also color plates)*

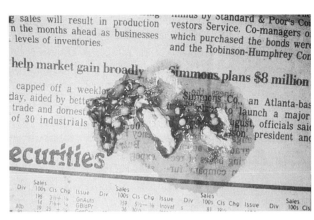

Plate 2.5. *Undigested seeds. (Photo courtesy of Dr. Sam Rivera) (See also color plates)*

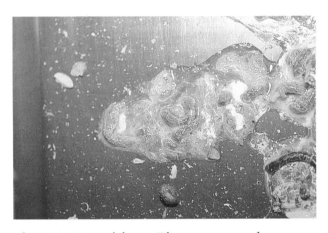

Plate 2.3. *Normal feces. (Photo courtesy of Ryan Cheek) (See also color plates)*

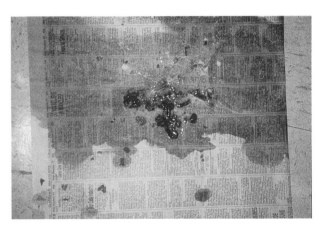

Plate 2.6. *Polyuria. (Photo courtesy of Dr. Sam Rivera) (See also color plates)*

Plate 2.4. *Hematuria and melena. (Photo courtesy of Dr. Sam Rivera) (See also color plates)*

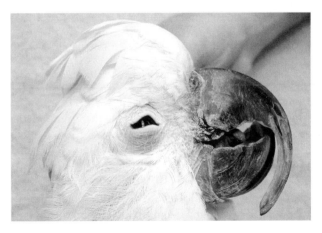

Plate 2.7. *Bird with PBFD. (Photo courtesy of Dr. Stephen J. Hernandez-Divers, University of Georgia) (See also color plates)*

There is no treatment. There has recently been described a PBFD-2 of lories in which birds recover from the disease (Ritchie et al. 2000). A DNA probe blood test for PBFD-2 is available. A diagnosis of PBFD-2 so far signifies a better prognosis.

Polyoma
The causative agent is polyomavirus. This is usually a disease of young birds, but can affect adult birds. Clinical signs are as follows: most parrots, except budgies, show delayed crop emptying, anorexia, lethargy, and subcutaneous hemorrhages.

While this disease may be suspected based on clinical signs, the definitive test is the DNA probe of feces or of necropsy tissues (kidney, liver).

There is no treatment. A killed vaccine is commercially available for parrots (Biommune Co., Lenexa, KS). Two vaccines administered 2 weeks apart are required for optimal protection (Ritchie 1995b). Birds are maximally protected 2 weeks after the second vaccination. The first vaccine is generally given at 35 days of age, although a series of vaccinations can be started at a younger age, if necessary.

Pacheco's Disease
The causative agent is a herpesvirus. Clinical signs include none or sudden death, or possibly an enlarged, darkened liver at necropsy.

A diagnosis is made by performing a fluorescent antibody test of liver at necropsy. A serum antibody test is available and if positive suggests the bird has been previously exposed, but a positive test does not differentiate between a latent or active infection. A negative antibody test may occur in a bird with the disease (Ritchie 1995a).

There is no treatment but the mortality may be decreased in an outbreak if the antiherpesvirus drug acyclovir is administered to the rest of the exposed flock.

Proventricular Dilatation Disease (PDD)
The causative agent is an unidentified 89 nanometer virus. Clinical signs include severe weight loss despite a ravenous appetite, whole pieces of food or seed found in the feces, delayed crop emptying, or little to no crop movements.

A diagnosis is made definitively with a crop biopsy with a histopathologic diagnosis of lymphoplasmocytic ganglioneuritis.

There is no treatment. A dilated proventriculus visible on radiographs is a suggestive diagnosis, but many diseases of birds can cause this and it is not definitive for PDD.

Unclassified Organisms

Cloacal Papillomatous Lesions
The causative agent is thought to be a herpesvirus. Clinical signs include a wartlike mass at the cloaca, and sometimes elsewhere in the gastrointestinal system such as the oral cavity.

A diagnosis is made visually or by biopsy.

There are many treatments including chemical cautery with silver nitrate on half the lesion, rotating sides weekly until gone as one suggested treatment, but the disease is not considered curable. If the disease is in fact caused by a herpesvirus, then acyclovir should help in treatment.

Megabacteria
The causative agent is an up to 90 micrometer long organism, thought to be a fungus. Clinical signs may include regurgitation or no signs at all.

A diagnosis is made by observing the organisms on a fecal gram stain or direct smear or from histopathology of a biopsy/necropsy.

The treatment for this disease is amphotericin-B.

NONINFECTIOUS DISEASES

Toxins

Lead
This is caused by ingested or inhaled exposure to lead. Sources include paints, fishing weights, bullets, champagne wrappers, fashion jewelry, hardware cloth used in homemade cages, venetian blinds, soft plastic twist ties, and ceramic glazes.

Clinical signs include a nondescript sick bird (bottom of cage, fluffed), neurological signs (falling off perch, seizure), or vomiting.

A diagnosis is made by the detection of metal dense foreign body in the ventriculus on radiograph or elevated blood lead levels.

This disease is treated with calcium EDTA or dimercaptosuccinic acid (DMSA).

Zinc
The causative agent is ingested exposure to zinc. Sources include paints, powder-coatings, anything galvanized to prevent rusting, hardware cloth, fashion jewelry, toy cars, and pennies.

Clinical signs include a nondescript sick bird (bottom of cage, fluffed), neurological signs (falling off perch, seizure), or vomiting.

A diagnosis is made by the detection of metal dense foreign body in ventriculus on radiograph or elevated serum zinc levels.

The treatment is Calcium EDTA or dimercaptosuccinic acid (DMSA).

Teflon Fumes

The cause is polytetrafluoroethylene (PTFE) gas, which is released when Teflon pans are burned (heated to above 530°F).

Clinical signs include death or dyspnea.

A diagnosis is suggestive based on history and hemorrhagic lungs at necropsy.

Treatment is typically unsuccessful but fresh air can be tried or the administration of steroids, however it is usually rapidly fatal.

Trauma

Dog/Cat Bites

The cause is an unsupervised bird out of its cage encountering a mammal.

Clinical signs include a visible bite wound or scratch, but may include a nonvisible puncture wound. See color plate 2.8.

A diagnosis is made based on the history and physical exam.

Treatment involves cleansing the wounds. These patients should ALWAYS be started on a broad-spectrum, bacteriocidal antibiotic even if no wounds are visible. Birds can die of septicemia within 12 to 24 hours after a mammal bite/scratch.

Ceiling Fans/Window Panes

The cause is an unsupervised bird out of its cage flying into an object.

Clinical signs include bruising or edema about the face, loss of consciousness, or neurological signs.

A diagnosis is made based on history and clinical signs.

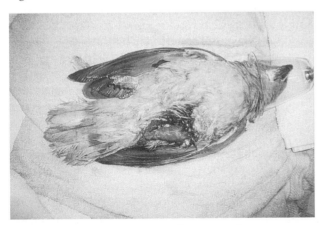

Plate 2.8. Amazon parrot with trauma from a cat. (Photo courtesy of Dr. Sam Rivera) (See also color plates)

Treatment includes keeping the patient in a dark, quiet cage without excessive heat. Steroids are also used.

NUTRITIONAL DEFICIENCIES

Vitamin A Deficiency

This is caused by a vitamin A-deficient diet, such as a seed diet.

Clinical signs include choanal papillae in the oral cavity that are blunted, plantar erosions on the feet, and poor quality skin and feathers (darkened areas on feathers of wings).

A diagnosis is made based on the history and clinical signs. Secondary bacterial or fungal infections involving the respiratory tract are common. Sometimes a Gram's stain of a choanal swab will show increased epithelial cells and basophilic staining.

Treatment includes an increase in vitamin A in the diet by providing the bird with dark yellow vegetables (sweet potato, carrot, commercial bird pellets). One can also administer an injection of vitamin A.

Hypocalcemia

The cause is a calcium-deficient diet or a diet high in phosphorus, which competes with calcium. Hypocalcemia is more common in African grey parrots (AGP) or those birds with a greater need for calcium such as laying hens.

Clinical signs in the laying hen include the bird being egg bound, laying soft-shelled eggs, or metabolic bone disease. In the African grey parrot signs may be neurological (falling off perch, seizures).

A diagnosis is confirmed by evidence of a low serum calcium level (less than 8.0 g/dl).

Treatment strategies include a change of diet, injectable calcium gluconate or oral calcium glubionate (also see below, "Egg Bound").

OTHER DISEASES

Crop Burn

The cause is a neonate being fed a high temperature gruel creating the burn or heating hand-feeding formula in a microwave, which creates uneven heating.

Clinical signs typically occur 10 days after the incident when a scab falls off and a fistulous tract is seen leaking gruel onto the bird's chest.

A diagnosis is made based on clinical signs.

Treatment involves surgery at 10–14 days after the burn to suture the hole in the crop and skin closed.

Hemorrhaging Blood (Pin) Feathers

This is caused by a developing feather called a blood or pin feather. The large wing and tail feathers obtain their blood supply near the bone, and if damaged they will bleed until the entire feather is removed from the follicle.

The clinical sign and diagnosis is the observation of a damaged developing feather that is bleeding.

The treatment is to remove the bleeding feather by gently grasping the follicle at the base, near the skin, and pulling in the direction of feather growth. The entire feather must be removed in order to stop the hemorrhage. The tip of the feather comes to a point called an umbilicus.

Egg Bound

There are many causes but usually this is due to hypocalcemia from a seed diet.

Clinical signs include straining at bottom of cage or a history of laying other eggs.

A diagnosis is made by palpating the egg or visualizing it on radiographs.

Treatment may include giving calcium gluconate IM, placing the bird in a warm, dark, quiet place, sometimes giving oxytocin, PGE2 alpha, ovocentesis (imploding the egg by removing its contents), or surgery if necessary.

TAKING THE HISTORY AND PERFORMING A PHYSICAL EXAM

History

Obtaining an adequate history on a bird patient is more time-consuming than obtaining a history on a dog or cat patient. Therefore, allow more time to complete this vital task.

Presenting Complaint

The following questions should be asked: How long has this been going on? When did it start? Is it progressive/getting worse? Are any other birds/animals/people sick?

The Bird

The following questions about the bird should be asked: How old is the bird? How was it obtained (pet store/breeder?)? Was the bird quarantined 3 months after acquisition? Has it been vaccinated against polyomavirus? Has it been tested for chlamydiosis and Psittacine Beak and Feather Disease? How long have you owned it? Have there been any previous prob-

lems? What is the diet? What brand and type of food do you give it? What is offered? What is consumed? How much and what kinds of people food are offered? Are supplements offered (cuttlebone)? Is fresh water available at all times? Does the bird bathe? What is the personality of the bird (phobic, easily stressed, playful, extrovert)? Has the bird's attitude changed? Has the voice changed? Has the weight changed? When was the last molt? Has there been a change in droppings? Has the bird been given any medications?

The Cage and Environment

The following questions should be asked: Is this the bird's regular cage or is this a travel cage? Where was the cage obtained? What is the brand of the cage? Does it have silver- or gold-toned metal? If painted or powder coated, what is its color? Is it chipping? What type of substrate is used? How often is it changed? How often are bowls cleaned? What are they made of? Describe the perches. Is the bird kept indoors or outdoors? What is the temperature of the enclosure? Is the bird let out of the cage? Is it supervised? Describe the toys. What is the light cycle? (i.e., Does the bird get 14 hours of darkness?) Are there other animals in the household? Is this bird housed alone or with another bird? When was the last bird added to this collection?

Physical Exam

First observe the bird from afar, perhaps while taking the history from the owner. Birds, having a flock mentality, tend to hide signs of illness so that members of their "flock" will not ostracize them for behaving in such a way as to attract a predator. It is only when a bird can no longer compensate for its illness (i.e., can no longer "put on a good show of looking normal") that owners recognize that their bird is ill. A normal bird in a strange place such as a veterinary hospital, should not be fluffed or closing its eyes (fig. 2.4).

Before restraining the bird, examine as much as possible from a distance, including the cage, substrate, droppings, food dishes, perches, and toys. Also, observe the bird's behavior, attitude, posture, breathing, symmetry of face, body, and wings, skin and feather quality, and neurological status. Dyspnea in a bird usually manifests as a "tail bob," a movement of the tail up and down with each breath. After observing the bird from a distance, a physical exam can be performed with the bird restrained in a towel (see below, "Restraint").

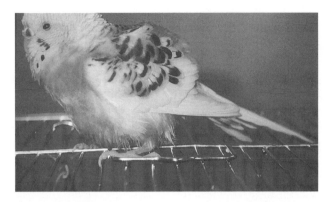

Fig. 2.4. A bird with fluffed up feathers. (Photo courtesy of Dr. Sam Rivera)

Abnormalities That Can Be Identified in a Physical Exam

Head—lack of symmetry, bruising, swelling

Eyes—lack of symmetry, discharge, opaque lens, blood, disruption of normal anatomy

Beak—lack of symmetry, elongated, severe flaking, fractures, pitting of the surface. Note: Some flaking of the beak is normal.

Ears—closed meatus, discharge, odor

Nares—lack of symmetry, discharge, mass, debris, blood. Note: It is normal for a structure to be present just inside the nares, called the operculum. It is important not to disturb this structure or it may bleed.

Skin—Excess flaking, pitting of the surface, blood, redness, swelling, masses. Note: It is normal for birds to bruise green, rather than purple, so it should not be mistaken for gangrene.

Feathers—unzipped barbules, dull, greasy, unkempt, stained, plucked or shredded feathers, lack of powder down, stress bars (horizontal lines of malformation along the feather, suggesting the bird encountered a stressful incident during the formation of that feather)

Crop—no movement within one minute, fistula, distended, empty

Pectoral muscle mass (thin or obese)—A body condition score is assessed by determining pectoral muscle mass. Normally, the edge of the keel can be palpated between the rounded pectoral muscles that slope slightly to either side.

Wings—feathers missing, damaged hemorrhaging blood feathers, masses, fractures, dislocations, feathers trimmed, ulcers in skin, lice

Abdomen—firm, distended, egg palpable, enlarged liver palpated or seen as a dark area through the skin that is extending caudal to the borders of the sternum

Cloaca—masses, dilated, irritated (hyperemic), prolapse of tissue, accumulation of feces, diarrhea on feathers

Feet—plantar erosions (pink areas on bottom of feet), flaky skin, necrotic areas, scab, swelling (abscess, or gout, which is an accumulation of white uric acid under the skin)

Assessing Hydration Status—A "vein refill time" can be performed on the basilic (cutaneous ulnar) vein of birds. In a normally hydrated bird, the basilic vein should instantaneously refill, and by the time a finger is off the vein to see it, it should have refilled. If the basilic vein can be seen to refill, then it is estimated the bird is approximately 5% dehydrated. If the vein requires one second to refill, then the bird is severely dehydrated (10%) or is in shock (low blood pressure).

PREVENTATIVE MEDICINE

Since birds are so adept at hiding signs of illness, any vague sign of illness in a bird should be taken seriously. Annual exams are ideal, but it is important to stress to clients to observe the bird carefully each day, and if any slight abnormality is identified, call the veterinary hospital. In the case of neonates, they should be weighed daily on a gram scale by the owner.

Ideally, a prepurchase exam should include a physical exam, CBC, fecal gram stain, chlamydiosis test, Psittacine Beak and Feather Disease (PBFD) test (in susceptible species), and polyoma vaccine. Some aviaries sell birds that are already PBFD tested, polyoma vaccinated, and chlamydiosis tested.

RESTRAINT

Above all do no harm. Since a bird does not possess a diaphragm, it moves its sternum up and down to move air through the lungs and air sacs. Therefore, do not press on the sternum or the bird could suffocate and die rapidly.

Finches and canaries can be grasped and restrained with a bare hand (fig. 2.5). Parrots on the other hand should not be grasped with a bare hand or glove since that may cause them to be apprehensive of stepping up onto a hand afterward. Parrots should be grasped and restrained in a towel. The parrot's weapon is its extremely powerful beak that can cause a severe crushing injury. The towel helps to some degree in protecting the fingers from being bitten.

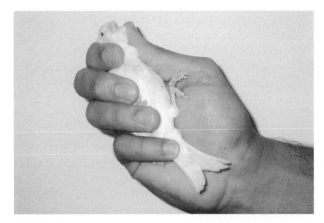

Fig. 2.5. Restraint of a small bird. (Photo courtesy of Dr. Sam Rivera)

Approach the parrot with a towel-covered hand and attempt to quickly wrap the fingers around the bird's neck. An ideal opportunity to grasp the neck is when the bird is attempting to move away from the towel and uses its beak to grasp the cage. Once the towel-protected fingers are around the parrot's neck (coming from behind), the towel is wrapped around the bird to control flapping of the wings. (See figure 2.6.) Speaking to the bird in a soothing voice will help reduce the stress during handling.

Restraint time should be kept to a minimum (preferably less than 2 minutes). Release the bird immediately at the first signs of stress including panting, eyes closing, weakness, and generally any change of behavior from when the bird was initially restrained, for example, cessation of biting the towel. Unhealthy birds have died while being restrained in a towel even for a brief period. If a bird loses consciousness while being restrained in a towel, rarely does it recover. It is the responsibility of the person restraining to determine if a bird is stressed and needs to be released (figs. 2.7 and 2.8).

RADIOLOGY

There are varying opinions as to whether a bird should be anesthetized or restrained for a radiograph. It is the author's opinion that birds, even most debilitated birds, can be anesthetized briefly with isoflurane for radiographs in order to produce good quality radiographs with good positioning of the patient and to produce them safely without exposure of personnel to radiation. There is absolutely no excuse for a human finger to be present on a radiograph of a bird. Occasionally, a severely debilitated

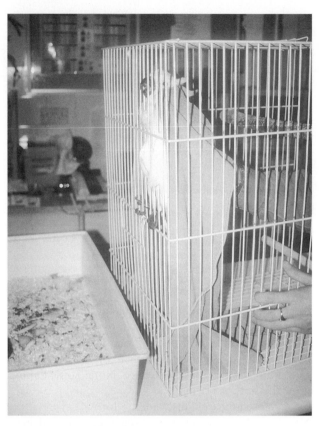

Fig. 2.6. Capturing a bird while in its cage. (Photo courtesy of Dr. Stephen J. Hernandez-Divers, University of Georgia)

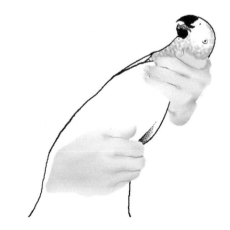

Fig. 2.7. Restraint of a bird. (Drawing by Scott Stark)

bird can be placed in a cardboard box and a radiograph taken if the reason is to determine if there is a metal foreign body or egg within the bird. A dorsoventral (DV) radiograph can be obtained utilizing this method, as well as an across the table (horizontal beam) lateral.

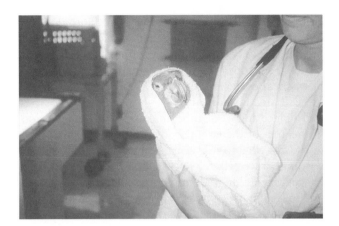

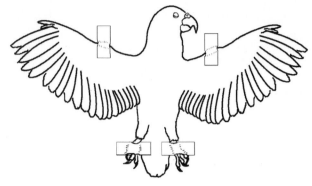

Fig. 2.8. *Bird restraint. (Photo courtesy of Dr. Sam Rivera)*

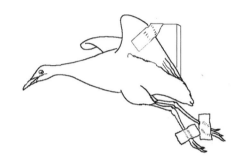

Fig. 2.9. *Positioning of an avian patient for radiographs. (Drawing by Scott Stark)*

Two views are obtained, a ventrodorsal view (VD) and a lateral view. The VD is obtained by placing the bird on its back, using nonradiopaque white or masking tape to position the laterally stretched wings evenly and gently to the table or cassette, and taping the caudally stretched legs evenly and gently. The tape is placed around the tarso-metatarsus. In order to pull the leg caudally without moving the body of the bird, a finger can be placed at the tip of the sternum for resistance, making sure not to press down (dorsally) on the sternum while doing so (see above, "Restraint"). Ideal positioning of a VD view results in the keel of the sternum lining up with the spine the entire length of each; the femurs should be parallel. The lateral view is obtained by placing the bird on its right side with the wings stretched gently and evenly dorsally and taped. Be gentle, because if forced, luxation of the shoulder can occur. If it is difficult to move the wing dorsally, the bird may be in a light plane of anesthesia and the muscles are not relaxed, or the bird may have an anatomical inability to move the wing into that position (i.e., arthritis or old fracture). The legs are pulled evenly and gently caudally straight behind the bird and taped. Ideal positioning of a lateral view results in the femoral heads being superimposed on each other (fig. 2.9).

Radiographic equipment, film, screens, and settings will vary with each hospital and each machine, therefore a technique chart will need to be developed for each hospital, or each machine if there are more than one. Generally, non-Bucky techniques are utilized with rapid film and techniques similar to obtaining a radiograph on an extremity of a dog or cat (lowest kVp, high mA, and a short exposure time; McMillan 1994). An example of what is utilized at one hospital for an African grey parrot is a kVp of 70, mA of 300 at $\frac{1}{120}$

second. Some practitioners prefer to use mammography film with birds for better soft tissue differentiation.

ANESTHESIA AND SURGERY

Anesthesia
Isoflurane and, more recently, sevoflurane are the inhalant anesthetic agents of choice for use in birds (Quandt & Greenacre 1999). Other inhalant and injectable anesthetic agents are not as safe and predictable in birds. Propofol has been shown to produce dramatic respiratory arrest in pigeons. Mask induction is common, starting at 2% and increasing in 0.5% increments until at desired plane of anesthesia. A high flow rate of 2 liter/minute of oxygen is utilized due to the large amount of dead space within the mask. Once intubated, the oxygen flow rate is set at approximately 1 L/min. The eyes of the bird should be lubricated as soon as possible (fig. 2.10).

Monitoring depth of anesthesia in birds is different than in dogs and cats since palpebral reflex, toe pinch, and jaw tone are unreliable. A Doppler, placed on the medial metatarsal artery or radial artery, and a pulse oximeter, placed over the femur (of cockatiels), foot,

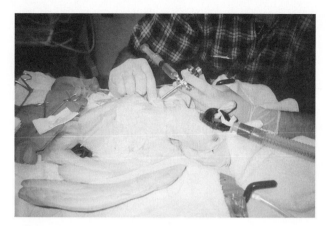

Fig. 2.10. Anesthesia via endotracheal intubation. (Photo courtesy of Dr. Sam Rivera)

toe, or humerus are helpful, but nothing replaces vigilantly and constantly observing breathing, and periodically ausculting the heart rate with a stethoscope. If a bird is shivering, the plane of anesthesia is very light.

Note: A bird requires a deep surgical plane of anesthesia to pluck feathers, especially those feathers attached to the periosteum (bone), such as the large wing and tail feathers. Lighten the plane of anesthesia after plucking.

Butorphanol is administered IM if a painful procedure is expected. A study has shown birds require a substantially higher dose than dogs (bird dose is 1–2 mg/kg; Paul-Murphy, Brunson, & Miletic 1999).

Supplemental heat is critically necessary. Depending on the species, a bird's normal temperature can be approximately 104–112°F. Water recirculating blankets have typically been utilized, but recently, forced heated air blankets have been shown to be superior in maintaining a bird's core body temperature (Rembert et al. 2001). In general, all attempts are made to prevent a bird from being under anesthesia for more than 1 hour.

Intermittent partial pressure ventilation (IPPV) should be performed at a rate of once every 30 to 60 seconds. It is possible to overinflate and rupture the air sacs or individual air capillaries, therefore pressure exerted on the bag should not exceed 15 mm H_2O (Sinn 1994).

Since birds possess complete tracheal rings, which are not distensible, it is necessary to place uncuffed endotracheal (ET) tubes. Inflation of cuffed ET tubes can cause pressure necrosis and sloughing of the tracheal mucosa.

Due to the unique respiratory anatomy of birds in which oxygen exchange occurs on both inspiration and expiration, an ET tube can be placed into the caudal thoracic air sac through the lateral body wall to provide not only oxygen but inhalant gas anesthesia as well. Air sac tubes are instrumental in emergency cases of tracheal occlusion, or when surgery of the trachea or head area is necessary.

To place an air sac tube, make a 2 mm skin incision in the area of the lateral body wall that is just caudal to the last rib and just ventral to the lateral process of the lumbar vertebrae. Push a fine hemostat through the relatively thin abdominal musculature taking care not to traumatize underlying organs. An ET tube is placed through the open jaws of the hemostat and sutured in place.

Sudden death has occurred in African grey parrots under isoflurane anesthesia and is thought to be due to a sudden drop in the blood calcium levels causing cardiac arrest. African grey parrots should be administered calcium gluconate IM at least 15 minutes prior to anesthesia to prevent a hypocalcemic incident. Further studies are needed to determine if there are other factors involved.

Surgery

Skin: Bird skin is relatively thin, therefore fine suture is commonly utilized such as 4-0 and 5-0 polydioxanone. Catgut is reactive and not recommended in birds.

Crop: Surgeries of the crop include a crop biopsy to diagnose Proventricular Dilitation Disease, crop fistula repair after a burn from being fed extremely hot hand-feeding formula, or a crop incision to remove a foreign body or to provide better access to more caudal GI structures.

Ceolom: Reasons to perform a celiotomy include a salpingohysterectomy to prevent egg laying in a hen, a proventriculotomy to remove a foreign body, a liver biopsy, and exploratory surgery.

Rigid Endoscopy: Commonly a rigid endoscope is utilized in birds for performing liver or kidney biopsies, exploratory evaluation and sexing by direct visualization of the gonads (fig. 2.11).

PARASITOLOGY

Giardiasis

The causative agent is *Giardia* spp. Clinical signs may include none to diarrhea.

A diagnosis is made by visualizing the trophozoites on a direct fecal smear or by a positive *Giardia* antigen ELISA test. Treatment involves the administration of metronidazole.

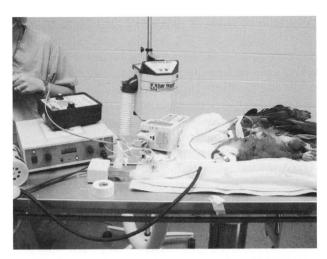

Fig. 2.11. *Avian patient in surgery. (Photo courtesy of Dr. Stephen J. Hernandez-Divers, University of Georgia)*

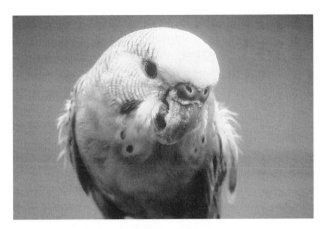

Fig. 2.12. *Deformed beak from* Knemidokoptes. *(Photo courtesy of Dr. Sam Rivera)*

Trichomoniasis

The causative agent is *Trichomonas* spp. Clinical signs include white plaques in oral cavity and regurgitation. A diagnosis is made by visualizing the trophozoites on a direct fecal smear. The treatment is metronidazole. This organism is usually observed in pigeons and doves or hawks that eat these species.

Ascaridiosis

The causative agent is *Ascaridia* spp. Clinical signs include none to regurgitation, anorexia, or intestinal obstruction. Diagnosis involves visualizing the typical ascarid egg on a fecal float. Treatments include piperazine, ivermectin, or fenbendazole. These nematodes can migrate to the liver.

Knemidokoptosis

The causative agent is the mite, *Knemidokoptes pilae*. Clinical signs include scaly legs and face, or pitting of skin about the face, beak, and legs. A diagnosis is made based on clinical signs and visualizing the mites from a skin or beak scrape (fig. 2.12).

Treatment involves giving ivermectin either topically or orally, not IM. The IM route of administration can cause death, especially in a small bird such as a budgie. Also, it is important to accurately weigh the bird on a gram scale and appropriately calculate the dose.

Severe cases can cause beak deformities.

HEMATOLOGY

Hematology for avian species is discussed extensively in chapter 15.

EMERGENCY AND CRITICAL CARE

In general the approach to emergencies in birds is similar to that of mammals with a few exceptions. House birds in a warm (85°F) quiet area (i.e., no barking dogs should be heard). As with mammals, fluids are administered at 50 ml/kg/day including lactated Ringer's solution or with 2.5% dextrose added. Administer fluids via the IV or intraosseous (IO) route (see below, "Catheter Placement"). An advantage that birds have over mammals is that if the trachea is obstructed making tracheal intubation impossible, a bird can still be delivered oxygen, even inhalant anesthesia through an air sac tube placed in the caudal thoracic air sac (see above, "Anesthesia and Surgery"; see also fig. 2.13).

The calculation for determining dehydration deficit and maintenance fluid requirement for birds is similar to that of mammals. Maintenance is 50 ml/kg/day.

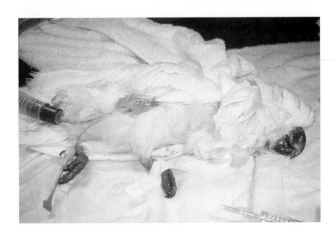

Fig. 2.13. *Anesthesia via air sac intubation. (Photo courtesy of Dr. Sam Rivera)*

The percentage of dehydration (under "Taking the History" above, see "Assessing Hydration Status") is represented as a decimal and multiplied by the weight of the bird in kilograms. The product is the deficit expressed in liters (there are 1,000 ml to 1 L).

Therefore, the fluid deficit for an 800 g bird that is 5% dehydrated is:

$$0.05 \times 0.800 \text{ kg} = 0.04 \text{ L} = 40 \text{ ml}$$

Therefore, the 24-hour maintenance requirement for an 800 g bird is:

$$50 \text{ ml/kg/day} \times 0.800 = 40 \text{ ml}$$

Figure 2.14 shows a parrot being weighed on a gram scale.

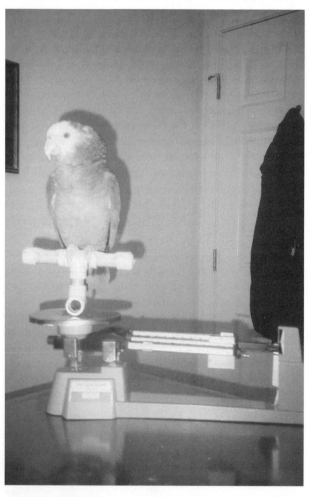

Fig. 2.14. *Weighing an avian patient. (Photo courtesy of Dr. Sam Rivera)*

NEONATOLOGY AND PEDIATRICS

Neonates need to be housed in a warmer (85–95°F or more) environment than adult birds since they lack the insulating feathers. Humidity should be at approximately 50–60%. Some species (macaws, eclectus) will develop constricted toe syndrome if housed in an environment that is too dry (fig. 2.15).

Most neonates are removed from the nest after a few days with the parent birds (10 days for African grey parrots), although others are removed as eggs. Once removed they must be hand-fed commercially available parrot hand-feeding formula. It is sold as a powder and mixed with heated water to a temperature of approximately 101–104°F for hand-feeding. Temperatures over 115°F have been associated with burns of the crop. More severe burns can injure other nearby tissue as well. Food should not be heated in the microwave, as this causes uneven temperature within the hand-feeding formula. (See above, "Other Diseases, Crop Burn.") Hand-feeding formula should be made fresh from the powder every feeding time. Leftover hand-feeding formula should be discarded. Each neonate should have its own feeding syringe (Luer tip) and cup that should not be used with other neonates.

Neonates should be weaned prior to sale. Some states require young animals, including birds, to be fully weaned prior to sale. Inexperienced hand-feeders can easily injure a nonweaned bird causing burns, aspiration, inappropriate intake due to amount fed or temperature of hand-feeding formula, temperature of environment or stress. Weaning is a stressful time for a bird and it does not need to be coupled with the added stress of moving to a new environment. Stress

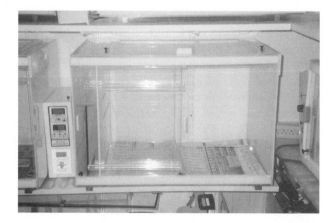

Fig. 2.15. *Hospital cage. (Photo courtesy of Dr. Sam Rivera)*

leads to immunosuppression and susceptibility to disease (see above, "Candidiasis").

SEX DETERMINATION

Since many parrots do not exhibit obvious signs of sexual dimorphism, a blood test or surgical sexing is necessary to determine the gender. Blood sexing involves drawing a blood sample and submitting it to one of the many laboratories that perform an ELISA gender determination test. If a client wishes to know the gender of a pet bird a blood test is recommended. Surgical sexing involving the use of a rigid endoscope to directly visualize the gonads carries the low risk of anesthesia, hemorrhage, and infection. It is recommended if a bird is to be utilized for breeding purposes, it be surgically sexed so that possible abnormalities of the gonad or other structures can be identified.

TECHNIQUES

Grooming (Nail, Beak, and Wing Trims)
Always thoroughly clean and disinfect instruments with a 1:10 bleach solution in order to prevent spread of disease, especially the virus Psittacine Beak and Feather Disease, which is a very stable virus. Thoroughly rinse with fresh water after disinfecting.

Nails
If the nail extends in an arc that is more than half a circle it is probably too long, but individual birds differ in the length of the quick. Owners may only want the nail points dulled so the bird does not traumatize the skin of their arm. A stone tip on a roto-tool, human nail clipper, or guillotine-type nail trimmers can be utilized. Always have available silver nitrate sticks or ferric subsulfate powder to stop hemorrhage if it occurs.

Beak
Some individual parrots maintain their beak length and never need a trim, while others require a trim every 6 months. Some species of parrots possess a longer beak (macaw) than other parrots (Amazon parrot), and these differences need to be learned before trimming. Beak trims are performed when the bird is either awake or under a light plane of isoflurane anesthesia. A roto-tool or a nail file is utilized. If the bill tip organ becomes visible (as a row of white dots on the occlusal surface of the beak) then the beak should be trimmed no further or hemorrhage and pain will occur. Some birds with an overgrown beak have underlying liver disease that needs to be addressed. In general, it is acceptable for a bird to have some flaking of the beak on the external surface.

Wing
Wing trims are performed in order to prevent the bird from flying freely and encountering danger, such as flying into a large paned window at high speed. A wing trim will not prevent a bird from flying away if taken outside. An ideal wing trim will be performed symmetrically and allow a bird to flutter down to the ground softly. Too severe of a wing trim can allow a bird to fall too fast and cause trauma, most commonly resulting in a laceration to the keel. Depending on the weight of the bird (i.e., some Amazon parrots become obese), the body type of the bird (i.e., African grey parrots are heavy bodied birds), and the number of pin (blood) feathers one is trying to avoid cutting, a wing trim consists of cutting three to ten primary feathers at the level of the tips of the lateral coverts (fig. 2.16). Budgies can still fly very well despite trimming all ten primary and all ten secondary feathers. It is not recommended to trim the feathers any shorter than described above since the cut end of the shafts may irritate the bird and possibly lead to feather picking (especially in African grey parrots). If a pin (blood) feather is encountered it is best to leave one feather before and after the pin feather to protect it as it grows out.

Catheter Placement (IV and IO)

Intravenous Catheter Placement
Some veterinarians prefer to have an IV catheter placed in the medial metatarsal vein. It is placed as any catheter would be and taped in place around the leg. This catheter works very well in long legged birds.

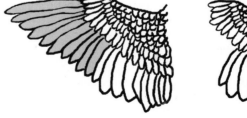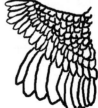

Fig. 2.16. Wing trim. (Drawing by Scott Stark)

Intraosseous Catheter Placement

The disadvantages of an IV catheter include potential trauma to flimsy veins and difficulty in stabilizing the catheter. The advantage of IO catheters is that they are easy to place and secure. The IO catheter should be placed in either the ulna or the tibiotarsus, but not the humerus or femur as these are pneumatic bones that directly connect to the air sacs of the bird. Fluid administration into a pneumatic bone would result in drowning the bird.

To place an IO catheter in the ulna, perform a sterile prep on the distal ulna (at the wrist of the bird) and instill a needle or spinal needle (25–20 gauge) into the lateral condyle pointing toward the elbow until the needle suddenly enters the intramedullary cavity. It should be sutured in place. Fluids, blood transfusions, and even total parenteral nutrition can be administered through an IO catheter.

Venipuncture

Right Jugular Vein

The right jugular vein is two-thirds larger than the left and is easily visualized by applying a small amount of alcohol to the featherless tract on the right side of the neck. Occlude the vein with a thumb or finger at the level of the thoracic inlet and use a 25- to 22-gauge needle to perform the phlebotomy. No more than 1% of the body weight in blood should be removed from a healthy bird. Less should be removed from ill birds.

For example, a maximum of 1.0 ml can be removed from a healthy 100 g (0.1 kg) cockatiel without any adverse affects. A maximum of 10 ml can be removed from a healthy macaw without any adverse affects.

Cockatiel $0.1 \text{ kg} \times 0.01 = 0.001 \text{ liters} = 1 \text{ ml}$
Macaw $1.0 \text{ kg} \times 0.01 = 0.010 \text{ liters} = 10 \text{ ml}$

Basilic Vein

Also known as the cutaneous ulnar vein, this vein courses over the medial surface of the proximal ulna. It is an excellent site for phlebotomy in hawks, pigeons, and chickens, but is very prone to forming a hematoma, especially in parrots.

Metatarsal Vein

This vein courses over the dorsal, then medial surface of the hock (the tibotarsal-tarsometatarsal joint) and is an excellent site for phlebotomy in pigeons, chickens, and ducks (fig. 2.17).

Bandaging and Wound Care

Birds lack an enzyme to liquefy pus, therefore their pus is very thick and caseated. Placement of drains in birds is generally not recommended for this reason. Most abscesses need to be lanced and managed as a wound that will heal by second intention, or be totally excised and the skin sutured.

Ball Bandage

A ball bandage is utilized on the foot of a bird to protect a lesion on the bottom of the foot (the plantar surface) and to redistribute the weight to other areas of the foot to relieve pressure on the affected area. A classic example for use of this bandage is a hawk with bumblefoot (ulcerative pododermatitis). Watch for problems in the other "good" foot if the bird is putting less weight on the "bad" foot. The bandage consists of placing medication on the wound, covering it with gauze or a nonstick bandage, then applying cast padding around the toes and tarsi to create a ball. Alternatively, a piece of cardboard or similar material can be placed under the foot to form what is called a snowshoe bandage (fig. 2.18). Also see chapter 14 for bandaging techniques.

Figure-eight Bandage

Appropriate uses of a figure-eight bandage include abnormalities of the distal wing such as needing to stabilize the ulna, radius, carpus, metacarpi, and phalanges. It is not appropriate to use a figure-eight bandage to stabilize the humerus, because it can only extend half way up the humerus and actually creates an area of pressure in this area. If you want to stabilize a humeral fracture, a temporary solution is to place a figure-eight bandage and wrap the bandage around the body of the bird (over the keel and back and under the wings). Sometimes a figure-eight bandage is utilized to stabilize a wing that has an ulnar IO catheter placed.

To place a figure-eight bandage, have the bird in lateral recumbency (preferably under light isoflurane anesthesia), hold the wing in its natural folded position, and create the figure-eight pattern by going around the carpus and then around the elbow of the bird, making sure to have bandage material cross the wing over the bones, not distally where there are only feathers (see fig. 2.19).

Also see chapter 14 for bandaging techniques.

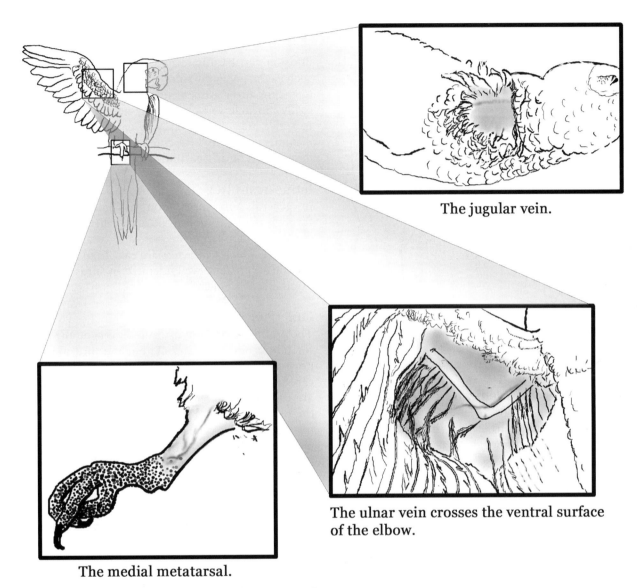

The jugular vein.

The ulnar vein crosses the ventral surface of the elbow.

The medial metatarsal.

Fig. 2.17. Venipuncture sites. (Drawing by Scott Stark)

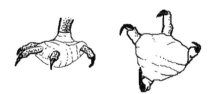

Fig. 2.18. Ball foot bandage. (Drawing by Scott Stark)

Elizabethan Collars

It is not recommended to place an Elizabethan collar on birds, since it prevents their normal preening behavior, is very heavy on their flexible necks, it does not allow them to eat or drink properly, easily creates chafing, causes them to act depressed, and is unkind if the bird is truly pruritic. If a bird is self-mutilating (i.e., biting at its muscle), then a hard plastic tubular collar especially made for birds can be applied. Note that picking at the feathers alone is not a reason to place a collar.

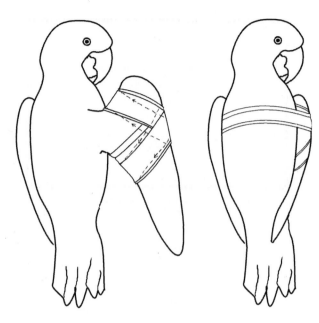

Fig. 2.19. Figure-eight bandage. (Drawing by Scott Stark)

Administration of Medications (IV, IO, PO, IC, ICe, SQ, IM)

Before administering medication, it is necessary to weigh the bird on a gram scale so as to accurately calculate the medication to be administered. Guessing a weight could be fatal to the bird.

In general, almost all medications utilized in birds have not been evaluated through pharmacokinetic studies and are considered extralabel use. The bird dose available in formularies for most all drugs is arrived at empirically, meaning others have utilized that dose in the past and it worked. Remember, there is no generic parrot. Each species, even each individual, is different, and all birds do not respond to medications equally. Of particular note, most macaws regurgitate and become severely depressed when administered trimethoprim-sulfa, whereas in most other species it causes little to no ill effects. Also, African grey parrots are extremely sensitive to the antifungal agent itraconazole, and become severely depressed after administration of just one dose. Therefore, it is recommended that you learn the species, and consult a current formulary published exclusively for exotics (Carpenter, Mashima, & Rupiper 2001). When choosing an antibiotic, it is recommended that you chose one that is broad spectrum and bactericidal. Most, but not all, bacterial infections in birds involve gram-negative bacteria.

Intravenous (IV)

Fluids, blood transfusions, and medications can be administered through the IV route either by bolus infusion, or via catheter and intermittent bolus infusion, or directly attached to an infusion pump. Bolus infusion can be administered in any accessible vein, such as the jugular, basilic, or metatarsal. It is difficult to secure an IV catheter in a bird since they possess easily movable veins with little nearby support tissue in active areas of the body. A catheter placed in the metatarsal vein can be secured fairly well, especially in long-legged birds (see above, "Catheter Placement").

Intraosseous (IO)

In general, any medication or fluid administered through the IV route can be administered IO, including fluids, blood transfusions, and totally parenteral nutrition. The IO catheters are easy to place, very stable and secure, and well tolerated by birds (see above, "Catheter Placement").

Oral (PO)

The oral route of administration is commonly utilized for liquid oral medications, but the bird must have normal gastrointestinal motility and absorptive capacities for the medication to be of use. Whole pills are not administered to birds since the covering on the pill may not be removed at the appropriate time for the bird to maximally absorb the medication. For medications that are not sold in a liquid form, a solution can be made by mixing the crushed pill with a sweet syrup, understanding the fact that this suspension may yield uneven dosing, needs to be refrigerated, and has not been evaluated as to its efficacy. To administer oral medications, the bird can be either restrained in a towel in a normal upright standing position (not on its back), or allowed to take the medication from the syringe unrestrained. The goal is to place the medication under the tongue one drop at a time, so as not to drown the bird. Birds have a relatively large glottis (opening to the trachea) and liquids can easily gain entrance, and aspiration and death can occur if the "squirt in the back of the mouth" method is followed. Some birds are very adept at not accepting oral medications. In that case, an oral medication can be administered via a crop lavage tube (see below, "Crop Sampling/Flush/Lavage"). It is generally not recommended to offer medicated water or feed to pet birds because this results in inappropriate dosing, loss of effectiveness of the medication, bacterial overgrowth in the water, and dramatically less water (or food) intake by the bird. It also can create resistant bacteria.

Intracardiac (IC)

It is not recommended at any time other than euthanasia (under anesthesia) to perform an IC injection. Emergency medications can be administered through the easily accessible jugular vein or intratracheally.

Intracoelomic (ICe)

The ICe route is not recommended in birds at any time since injections could easily enter the air sacs and drown the bird.

Subcutaneous (SQ)

The SQ route is generally utilized for administering fluids to a bird. The SQ route is not recommended in birds that cannot absorb fluids from this site, such as severely debilitated birds, or birds that are in shock. Such birds require IV or IO fluids. The best site for SQ fluid placement in a bird is in the inguinal region. There is little SQ space elsewhere in birds other than perhaps a small area over the scapula.

Intramuscular (IM)

Any medication administered IM should be labeled for IM administration. This route is often the best route available in debilitated birds because it is known the bird received the entire dose and administration is fast resulting in less restraint time. Some commonly utilized IM medications (enrofloxacin) can cause severe muscle necrosis and it is recommended to switch to the oral form of the medication as soon as the bird is able. The IM injections are administered with a 27- or 25-gauge needle into the pectoral muscle mass on either side of the sternum. Always aspirate before injecting and if blood is aspirated remove the needle and move elsewhere. Ideally, record on which side the drug was administered and alternate sides. Avoid administering more than 0.5 ml/kg in any one IM location. It is not recommended to administer medications in the leg, since birds possess a renal-portal system that may shunt blood from the caudal half of the body to the kidney (see above, "Anatomy and Physiology, Cardiovascular Lymphatic System").

Cloacal Sampling

A premoistened cotton-tipped applicator or sterile culture swab can be gently inserted into the cloaca to obtain a sample of organisms residing or passing through the cloaca (i.e., feces). Uses include bacterial culture, gram or other special stains, or for DNA probe tests or ELISA tests (i.e., *Chlamydophila*). Sterile swabs placed in a sterile container should be utilized for the very sensitive DNA probe tests, to prevent contamination.

Choanal Sampling

A culture swab inserted into and moved along the choanal slit of a bird can be submitted for bacterial culture or DNA probe tests (i.e., *Chlamydophila*).

Crop Sampling/Flush/Lavage (i.e., tube feeding)

A premoistened cotton-tipped applicator or sterile culture swab can be gently inserted into the crop via the mouth to obtain a sample of organisms residing in the crop. Uses include bacterial or fungal culture or gram stains. Indications for performing a crop flush include removing crop material that is unwanted (high in bacteria or yeast, dry, contains foreign material), or obtaining a representative sample of crop contents for evaluation. A crop flush is accomplished with a syringe of warm fluid (LRS) being instilled into the crop and immediately removed by suction on the syringe and repeating the process as needed or is safe. Crop lavage is accomplished with a syringe of warm (90–101°F) material such as hand-feeding formula, oral fluids, and oral medication. It is important to suction hand-feeding formula through the tube that is going to be passed into the bird to avoid clogging the tube with material that is too big to pass.

To flush/lavage/tube feed, the syringe is attached to either a ball-tipped metal feeding tube or a red rubber catheter placed through a mouth speculum (figs. 2.20 and 2.21). Before insertion, the tube should be filled with material (fluid, food, medication, etc.), not air. The tube is inserted at the bird's left commissure of the beak and gently pushed over the tongue and then angled down toward the bird's right shoulder (fig. 2.20). The esophagus and crop lie on the right side of the bird's neck. Palpate the tube to be certain it is in the crop before instilling material. It is best to use a tube that is bigger than the bird's trachea to prevent inadvertent placement and aspiration and death. Another complication of passing a tube into the crop is overzealous placement and puncture of the thin esophagus and deposition of material into the neck tissues of the bird.

Nasal Flush

A syringe of warm saline or LRS is flushed through a bird's nostril for diagnostic (culture, cytology) and/or therapeutic purposes. Most prefer to perform this procedure in an awake patient, but others prefer to perform this in an anesthetized, intubated patient. In either case it is important to have the bird completely upside down for the procedure or life-threatening aspiration could occur. The syringe's Luer tip is used to cover the opening of one nostril and the warm fluid is flushed in and should be seen exiting the opposite nostril and out the mouth via the choana. Normally

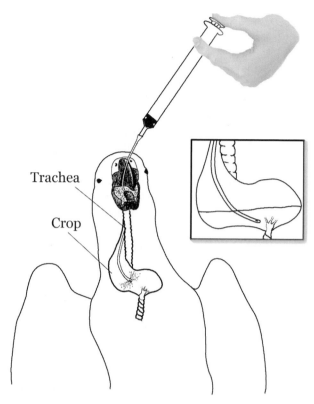

Trachea

Crop

Fig. 2.20. *Crop lavage. (Drawing by Scott Stark)*

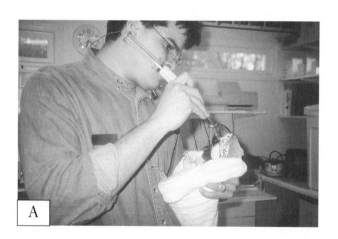

A

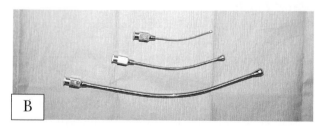

B

Fig. 2.21. A. *Tube feeding. (Photo courtesy of Dr. Sam Rivera).* **B.** *Ball-tipped metal feeding tubes (also called lavage or gavage needles).*

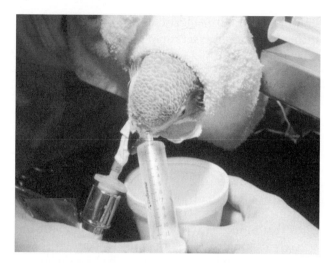

Fig. 2.22. *Nasal flush. (Photo courtesy of Dr. Stephen J. Hernandez-Divers, University of Georgia)*

the exiting fluid is relatively clear and thin. Birds with sinus irritation or infection will often have a very mucoid, cloudy material removed by this procedure.

EUTHANASIA

Birds should be anesthetized and unconscious prior to injection of euthanasia solution into the jugular vein, heart, metatarsal vein, basilic vein, liver, or occipital sinus. Realize that injections into the heart will alter the heart tissue, making a diagnosis of heart disease more difficult for the pathologist. Typically, birds require a relatively higher dose of euthanasia solution than mammals. After administration of the euthanasia solution be sure to auscult the heart with a stethoscope to determine that the bird has been properly euthanatized.

REFERENCES

Brue, RN. 1994. Nutrition. In *Avian Medicine: Principles and Application*, edited by Ritchie, BW, Harrison, GJ, Harrison, LR. Lake Worth: Winger's Publishing.

Carpenter, JW, Mashima, TY, Rupiper, DJ. 2001. *Exotic Animal Formulary*. 2d ed. Philadelphia: W.B. Saunders Co.

Flammer, K, Clubb, SL. 1994. Neonatology. In *Avian Medicine: Principles and Application*, edited by Ritchie, BW, Harrison, GJ, Harrison, LR. Lake Worth: Winger's Publishing.

Forshaw, JM, Cooper, WT. 1989. *Parrots of the World*. 3d ed. Willoughby, Australia: Landsdown Press.

Harrison, GJ, Ritchie, BW. 1994. Making distinctions on the physical examination. In *Avian Medicine: Principles and Application*, edited by Ritchie, BW, Harrison, GJ, Harrison, LR. Lake Worth: Winger's Publishing.

Joyner, KL. 1994. Theriogenology. In *Avian Medicine: Principles and Application*, edited by Ritchie, BW, Harrison, GJ, Harrison, LR. Lake Worth: Winger's Publishing.

King, AS, McLelland, J. 1984. *Birds, Their Structure and Function*. 2d ed. Eastbourne, England: Bailliere Tindall.

McMillan, MC. 1994. Imaging techniques. In *Avian Medicine: Principles and Application*, edited by Ritchie, BW, Harrison, GJ, Harrison, LR. Lake Worth: Winger's Publishing.

Paul-Murphy, J, Brunson, DB, Miletic, V. 1999. Analgesic effects of butorphenol and buprenorphine in conscious African grey parrots (*Psitticus erithacus erithacus*) and (*Psittacus erithacus timneh*). *Am J Vet Res* Oct. 60(10):1218–21.

Perry, RA. 1994. The avian patient. In *Avian Medicine: Principles and Application*. Ritchie BW, Harrison GJ, Harrison LR, Lake Worth: Winger's Publishing.

Quandt, JE, Greenacre, CB. 1999. Sevoflurane anesthesia in Psittacines. *Journal of Zoo and Wildlife Medicine* 30 (2): 308–309.

Rembert, MS, Smith, JA, Hosgood, G, Marks, SL, Tully, TN. 2001. Comparison of traditional thermal support with the forced air warmer system in Hispaniolan Amazon parrots (*Amazona ventralis*). Assoc Avian Vets Annual Conf, 215–217.

Ritchie, B, Dreesen, D. 1998. Avian zoonoses: Proven and potential diseases, Part II. *Comp Cont Ed* 10(6):688–696.

Ritchie, B, Harrison GJ, Harrison, LR. 1994. *Avian Medicine: Principles and Application*. Lake Worth: Winger's Publishing.

Ritchie, BW. 1995a. Herpesviridae. In *Avian Viruses, Function and Control*. Lake Worth: Winger's Publishing.

Ritchie, BW. 1995b. Papovaviridae. In *Avian Viruses, Function and Control*. Lake Worth: Winger's Publishing.

Ritchie BW, Gregory CR, Latimer KS, Campagnoli RP, Pesti D, Ciembor P, Rae M, Reed HH, Speer BL, Loudis BG, Shivaprasad HL, Garner MM. 2000. Documentation of a PBFD virus variant in lories. Assoc Avian Vets Annual Conf, 263–268.

Sinn, LC. 1994. Anesthesiology. In *Avian Medicine: Principles and Application*, edited by Ritchie, BW, Harrison, GJ, Harrison, LR. Lake Worth: Winger's Publishing.

Van Sant, F. 1998. Zinc and parrots: More than you ever wanted to know. Assoc Avian Vets Annual Conf, 305–312.

CHAPTER THREE

The Lizard

Brad Wilson

INTRODUCTION

From the seemingly impenetrable spines of *Moloch horridus*, the gliding pseudo-wings of *Draco* spp., the color-changing chromatophores of *Chamaeleo* spp., the cryptic cutaneous fimbriations of *Uroplatus* spp., the venomous bite of *Heloderma* spp., to the bipedal water-walking *Basiliscus* spp., the adhesive glass-climbing Gekkonidae, and the legless snakelike Anguinidae lizards of the order Squamata in the class Reptilia exhibit tremendous anatomic, physiologic, nutritional, and behavioral variation that makes them the hallmark of diversity among all modern reptiles. When distributed among 3,800 known species (Barten 1996a; de Vosjoli 1992), it becomes obvious that the diagnostic challenge presented to the veterinary clinician and technician can be overwhelming. See color plates 3.1, 3.2, 3.3, 3.4, 3.5, 3.6.

Though the details may seem overwhelming, the basic categories of differentiating lizards based on natural history lead to a basic understanding of husbandry requirements. Technicians familiar with reptile medicine soon learn that many health disorders arise from improper husbandry. Therefore, recognizing and correcting improper husbandry techniques may hasten the recovery from disease and prevent unnecessary medicating of debilitated patients.

Representatives of many families of lizards are commonly seen in the pet trade (table 3.1). The green iguana (*Iguana iguana*) is one of the most popular of all reptile pets and historically has been the first reptile pet of many people new to the hobby of herpetoculture, the care and maintenance of captive reptiles and amphibians. In the past 15 years, the reptile pet industry has exponentially increased in popularity and in recent years the author has observed the popularity of lizards approach, if not exceed, that of snakes as reptile pets. This leads to the question: why keep reptiles as pets? To the dedicated pet owner, the answer is the same as if the question were why keep a spider, fish, bird, cat, dog, goat, or horse as a pet. For avid reptile pet owners, however, a quote from de Vosjoli (1997) is most appropriate: "the current philosophy in herpetoculture strives towards establishing viable self-sustaining captive-breeding populations through managed field culture and/or through more controlled systems of indoor and outdoor vivaria."

ANATOMY AND PHYSIOLOGY

Integument

Lizard scales commonly overlap and are created by a many-layered epidermis that is shed at regular intervals during the life of the lizard. The shedding of skin, ecdysis, occurs in multiple pieces in lizards as opposed to snakes in which the skin is usually shed in one piece. Many lizard species will eat the shed skin. Factors that influence ecdysis are age, growth rate, temperature, humidity, and nutrition (Barten 1996a; Goin, Goin, & Zug 1978). Dysecdysis is commonly associated with low humidity and poor nutrition among other health abnormalities.

Reptilian epidermis does not have a respiratory function and contains very few glands (Goin et al. 1978). The skin and scales are relatively impermeable in normal health. The mucous membranes (oral cavity, cloaca, conjunctiva), however, are quite permeable. This consideration is of importance when considering potential absorption of topical medications applied to these regions (Mader 2000a; Klingenberg 1996). Some reptile vitamin supplements are marketed as sprays to be applied to the skin. These products, though not likely harmful, have little to no systemic physiologic value to reptiles.

Chamaeleo spp. and *Anolis* spp. have chromatophores in the skin that allow change in the reflectivity of visible light resulting in color change. These changes are influenced by light, heat, and social influences, and not by surrounding environmental color (Barten 1996a; Goin et al. 1978). Many herpetoculturists who raise chameleons can predict color

31

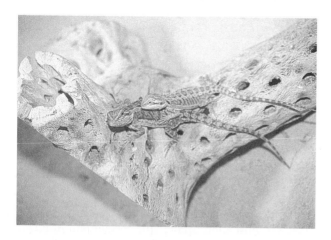

Plate 3.1. *Bearded dragon. (Photo courtesy of Ryan Cheek) (See also color plates)*

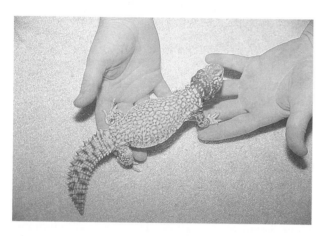

Plate 3.2. *Mali uromastyx. (Photo courtesy of Ryan Cheek) (See also color plates)*

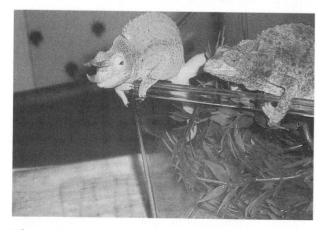

Plate 3.3. *Jackson chameleon. (Photo courtesy of Dr. Sam Rivera) (See also color plates)*

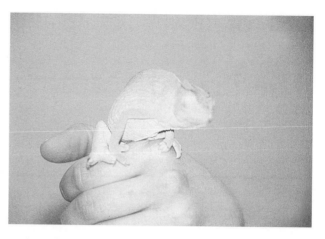

Plate 3.4. *Chameleon. (Photo courtesy of Ryan Cheek) (See also color plates)*

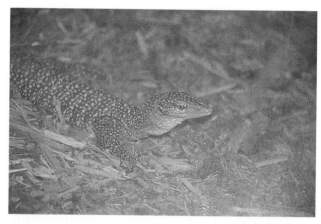

Plate 3.5. *Mangrove monitor. (Photo courtesy of Ryan Cheek) (See also color plates)*

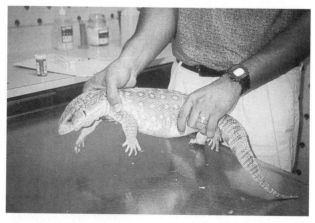

Plate 3.6. *Savannah monitor. (Photo courtesy of Dr. Sam Rivera) (See also color plates)*

changes of particular species or individuals based on a variety of environmental or behavioral influences.

Some gecko species can autotomize, tear or release, the entire skin in response to capture by a predator. These include the fish-scale geckos (*Geckolepis* spp.) and the day geckos (*Phelsuma* spp.; Glaw & Vences 1994; McKeown 1993). Skin regeneration does occur in these species, but may result in unsightly scars and may result in secondary bacterial or fungal infections.

Foot and toe adaptations are diverse. Integument specialization is quite notable in the fanlike adhesive discs of Gekkonidae. These species are capable of climbing glass and inverted smooth surfaces. Large arboreal and terrestrial lizards usually possess sharp sturdy claws. Lizard claws are similar to those of birds in having a pulp containing a blood vessel and nerve that is sensitive to short trimming.

Skeletal System

The general lizard skeletal system is quadruped consisting of an ossified skull, vertebral column, ribs, and pelvic and pectoral girdles (fig. 3.1). The ribs of lizards connect ventrally to a cartilaginous sternum that is absent in snakes and turtles (Goin et al. 1978). Lizard teeth are either acrodont or pleurodont. Acrodont teeth attach to the masticating surface of the mandible or maxilla and have no socket. These teeth are not replaced when lost and are characteristic of true chameleons. Pleurodont teeth are attached to the inner or lingual surface of the mandible or maxilla and have no socket. These teeth are replaced through the life of the lizard

and are characteristic of iguanas and monitors.

Locomotion for lizards is apodal, bipedal, or quadrupedal. Most lizards have four legs and five toes, though there are species that are snakelike with no functional legs (*Anguis* spp., *Anniela* spp., *Lialis* spp., *Ophisaurus* spp.) and others with greatly reduced limbs (*Chalcides chalcides*, *Neoseps reynoldsi*, *Chamaesaura* spp.). Bipedal locomotion is observed in basilisks (*Basiliscus* spp.) and frilled dragons (*Chlamydosaurus kingii*) when excited or during escape behavior. This behavior is rarely observed in small enclosures. Old World chameleons (*Chamaeleo* spp.) are zygodactylous, having two toes and three toes fused into a clawlike foot, creating a strong gripping foot for climbing on limbs and branches (Goin et al. 1978).

Tail autotomy, the loss or release of the tail, occurs in many species (Iguanidae, Gekkonidae, some Scincidae). This adaptation (coupled with certain behaviors) creates distraction and allows the tailless lizard to escape as a potential predator investigates the released, yet still moving tail. Transverse cleavage plates are present in each caudal vertebrae of these species allowing release of the tail at multiple locations (Barten 1996a; Goin et al. 1978). Hemorrhage is minimal with tail loss as vertebral vessels are quick to constrict. If the tail stump is undamaged, species capable of autotomy can regenerate tails that are usually smaller with irregular scalation and darker color than the original tail. If species that are not capable of autotomy (Chamaeleontidae, Varanidae) suffer traumatic

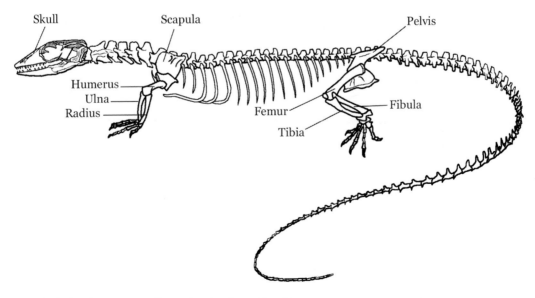

Fig. 3.1. *Lizard skeletal anatomy. (Drawing by Scott Stark)*

Table 3.1. Lizards Commonly Seen in Captivity

Common name/species name	Origin	Habitat	Size (cm)[1]	Temp (d/n)[2]	Repro[3]	Feed[4]	Rest[5]	Handling concerns[6]
Agamidae								
Agamas, *Agama* spp.[10]	Africa	Arid, desert, terrestrial	30–40	30C/20C	oviparous	O/a	yes, no	Occas. aggressive, sturdy
Bearded Dragon, *Pogona* spp.[10,16]	Australia	Arid, terrestrial	to 50	30C/20C	oviparous	O/a	yes	Docile, surdy
Frilled lizard, *Chlamydosaurus kingi*[10,16]	Australia	Dry, forest, terrestrial	to 100	30C/20C	oviparous	C/a,v	yes	Occas. aggressive, sturdy
Water dragon, *Physignathus coccinus*[10]	SE Asia	Humid, rain forest, arboreal	100	26C/20C	oviparous	O/a,v,n	no	Occas. aggressive, sturdy
Uromastyx, *Uromastyx* spp.[12]	NW Afr, SW Asia	Arid, desert, terrestrial	30–50	37C/22C	oviparous	H,O/a	yes	Docile, sturdy
Anguidae								
Glass lizards, *Ophisaurus* spp.[10]	Worldwide	Dry, rocky forest, terrestrial	to 140	26C/20C	oviparous	C/a,g	yes	Docile, fragile, tail autotomy+
Chamaeleontidae								
Veiled chameleon, *Chamaeleo calyptratus*[13]	E Africa	Montane forest, arboreal	50	30C/20C	oviparous	I	no	Docile, fragile to sturdy
Flapneck chameleon, *Chamaeleo dilepis*[10,14]	Africa	Tropical savanna, arboreal	30	30C/20C	oviparous	I	no	Docile, fragile to sturdy
Three-horned chameleon, *Ch. jacksonii*[13]	E Africa	Montane forest, arboreal	30	25C/20C	viviparous	I	no	Docile, fragile to sturdy
Panther chameleon, *Chamaeleo pardalis*[13]	Madagascar	Coastal forest, arboreal	60	30C/20C	oviparous	I	no	Occas. aggressive, sturdy
Gekkonidae								
Day geckos, *Phelsuma* spp.[8]	Indian Ocean Islands	Tropical rain forest, arboreal	to 25	30C/25C	oviparous	O/a,n	no	Docile, tail autotomy, skin slough
Leaf-tailed geckos, *Uroplatus* spp.[6,10,14]	Madagascar	Tropical rain forest, arboreal	to 25	28C/22C	oviparous	I	no	Docile, fragile, tail autotomy+
Leopard gecko, *Eublepharis macularius*[9]	Asia	Desert, terrestrial	to 20	30C/25C	oviparous	I	yes	Occ. aggressive, tail autotomy+
Tokay gecko, *Gekko gecko*[10]	SE Asia	Tropical rain forest, arboreal	to 30	27C/20C	oviparous	C/a,v	no	Aggressive, sturdy
Iguanidae								
Green anole, *Anolis carolinensis*[10]	N America	Temperate forest, arboreal	20	26C/20C	oviparous	I	yes	Docile, tail autotomy
Green iguana, *Iguana iguana*[7]	Central, S America	Tropical rain forest, arboreal	200	31C/22C	oviparous	H	yes	Very aggressive, tail autotomy
Horned lizards, *Phrynosoma* spp.[10]	Central, N America	Arid, desert, savanna, terrestrial	to 20	35C/20C	vivi-,ovi-	I/t	yes	Docile, sturdy
Spiny lizards, *Sceloporus* spp.[10,14]	N, S, Central America	Dry, rocky, forest, arb/terrestrial	to 30	26C/20C	vivi-,ovi-	I	yes	Docile, sturdy

Family / Common name, Genus	Distribution	Habitat	Size[1]	Temp[2]	Repro[3]	Diet[4]	Brumate[5]	Response[6]
Lacertidae								
Jeweled lizard, *Lacerta* spp.[10]	Europe, Africa	Dry, forest, arboreal/terrestrial	to 40	25C/15C	vivi-,ovi-	O/a,n	yes	Occas. aggressive, sturdy
Scincidae								
Skinks, *Eumeces* spp.[10]	Worldwide	Forests, terrestrial, occas. arboreal	to 30	26C/20C	vivi-,ovi-	I	yes	Docile, tail autotomy
Blue-tongued skinks, *Tiliqua* spp.[10,14]	Australia	Forest, desert, terrestrial	to 50	30C/20C	viviparous	O/a,g	yes	Docile, sturdy
Prehensile-tailed skink, *Corucia zebrata*[15]	Solomon Islands	Topical forest, arboreal	to 60	30C/24C	viviparous	H	yes	Occas. aggressive, sturdy
Teiidae								
Ameivas, *Ameiva* spp.[10]	Central, S America	Forest, fields, terrestrial	to 50	26C/20C	oviparous	O/a,n	yes	Docile, sturdy
Tegus, *Tupinambis* spp.[10,11]	S America	Forests, terrestrial	to 140	30C/20C	oviparous	C/a,v,e	yes	Occas. aggressive, sturdy
Varanidae								
Nile monitor, *Varanus niloticus*[11]	Africa	Stream, riverbanks, terrestrial	to 200	30C/20C	oviparous	C/e,g,v	yes	Very aggressive, sturdy
Savannah monitor, *V. exanthematicus*[11]	Africa	Desert, dry grassland, terrestrial	to 100	30C/20C	oviparous	C/a,g,e,v	yes	Occas. aggressive, sturdy

[1] Average maximum adult size.

[2] Average day and night temperatures for adults of species or typical of genus.

[3] Oviparous (ovi-)= egg laying; viviparous (vivi-) = live birth; parthenogenic (partheno) = produces offspring without mating.

[4] Diet of the adult lizard *in nature*: O = omnivore, I = exclusive insectivore, C = primary carnivore, H = exclusive herbivore, H,O = some spp. exclusively herbivorous, some spp. omnivorous. Specializations or primary food consumed listed in order of importance for each sp.: a = arthropods, e = eggs, g = gastropods, n = nectar or ripe fruit, t = termites and ants, v = vertebrates.

[5] Does lizard seasonally hibernate or brumate? Yes = successful captive breeding may require cooling/rest period. No = successful breeding does not require cooling/rest period.

[6] Typical response of patient to handling:

  Docile: lizards will allow handling with minimal resistance.

  Occasionally aggressive: lizards may attempt to bite or claw when handled and can inflict injury upon handler.

  Aggressive: lizards will routinely bite, claw, or struggle during or before handling. The Tokay gecko is not particularly dangerous to handle, but is aggressive.

  Very aggressive: lizards may bite, scratch, or whip tail *prior* to handling. Large monitors and iguanas should be considered dangerous at all times and handled only by experienced staff.

  Sturdy: little to no stress or trauma results from routine handling when healthy.

  Fragile: may stress easily when handled for routine examination. Bodily injury to lizard may result from routine restraint or handling.

  Tail autotomy: lizards may lose tail when handled (not all spp. capable of autotomy are marked). [+]Tail autotomy in some species may occur even if lizard is not handled, but merely stressed.

  Skin slough: lizards with skin that tears easily when minimally restrained or touched.

[7] de Vosjoli, 1992.
[8] McKeown 1993.
[9] de Vosjoli et al. 1997.
[10] Obst et al. 1988.
[11] Balsai 1997.
[12] de Vosjoli 1995.
[13] de Vosjoli &Ferguson1995.
[14] de Vosjoli1997.
[15] de Vosjoli1993.
[16] de Vosjoli 2001.

tail loss, the tail usually cannot regenerate completely. Some lizards (some Chamaeleontidae and *Corucia zebrata*) utilize a prehensile tail for stabilization or movement between branches.

It is important to note that touching or manipulating the tail is not necessary to cause its release in some species! The leaf-tailed geckos, *Uroplatus* spp., can only autotomize the entire tail from the first one or two caudal vertebrae so the entire tail is always lost (Glaw & Vences 1994). A common escape behavior in these species is to wave the tail to distract the potential predator and then release it from the body without the lizard being touched or manipulated. Similar behavior can occur in the terrestrial leopard and African fat-tailed geckos (*Eublepharis macularius, Hemitheconyx caudicinctus*) (de Vosjoli 1997).

Cardiovascular System

The heart has three chambers consisting of two atria and one ventricle. Despite the absence of an interventricular septum, the majority of deoxygenated blood is directed to the lungs via the pulmonary aorta and oxygenated blood is directed to the right and left aortic arches to perfuse the body tissues (Goin et al. 1978).

Lizards, like amphibians, possess a large ventral abdominal vein that is intracoelomic along the ventral midline several millimeters dorsal to the body wall. This vein is secured by a thin mesovasorum and travels adjacent to the ventral midline from one-fourth the distance from the cranial aspect of the pubis cranially to the umbilicus and then courses dorsally to join the hepatic vein. Venous collateral circulation parallels the ventral abdominal vein via the caudal vena cava. The ventral abdominal vein is routinely avoided during coelomic surgery, though accidental or intentional transection and ligation of this vessel would be compensated by collateral circulation (Mader 2002b).

The caudal tail vein is the optimal site for blood collection from lizards. This vein is located along the ventral midline of the tail and is accessed approximately one-third (or less) the distance from the cloaca to the tail tip.

Respiratory System

The respiratory system of lizards consists of external nares, internal nares, glottis, trachea, and lungs. The internal nares are located rostrally in the dorsal oral cavity and are contiguous with the external nares. The glottis, located at the base of the tongue, fits into the common opening of the internal nares when the mouth is closed to enable nasal respiration.

The trachea of most lizards bifurcates into the lungs that in some lizards may more resemble air sacs of birds than the familiar mammalian lung. Lizards do not have a diaphragm and therefore have a common coelomic cavity rather than separate thoracic and abdominal cavities. Ventilation in lizards is accomplished with rib expansion by contraction of intercostal muscles.

The lungs of lizards are not as highly derived as mammals. The cranial portions of the lungs are more vascular and serve for most respiratory functions and the caudal lungs are more saclike and may extend to the pelvis (Murray 1996). Unlike birds, lizards do not have pneumatic bones.

Digestive System

The digestive system of most lizards is quite basic and, with the exception of the teeth, follows the design of higher vertebrates. The oral cavity contains several glands that aid in the lubrication of food items for swallowing. The Gila monster and Mexican beaded lizard (*Heloderma suspectum, H. horridum*) have modified bilateral sublingual glands that produce poisonous saliva that is chewed into the prey item rather than hypodermically injected as with venomous snakes (Barten 1996a; Goin et al. 1978).

The tongue of some lizards serves both in scent collection and swallowing. The tongue of anguimorph (legless) lizards serves, almost exclusively, a sensory function and the tongue of some Chamaeleontidae serves an exclusive food prehension and swallowing function (Goin et al. 1978). Most carnivorous lizards (Varanidae) have snakelike tongues to track prey items, and the majority of herbivorous lizards have thick fleshy tongues to aid in swallowing. The sensory tongue retracts into a lingual sheath that lies ventral to the glottis.

The alimentary tract consists of an esophagus, stomach, small and large intestines, and cloaca. The alimentary, respiratory, reproductive, cardiovascular, and reproductive tracts are not separated by a diaphragm and are contained within a pleuroperitoneum or coelomic cavity (coelom). The proximal portion of the esophagus is the only opening to the back of the oral cavity. Thus, by visualizing and avoiding the opening to the glottis on the floor of the mouth, feeding or sampling tubes may be safely passed into the digestive tract with no risk of accidental respiratory intubation. The stomach in most lizards is quite large and does not serve as a gizzard or grinding organ (Barten 1996a; Goin et al. 1978). The small intestine has histologically discrete duodenum, jejunum, and ileum (Frye 1991). A cecumlike sacculation of the colon is present in herbivorous lizards (*Corucia zebrata, Iguana* spp., *Uromastyx* spp., and others). The cloaca is the common collecting chamber of the digestive and genitourinary tracts. These openings are the coprodeum and urodeum, respectively. The proctodeum is the common chamber opening to the vent (figs. 3.2 and 3.3).

The liver and gall bladder are present in lizards and located cranial to the stomach in the cranioventral abdomen. The gall bladder in anguimorph lizards is observed in a more caudal position, and is usually found in close proximity to the pancreas as seen in snakes. The pancreas in lizards has both endocrine and exocrine glandular functions.

Large paired fat bodies in the left and right caudal coelomic cavity are not digestive structures, but may be commonly confused with pathologic lesions. These are particularly palpable in bearded dragons and are commonly observed in dorsoventral radiographs.

Excretory System

Paired kidneys are located in the caudodorsal coelom and the caudal poles commonly extend into the pelvic canal. Lizards are uricotelic; the majority of nitrogenous waste from purine digestion is excreted from most lizards as insoluble uric acid (Frye 1991). A mesonephric duct collects and transports nitrogenous wastes from each kidney to a urinary bladder. The urinary bladder empties into the cranioventral urodeum. In larger lizards the urinary bladder may be catheterized from the cloaca via this opening.

The renal-portal system in reptiles is well documented (Barten 1996a; Frye 1991; Innis 2000). The system allows blood to flow from the caudal portion of the body directly to the kidneys prior to returning to the heart. Historically this physiology has led to the conclusion that the reptile kidney may reduce the concentration of chemotherapeutics injected into the caudal body prior to their entry into the general circulation, thus leading to a decreased concentration in the blood and tissues. Also, suspicion was raised that injections of potentially nephrotoxic drugs should be avoided in the region. Several pharmacologic studies in turtles have revealed that the presence of this system does not necessarily indicate that all blood flow follows this theorized pathway and there may be no impact on drug metabolism when injected into the caudal body of tortoises (Innis 2000).

Reproductive System

Lizards have intracoelomic paired testes or ovaries, and oviducts. Female lizards have no true uterus, but in livebearing (ovoviviparous or viviparous) lizards, the oviduct may serve a similar function to the nonplacental uterus of mammals by providing nutrients for the

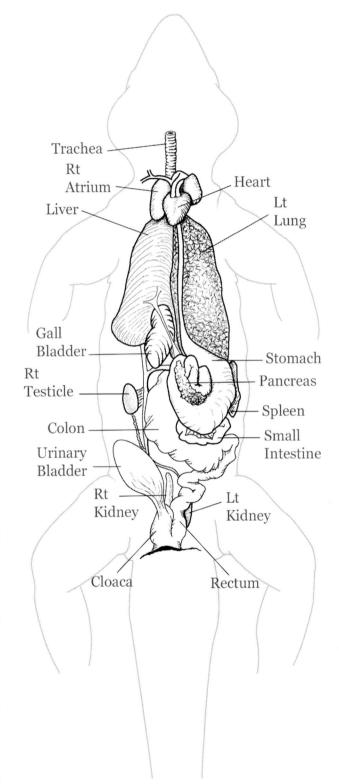

Fig. 3.2. *Lizard visceral anatomy. (Drawing by Scott Stark)*

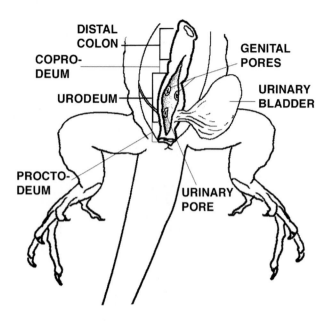

Fig. 3.3. Lizard cloaca. (Drawing by Scott Stark)

Labels in figure:
DISTAL COLON
COPRODEUM
URODEUM
PROCTODEUM
GENITAL PORES
URINARY BLADDER
URINARY PORE

developing nonshelled embryo (DeNardo 1996a). DeNardo (1996a) refers to all ovoviviparous reptiles as viviparous. The eggshell is secreted in the oviduct of oviparous lizards and is occasionally referred to as the "shell gland." The eggshell of many lizards (except Gekkonidae) is somewhat pliable as seen in snakes rather than rigid as seen in tortoises and birds.

Male lizards have paired hemipenes that are invaginated into the proximal ventral tail slightly lateral and caudal to the vent. During mating one hemipenis is everted by relaxation of the retractor muscle and the filling of vascular spaces of the hemipenes with blood. Following mating fertilization is internal and occurs within the oviduct. No urinary structures are present within the hemipenes of lizards.

Sexual dimorphism occurs in some species of lizards, while in others determining sex may be difficult. For most juvenile lizards of all species, there is no reliable method to determine sex. For adult lizards, the technique of sex determination differs by species (see table 3.2).

External sex characteristics may be applied to many lizards. These characteristics include the presence of obvious sexual dimorphism such as the horns of *Chamaeleo jacksonii*; precloacal pores of many Gekkonidae; femoral pores of many Iguanidae; and postcloacal tail bulging of the hemipenes in many species. Researching the anatomy of the species in question is the best method to determine if external sex characteristics are applicable.

Cloacal probing, the primary technique used in sex determination of snakes, may be applied to monitors (Varanidae), but is not 100% accurate in all species. A blunt or ball-tipped smooth metal sexing probe designed exclusively for this purpose is used. The only other acceptable instrument may be a sovereign red rubber urinary catheter or feeding tube. This procedure carries risk of causing trauma to the patient; therefore, proper restraint and proficiency are required. The probe is inserted into the vent and directed caudally just lateral to the ventral midline in a position parallel to the surface of the tail. In males, the probe will enter the inverted sheath of the hemipenis and travel a distance into the tail. This distance is subjective and variable by species. In some female monitors, the distance the probe travels is shorter when compared to the male.

Radiographic sex determination is possible in some monitors. This technique is based on the presence of calcifications in the hemipenes of some species. These mineralizations are absent in males of both Nile and savannah monitors.

Surgical or endoscopic sex determination is obviously definitive. Surgical scar tissue formation, difficult visualization, and availability of equipment are potential complications. Sedation is required for either procedure.

Manual eversion of the hemipenes is advocated for some species (*Pogona* spp., *Corucia zebrata*) (de Vosjoli 1993; de Vosjoli et al. 2001). This method is commonly used in juvenile snakes. The procedure involves bending the tail slightly dorsally distal to the cloaca while simultaneously applying light pressure with the thumb in a rolling motion proximally toward the cloaca. This process in some male lizards will evert the hemipenes. This method will definitively identify males by the presence of the hemipenes, but only identifies the females by exclusion. Males that do not evert a hemipene may be mistaken for females.

Hydrostatic eversion of the hemipenes is a definitive method to sexing monitors, but carries moderate to great risk of injury to the lizard. Proper restraint and mastery of technique are paramount. The principle is that injection of sterile saline caudal to the retracted hemipenis will evert the organ through its cloacal opening. In female lizards, with proper technique, no hemipenis will evert and the oviductal papillae of the female may be visualized. This technique should be performed in sedated patients and restricted only to those animals in which no other method of sex determination is available.

Table 3.2. Sex Determination in Selected Captive Lizards

Species	Anatomic	Probe	Manual eversion	Hydrostatic eversion
Bearded dragon, *Pogona* spp.	A		J	
Frilled lizard, *Chlamydosaurus kingi*	A			
Uromastyx, *Uromastyx* spp.	A			
Veiled chameleon, *Chamaeleo calyptratus*	A			
Three-horned chameleon, *Ch. jacksonii*	A,J			
Day geckos, *Phelsuma* spp.	A,j			
Leopard gecko, *Eublepharis macularius*	A,j			
Green iguana, *Iguana iguana*	A,j			
Blue-tongued skinks, *Tiliqua* spp.	a		j	A
Prehensile-tailed skink, *Corucia zebrata*	a		A,j	
Tegus, *Tupinambis* spp.	a	A		
Nile monitor, *Varanus niloticus*		a		A
Savannah monitor, *V. exanthematicus*		a		A

Note: A = preferred method, adult; a = inconsistent method, adult; J = preferred method, juvenile; j = inconsistent method, juvenile.

Nervous System

The central nervous system consists of a cerebrum, cerebellum, brainstem, and spinal cord. The spinal cord extends to the tip of the tail as opposed to mammals in which the cord terminates proximal to the sacral vertebrae. The peripheral nervous system consists of 12 cranial nerves and numerous peripheral nerves to the viscera, trunk, and limbs.

Pain receptors and pain responses in reptiles are still poorly understood (Bennett 1996a). It is apparent that lizards have a withdrawal response or reflex from traumatic wounds such as punctures, lacerations, or surgical incisions; however, expected withdrawal reflexes and responses from potentially traumatic heat are not observed (Mader 2000b). Captive management of lizards must take into account these apparent behavioral and/or neurologic reflex differences from mammals with regard to cage heating (see below, "Husbandry").

Sense Organs

The majority of lizards have movable eyelids and a nictitating membrane. Those without movable lids (some Gekkonidae, and *Ablepharus* spp.) have a clear spectacle as seen in snakes. The spectacle is a scalelike structure formed by the fusion of the upper and lower eyelids. As with snakes, the spectacle is impermeable to topical medications. True chameleons possess turretlike eyelids and eyes that are capable of independent movement. Glands are present in the eyelids of lizards and may become swollen in cases of hypovitaminosis A.

The muscles of the iris are striated and under conscious control; thus, pupillary light reflexes are not predictable and the use of standard mammalian mydriatics is not possible (Williams 1996). The pupil may be circular or elliptical.

The parietal eye, or "third eye," is apparent in some species (Iguanidae; Tuatara, *Sphenodon punctatus*). This structure is located on the dorsal head and is connected via the parietal nerve to the pineal body in the brain. The parietal eye is a photoreceptor that is integral in hormone production and thermoregulatory behavior (Goin et al. 1978).

The lizard ear consists of an external acoustic meatus, tympanic membrane, middle ear cavity, and inner ear cavity. Within the middle ear cavity is the columella bone that receives vibrations from the tympanic membrane via the extracolumella cartilage (Rossi 1998b). The tympanic membrane of some lizard species is clear and in others it is covered with scales and not visible.

The vomeronasal organ, or Jacobson's organ, is present in many lizards and located in the dorsal oral cavity ventral to the nasal cavity but not continuous with the nasal cavity (Goin et al. 1978). Scent particles collected on the tongue are transferred to sensory cells when the tongue is retracted into the mouth. This organ is primarily used by lizards to track prey items and possibly to detect mates or enemies by detecting pheromones.

HUSBANDRY

Understanding the natural history (anatomy, physiology, habitat requirements, reproductive habits, behavior, longevity) of the patient in question is the greatest diagnostic tool in differentiating between normal health and disease. Combining this knowledge with the presenting complaint, medical history, physical examination, and laboratory data is necessary for the treatment and rehabilitation of the diseased patient. For instance, understanding the differences in dietary and habitat requirements of two common similarly sized lizard pets, the green iguana (*Iguana iguana*) and the savannah monitor (*Varanus exanthematicus*), is essential even to obtain an appropriate history. It is not possible for even the most educated zookeeper to know every aspect of natural history of every lizard, nor is it expected that the veterinary technician can become educated in the feeding habits of every species of lizard kept in captivity. There are, however, several fundamental aspects of knowledge regarding lizards with which to simplify the approach to understanding natural history.

The following are general categories and associated specific questions with which the technician and practitioner should be familiar regarding every lizard patient:

1. Native habitat and microhabitat
   Does the patient inhabit tropical rain forest, desert, mountain slope, estuary, beach, etc.?
   Is the patient arboreal, terrestrial, aquatic, or subterranean?
2. Anatomy and physiology
   What is normal coloration and can the patient change coloration in response to environmental, seasonal, health, reproductive, or behavioral influences?
   Are there size or other physical differences based on sex?
   What is the normal mucous membrane color?
   Does the patient normally have four limbs and a certain number of digits?
   Does the patient normally have secretions from the eyes or nostrils?
   What are the characteristics of normal feces and urates?
   How long does the patient normally live?
3. Diet
   Is the patient insectivorous, carnivorous, herbivorous, or omnivorous—does the diet change with respect to life stage or seasonality?
   If insectivorous, does the patient have a preferred food item or size of food item? (i.e., ants, centipedes, spiders, etc.)
   How does the patient prehend food and at what time of day does it normally feed?
   How does the patient normally obtain water?
4. Behavior
   Is the patient diurnal, nocturnal, or crepuscular?
   Is the patient solitary or communal?
   Does the patient experience climatic seasonality?
   Does the patient hibernate or aestivate?
   Does the patient utilize different microhabitats during different seasons or life stages?
   How does the patient reproduce and how often?

These natural history parameters for all species of lizards would fill volumes, and these are questions for which the technician or veterinarian may not always know the answer. There are many similarities among genera, but even within the same genus there are marked differences between species in husbandry requirements.

Looking again at the green iguana and the savannah monitor: the green iguana is a tropical, arboreal, diurnal, somewhat communal (though not in captivity), generally nonseasonal, and nonhibernating lizard (de Vosjoli 1992; Obst et al. 1988), whereas the savannah monitor is a temperate, semiarid, terrestrial (and burrowing), crepuscular (to diurnal), solitary, somewhat seasonal, and occasionally hibernating lizard (Obst et al. 1988; Balsai 1997). For the green iguana the diet is generally herbivorous, though as with other species, in their native habitat they may be opportunistically insectivorous. For the savannah monitor the diet is carnivorous or insectivorous (depending on the life stage and food availability). Remember, however, that one can only speak of living systems in generalities; adaptation is the key to survival and many captive lizards "adapt" to the captive environment. Thus, behavior observed in nature may not occur in captivity.

Reptile hobbyists who pride themselves on maintaining and breeding common and rare lizards in captivity have learned that re-creating the native environment in almost every aspect is the key to success. These achievements are accomplished by observing the animals in their native habitat, corresponding with other hobbyists or zoologic professionals, and countless hours of trial and error. Occasionally substantial investment is made in the construction of suitable habitats that far exceeds the monetary value of the lizard in question.

Enclosures and Environment

Cages

There is no way to generalize a "basic lizard cage." There are, however, categories of habitats from which the foundation for housing most species can be derived. In general terms lizards are categorized as arboreal or terrestrial. Remember that some arboreal lizards are occasionally both terrestrial and arboreal. Therefore, suitable cage design may not be exclusive for either habitat. Native habitat utilization is listed in table 3.1 for common species. Key requirements for all enclosures include security from escape; protection from injury; access for cleaning; environmental control of light, heat, humidity, ventilation; and water and food availability.

True chameleons (*Chamaeleo* spp.) and day geckos (*Phelsuma* spp.) are good examples of primarily arboreal lizards. Though these species vary greatly in size and in microhabitat distribution, most species benefit from a vertically spacious cage that offers visual security on three sides and from above. Typically, enclosures for arboreal lizards contain numerous limbs, branches, or plants in both a vertical and horizontal orientation. The cage is typically rectangular and may range from 0.3 m by 0.3 m by 0.5 m to 1.0 m by 1.0 m by 2.0 m. The primary, if not exclusive, construction material should be plastic screen with metal or plastic frame for chameleons and a glass or plastic aquarium for geckos. Screen allows for good ventilation and is relatively nonabrasive to the lizard. Wire mesh can lead to skin abrasions and may be more difficult to clean. Glass or plastic (Plexiglas) offers no ventilation and may lead to overheating, but allows for maintenance of higher humidity. The cage floor may be solid (wood, glass, or plastic) or mesh. Though a mesh floor with removable tray beneath may be most accessible for cleaning, it potentially allows escape of insect food items or may cause injury to the lizard. A solid floor with removable indoor/outdoor carpet is relatively easy to clean and provides security for chameleons. A well-sealed cage and lid are required for geckos as they are masters of escape. The cage ceiling is typically screen for both chameleons and geckos to allow adequate ventilation and humidity control (fig. 3.4).

Substrate for chameleons should be simple: newspaper or indoor/outdoor carpet is best. Soils, mulches, and shavings are messy and not essential for housing chameleons. Glass enclosures for arboreal lizards requiring higher humidity, such as day geckos, may contain soil in which plants are grown. The great

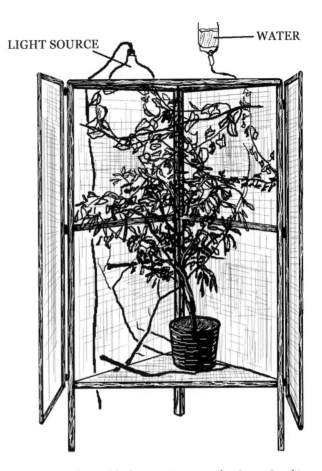

Fig. 3.4. Arboreal habitat. (Drawing by Scott Stark)

majority of arboreal captive lizards do not utilize the substrate except to oviposit and this substrate may be provided in the form of a nesting box or potted plant when required. Though aesthetically pleasing, particulate substrates such as soil, sand, gravel, and wood chips pose a great risk to small (<20 cm) lizards as accidental ingestion may result in gastric or intestinal obstruction or impaction.

The leopard gecko (*Eublepharis macularius*) and the savannah monitor (*Varanus exanthematicus*) are good examples of primarily terrestrial lizards. As opposed to the arboreal cage design, terrestrial enclosures are horizontally spacious to accommodate a large cage floor and may contain one or several diagonal or horizontal perches of relatively large diameter. Smaller cages range from 0.2 m by 0.3 m by 0.5 m to many meters in length, width, and height. Because many terrestrial lizards are relatively strong, more durable construction materials may be required for cage design. The glass aquarium is the standard enclosure for most small terrestrial lizards. Larger lizards, such as monitors, commonly require custom-built enclosures made from wood, glass or plastic, or wire mesh. Commonly these larger lizards are housed in outdoor enclosures where climates are favorable (figs. 3.5 and 3.6).

Lighting

Lighting requirements vary greatly among species. Some lizards require ultraviolet light (specifically UV-B) for vitamin D_3 (cholecalciferol) synthesis and subsequent calcium absorption from the gastrointestinal tract (Frye 1991; Donoghue & Landenberg 1996; Boyer 1996). A general rule is that primarily insectivorous (Gekkonidae), primarily herbivorous lizards (*Iguana* spp., *Uromastyx* spp.), and omnivorous lizards (*Pogona* spp.) require supplemental UV-B light and most primarily carnivorous lizards (monitors) do not. Many lizard owners provide artificial lighting in the form of various incandescent and fluorescent fixtures. It is important to understand that ultraviolet light will not penetrate glass or plastic; therefore, sunlight through windows and fluorescent lighting filtered by glass is inadequate to meet ultraviolet light requirements. Direct sunlight is the best source of ultraviolet light for lizards and may be provided periodically (once or twice weekly for 15 minutes) to lizards that otherwise are maintained indoors (Ritchie 1992). Most if not all lizards become stimulated when exposed to direct sunlight and may become aggressive and very quick, making escape possible. Also, lizards should never be housed in enclosed or open-top glass or plastic containers when in direct sunlight to avoid life-threatening hyperthermia. Some nocturnal lizards, such as leaf-tail and flat-tail geckos (*Phyllurus* spp., *Uroplatus* spp.), avoid bright light and are not active by day when in good health.

Light fixtures for lizards should be mounted outside the enclosure so that the lizard cannot directly contact the light (or heating element). Ultraviolet light sources should be within 18 to 24 inches of the closest basking surface. Many UV-B light bulbs are available as fluorescent bulbs and black lights (BL), and are available through pet shops and lighting retailers. Vita-Lites (Duro-Test Corp.) used in conjunction with BL lighting provides a satisfactory UV output for most captive lizards (Gehrman 1994).

Heating

Most common pet lizards require additional heating during some portion of their captive existence. Because lizards are ectothermic they seek microhabitats that meet their preferred optimal temperature zone (POTZ). The POTZ is the temperature range in which normal physiology is most efficient (Barten 1996a). It is important for the client to understand that a lizard utilizes a range of temperatures to create the POTZ, not a uniform cage temperature. In the cage setting this range is commonly referred to as the thermal gradient. It is also important to understand that various physiologic conditions such as pregnancy or disease may change the POTZ for a given animal. Observing the natural history and behavior and the study of lizard physiology is important for deriving the POTZ of each species. These values are available in many books, manuals, and journals for the species in question (see table 3.1). Lizards achieve their POTZ by thermoregulation. By altering their exposure to light, orientation to light, reflectivity of light (coloration), and by radiating heat (gaping, respiration) lizards are able to regulate body temperature within a few degrees.

Heating a lizard cage is generally not as difficult as providing an adequate thermal gradient. The ideal heat sources should be located outside the cage so that the

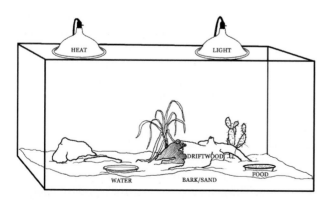

Fig. 3.5. Terrestrial habitat. (Drawing by Scott Stark)

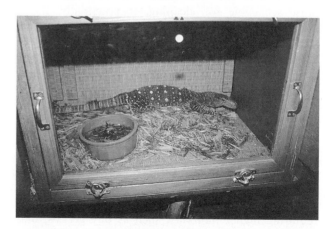

Fig. 3.6. An inappropriate size cage for a lizard. (Photo courtesy of Ryan Cheek)

lizard cannot directly contact the heating element. In-cage heating elements such as hot rocks are poor choices for heating reptiles and should never be recommended by veterinary staff. Similarly, ceramic radiant heating elements and light bulbs, which mount into incandescent fixtures, should not be placed inside the enclosure. All in-cage fixtures may cause thermal burns to lizards through prolonged direct contact (plate 3.7). Lizards have a poor sense of conductive heat and do not necessarily avoid contact with hot surfaces (Mader 2000b). Ideally cage heating should be provided through radiant heat from an overhead light or ceramic heating element. Commonly heating tape or heating blankets are placed outside and beneath the cage. Care must be exercised to avoid regions of the substrate or cage floor where heat is excessive. Additionally, below cage heating may lead to increased evaporation of water sources and increased cage humidity.

Some desert species, such as *Uromastyx* spp., may require daytime basking temperatures that range from 37° to 43°C (100° to 110°F) to nighttime temperatures of 25°C (77°F) (de Vosjoli 1995). Montane forest lizards such as Jackson's chameleon (*Chamaeleo jacksonii*) require daytime temperatures of 25°C (77°F) and night temperatures near 17°C (62°F) (de Vosjoli & Ferguson 1995). Arboreal lizards generally do not benefit from undercage or substrate heating. Certain temperate and some subtropical lizards may require cooler temperatures during winter months to induce brumation or hibernation that is essential for successful breeding. Temperature is best measured with thermometers or temperature probes, which are placed inside the enclosure at various locations.

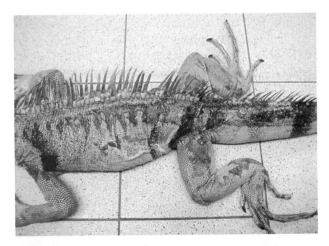

Plate 3.7. Thermal burns. (Photo courtesy of Dr. Stephen J. Hernandez-Divers, University of Georgia) (See also color plates)

Humidity can be a difficult parameter to regulate in the lizard enclosure. In a smaller enclosure, humidity is more difficult to regulate. As with temperature, many lizards benefit from a "humidity gradient"—another example of microhabitat utilization by lizards. In larger cages this gradient is created by the interface between substrate and cage ornaments such as rocks or logs. Small covered plastic containers containing moistened substrate such as vermiculite or moss may be provided. These are called "humidified shelters" (de Vosjoli 1997) and are particularly useful to assist shedding in some desert species such as leopard geckos and juvenile bearded dragons.

In well-ventilated cages, such as those for true chameleons, hand misting or electronic misters, vaporizers, or nebulizers are useful for increasing humidity. These are easily regulated by automatic timers. Regulating ventilation with screen lids or the addition of small fans is helpful to control humidity for glass aquariums or terrariums. Humidity is an important factor in both the respiratory epidermal health of some lizards. Hygrometers are used to measure humidity in the lizard cage.

Ventilation is primarily controlled to indirectly regulate heat and humidity. Ventilation can be modified by cage design or may be controlled by external and internal cage accessories. Small fans, such as computer cooling fans, are quiet and capable of moving large quantities of air. To a lesser extent, moving water, such as small waterfalls, misters, and passive evaporation, creates some air circulation for more humid enclosures. It is important with any electrical devices that all wires be fully insulated from contacting water or metal in or on the cage and that they cannot be altered by cage inhabitants. Also, fans must be housed outside the enclosure so that the lizard cannot contact the turning blades.

Water availability and water quality must be closely controlled. Some desert species, such as *Uromastyx* spp., do not require standing water in the cage (de Vosjoli 1995). Instead, these animals may be removed from the cage and soaked in water once weekly or they may be misted in an enclosure separate from their cage once weekly. Some tropical lizards such as true chameleons may drink only dripping water off leaves or other cage ornaments. In time these lizards may learn to drink from containers or from hand misting. The client should be educated that not all lizards readily accept water from containers or they are not physically capable of ingesting standing water. If water is not provided in the form that these lizards typically drink, they will dehydrate rapidly. Water containers for all lizards should be cleaned at least weekly.

Soaking with a 10% bleach solution for 15 minutes is sufficient for disinfection. Because some lizards may defecate in or otherwise contaminate larger water containers, more frequent cleaning of water containers may be required.

Feeding stations for lizards are preferred over the random introduction of food items into the enclosure. Carnivorous lizards should be fed prekilled food items such as small mammals from a container within the cage, or the lizard may be moved to a separate cage for feeding. Most insectivores will eat only moving insects and therefore must be fed live food items such as crickets, mealworms, and wax worms. These food items may be introduced into small bowls within the enclosure. Many lizards will readily adapt to eating from containers. Invariably some food items will escape into the cage and are usually consumed by the lizard. Presenting food in containers can reduce the risk of accidental substrate ingestion. It also may provide a central location at which the lizard may be observed while feeding to evaluate appetite and health. Feeding live foods such as small mammals and crickets increases the risk of bodily damage to the lizard by the food item. Crickets, just as mice and rats, may feed on the flesh of lizards if deprived of food for more than a day in the enclosure.

Herbivores are generally fed prepared meals in containers. Most healthy herbivorous lizards will consume their daily share of food at one feeding though in nature these animals generally browse throughout the day. Uneaten food should be removed from the cage on the day of feeding to prevent spoiling. Prepared foods, such as powdered, frozen, or otherwise processed herbivore foods, should be provided with strict attention to the manufacturer's recommendations for rehydration, thawing, and feeding frequency. For herbivorous lizards, freshly prepared vegetable diets are preferable over processed diets.

QUARANTINE

The most important consideration often overlooked by the owner of new pet lizards is quarantine. Many clients who own one lizard eventually increase their collections, establish breeding colonies, or expand their interests to other reptiles. In their excitement to introduce new pets to the home, they ignore the potential for contagious infectious diseases that may affect their entire collection of animals.

A significant contagious disease seen in reptile collections is acariasis (see below, "Parasitology"). Mite infestations can lead to reduced fertility, multisystemic disease, and death in captive reptile collections and may be extremely difficult to eradicate once established in large collections (Mader 1996a). In lizards housed together, intestinal parasitism is a prime concern. Other diseases that are generally not contagious, but may opportunistically spread, are bacterial and fungal dermatitis, pneumonia, and infectious stomatitis (primarily from fighting).

Though recommendations on quarantine vary, a minimum of 30 days of isolation in addition to physical exam and clinical laboratory tests are required. Wild-caught lizards should have the quarantine period extended to 60 to 90 days with serial fecal exams performed monthly. In the absence of fecal parasites, prophylactic deworming may be indicated in wild-caught animals and many herpetoculturists routinely medicate new animals without the diagnosis of parasitism. Clients who prophylactically deworm their pets should be thoroughly informed of the potential side effects of medications and the potential side effects of killing parasites in the patient's body. Prophylactic treatment with antibiotics is not recommended unless clinical signs of bacterial or protozoal infections are observed or clinical disease is diagnosed.

Housing during quarantine should consist of an enclosure that provides comfort and visual security for the lizard, but also provides visualization of every aspect of daily (or nightly) activity. Substrate, when possible, should be paper to visualize and collect feces, urates, and urine. Feedings should be provided at a consistent feeding station and supervised to observe all aspects of feeding behavior and quantify food intake. Impeccable sanitation and cage hygiene are essential.

Ornaments, hide boxes, and water bowls should be simple and either disposable or easily cleaned. Minimizing accessories and having duplicates for each cage will aid in cleaning. Safe and effective disinfectants for home use are chlorine bleach at a 1:10 dilution of the commercially available concentration and ammonia at 5% solution (McKeown 1996). The two products should never be mixed to prevent the release of poisonous chlorine gas! Soaking surfaces for 15 minutes is adequate for disinfection with chlorine bleach at a 1:10 dilution (Ritchie 1992). In cases where cryptosporidiosis is a concern, soaking accessories with ammonia 5% and allowing them to dry for a minimum of 3 days is advised (Bennett 1996d).

Record keeping by the client is essential both for long-term captive lizards and new arrivals. Recording dates of feeding and ecdysis, environmental parameters, and especially weekly or monthly weight (in grams) are all helpful in monitoring for disease. With the exception of hibernation or parturition, lizards rarely lose weight as part of normal physiology. Juvenile lizards that fail to grow or adults that progressively lose weight are usually diseased. Casual observations such as the frequency and consistency of defecation and urination and daily activity patterns should also be recorded.

NUTRITION

One adaptation that has allowed lizards to colonize nearly every terrestrial (and some aquatic) habitat on earth is their variation in dietary preference. Consequently, their prime vulnerability in captive management becomes nutritional related disease when proper diet is not provided. Lizards are commonly classified as herbivorous, insectivorous, carnivorous, or omnivorous. Though the differentiation between insectivorous and carnivorous may seem subtle, some species are so highly specialized to eat specific arthropods and gastropods that they refuse to eat and fail to thrive in captivity if offered any substitutes. Additionally, when fed proper whole animal meat diets, carnivorous lizards generally do not require supplemental ultraviolet lighting whereas the great majority of insectivorous lizards do require routine ultraviolet light exposure even when fed calcium enriched or supplemented insect diets (Donoghue & Landenberg 1996).

Just as there is no way to describe the "basic lizard cage," it is impossible to generalize lizard diets. Each species has specific dietary requirements and variation in food availability in its native habitat that dictate diet preferences on a seasonal or even monthly basis. Carnivorous lizards (monitors, tegus) ingest other vertebrates (fish, reptiles, birds, and mammals) as their primary diet, but remain opportunistic and will usually attempt to eat anything that moves and anything that will fit into their mouths. Some carnivorous and omnivorous species may also eat carrion or may be cannibalistic (Balsai 1997; Donoghue & Landenberg 1996). Carnivorous lizards that are not fed whole animal meat products are more likely to develop nutritional disease (Donoghue & Landenberg 1996). Some herbivorous lizards will be opportunistically carnivorous or insectivorous, which, with some species in captivity, may cause serious nutritional disease when animal protein is fed in abundance (see below, "Common Disorders"). The ultimate paradox with the cause of some nutritional diseases in lizards, however, is that the causes of disease may have nothing to do with food. Temperature, humidity, landscape,

water, infectious organisms (intestinal endoparasites, bacteria), and especially light (specifically, ultraviolet light) commonly factor into nutritional health despite the provision of proper diet. Thus, proper husbandry becomes the key to providing proper nutrition.

There are nutritional requirements that pertain to all lizards. Feeding behavior, digestion, the absorption and assimilation of nutrients, and cellular physiologic activity are all somewhat dependent on temperature for all reptiles (Barten 1996a; Donoghue & Landenberg 1996). The POTZ (preferred optimal temperature zone) and thermal gradient must be provided for each species to optimize nutritional value of foods. Improper humidity also impacts overall patient health and may lead to decreased feeding response. Donoghue and Landenberg (1996) provides an excellent discussion of the nutrient requirements and daily energy needs of various reptiles and the nutrient values of various animal, plant, and commercial food items.

The quality and variety of food offered is important for all lizards. Food items should be fresh or provided promptly after thawing if frozen. Foods offered once to lizards should be disposed and not refrozen or preserved and offered again. Protein content and quality are generally met with whole animal diets and insects. For herbivores, the entire protein requirement should be of plant origin. Good plant protein sources include romaine lettuce, spinach, alfalfa sprouts, clover, dandelion, bean sprouts, and bamboo shoots (Donoghue & Landenberg 1996).

Calcium is an essential element for all captive lizards and its deficiency is the cause of metabolic bone disease (MBD) that encompasses a vast syndrome of physiologic disorders. Calcium absorption and excretion is regulated by several factors. Calcium absorption in the small intestine is regulated by an activated metabolite of vitamin D_3, cholecalciferol, which occurs in some animal tissues (Frye 1991). Vitamin D_2, ergocalciferol, occurs in plants, does not apparently facilitate the uptake of calcium in the gut of lizards, and does not appear to be beneficial as a dietary supplement for reptiles regarding calcium metabolism (Boyer 1996). Therefore, supplements claiming to contain vitamin D should be scrutinized as to which form of vitamin D is provided. Vitamin D_3 may be exogenously consumed in the form of dietary animal tissues and some dietary supplements or it may be endogenously produced when the lizard is exposed to appropriate ultraviolet (UV) radiation. Cholecalciferol is synthesized in the skin of lizards, and then is hydroxylated first in the liver and then the kidney to become 1,25 dihydroxycholecalciferol, the active metabolite of vitamin D_3 (Frye 1991). The consequence of this pathway is that in spite of adequate calcium in the diet, lizards may be prone to MBD in the absence of adequate vitamin D_3. Clinically, this is most commonly the result of insufficient exposure to UV-B radiation.

Ultimate control of blood calcium homeostasis rests with the parathyroid glands and their production of parathyroid hormone (PTH). The occurrence of hypocalcemia or hyperphosphatemia results in increased production of PTH. Calcium is removed from bone (calcium resorption) to increase calcium ions in the blood. Additionally, PTH stimulates the production of the active metabolite of cholecalciferol (vitamin D_3) to increase intestinal calcium absorption. When calcium levels in the blood are adequate, the thyroid hormone calcitonin inhibits the effects of PTH and bone resorption slows or reverses.

Excess phosphorus in the diet is also a nutritional concern. High-phosphorus diets can induce nutritional secondary hyperparathyroidism that ultimately depletes calcium stores in bone (Frye 1991; Mader 2002a). In addition to the overall content of calcium in the diet, attention must be given to the calcium to phosphorus ratio (Ca:P). This ratio should be 1:1 to 2:1 for the entire diet (Frye 1991; Donoghue & Landenberg 1996). Whole-animal diets (rodents and chicks) provide this ratio. Organ meats such as heart, liver, and muscle without bone are excessively high in phosphorus. Most commonly fed insects have a Ca:P of 1:9 and thus require periodic to routine vitamin and mineral supplementation (Donoghue & Landenberg 1996). Salads containing leafy greens such as beet greens, broccoli leaves, outer green cabbage leaves, collards, dandelion leaves, and mustard greens are calcium-rich (Donoghue & Landenberg 1996; Boyer 1996).

Nutritional supplements abound for reptiles and are required for optimal nutritional health of insectivorous and herbivorous lizards (Donoghue & Landenberg 1996). Calcium with vitamin D_3 (Rep-Cal, Los Gatos, CA) or calcium and phosphorus-containing powdered supplements are preferred. Some vitamin and mineral supplements contain no calcium (Nekton-Rep, Clearwater, FL) or very low calcium (Herptivite, Rep-Cal, Los Gatos, CA) and additional calcium must be mixed or given separately. Supplements are applied to insects by "dusting" in which the prey items are placed in a container and the powder added. With gentle swirling of the container the supplement is attached to the insect and then fed to the lizard. For herbivores the supplements are sprinkled over or mixed with the salad. Supplements should be provided once weekly for adult lizards that are fed well-balanced diets. Juvenile or growing lizards should be supplemented two to three times weekly. Problems associated with mineral supplements include decreased palatability or refusal of supplemented food items; disproportionate distribution, improper ratio, or decomposition of nutrients within supplements; toxicities from overdosing or ingestion of high levels of certain nutrients; and false claims made by manufacturers. Supplements will not compensate for the feeding of imbalanced or poor quality diets.

Herbivorous Lizards

The dietary requirements of the captive herbivorous lizard diet have been well documented in literature and the veterinary staff is responsible for informing clients of these requirements (Barten 1996a; de Vosjoli 1992; Rossi 1998b; Donoghue & Landenberg 1996; Boyer 1996; de Vosjoli 1995; de Vosjoli 1993). For years the diet of the green iguana has been the standard after which all herbivorous diets have been modeled, but the natural history of various species necessitates modifying the approach to feeding for optimal health. Barten (1996a) presents the best summary of the green iguana diet in current literature. Several of the primary to exclusive herbivorous lizards seen in practice include green iguanas (*Iguana iguana*), rhinoceros iguanas (*Cyclura* spp.), desert iguanas (*Dipsosaurus* spp.), spiny tailed iguanas (*Ctenosaura* spp.), chuckwallas (*Sauromalus* spp.), prehensile-tailed skinks (*Corucia zebrata*), and spiny-tailed agamids (*Uromastyx* spp.). The green iguana is highly adaptive in its dietary preferences in a captive environment and is known to eat commercial dog and cat foods, rodent diets, insects, fish, mice, and a wide variety of plant materials (de Vosjoli 1992).

Several beliefs regarding the feeding of iguanas have been modified over the past few years. Hatchling and juvenile iguanas do not eat insects as a substantial portion of their diet and then switch to primarily vegetarian diets as adults (Barten 1996a). Contrary to popular belief, leaf lettuce is an acceptable source of protein and calcium for herbivorous reptiles (Donoghue & Landenberg 1996). Iguanas of any age *do not require animal protein in the diet*; this includes insects, whole animal or organ meat, and commercial pet foods for dogs, cats, primates, and fish (Barten 1996a). All protein in the diet of the green iguana should be derived from plant sources.

Herbivorous lizards at all life stages are generally fed more often than carnivorous lizards and in many cases daily feeding is indicated. Adult herbivores are commonly fed every other day. Most herbivores conserve water well and will obtain the majority of their water needs from plants. Tropical lizards such as green iguanas and particularly juvenile green iguanas should have constant access to water. Desert species need to be soaked in water in buckets or other containers once weekly to meet their water requirements. This treatment helps reduce the risk of certain respiratory and skin diseases that may occur from elevated enclosure humidity.

Insectivorous Lizards

Insectivorous lizards, among the most popular pet lizards today, have nutritional and feeding needs similar to herbivorous lizards. The insectivores comprise the majority of all modern lizards and because of their dietary diversity their nutritional needs are the least known of captive lizards. The likely key to understanding insectivorous lizard nutrition is likely not in the food items themselves, but in the food *of* the food items themselves (Donoghue & Landenberg 1996; de Vosjoli 1997). Lizards in nature eat insects that browse on numerous plants, detritus, feces, soil, and other animals. The assimilation of these nutrients may be crucial for the health and survivability of some species. For example, in amphibians, poison dart frogs derive skin toxins secondarily from alkaloids and other chemicals originating in plants through the insects that they ingest in their native habitat. In captivity, when wild-caught frogs are fed similar insects that are not exposed to native plants, the skin toxins are greatly reduced or absent (Daly et al. 1994).

Herpetoculturists of insect-eating lizards are becoming aware of the importance of "prey item nutrition," and specialty diets to feed to crickets have appeared on the market (Ziegler, Gardners, PA). Some research suggests that some high-calcium diets are inappropriate for crickets and may affect the growth and reproduction of these insects (Donoghue & Landenberg 1996).The diet for captive insectivorous lizards should be varied and supplemented with vitamin and mineral powders. Because most domestically raised insects are low in calcium and have improper Ca:P ratio, calcium supplementation is crucial. Little is known about the dietary needs for amino acids, vitamins, other minerals, and trace elements. Generally these are supplemented in addition to calcium.

Insectivorous lizards as a group have the same light requirements for vitamin D_3 synthesis as do herbivores (Frye 1991; Donoghue & Landenberg 1996; de Vosjoli 1993). This is particularly true of juvenile insectivorous lizards. The author has observed numerous juvenile to young adult *Chamaeleo* spp. present with MBD that are fed a varied diet routinely supplemented with calcium. The deficiency arises from insufficient UV light exposure. Questions must arise, however, regarding the required light exposure of nocturnal insectivorous Gekkonidae, such as *Phyllurus* spp. and *Uroplatus* spp., that hide by day.

The patterns by which animals choose their prey are described under the optimal foraging theory (OFT) (Helfman 1990). It is theorized that animals choose between energetic costs and energetic gains when selecting food items. Insectivorous lizards have been observed to choose certain species of insects even when multiple species of a similar size of insect are present or the lizard chooses a certain size of insect when different sizes of the same species of insect are available. For example, the energetic costs involved in prehending, swallowing, and digesting ten 10 mg crickets may exceed the energetic costs of capturing and eating a single 100 mg cricket for a particular lizard. Therefore, the lizard ignores the smaller food items and searches or waits for a larger item. This behavior is seen in captivity as the refusal of certain size foods. Lizards that are incapable of dismembering or shredding large food items will usually avoid catching and eating them. Similarly, large lizards will typically ignore small food items that the lizard may have eaten as a juvenile. Both the size and type of food items must be considered when feeding captive lizards.

Some lizards will eat only one or two specific prey items and may or may not accept crickets or other domestic insects at the expense of anorexia (*Moloch horridus* and some *Phrynosoma* spp., ants; *Dracaena* spp., snails; Obst & Jurgen et al. 1988). Most other insectivores will accept domestic insects such as crickets, mealworms, wax worms, superworms, and roaches. Field sweepings for wild insects can also be offered to smaller insectivores, though the owner must be cautious of pesticides and potentially venomous or dangerous insects. Insects are offered in an amount that the lizard can consume in one feeding, which is typically several hours in a day or overnight in the case of nocturnal lizards.

Insects loose in a cage can be as much a hazard to insectivorous lizards as live rodents are to carnivorous lizards. Adult crickets are capable of chewing through skin, digits, and eyes of lizards that cannot escape from the enclosure. Mealworms are also similarly implicated in trauma or death to otherwise healthy lizards (de Vosjoli 1997). Feeding stations that restrict the movement of these insects can reduce the possibility of health risk to caged lizards. Most insectivorous lizards should be fed daily, though as with adult herbivores, every other day feedings are appropriate (de Vosjoli 1992; de Vosjoli 1997). Dusting food with vitamin and mineral supplements is done as with various life stages of herbivorous lizards.

Carnivorous Lizards

Clinically, carnivorous lizards typically present less often with nutritional diseases than do herbivorous or insectivorous lizards. Carnivores are generally fed whole animal vertebrates such as small mammals or birds which, when fresh, are generally well balanced with nutrients (Donoghue & Landenberg 1996). Also, these lizards are more likely to accept a wide variety of food items, which allows for more variety in nutrients. Several reasons based on natural history for the nutritional stability of carnivorous lizards in captivity include: a generally wider POTZ than herbivores and insectivores, less specific humidity requirements, and, with proper diet, less specific light requirements, all of which make habitat management less time-consuming and less expensive for the owner. Two intangible reasons for the nutritional stability of carnivorous lizards are that they are less shy about eating in captivity; and the availability of food as a whole animal requires less work by the owner to prepare the meal and provide balanced nutrition. Though several of these reasons suggest owner noncompliance, they are unfortunately substantial causes for the prevalence of nutritional disease in many herbivorous reptiles in the pet trade.

Consideration must be given to the quality of the carnivore diet. Live foods should never be fed to carnivorous lizards to prevent rodent bites. Similarly, live wild-caught vertebrates and most purchased "feeder" reptiles and amphibians should not be fed to prevent the transmission of some parasitic, bacterial, and viral diseases. Fresh-killed prey items have equal nutritional value to live prey (Donoghue & Landenberg 1996). Frozen vertebrate food items are commonly offered after complete thawing. These items should have been frozen immediately after death, thawed only once, and disposed of if not consumed within hours after feeding. Thawed frozen tissues decompose rapidly after thawing and the author has observed regurgitation by lizards within days after the ingestion of apparently rancid food items. Adult monitors and tegus are fed several adult mice or small rats several times weekly. This feeding schedule may be adjusted for obesity or leanness.

Prepared foods, such as poultry meat, beef, dog and cat foods, are not substitutes for whole animal meals and should not be offered. Exceptions may be made for short periods if rodents are unavailable or if assisted feeding is required for health-compromised individuals. In these cases canned cat foods are the better choice for feeding these patients. A variety of prepared diets specifically for lizards is available through pet suppliers. Veterinarians and herpetoculturists should thoroughly research dietary claims and scrutinize research for these products before recommending them as a sole source of nutrition. Lizards fed diets of primarily fish may be susceptible to thiamin and vitamin E deficiencies (Donoghue & Landenberg 1996; Barten 1996a).

Hatchling and juvenile carnivorous lizards can present a few nutritional challenges to their owners. Because of their smaller size, these lizards may not accept whole vertebrate food items early in life. Therefore, insects are commonly offered to smaller lizards and newborn or "pinkie" mice are offered to larger juvenile lizards. Because insects have a relatively poor Ca:P (1:9) ratio, dusting these insects with calcium powders is recommended. Pinkie mice (1:1) have a lower calcium content than do weanling (1.1:1) or adult mice (1.4:1), though the Ca:P ratio is suitable and due to the relatively short term that these food items are offered, calcium supplementation is not likely required (Donoghue & Landenberg 1996). Hatchling and juvenile carnivorous lizards should be fed at least every two to three days.

Finally, never feed large adult carnivorous or herbivorous lizards by hand! The potential consequence to fingers and hands is obvious, but more serious is the conditioned response that is created by this behavior. Lizards are wild animals whose behavior is driven by instinct and conditioning, not by reasoning. A lizard cannot discern between the end of the food item and the beginning of the human hand until after the bite occurs. The client should also be instructed to exercise caution when removing uneaten food items from cages.

COMMON DISORDERS

Diseases of lizards include many diseases common to reptiles in general and a few that are unique to particular species or families of lizards. Many disorders are husbandry related. Some diseases are more common in imported lizards than in domestically captive-raised lizards; therefore, it is important to inquire or discern the origin of the patient.

Not all disorders require medications! Many diseases require correction of improper husbandry and supportive care. The author advocates increasing quality caloric intake for all traumatic injuries and many infectious diseases to strengthen immune response and speed tissue repair in reptiles. Observation of POTZ and humidity is essential for the healing of all reptilian diseases.

Integument

Rostral abrasions are a common skin disorder of many lizards including *Iguana* spp., *Physignathus* spp., *Chlamydosaurus kingii,* and some *Varanus* spp. Abrasions are less common in Gekkonidae or in deliberate or slow-moving species such as *Uromastyx* spp. and *Chamaeleo* spp. The most common cause of rostral abrasions is facial impact with glass walls of aquariums or pacing and rubbing the nose on cage walls. Many larger imported iguanas and water dragons develop these abrasions from handling during the importation and distribution process to pet stores. Animals not adjusted to captivity commonly attempt escape by incessantly rubbing on cage walls or lids or crash into walls when startled by movement in the room around them. See color plate 3.8.

Recovery from rostral abrasions may be prolonged and the patient may be subject to recurrent injury. Treatment must include altering the enclosure to prevent further injury. Creating visual security such as a paper covering or the painting of glass walls or adding other visual barriers, even if temporary, is mandatory. Various antibiotic ointments may be used if indicated for infection. *Inform the client that treatment through habitat or behavioral modification is more important than medicating the lesion.*

Traumatic injury may occur from bite wounds, thermal burns, and skin autotomy. Both burns and bite wounds (cage mate or prey item) commonly require surgical debridement of damaged or necrotic tissue and primary or delayed secondary closure. Secondary bacterial and/or fungal infections are common and systemic antibiotics are indicated in most cases. Bacterial culture and sensitivity are indicated for all slow-healing or nonhealing wounds that do not respond to empiric therapy. Topical cleansers such as

chlorhexidine (Rossi 1996; Barten 1996c) or chloroxylenol (personal observation) (Vet Solutions, Fort Worth, TX) are excellent topical antimicrobial agents. These injuries invariably result in scar tissue formation and occasionally disfiguration. Reptile skin is slow to heal and open wounds require sequential shedding to fully close. Proper nutrition is vital for wound healing and the author recommends increased quality caloric intake for these patients to increase the rate of shedding and repair. *Inform the client to expect prolonged (months) healing and to expect permanent scarring to the affected skin.*

Bacterial and fungal dermatitis may occur as primary or secondary infections and are typically the result of improper husbandry. It is essential to know if the patient is captive-raised or wild-caught and if any cage mates are similarly affected. Clinically these diseases are more common in terrestrial species. Improper hygiene and increased humidity are suspected as the primary causes of infection (Rossi 1996). Other potential causes include acariasis, trauma from cage ornaments or accessories, immunosuppression from a variety of factors (temperature, nutrition, metabolic disease, overcrowding, capture and importation), prolonged exposure to water or sitting in water bowls, and dysecdysis. Histologic microscopy, fungal culture, and bacterial culture are all indicated for diffuse or focally extensive disease. Treatment is based on diagnostic testing and may include enteral or parenteral antibiotics, topical antibiotics or antifungal agents, and most importantly identification and correction of improper husbandry. *Inform the client of prognosis based on diagnostic testing and response to treatment. Correcting any existing husbandry is essential for both healing and prevention of reoccurrence.*

Dysecdysis is more a clinical sign of disease than a disease itself. Shedding problems are most commonly the result of underlying diseases or improper husbandry, particularly low humidity and malnutrition. Low humidity may not be an entire enclosure phenomenon as much as a lack of humidity gradient. Even some desert dwelling lizards benefit from microenvironmental humidified shelters to aid in shedding. Occasional misting for some species is beneficial. Other diseases that may contribute to dysecdysis are external parasitism and possibly thyroid disorders (Rossi 1996).

Complications that arise from dysecdysis are extremity necrosis, particularly toes and tails. This process arises from portions of the extremities that shed incompletely (occasionally more than once in several layers) and form a tourniquet on the distal extremity. Devitalization is quick and necrosis follows

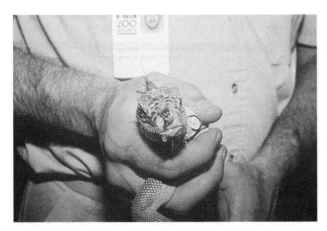

Plate 3.8. *Rostrum abrasion. (Photo courtesy of ZooAtlanta) (See also color plates)*

slowly over days or weeks. Lizards with thick skin or heavy scales may show no apparent signs of necrosis for weeks. Amputation of the affected extremity to the next proximal viable joint is required. Similar treatment is required for tails (see ascending tail necrosis below).

Broken tails resulting from tail autotomy and not from traumatic amputation usually do not require medical treatment. In rare cases hemorrhage may be profound or extend beyond one minute. In these cases pressure bandaging may be used. An appropriate size syringe casing packed with gauze is taped to the tail for one day if needed. The lesion should be cleaned if indicated and the patient maintained on a clean surface with no substrate for several days following the injury. Topical or systemic antibiotics are indicated only if wound contamination has occurred and only then for several days. Surgical repair is contraindicated in autotomous species as this will inhibit or prevent tail regeneration. *Inform the client to maintain a clean environment and report any signs of inflammation; the less manipulation of the wound, the better. Regeneration will occur over months resulting in a smaller and often darker regenerated tail.*

Tail amputation in nonautotomous species or ascending tail necrosis in all species may require surgery and antimicrobial therapy. Traumatic tail amputation, though uncommon, may occur in chameleons, prehensile-tailed skinks, and (rarely) monitors. Also common is ascending tail necrosis that results from trauma to the tail, such as bite wounds, handling injuries, enclosure injuries, or dysecdysis. Gradually ascending darkening and devitalization of the tail proximal to the injury characterize this disease. Skin may slough at times revealing devitalized vertebrae. Surgical tail amputation at a level proximal to the devitalized tissue is required. The gangrenous nature of this disease may lead to sepsis, and systemic antibiotics are indicated. For nonautotomous lizards, the tail stump can partially regenerate and is generally not sutured though hemorrhage control with pressure is essential. *Inform the client to observe diligently for any signs of continued ascending devitalization and to be aware of signs of lethargy or anorexia that may result from sepsis.*

Skeletal System

Metabolic bone disease (MBD) is a somewhat overwhelming and confusing disorder that might be best described as a syndrome with variable manifestations. The pathophysiology of nutritionally derived MBD is described above in "Nutrition." Clinically, one of the most common signs of MBD is generalized or hindleg weakness or paralysis. Therefore, it might best be considered a neurologic disorder. MBD is the primary ruleout for lizards presented with this clinical sign. Other common signs include failure to grow, generalized weakness, anorexia, soft or pliable mandible on palpation, palpably swollen or thickened long bone(s), fractures of long bones, and occasionally tremors or fine-muscle fasciculations. In profoundly weak lizards, the pupils may appear to dilate and constrict erratically, possibly an ocular manifestation of muscle fasciculations (personal observation). Presentation of a lizard with flaccid paralysis is an emergency. These clinical signs are most common in species of Iguanidae and Varanidae.

In species of Chamaeleontidae clinical signs are commonly generalized weakness, anorexia, the inability to grasp or climb, loss of balance, swollen joints, soft mandibular bones, crest deformities (*Chamaeleo calyptratus*), and occasionally flaccid tongue paralysis. Clinically, MBD is related to inadequate exposure to UV light. Prognosis for recovery for severely affected juvenile chameleons with MBD is poor at best. Tremendous nutritional support and great care in handling is required for rehabilitation.

A detailed history of diet, dietary supplementation, and lighting are essential. Diagnostic testing includes blood chemistry and radiographs (if fractures are suspected). If hypocalcemia is detected, the patient should be considered critical and intramedullary (via catheter) or intracoelomic calcium gluconate 10% is administered at a dose of 100 mg/kg every 6 hours until weakness and/or muscle tremors resolve (Boyer 1996). Blood calcium levels are monitored routinely. Advanced cases of hypocalcemia with paresis carry a grave prognosis. Assess hydration and treat as indicated. Nonhypocalcemic patients are treated with oral calcium glubionate (Neo-Calglucon) at a dose of 1.0 ml/kg PO every 12 hours. This treatment may continue for several weeks to months until normal appetite returns. Nutritional support is required in hypocalcemic patients (see Techniques). Exposure to unfiltered sunlight for 15 minutes once or twice weekly and oral vitamin D_3 supplementation is indicated. Fracture management is conservative for patients with MBD. Traction and immobilization of forelimb and hindlimb fractures with external coaptation is performed (see below, "Techniques").

MBD is physiologically a gradual onset disease. From the client's perspective the clinical signs of MBD are rapid. *Educate the client about the basics of MBD pathophysiology with emphasis on the interrelationships among diet, dietary supplements, and UV-light exposure. Explain that a deficiency in one of these fac-*

tors can lead to MBD. Most important, stress the fact that recovery from MBD may require months and may result in some permanent debilitation or disfiguration in the patient that presents with advanced disease.

Cardiovascular System

Cardiovascular diseases are rarely reported in literature. The author has observed one case of suspected heart failure in an adult savannah monitor. The patient presented with generalized limb and coelomic swelling. Aspiration of the coelomic cavity revealed straw-colored amber serous fluid that was relatively devoid of cells. Cardiac auscultation revealed a grade III-IV/VI holosystolic murmur. Pulmonary auscultation was unremarkable. Unfortunately, workup of the case was not permitted and the deceased animal was not available for necropsy.

Respiratory System

The most common true respiratory disease in lizards is pneumonia. In lizards etiologic agents of pneumonia are bacteria, fungi, and parasites (see below, "Parasitology"). Clinically, pneumonia develops with improper husbandry and rarely as contagious disease and generally presents in the advanced stages of the disease. Pneumonia associated with pulmonary parasitism commonly occurs as a secondary bacterial infection (Murray 1996).

The most prominent clinical sign of pneumonia is dyspnea. The posture may be altered with the neck held in extension and the mouth held open. Occasionally, oral and nasal mucoid secretions are observed, though neither of these signs is pathognomonic for respiratory disease. Secretions originating from the mouth or esophagus can appear foamy in lizards with normal respiratory health. Thoracic auscultation may reveal crackles or popping sounds with pneumonia. These sounds in the absence of oral secretions are highly suggestive of pneumonia. The absence of any air sounds may indicate lung consolidation and advanced disease.

Radiographs are the diagnostic test of choice for pneumonia. Transtracheal wash (see below, "Techniques") with cytology and bacterial culture with sensitivity of the wash are diagnostic for the etiology of pneumonia. For seriously compromised patients, a swab of the glottis or aspiration of tracheal exudate without flushing is recommended. A fecal exam is indicated in cases where a tracheal wash is not possible to diagnose lungworm infection.

Treatment is initiated upon diagnosis of pneumonia and modified based on cytology and culture and sen-sitivity results if indicated. Pneumonia in lizards many times presents as an emergency and treatment must not be delayed. Antibiotics commonly used are broad-spectrum and bactericidal. These include aminoglycosides, beta-lactam antibiotics (cephalosporins), fluoroquinolones, and advanced generation semisynthetic penicillins, all of which should be administered parenterally either IM or SC (Murray 1996).

Recovery from pneumonia is prolonged physiologically by the accumulation of pulmonary exudates in recesses of the lungs (particularly caudally) and an inability of achieving the MIC of antimicrobial agents in these relatively poorly vascularized regions. Nebulization with bacterial antimicrobial agents may be beneficial. Aerosolized particles must be 3 microns or smaller to reach the lungs (Murray 1996). Treatment periods are 10 to 30 minutes at a frequency of every 6 to 12 hours. Duration of treatment may be several days to one week pending clinical improvement.

Meticulous investigation of all aspects of husbandry and correction of improper husbandry are required to develop a complete treatment plan. Inform the client of the seriousness of the disease and be realistic regarding prognosis. Treatment of pneumonia often requires protracted hospitalization, repeated diagnostic testing, moderate to marked financial investment, and tremendous patience.

Digestive System

Anorexia is one of most common presenting complaints for digestive disorders, and its cause can be a challenge to diagnose. Though anorexia is not a disease, it is both a clinical sign of nearly all reptilian diseases and a contributor to several others diseases. Comprehensive history is required as improper husbandry often contributes to the cause of anorexia. If history and physical exam fail to uncover improper husbandry issues or clinical disease, a series of diagnostic tests are indicated including fecal exam, blood chemistry, complete blood count, and radiography (including positive contrast). Treat the diagnosed underlying disease and provide nutritional support.

Infectious stomatitis occurs as a secondary disease in lizards (Mader 1996d; Barten 2002). This disorder may be unobserved by clients as the patient is presented for anorexia, lethargy, weight loss, or occasionally oral or nasal exudate. Oral exam may reveal focal or diffuse gingival erythema, petechia, swelling, erosion, ulceration, and mucoid or purulent exudate (fig. 3.7).

The glottis mucosa may be involved in diffuse disease. In severe cases, aspiration of infectious exudates may lead to pneumonia (Mader 1996d; Murray

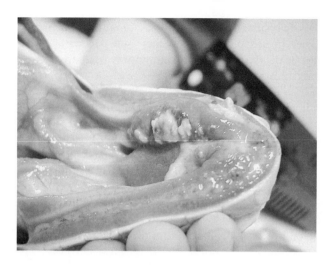

Fig. 3.7. Stomatitis in a lizard. (Photo courtesy of Dr. Stephen J. Hernandez-Divers, University of Georgia)

1996). Because the oral cavity communicates with the nasal cavity dorsally through the choana, exudates may be observed bubbling from the nose in the absence of true respiratory disease.

Immunosuppression resulting from a myriad of underlying causes contributes to the development of infectious stomatitis. Improper temperatures, poor nutrition, and trauma from fighting with cagemates or oral cavity manipulation may be implicated. The infectious agent is determined through bacterial culture and sensitivity and is commonly identified as normal oral cavity bacterial flora including *Aeromonas* spp. or *Pseudomonas* spp., bacteria that are opportunistic pathogens.

Treatment is based on degree of involved tissues, husbandry parameters, and sensitivity values. Small (2–3 mm) focal regions of stomatitis may require only warming the environment and no antibiotic treatment or a single topical antiseptic or antibiotic application. Generalized or deep infections may require sedation, debridement, and a combination of topical and systemic therapy. Aminoglycosides (gentamicin, amikacin) and fluoroquinolones (enrofloxacin) are most commonly administered. *Inform the client that recovery may be protracted in severe cases of stomatitis. Routine rechecks are necessary to monitor progress of healing of infection. Correcting improper husbandry is of primary importance.*

Obstruction and impaction are common and may present days or weeks after the onset of the actual disease. The usual presenting complaint is anorexia, but bloating, lethargy, weight loss, diarrhea, constipation, and (rarely) regurgitation may be observed. Diagnosis may be suspected based on history alone. Investigating the patient's enclosure substrate, feeding habits, and normal defecation habits is important. Confirmation of obstruction can occasionally be made on physical exam, but commonly radiographs or exploratory surgery are required for definitive diagnosis. Complete foreign body obstruction commonly results in gas bloating, which is evident radiographically; the causative item, however, may not be radiographically visible. Complete obstruction with gas bloating is an emergency.

Impaction is the result of fine particulate substrate, rodent hair, arthropod exoskeleton, or other food item accumulation in the intestines and may develop independently, in association with, or secondary to foreign body obstructions. Impactions are commonly palpable and visible on radiographs. If the lizard is alert and marked gas accumulation is not observed on radiographs, enemas and/or oral laxatives are indicated (see below, "Techniques"). Soaking in tepid water for 10–15 minutes may also stimulate defecation. Assess for dehydration and treat as indicated. Impaction may occur secondary to a number of husbandry issues, dehydration, improper diet, and hypocalcemia. Weak lizards with diagnosed or suspected obstruction should have blood chemistry analyzed. Surgical correction is required when laxatives, enemas, or other conservative therapy fails.

Intestinal parasitism is very common if not ubiquitous in imported lizards (Klingenberg 1993; Lane & Mader 1996). Signs of intestinal parasitism include anorexia, diarrhea, weight loss, failure to gain weight, and weakness. Treatment is based on diagnosis (see below, "Parasitology"). Quarantine, fecal screening, and cage hygiene are essential in limiting reinfection. Some parasites are zoonotic (see below, "Zoonoses") (Johnson-Delaney 1996).

Cloacal prolapse may occur as a digestive, reproductive, or excretory disorder. The prolapse may occur secondary to straining from enteritis, egg laying, and uroliths and may comprise colon, oviduct, urinary bladder, or a combination of the three. Treatment is based on which organ is prolapsed and the duration of the prolapse and resultant trauma to involved tissues (fig. 3.8).

The colon is a tubular, smooth structure with a lumen. Fecal material may or may not been seen within the lumen. The oviduct is a thin-walled, longitudinally banded structure with a lumen and no fecal material will be present. The urinary bladder is globular, thin-walled, smooth structure with no lumen and may be fluid filled. Prolapse of these organs originates from the coelomic cavity cranial to the vent.

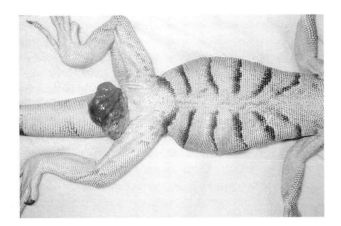

Fig. 3.8. *Cloacal prolapse in an iguana. (Photo courtesy of Dr. Sam Rivera)*

Paraphimosis, or prolapse of the hemipenes, originates from the proximal aspect of the tail caudal to the vent. The prolapsed hemipenis is a solid, fleshy structure with no lumen. All organs may be darkened in color from devitalization or necrosis. Cloacal prolapse of coelomic structures is an emergency.

In cases where prolapse is recent, tissues may be cleaned and lubricated with a water-based lubricant and gently reduced through the cloaca (Bennett 1996d). A single transverse cloacal suture is loosely applied to maintain the reduction yet still allow the passage of urates and feces. If swelling of the tissue is present in the absence of necrosis, swelling may be reduced with hypertonic sugar solutions followed by manual reduction. Necrosis of prolapsed tissue requires surgical resection in the case of coelomic structures or amputation of the hemipenis (see below, "Surgery and Anesthesia").

Excretory System

Renal failure is generally a secondary disease caused by either improper nutrition in primarily herbivorous lizards or by aminoglycoside toxicity in all lizards. Clinical signs and diagnostic test results may mimic those seen with MBD with the absence of bony lesions. History may indicate polyuria, anorexia, weakness, and weight loss. Blood chemistry commonly reflects hyperphosphatemia, normo- or hypocalcemia, and normal or elevated uric acid. Radiographs may reflect enlarged kidneys that appear as masses within and slightly cranial to the pelvic canal. Renal enlargement is occasionally palpable.

The dietary etiology is theorized to be a result of excessive dietary animal protein. Aminoglycoside toxicity is well documented as a cause of renal insuffi-

ciency in mammals and reptiles. Treatment consists of fluid support and diuresis, though prognosis is typically poor for recovery and long-term survival. Other renal diseases seen in lizards include pyelonephritis and neoplasia.

Reproductive System

Lizards are presented with several reproductive abnormalities. Dystocia in females and paraphimosis in males are most common. Other disorders include cloacal prolapse of oviducts, ectopic eggs, and neoplasia. It is possible for lizards to ovulate and deposit infertile shelled eggs in the absence of a male. When gravid or pregnant, most lizards will not eat but remain alert and active for a period of several days prior to egg laying and many will retain eggs until a suitable substrate or nest box is provided. Any dystocia accompanied by weakness or nonresponsiveness despite the presence of a suitable nesting area is a critical emergency.

Dystocia in lizards can be pre-ovulatory (as follicles on the ovary) or post-ovulatory (as follicles or shelled eggs in the oviduct) (Stahl 2000). Differentiation of the two is made by radiography as the pre-ovulatory eggs are nonshelled and located dorsally in the abdomen and post-ovulatory eggs may be shelled and are more caudoventral in the abdomen. Conservative management is advised when the lizard is alert and active with pre-ovulatory or post-ovulatory dystocia. Environmental modification such as providing a suitable nesting area or more visual security may be curative.

Traditional mammalian treatments for post-ovulatory dystocia refractory to conservative management include oxytocin and calcium injections to stimulate smooth muscle contractions. Calcium gluconate at a dose of 100 mg/kg IM or ICe followed in 1 hour by oxytocin at a dose of 5 to 30 IU/kg IM or ICe is given (Stahl 2000; DeNardo 1996b). Oxytocin may be repeated within 30 minutes of the first injection. Efficacy is unpredictable and may only approach 50% effectiveness in lizards (DeNardo 1996b). Manual reduction of retained eggs may be attempted for one or two eggs in close proximity to the cloaca and distal to the pelvic canal. Tremendous care must be exercised to avoid prolapse, oviductal rupture, or trauma to the kidneys. If the eggshell is not clearly visible emerging from the cloaca, manual reduction is contraindicated. Lizards with distal oviductal or cloacal dystocias following normal oviposition may be hypocalcemic.

Many cases of dystocia require surgical management. These are weakened and visibly distressed animals or those in which a radiographic diagnosis of obstruction is diagnosed. Obstruction may result from eggs too large to pass through the pelvic canal or from coelomic masses or enlarged kidneys that prohibit the passage of eggs.

Paraphimosis is managed similar to cloacal prolapse (Barten 1996d). The prolapsed hemipenis is assessed for viability and replaced or amputated as indicated. Transverse cloacal suturing is indicated with reduction of paraphimosis.

Nervous System

Diseases of the lizard nervous system are typically secondary to systemic, metabolic, or nutritional disease or trauma. Hypocalcemia from the various forms of MBD is one of the most common causes of neurologic weakness or paralysis in captive lizards (Barten 1996b). The pathophysiology of hypocalcemia is described above in "Nutrition." All lizards presented with weakness, tetany, or muscle fasciculations should have blood calcium levels assessed immediately.

Trauma is a common cause of neurologic disorders in lizards and is common in lizards that are free-ranging in homes or traveling with the owner (fig. 3.9). Both cerebral and spinal trauma occur and are treated empirically with corticosteroids and time. Prognosis for even apparently severe injuries may not be grave if the client is able to provide adequate supportive care (see below, "Emergencies").

Ophthalmology

Periocular inflammatory diseases are clinically the most common ophthalmic disorders in lizards. Infectious agents do not cause all periocular diseases.

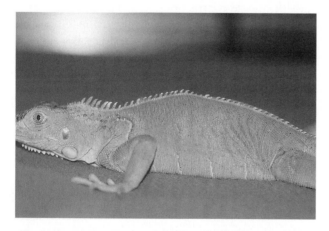

Fig. 3.9. *Spinal cord injury with vertebral column fracture due to trauma. Note the dorsal deviation caudal to the forelimbs. (Photo courtesy of Ryan Cheek)*

Many inflammatory diseases, however, result from or give rise to secondary bacterial infections. Williams (1996) reports that the majority of ocular diseases are a sign of more generalized infection. One nutritional disorder that affects the eye is hypovitaminosis A. This disease is not specific to the eye, but also affects glandular mucous membrane epithelium including the respiratory and digestive tract. Clinically, hypovitaminosis A is most commonly seen in turtles and occasionally in lizards. Clinical signs include blepharitis, chemosis, and epiphora. Secondary bacterial infection is commonly observed in these cases and topical ophthalmic antibiotics are commonly indicated in addition to weekly vitamin A injections (Williams 1996). Recovery may be prolonged to several months. A thorough review of diet is recommended.

Several species of geckos have spectacles (see above, "Anatomy and Physiology"). Subspectacular abscesses and retained spectacles occur as in snakes. The abscesses may be unilateral or bilateral and often are the result of ascending bacterial infection from the mouth. Treatment consists of surgical drainage and irrigation of the abscess along the ventral margin of the spectacle as well as treatment of associated stomatitis. The surgical incision remains open to drain, but commonly seals in a matter of days. Subsequent shedding of the spectacle results in complete closure of the surgical incision and resolution of the abscess. The spectacle revealed following shed may appear wrinkled and typically requires several shed cycles to return to normal appearance.

Foreign bodies and trauma commonly result in blepharospasm. Evaluation of the globe and periocular tissues may require sedation. Treatment of lesions depends upon thorough examination of the globe, eyelids, and conjunctiva (fig. 3.10).

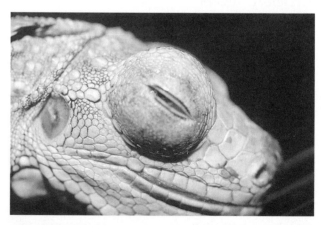

Fig. 3.10. *Retrobulbar abscess in an iguana. (Photo courtesy of Ryan Cheek)*

Behavior

The primary reported behavior disorder of lizards is aggression and is categorized as dominance or fear aggression as seen in dogs and cats. Dominance aggression may be conspecific (same species) or intraspecific (different species) among lizards housed together and it may be difficult to separate from fear aggression in cases of lizard-human interactions. Aggression is most often observed against humans in cases of large lizards such as iguanas, monitors, and tegus especially during breeding season and is likely hormonally induced. This behavior is variable and may be directed at only one person in the household (personal observation). The author suspects the possibility of pheromonally induced aggression in iguanas against women who may be in their menstrual cycle. Aggression in large lizards directed against humans is a serious and dangerous problem (see below, "Zoonoses"). Seasonal aggression is treated with ovariectomy or orchiectomy.

Toxicity and Miscellaneous Nutritional Disorders

Toxicities occur from a variety of substances including pharmaceuticals, insecticides, dietary supplements, chemicals, and cigarette smoke (Williams 1996). Pharmaceutical toxicities are most commonly seen from injectable aminoglycosides and ivermectin, oral metronidazole, and topical pyrethrin or organophosphate compounds. The author is unaware of Teflon toxicity in lizards as reported in birds, but this possibility should be considered. A thorough history is required for diagnosis of toxic exposure, as there are rarely pathognomonic clinical signs for exposure to any of these compounds. Treatment is supportive depending on the underlying exposure. Mader (1996a) recommends standard atropine, diazepam, and isotonic fluid therapy for lizards with pyrethrin toxicity (see below, "Emergencies").

Nutritional disorders leading to neurologic signs of disease include vitamin B_1, vitamin E, and selenium deficiencies. Thiamine (B_1) deficiency is seen in carnivorous lizards fed raw egg diets in which the compound avidin inhibits vitamin B. Vitamin E deficiency is seen in lizards fed high fatty fish diets (Donoghue & Landenberg 1996). Treatment consists of dietary correction and injectable vitamins as indicated.

Gout is a disease of lizards and other animals with several potential etiologies. In lizards, gout can originate both from improper nutrition or secondary to pharmaceutical toxicity. In vertebrates, the pyrimidine amino acids are metabolized into CO_2 and NH_3 and eliminated from the body. Purine amino acids are metabolized into various degradation products of which uric acid is the final product in reptiles (Mader 1996c). Uric acid in high concentrations in the blood becomes insoluble. Simplistically, gout is the result of excessive uric acids in the blood that crystallize and precipitate in tissues prior to elimination from the body via the kidneys. Common sites of this deposition are serosal surfaces of internal organs and synovial membranes. A common presenting complaint of gout is swollen joints or white to yellow nodules of the oral mucous membranes.

Gout is seen in lizards on diets high in purines, most commonly in herbivorous lizards fed a primarily animal rather than plant protein diet. Gout may also be renally induced secondary to dehydration or renal disease most commonly in association with renal tubular toxicity from aminoglycosides or sulfonamides. Even at proper dosages these antibiotics can induce renal disease if the patient is or becomes dehydrated during treatment. Gout is a managed disease and not a curable disease in most cases. Medications to lower blood uric acid concentrations and anti-inflammatory agents are recommended (Mader 1996c). In cases of advanced gout, palliative therapy may be insufficient. This disease is best prevented before it occurs with proper client education regarding diet and the judicious use of potentially nephrotoxic medications.

ZOONOSES

Client education regarding zoonotic diseases must be a priority for all veterinary health professionals. Unfortunately, popular literature, television/radio, and the Internet are saturated with misinformation regarding reptile zoonotic diseases. The threats posed to humans, however, should not be underestimated. Unfortunately, this information gap is prevalent within human medicine as well, and human physicians fall victim to the lack of education reflected by the popular press regarding disease in many domestic pets.

All veterinary staff should have the following knowledge about zoonotic disease:

1. A complete understanding of the pathophysiology and method of transmission (direct or indirect and vector) of the disease in question both in the potential source animal and in humans
2. A complete understanding of risk factors for humans to contract the disease in question including immunosuppression and human behaviors when handling the pet

3. Which pet species are more likely to harbor particular zoonotic pathogens 4. A thorough knowledge of laws governing the possession and treatment of exotic species in a given jurisdiction

Human behavior is likely to be a primary cause or facilitator of contracting zoonotic diseases from reptiles. Because many lizards are particularly sociable and exhibit behaviors that are commonly anthropomorphized, their owners form a human-animal bond that is similar to that seen with other domestic animals. Therefore, reasoning regarding the potential for zoonotic diseases is commonly ignored because of emotional considerations.

Behaviors that greatly increase the risk of contracting infectious diseases from lizards include:

1. Housing or handling lizards in or near food preparation or storage areas
2. Allowing lizards to soak in bathtubs, basins, or containers used for human hygiene
3. Allowing any part of the lizard to contact a human mouth or face
4. Allowing lizards to roam free in any facility of human habitation
5. Allowing young children to handle or have access to pet lizards when not under direct adult supervision
6. Handling lizards by any person under treatment of immunosuppressive medication(s) or having contracted any immunosuppressive disease
7. Not washing hands and exposed skin following handling of pet lizards.

   Other risk factors include possessing aggressive or potentially dangerous lizard species, disregard for proper handling techniques of any lizard, feeding pet lizards by hand, and not maintaining proper cage sanitation.

Bacterial diseases are most commonly implicated among reptilian zoonoses. Of these diseases, salmonellosis (*Salmonella* spp.) is most notorious for causing disease in humans.

See Johnson-Delaney for a comprehensive discussion of salmonellosis (Johnson-Delaney 1996). Salmonellosis is directly transmitted by a fecal-oral route. Transmission of infective serotypes does not require the direct contact of fecal material by a human. Because lizards are commonly maintained in enclosures where they defecate, invariably bacterial organisms from feces may contact the skin of the pet. Handling of the pet can transfer infective organisms to human skin. It is likely that disease transmission will

not occur given the combination of a relatively low number of infective organisms and an immunocompetent host; with zoonotic diseases, however, there is no acceptable level of risk.

Other bacterial infections may occur in humans from fecal-oral contamination or from penetrating wounds such as bites or scratches. *Aeromonas* spp., *Pseudomonas* spp., and other gram-negative bacteria may be normal flora in the mouths of lizards. *Mycobacterium* spp. infections may occur in reptiles and are potentially infectious to humans through direct contact with skin defects and inhalation. This infection in reptiles may appear in any organ. *Chlamydophila psittaci* has been identified in infections of various species of lizards (Jacobson 2002). Direct transmission of *Chlamydia* from reptiles to humans is unknown. Several fungal infections, mycoses, have been reported in reptiles that would have the potential to infect humans.

Reptiles are the definitive host for tongueworms, pentastomids, of various genera that are know to infect humans incidentally (Lane & Mader 1996; Johnson-Delaney 1996). Transmission is direct and fecal-oral by ingesting eggs or larvae. Because humans are incidental "dead-end" hosts, they do not pass infective stages of pentastomids. Larval forms of these worms may migrate and then die in humans resulting in localized immune response and calcification or granulation of lesions.

There are a variety of indirectly transmitted diseases for which lizards may be reservoirs of disease or carry the vectors of zoonotic disease. A variety of ticks, mites, and biting insects are implicated in transmitting disease such as viral, rickettsial, and bacterial diseases. Lizards have not been implicated in acting as a reservoir host for these diseases, but they may harbor ticks and mites that can bite and infect humans (Johnson-Delaney 1996).

An often overlooked yet significant risk to humans from captive reptiles is trauma from bites and scratches. With all infectious diseases aside, there is no excuse for humans to incur bite wounds from pet lizards. Some species are simply poor choices for the average hobbyist. These include *Heloderma* spp., adult green iguanas, large monitors, and some adult tegus. There is risk of bite wounds or other injuries from these species when simply performing routine maintenance and a minimal amount or even no handling. Generally, however, injuries occur from careless interaction with the animals.

The importance of this issue becomes evident when legal authorities attempt to strip the rights of pet owners to possess these animals because of accidental bites or the irresponsible behavior of a few people. Many local ordinances exist that restrict or prohibit the sale or possession of certain exotic animals, particularly venomous reptiles and large snakes or lizards, because of perceived danger to humans. Accidental bites that occur at zoological parks and large snake escapes that are reported by the media contribute substantially to the hysteria that enables much knee-jerk improper legislation. Veterinary staff have a critical role in educating clients about the proper handling of exotic animals and in advising clients about exotic animals which are unsuitable as pets.

Additionally, however, veterinary staff must be aware of these laws when admitting or treating pets that are illegal to possess. Injuries sustained to staff or clients by these pets (and others) are the responsibility of the practice owners when on the premises. Similarly, advising clients regarding the home treatment of potentially dangerous animals should be approached with great discretion. For a somewhat complete but already outdated overview of laws regarding reptiles in the United States, see Levell (1998).

HISTORY AND PHYSICAL EXAM

History

In the practice of exotic animal medicine, as much can be learned about a patient from the history as from any other diagnostic procedure. With lizards, a veterinary technician or receptionist educated with a basic understanding of the patient's husbandry needs can often develop a working diagnosis well before the veterinarian examines the patient. It is the very diversity of husbandry requirements among species of lizards that demands a fundamental knowledge of all natural history aspects of the patient.

It is essential to not dismiss any observation by the client as trivial or inconsequential. The client may be the most educated person in the exam room with regard to the natural history of the patient, and with long-term captive lizards, the client is usually aware of a pattern of "normal" behavior. Discovering the deviations from normal behavior is essential to obtaining a complete history.

These are several fundamental questions for clients to answer regarding their lizard pets:

1. What is the presenting complaint(s), what is the duration of the problem, how rapidly has the problem developed, and does the client believe that the problem is related to any external influence(s) on the lizard?

2. What is the species, age, sex; how long in client's possession; and any known previous disease or health problems?

   Has the client or anyone else medicated the lizard or been instructed to medicate the lizard, and if so, by whom and for what reason?

3. Is the lizard captive-born or wild-caught? This is not essential to the diagnosis, but can be very helpful in developing a diagnostic plan for infectious disease.

4. General husbandry. In addition to obtaining a general overview of housing, lighting, temperature and heating, humidity, substrate, water availability, cage cleaning, and cage accessories, it is essential to ask the following:

   Does the lizard ever roam free in the house or in any area other than the cage or enclosure or has the lizard ever escaped from its enclosure?

   Does the lizard have any direct or indirect exposure to any other animals presently or in the past and are those animals similarly affected?

   Is the lizard ever handled or observed by anyone except the client?

   Where is the cage located in the house; is it ever moved; what are potential exposures to noxious materials such as cleaning agents, cigarette smoke, fuel exhaust, etc; are there temperature, light, humidity, or ventilation fluctuations?

5. Nutrition. Determine *exactly* what the lizard is fed and what is the origin of the food (i.e., Does the client collect food in the environment to feed or purchase the food at a pet store or grocery store?)

   How often is food offered, at what time of day is food offered, and in what quantities is food consumed?

   In cases where a variety of food items are offered, which portions are usually consumed?

   Does the client use any commercially available foods or vitamin and mineral supplements and, if so, how often and in what quantity?

   Does the client *actually observe* the lizard eating the food items or just notice that food is missing after a period of time?

Restraint

Portions of the physical exam, most diagnostic procedures, and many treatments require restraint (fig. 3.11). The veterinary staff must be aware that every species of lizard can bite. Most, however, will not bite or scratch unless restrained and the more firmly they are restrained, the more they will struggle and attempt to bite or scratch the handler. Lizards with delicate skin should not be handled for physical examination

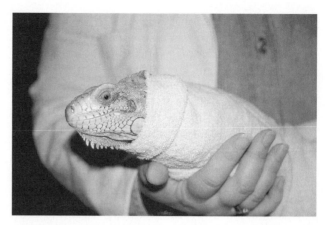

Fig. 3.12. *Lizard restraint using a towel. (Photo courtesy of Dr. Stephen J. Hernandez-Divers, University of Georgia)*

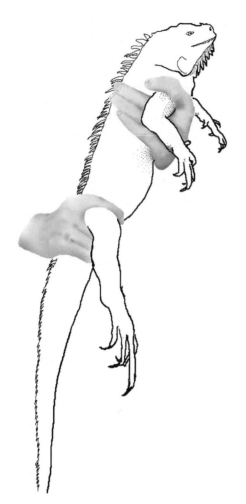

Fig. 3.11. *Proper restraint of a lizard. (Drawing by Scott Stark)*

unless absolutely necessary. These species include the Malagasy geckos, *Geckolepis* spp. (fish-scale geckos), and *Phelsuma* spp. (day geckos) that may autotomize both tails and skin with minimal physical restraint. This behavior rarely results in death of the lizard, but it may cause permanent disfigurement. These patients can be observed through clear enclosures such as plastic pet carriers or they can be placed inside a 5–6 cm diameter, clear plastic tube for examination (Barten 1996b).

There are some lizards that *at all times should be considered dangerous* to handle. These include all lizards greater than 1.0 m length, especially all large species of iguanas and monitors. Large lizards may be calmed by covering the head and eyes with a towel in addition to wrapping the body in a large towel or blanket to prevent clawing (fig. 3.12). The head, however, must be fully and firmly immobilized at all times. Occasionally, these lizards cannot be safely restrained

and examined without sedation (see below, "Surgery and Anesthesia"). Other species, though smaller and typically docile, are capable of producing digit amputating, disfiguring, or extremely painful bites to humans. These include prehensile-tail skinks (*Corucia zebrata*), and some adult tegus (*Tupinampis* spp.). Some smaller lizards such as the Tokay gecko (*Gekko gecko*) tend to be aggressive and will attempt to bite without being handled. Even small lizards such as fat-tailed geckos (*Hemitheconyx caudicinctus*) are capable of producing painful bites when handled and may be reluctant to release when biting a hand or finger (fig. 3.13).

The veterinary staff should refrain from inappropriate contact with pet lizards. This includes kissing the patient, placing the patient near a human face, placing fingers or hands within the mouth of the patient, or allowing the patient to cling to clothing or hair in an unrestrained fashion. This behavior is both irresponsible and unprofessional and may result in serious injury to either the patient or veterinary staff. Clients should also be informed of the potential health risks that may result from these behaviors. The veterinary staff should never allow the client to assist in the restraint of a potentially dangerous patient during examination or when performing a treatment or diagnostic procedure. Though lizards may become somewhat tame, there are no domesticated lizards and their behavior may not be predictable.

Physical Exam

The traditional physical exam for most companion animals is a hands-on affair. More can be learned, however, by simple observation of the lizard patient at rest in a cage while in the exam room or waiting area.

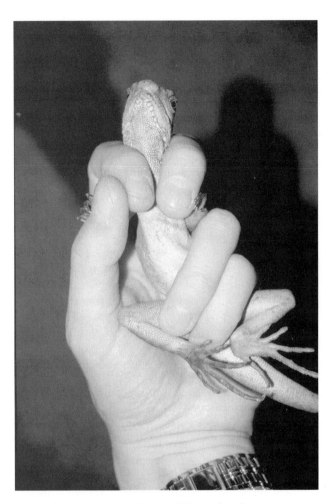

Fig. 3.13. Restraint of a small lizard. (Photo courtesy of Dr. Stephen J. Hernandez-Divers, University of Georgia)

These observations can commonly be made during the traditional question and answer session and may quickly uncover potential emergencies that have not been realized by the client. First observe the posture (again, the technician must first be familiar with normal posture of a particular species). Quadruped lizards will generally hold the head somewhat erect and may have a portion (if not all) of the body held suspended above the ground. For diurnal lizards, assess alertness. Does the lizard follow the observer in the room with eyes or head? Healthy chameleons, for example, are constantly surveying their environment with turretlike eyelids and generally do not sit still except when restrained or confined. For lizards with movable eyelids (all but some geckos), are both eyes open and are they clear?

Observe general body condition paying particular attention to muscle mass of the dorsal tail, dorsal pelvis, and dorsolateral scapular region. Emaciation results in diminished subdermal fat and muscle mass and the skin may have a concave contour to one or all of these body regions. Additionally, the eyes may have a sunken or recessed appearance from diminished retrobulbar fat or from dehydration. Species that routinely present with signs of emaciation include the green iguana, spiny-tailed lizards (*Uromastyx* spp.), prehensile-tailed skinks (*Corucia zebrata*), bearded dragons (*Pogona* spp.), and monitors (*Varanus* spp.). It is important to understand that the physical changes associated with emaciation are chronic and do not occur over several days. Some lizards, which are laterally or dorsally compressed, may appear thin or underweight but they are in fact normal. Some of these species include leaf-tailed geckos (*Uroplatus* spp.), some true chameleons (*Chamaeleo* spp.), and spider geckos (*Agamura* spp.). Observe for symmetry, particularly of skeletal structures. Except for some skin appendages, the external and skeletal anatomy of lizards is bilaterally symmetric.

As with general body condition, the skin can be observed without handling the lizard. There is great structural variation among lizards in skin and scale texture. Lizards such as bearded dragons and horned lizards (*Phrynosoma* spp.) have roughly textured and armored skin. Others such as some geckos (*Phelsuma* spp.) have relatively small granular scales and thin skin which is delicate. Observe for missing scales, abnormal skin coloration, crusts, dysecdysis (incomplete shed skin), subdermal swellings, and external parasites including mites and ticks. Pay particular attention to skin folds, flaps, nostrils, eyelids, axillae, and ears for mites and ticks. Observe for signs of trauma such as rostral abrasions, necrotic or missing toes, damage to the tail, bite wounds, and signs of thermal or chemical burns that may appear as erythema or tissue necrosis. Inspect for missing, damaged, or discolored toes or toenails. Remember that not all lizards have four legs and five toes per leg. *Ophisaurus* spp. and *Lialis* spp. are two examples of legless lizards. *Chamaeleo* spp. have five toes, which are fused into two gripping bundles per foot.

While observing the lizard systematically, pay attention to respiration and the respiratory effort. As with caged birds, respiration for most lizards at rest is relatively effortless and nearly imperceptible from a distance. Gaping (holding the mouth open) associated with dyspnea may be the result of upper or lower respiratory disease. Overheating, defensive posturing, and stress or anxiety may also lead to this behavior. Similarly, mucoid oral and nasal secretions are not normal, though crystalline or salt secretions may be normal in some species such as *Uromastyx* spp. and *Iguana* spp. Thoracic auscultation should be performed over the entire dorsal and lateral thoracic regions. When performing auscultation, a moistened paper towel or thin cloth may be wrapped over the diaphragm of the stethoscope to reduce noise from rough skin or scales.

An essential part of the physical exam for most lizards is the oral exam. This examination may require physical or chemical restraint and must be performed with consideration to safety of the veterinary staff and health risk to the patient. Some lizards (*Iguana* spp., *Varanus* spp., *Chamaeleo* spp., *Pogona* spp., some *Gecko* spp.) may voluntarily open the mouth when approached in the cage or when restrained making oral examination less physically challenging. In these species (excluding *Gecko* spp.) the mouth may be opened with gentle retraction of the dewlap while the maxilla is secured with the other hand. This approach is contraindicated in patients that have normally fragile skin (most species of Gekkonidae) or those with diseased skin as with hypovitaminosis C. The author has observed the dewlap skin easily tear in malnourished *Chamaeleo* spp. suspected of having hypovitaminosis C among other malnourishment-related diseases. The gentle introduction of a rubber spatula into the mouth is useful as a speculum. Metal and wood speculums should be avoided as they may result in damage to gums and teeth as well as damage to or accidental ingestion of the speculum (or portions thereof) with stronger lizards. For very small lizards plastic spoons or plastic credit cards may be used as a speculum. For large lizards or those with dark pigmented oral epithelium, an otoscopic or laryngoscopic illuminator is useful to visualize the oral anatomy.

Chemical restraint is required to examine the oral cavity with some species because of strong jaws and a reluctance to open the mouth. These species include spiny-tailed lizards, prehensile-tailed skinks, some monitors, some tegus, and occasionally bearded dragons. Similarly, lizards with metabolic bone disease or those with thin mandibles may suffer traumatic iatrogenic fractures from manipulation of the mouth. Tremendous caution and attention must be used when manipulating the mouth of adult iguanas and monitors. Any distraction or a mistake in handling may result in serious injury or amputation of a digit to the handler. The body of larger lizards must be fully immobilized prior to opening the mouth to prevent the patient from exerting any leverage by thrashing or spinning the body should an accidental bite occur.

Examination of the oral cavity includes observation of the choana, dentition, glottis, and mucous membranes. While manipulating the head, palpate for the firmness and symmetry of the mandible and maxilla. Bones that compress or bend in a lateral fashion may signify metabolic bone disease. The mandibular symphysis is fused in lizards. Abscesses and granulomas may occur in the mandible with no apparent mucous membrane abnormalities. The oral cavity should be bilaterally symmetric. The mucous membranes of the oral cavity are generally uniform in color. Many lizards have a pink to pinkish white color to the oral epithelium with a somewhat glistening surface. Some lizards may have pigmented oral epithelium. The oral mucous membranes of some Old World chameleons (*Chamaeleo* spp.) and bearded dragons (*Pogona* spp.) are yellow and should not be interpreted as icteric or jaundiced. In a healthy lizard there is little to no mucous, blood, pus, or other exudates in the mouth. The glottis should be observed through several respiratory cycles of inspiration both to observe normal movement of glottis cartilages and to observe for any exudates from within the glottis. The choana should be clear of any exudate. The dentition and gingiva should be free of erythema or exudate. Similar to snakes, some *Gecko* spp. have a spectacle, which covers the eye. Subspectacular abscesses are commonly observed in conjunction with and may arise from infectious stomatitis (Mader 1996d); an oral exam is always warranted with the presence of subspectacular abscesses.

Examination of the external cloaca or vent also requires physical restraint. The vent should have an appearance consistent with that of the remaining dermis with the exception of specialized scales that vary among species. Some lizards possess femoral pores that extend laterally from the vent onto the ventral aspect of the hind legs and prefemoral pores cranial to the vent. The vent and surrounding integument should be bilaterally symmetric. As with the integument, observe for signs of trauma, swelling, exudates, crusts, and observe for prolapse of cloacal tissue or hemipenes.

Abdominal palpation is a noninvasive method to evaluate gastrointestinal, reproductive, and urinary systems. Palpation is performed gently with the fingertips to create minimal stress and reduce the risk of internal damage to delicate or diseased patients. Caution must be exercised if gastrointestinal obstruction or bloating is suspected to prevent iatrogenic rupture to dilated gastrointestinal structures. In dorsally compressed lizards, such as bearded dragons and uromastyx, the kidneys may be palpable in the dorsal caudal coelom. It is difficult to differentiate the kidneys from other abdominal structures in laterally compressed or very large lizards without forceful palpation. Uroliths may be palpable as in dogs and cats. It is also difficult to impossible to differentiate gastrointestinal structures on palpation other than by extrapolating their location. Paired fat bodies are present in the caudal coelom. These are bilateral and may be confused with kidneys or masses in the coelom. The fat bodies are particularly evident in dorsally compressed lizards such as bearded dragons and *Uromastyx* spp.

Small lizards, particularly many Gekkonidae, have semitransparent ventral abdominal walls and skin. This allows for visualization of some abdominal structures while the lizard is contained in a clear plastic or glass container. This technique is particularly useful for visualizing eggs in these species. An oviparous lizard carrying eggs is termed gravid and a viviparous lizard carrying embryos is termed pregnant. Both terms are used interchangeably for both conditions. Eggs are generally visible against the body wall or palpable in many gravid oviparous lizards. Pregnancy in a viviparous lizard is suspected with generalized coelomic swelling, though developing embryos may not be palpable.

RADIOLOGY

Radiographic imaging is particularly useful in evaluating skeletal disorders in lizards. Evaluation of respiratory disorders and gastrointestinal disorders is also possible, though gastrointestinal imaging must commonly employ contrast media. Other coelomic structures that are evident on radiographs are kidneys, liver, coelomic masses, fat bodies, and occasionally uroliths. During ovulation, ovaries and shelled or nonshelled eggs as well as developing embryos may be observed; otherwise, gonads are not visible on radiographs in lizards.

Radiographic equipment should have several capabilities. A milliampere (mA) setting of 300 mA and exposure times approaching $\frac{1}{60}$ sec (5 mA) with relatively low kVp (45 to 60 kVp) produce excellent exposures on high-detail, rare-earth intensifying screens work best (Silverman & Janssen 1996). A collimator is essential as multiple exposures are commonly made on a single film for relatively small patients. The radiographic machine should have horizontal beam capabilities, though without this, and through creative positioning of the patient, acceptable imaging is possible.

A minimum of two exposures is desired of the coelomic cavity: dorsoventral and laterolateral (lateral). Similarly, extremities should be imaged in at least two planes.

For many lizards, a table-top technique is employed without a grid. Exposure techniques vary widely with different radiology units. For most small lizards (5 cm or less in thickness), small animal extremity techniques work well. For lizards larger than 5 cm, small animal thoracic techniques yield good exposure remembering that the lungs of many lizards, in part, may extend caudally to the pelvis. The author commonly uses small animal extremity techniques even for larger iguanas with satisfactory results. Generally, settings of lower kVp are desired as bone density is relatively lower in reptiles than mammals (Silverman & Janssen 1996). Similarly, the coelomic body fat of reptiles is typically lower than that of adult domestic animals, making the contrast of viscera more difficult to obtain with higher kVp. The standard dorsoventral and lateral positioning techniques may not reveal the true nature of coelomic structures or abnormalities. Therefore, partial rotation of the patient to a 30° or 45° lateral exposure can be useful as a third exposure when evaluating the coelom.

The difficulty with radiology in lizards is restraint and positioning. Large healthy or aggressive lizards should be sedated without exception. This minimizes bite risk and radiation exposure risk to the handler(s). Small lizards that are slow moving or calm may be allowed to rest unrestrained on the cassette for the dorsoventral vertical beam exposure. Lateral horizontal beam exposures are possible without restraint for some still or chemically restrained lizards. Small fast-moving or delicate lizards may be placed inside a clear plastic container or tube or cloth bag and positioned appropriately for exposure. Though some detail of the image may be lost, this may be the only option to obtain radiographs of these patients. When patients are sedated, gauze ribbons may be used to extend limbs as needed. Tape should be avoided as it may remove scales or otherwise damage skin.

Contrast media are commonly employed when nonskeletal imaging is required. Gastrointestinal contrast studies are not only beneficial for evaluating complete or partial obstructions, but also particularly useful for evaluating extraintestinal coelomic masses. Barium sulfate is the standard contrast material for gastrointestinal contrast imaging. Frye (1991) recommends the use of 10% barium sulfate at a maximum dose of 20 ml/kg. Barium for gastric and small intestinal imaging is administered via an oral ball tip dosing needle or flexible, nonrigid rubber catheter (see below, "Techniques"). Unless the imaging of the esophagus specifically is required, administration of barium via a gastric tube is best. Oral cavity dosing may result in partial aspiration and loss of barium through the mouth or nostrils. In diseased lizards, gastric to colonic transit times may be delayed substantially, though the author experiences partial to complete transit of barium within 24 hours in nonobstructed patients.

Retrograde or percloacal barium administration is indicated when distal intestinal obstruction or caudal abdominal coelomic masses are suspected. Barium is administered via a flexible, nonrigid rubber catheter. In small lizards (<200 grams) rigid or metal catheters should be avoided to prevent iatrogenic cloacal or colonic perforation (see below, "Techniques"). The clinician should approximate the amount of barium required for the desired image. Diseased colon or intestine may rupture with even the slightest pressure; therefore, resistance on the syringe is not a good practice for approximating dosing for administration of oral or percloacal barium.

SURGERY AND ANESTHESIA

Once uncommonly performed, coelomic cavity surgery, or celiotomy, is now routine for many pet lizards. These include ovariectomy, orchiectomy, salpingotomy, gastrotomy, enterotomy, cystotomy, biopsy, and tumor excision. Other surgeries that do not require celiotomy include amputation (digits, limbs, tails, hemipenis), enucleation, fracture repair, laceration repair, prolapse (intestinal, oviductal) repair, and reconstructive surgeries.

Anesthesia

Injectable and inhalant anesthetics are commonly employed both for surgery and sedation for diagnostic or treatment procedures. The most common injectable anesthetics are the dissociative agents ketamine and Telazol (tiletamine plus zolazepam). Ketamine is administered IM or SC at a dose of 22 to 44 mg/kg. A dose of 55 to 88 mg/kg is reported for surgical anesthesia (Bennett 1996a). Telazol is more potent than ketamine and is the preferred injectable anesthetic by the author. Telazol is administered IM or SC at a dose of 4 to 5 mg/kg (Bennett 1996a). Its potency allows for the administration of substantially less volume of injection, the effects are rapid, and recovery is typically quicker than with ketamine. Telazol is best used as a pre-intubation anesthetic for surgical procedures or as a sedative for diagnostic or treatment procedures. Intramuscular administration, when possible, is preferred for injectable anesthetics, as induction of anesthesia is typically more rapid than with subcutaneous administration. This is likely the result of quicker or more complete venous absorption. For procedures more invasive than cutaneous lacerations, inhalant anesthesia should be employed as movement of the anesthetized patient may continue with either ketamine or Telazol.

An additional injectable anesthetic, propofol (Diprivan, Rapinovet), is also in reptiles used for anesthetic induction and restraint. Propofol must be administered IV or via intraosseous catheter (IO) at a dose of 3 to 10 mg/kg (Schumacher 2002a). The drug is administered slowly over 30 to 60 sec or until the desired sedation is achieved. Propofol is eliminated rapidly from the blood and therefore is suitable for short diagnostic procedures or to achieve intubation for inhalant anesthesia. Its anesthetic effects may be extended by slow constant rate or intermittent infusion. Unless an indwelling catheter exists in the patient to be sedated, other injectable or inhalant anesthetics are preferred. Propofol is an ideal anesthetic when repeated daily sedation is required.

Opioids such as butorphanol (Torbugesic) provide a smoother induction when administered as a premedication for injectable or inhalant induction. Butorphanol is administered IM at a dose of 0.4 to 2 mg/kg (Bennett 1996a). The author uses 1 mg/kg IM routinely for reptile presurgical anesthesia.

The benefits of the anticholinergic atropine or glycopyrrollate (Robinul) as preanesthetic medications in lizards are questionable. Atropine is administered IM at a dose of 0.01 to 0.04 mg/kg and glycopyrrolate is administered IM or SC at a dose of 0.01 mg/kg (Bennett 1996a). In mammals, anticholinergics are administered to decrease salivary and respiratory secretions and for counteracting bradycardia during general anesthesia. These drugs may thicken respiratory secretions in reptiles (Murray 1996) causing tracheal or endotracheal tube occlusion and their efficacy at reducing the incidence of bradycardia is uncertain.

Inhalant anesthetics are preferred for maintenance of general anesthesia in lizards. The inhalant anesthetic of choice for lizards is isoflurane (Aerrane). Another recently introduced inhalant anesthetic is sevoflurane (Schumacher 2002a). Halothane and methoxyflurane are not recommended. Isoflurane provides relatively rapid induction if used alone for short sedation procedures. Because ventilatory suppression is common during anesthesia, recovery, though smooth, is prolonged (up to 15 minutes) compared to the typical recovery of mammals of similar size induced and maintained on isoflurane. The author has observed no benefit of quicker induction with sevoflurane in lizard patients. Additionally, recovery is typically as long or longer with sevoflurane compared to isoflurane for both healthy and health compromised lizards. Based on the dramatic price difference between these inhalants, isoflurane is still the inhalant anesthetic of choice for lizards (fig. 3.14).

Lizards should be intubated for inhalant anesthesia whenever possible. Intubation is relatively easy for the sedated lizard. The glottis is visible in the floor of the mouth at the base of the tongue. Minimal lubricant, if any, is applied to avoid obstruction of the small diameter tracheal tube (2 mm to 4 mm). Lizards that are too small for intubation may be maintained on a mask. A cone constructed of appropriate size syringe casing covered by a rubber glove, similar to that used for rodents, is ideal.

Reptilian respiratory physiology differs from that of mammals. In reptiles the spontaneous ventilation rate is directly related to temperature and the partial pressure of oxygen (PO_2) and in mammals respiration is driven by carbon dioxide (PCO_2) (Murray 1996). Thus, in high-oxygen environments, spontaneous ventilation is suppressed as the demand for oxygen by tissues is met by the oxygen saturation of inhalant anesthesia. As with mammals, control of the airway during anesthesia is helpful for the control of depth of anesthesia and is essential for assisted ventilation. Breath holding is a common problem during the induction phase of inhalant anesthesia in some lizards. Because lizards experience profound respiratory depression during general anesthesia, assisted or intermittent positive pressure ventilation (IPPV) is commonly required.

IPPV is performed at 2 to 4 breaths per minute at a pressure of less than 10 cm water in medium to large lizards and much less in smaller lizards (Bennett 1996a). Ideally the anesthetist should visualize rib expansion for several cycles of IPPV to discern the ideal pressure or ventilatory volume before the patient is draped. To avoid excessive pulmonary pressure and possible pulmonary rupture, the pop-off valve should never be fully closed when ventilating reptile patients. The great majority of lizards are maintained on a non-rebreathing anesthetic circuit. An oxygen flow rate of 300 to 500 ml/kg/min is indicated. Lizards over 5 kg can be maintained on a closed or circle circuit (Bennett 1996a). Isoflurane is typically maintained at 1.5 to 3% depending on the sedation obtained by injectable anesthetics.

Anesthetic monitoring is essential during reptilian sedation. Unlike snakes, cardiac movement may not be detectable through the chest wall because of the presence of a cartilaginous sternum. The author has found pulse oximetry to be satisfactory in monitoring at least the heart rate of sedated lizards, contrary to some reports. For small lizards, the finger probe may be placed across the dorsal head with the infrared transducer above the head and the receiver in the mouth. For larger lizards, the orientation is reversed on the mandible, or may be placed across the tongue. The advantage of pulse oximetry is the detection of blood flow that is reflective of mechanical cardiac activity as opposed to simply the detection of cardiac electrical activity that may continue after mechanical activity is compromised. Electrocardiography (ECG) is also valuable and is used with a three-lead system. A Doppler blood flow probe may be taped to the thorax over the heart for audible blood flow monitoring.

Reptile patients are warmed during surgical anesthesia with water recirculating heating pads. Electrical heating pads put the patient at risk for thermal burns. Surgical temperature should match the POTZ for a given species, but a range of 78° to 85°F is sufficient for most patients. Supplemental heating is also indicated during the entire phase of anesthetic recovery. Lizards sedated with injectable anesthetics may require hours to recover. In debilitated animals, this time is prolonged. For ketamine and Telazol, recovery times from 1 to 96 hours are reported in reptiles.

Surgery

Celiotomy is commonly performed in lizards for the variety of surgical procedures already listed. Surgical preparation for lizards is similar to that of small mammals. The lizard is placed in dorsal recumbency with legs and tail restrained by tape to the surgical table. The surgical site should be scrubbed with mild detergent if necessary to remove dirt or debris. Standard surgical preparation is performed. The author uses chloroxylenol 2% (Vet Solutions, Fort Worth, TX) as the sole surgical preparation. This agent, similar to chlorhexidine, provides excellent antibacterial and

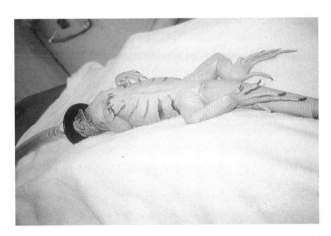

Fig. 3.14. Mask anesthetic induction of an iguana. (Photo courtesy of Dr. Sam Rivera)

antifungal activity on contact. Surgical draping is required. A fenestrated paper drape or a combination of clear plastic and fenestrated paper drape is used. The benefit of clear plastic drape is visualization of the patient for anesthetic monitoring during the surgical procedure (Bennett & Mader 1996).

Surgical incisions are made with consideration for skin and abdominal musculature lines of force, trauma to tissues, visualization of the desired surgical field, and wound healing. The long-accepted standard approach to celiotomy is the ventral paramedian incision in an effort to avoid transection or manipulation of the large ventral abdominal vein (see above, "Anatomy and Physiology"). This incision requires the transection of ventral abdominal muscle, which increases surgical bleeding, may decrease surgical field visibility (both from bleeding and from left versus right coelom access), and may increase postsurgical pain when compared to a ventral midline incision through the linea alba. In larger lizards the ventral abdominal vein may be gently retracted during the ventral midline incision.

The most common procedures performed during celiotomy are ovariosalpingectomy or salpingotomy for dystocia, ovariectomy, orchiectomy, and enterotomy. In most cases hemostatic clips are used for ligation of ovarian and oviductal vessels as indicated by surgical procedure. Great care must be exercised when handling all reproductive and mesenteric tissues in lizards, as they are delicate and quite friable. Closure of the celiotomy incision is two layers consisting of abdominal musculature or linea with absorbable suture, followed by the skin. The skin is closed in an everting pattern with absorbable or nonabsorbable tissue or skin staples. Reptilian skin heals significantly slower than mammalian skin. Suture removal is delayed until a minimum of 4 to 6 weeks post surgery (Bennett & Mader 1996).

A common nonceliotomy surgical procedure is digit or limb amputation. This procedure is indicated when trauma sustained from bites of cagemates, bites from rodents, or fractures result in nonhealing wounds or ascending limb infection. Surgical preparation is standard as in celiotomy. Amputation is performed at the most distal noninfected joint for limbs and preferably at the metacarpal or metatarsal-phalangeal joint for digit amputation. General anesthesia is required for limb amputations. Peripheral nerve block may be performed for some digit amputations.

Amputation of the hemipenes is indicated in cases of paraphimosis complicated by trauma, infection, or necrosis. This procedure may be performed with appropriate sedation using only injectable anesthetics such as ketamine, tiletamine/zolazepam, or Propofol. Aseptic preparation is standard. Amputation of one hemipenes does not sterilize the lizard as the hemipenes are paired. No compromise of urinary function will result from amputation, as there is no incorporation of urinary structures in the hemipenes or penis of reptiles (Barten 1996d).

Percloacal prolapse of the colon, oviducts, or urinary bladder may require amputation or resection of the affected tissues. Exposure of affected tissues or severe trauma may result in necrosis if the prolapse is not reduced promptly after occurrence. Necrosis of large portions of these tissues may require celiotomy to evaluate viability and repair the affected organ.

Open reduction and internal fixation of long-bone fractures in reptiles are performed following surgical approach and principles applied to mammals. Intramedullary pins, orthopedic wire, external skeletal fixation, and bone plating are employed as indicated.

Orthopedic devices are removed following the principles used in mammals, though healing of fractures in reptiles is slow and hardware may require removal prior to radiographic evidence of complete bone healing (Bennett 1996b).

PARASITOLOGY

Many reptile owners are unaware of the prevalence of parasitism in their animals. It is safe to assume that all wild-caught reptiles are parasitized (Lane & Mader 1996). Commonly, many captive-born reptiles are subclinically parasitized. In wild animals, internal parasites maintain a homeostasis with the host animal, as the host is essential for the survival of the parasite and a means of transporting future generations of the parasite to suitable areas for transmission to another host. Factors that maintain homeostasis include the host's immune system and the dilution of infective stages of the parasite in the environment that the host occupies. Thus, in many cases the captive environment offers a prime opportunity for imbalances in favor of the parasite through the stress and subsequent immunosuppression of the host and through the increased risk of reinfection of the host due to concentration of infective stages of the parasite.

Based on an awareness of parasites in some reptiles, however, some herpetoculturists advocate the prophylactic treatment of all reptiles with antiparasiticides for the more common intestinal parasites (de Vosjoli & Ferguson 1995). It is interesting, however, that the majority of hobbyists do not prophylactically treat for external parasites. This is perhaps because of an understanding of the potential side effects of pesticides applied to the animals. The side effects of oral deworming are similar. Though some therapeutics may be relatively safe at high doses, the potential effects of killing massive loads of intestinal parasites in an already immunocompromised animal can be severe. The safer alternative to prophylactic treatment of parasites is quarantine, serial parasite screening, and treatment of specific clinically identified diseases.

Techniques for identification of reptilian endoparasites are the same as those for small mammals. Fecal floatation of fresh fecal material in concentrated salt or sugar solutions and wet mount direct smears in saline are essential to screen for reptilian endoparasites. Smaller infective stages of some parasites may only be observed by direct smear. Stains such as Lugol's iodine solution (5.0 grams iodine crystals and 10.0 grams potassium iodide in 100.0 ml distilled water) both kills motile protozoans and stains cysts to make identification easier. Lane and Mader (1996) recommends examining both stained and unstained direct smears in addition to the fecal floatation.

External Parasites

External reptilian parasites consist of ticks, mites, chiggers, leeches, and biting flying insects. Acariasis, or mite, tick, or chigger infestation, is a serious disease of reptiles. Clinically, tick infestations are most common in imported lizards. Mader (1996a) reports that there are 7 genera of ticks and more than 250 species of mites that parasitize reptiles. Chiggers, also called red bugs, are the larval stage of Trombiculid mites and are generally self-limiting in lizards. Reptile mites (*Ophionyssus natricis*) are mobile and highly transmissible between reptiles and are capable of infesting multiple animals in a room or household without direct contact between hosts. These mites may be transmitted between hosts on the skin or clothing of people, though human infestation is supposedly rare.

Reptile skin provides many sites for attachment and protection for both mites and ticks. Ticks are commonly found beneath scales or in crevices such as the junction of the limbs and body or around the eyelids. Mites may be seen crawling freely over the lizard, but commonly concentrate in protected skin folds. It is not uncommon to diagnose mites after handling a lizard and then observing them on the human skin or seeing dead mites in water bowls of lizards that soak themselves routinely. Lizards that increase soaking behavior are commonly infested with mites.

Eradicating mites from individual animals is easier than eradicating them from the premises. Infestation of one animal indicates the possibility and likelihood of widespread infestation. Thus, prevention through quarantine of new animals is imperative (see above, "Husbandry"), and treatment of the cage and cage accessories and maintaining cleanliness of the surrounding environment are imperative.

Treatment consists of physical removal of ticks and inspection for the presence of ticks over several weeks. For mites the best treatment is pyrethroid flea sprays such as flea sprays for dogs and cats. Pyrethroids are synthetic pyrethrins and are less toxic to reptiles than pyrethrins. Allethrin is a common example of a pyrethroid. *Sprays containing pyrethrins or organophosphates should be avoided* (Mader 1996a). Prior to spray application, mineral oil or ophthalmic lubricant should be placed on the eyes of lizards. The pyrethroid spray is then applied to the entire lizard and rinsed immediately. Avoid spraying in the mouth or onto exposed wounds or mucous membranes. Oral exposure increases the risk of toxicity. The spray must be applied in a well-ventilated area and not into partially enclosed vivaria containing animals. All exposed mites are killed on contact. Pyrethroids are effective against mites in the environment, but not against eggs; therefore, reapplication on a weekly basis for two to three weeks is advised. The author is unable to confirm reports on the safety of fipronil spray as a miticide in lizards.

Ivermectin (Ivomec, Merck; and generics) is reported as both a topical and systemic treatment for mites in reptiles (Klingenberg 1993). The topical formulation is 0.5 cc ivermectin 1% (5.0 mg) added in 1,000 cc water and applied as a spray. The systemic administration is 0.2 mg/kg ivermectin 1% SC or PO. Clinical experience reflects unpredictable results and variable degrees of toxicity or side effects on a species-to-species basis with the injectable protocol, though no lethality has been observed in lizards by the author. Topical administration is absolutely not reliable. The miscibility and stability of ivermectin in water as a spray is questionable.

Many over-the-counter pet industry products are available for mites. These are generally "soap and water" mixtures designed to reduce the surface tension of water and to allow water to penetrate the spiracles or airways of mites, which essentially drowns the mites. The active ingredients are generally fatty acids (listed by scientific name) in an aqueous base.

Other home remedies include the use of pest strips: organophosphate impregnated resins designed to kill flying insects. These products are also quite effective in killing reptiles. If used in a safe manner (or by sheer luck), these products have been effective in environmental control of mites in large collections. However, the narrow safety margin prohibits recommendation of these products.

Finally, some insecticidal powders (Sevin dust, Ortho) have been effective in environmental control (Mader 1996a). Their use on the floor of well-ventilated cages of large terrestrial lizards beneath paper or carpet substrate is effective. This treatment is particularly effective against infestations refractory to other topical and environmental treatments. The enclosure is typically treated continuously for a period of one month and possibly repeated in one month if indicated. *Prepare the client for a long duration of treatment and for the strong possibility of both the contagious nature and high relapse rate of reptilian mite infestations. Also inform of the potential side effects of treatments both to lizards and to humans from pyrethrins, pyrethroids, and organophosphates.*

Internal Parasites

Internal parasites comprise many families and induce the majority of parasitic diseases in lizards. It is possible for many parasites to remain latent in the body and manifest disease during host immunosuppression from stress or other concurrent disease. Intestinal parasites consist of protozoa, nematodes, and trematodes.

Protozoans

Many protozoa inhabit the gastrointestinal tract of lizards as nonpathogenic or commensal organisms. The amoeba *Entamoeba invadens*, various species of coccidia, and specifically the coccidia *Cryptosporidium* spp. are responsible for the diseases amoebiasis, coccidiosis, and cryptosporidiosis respectively.

Amoebiasis is directly transmitted by a fecal-oral route in reptiles and is pathogenic and highly virulent to some snakes and lizards. Amoebiasis is nonpathogenic in turtles and crocodilians, but may be transmitted by both (Lane & Mader 1996). The life cycle of amoebiasis is as follows: the passing of infective cysts from a host, ingestion of cysts by a suitable host, multiplication into trophozoites in the intestinal tract, invasion of trophozoites into host tissues, formation of infective cysts, and shedding of infective cysts.

The pathogenesis of clinical disease is multifactorial and is caused by the tissue invasion of trophozoites and cellular destruction and from secondary bacterial infection. Clinical signs include diarrhea or loose mucoid stools, anorexia, dehydration, and weight loss. Infective trophozoites may spread to other organs hematogenously causing inflammation and, potentially, organ failure (Lane & Mader 1996).

Diagnosis is made by fecal examination. Cysts are identified by fecal floatation or direct saline smear and trophozoites are identified only by direct smear. For direct saline smears, a drop of Lugol's iodide is helpful to immobilize and stain the organisms.

Treatment of amoebiasis consists of antibiotics and antiprotozoal medications. Antibiotics are administered to treat potential secondary bacterial infections or potential septicemia. Aminoglycosides such as amikacin at a dose of 2.5 mg/kg IM or SQ every 72 hours for three to five treatments are appropriate. Metronidazole is administered at a dose of 50 mg/kg once weekly for two to three weeks while checking fecal samples for cysts or trophozoites (Lane & Mader 1996). Strict hygiene and sanitation are required to prevent horizontal transmission.

Coccidiosis is directly fecal-oral transmitted and is caused by protozoans of the genera *Eimeria*, *Isospora*, and *Caryospora*. The life cycle of coccidia is similar to that seen in mammals: oocysts passed in the stool sporulate outside the body and are ingested by a suitable host; sporozoites are released to invade host epithelial cells and mature; the epithelial cell ruptures and releases merozoites, which infect other cells and then can either multiply to infect other cells or form intracellular gametocytes, which eventually become infective oocysts to pass in the stool. Clinical disease results from cellular destruction and from secondary bacterial infection. Detection of oocysts is made by fecal floatation or direct smear.

Understanding the pathophysiology is important because infective oocysts are shed intermittently, thus clinical disease can occur in the absence of a detectable infectious agent. Clinically, lizards may be asymptomatic or have diarrhea, anorexia, weight loss, or failure to gain weight. The author has observed a higher incidence of coccidiosis in bearded dragons (*Pogona* spp.) than in other species of lizard with routine fecal examination. This phenomenon is also reported in popular literature (de Vosjoli et al. 2001). Many adult lizards with coccidiosis appear to be asymptomatic carriers, but neonates and juveniles with coccidiosis are usually clinically diseased. Coccidiosis can cause death in small or young lizards if undetected and untreated.

Treatment consists of trimethoprim-sulfamethoxazole (Sulfatrim) at a dose of 30 mg/kg PO once daily for 14 days or sulfadimethoxine (Albon) at a dose of 90 mg/kg on day one, then 45 mg/kg PO once daily for 14 days (Klingenberg 1996; Donaghue & Landenberg 1996; Lane & Mader 1996). Strict hygiene and sanitation are required to prevent horizontal transmission. Repeat fecal examinations are imperative.

Cryptosporidiosis is a highly virulent pathogen of snakes and lizards. Speculation exists regarding zoonotic potential, but at this point this potential is unknown (Cranfield & Graczyk 1996). Because cryptosporidiosis is considered untreatable in all animals, caution should be exercised when handling infected animals. The pathogenesis of Cryptosporidium in reptiles is not fully understood. Direct fecal-oral transmission is known to occur and the possibility of indirect transmission through an intermediate prey item is speculated. Cryptosporidiosis is reported in *Lacerta* spp., *Chamaeleo* spp., *Iguana iguana*, and two species of geckos (Cranfield & Graczyk 1996).

Oocysts are diagnosed by direct smear. Oocysts are 4 to 5 μm in size and are best identified by modified acid-fast staining (see Cranfield & Graczyk 1996). Serial fecal tests should be performed because of the intermittent shedding of oocysts. Diagnosis may be achieved through histopathology from gastric mucosal biopsy or by cytology of gastric lavage.

Though no treatments are known to be 100% effective, Sulfatrim as dosed for coccidia and the human drugs spiramycin and paromomycin have been used. Suspected or known positive animals are best isolated, not bred, and handled last in the maintenance of a collection of animals. Many traditional disinfectants have proved to be ineffective in environmental control. Ammonia solutions at 5% for a period of 3 days are effective for disinfection (Cranfield & Graczyk 1996).

Nematodes

Various nematodes infect lizards. Those infecting the gastrointestinal and respiratory tracts include various species of the familiar roundworms and hookworms; pinworms, *Oxyurus* spp.; hepatic worms, *Capillaria* spp.; strongyles, *Strongyloides* spp.; and lungworms of the genus *Entomelas*. Treatment for all intestinal and respiratory nematodes follows descriptions.

Roundworms in lizards are similar to those in mammals. Transmission is indirect and diagnosis is made by fecal floatation and identification of the typical thick-walled, round to ovoid oocysts. Diagnosis may also be made by identification of the adult worm in feces or vomitus. Because they require an indirect life cycle, these parasites are most commonly observed in carnivorous lizards and occasionally in omnivores.

Hookworms (*Oswalsocruzia* spp.) have direct transmission by fecal-oral route or through skin penetration. Diagnosis is made by fecal floatation and identification of the typical thin-walled oval eggs. Hookworms are responsible for more clinical disease in lizards than are roundworms because of the mucosal attachment of adult worms in the intestines. Clinical signs may include diarrhea, anorexia, and weight loss.

Pinworms (*Oxyurus* spp.) have a direct transmission by fecal-oral route and are found as adults in the large intestine of lizards. Diagnosis is made by fecal floatation and identification of the typically embryonated cigar-shaped larvae. Mammal pinworm ova or larvae may be passed in the stool of carnivorous lizards, but do not infect the lizards themselves. Typically, pinworms are an incidental finding on fecal examination, though diagnosed infections should be treated.

Hepatic worms (*Capillaria* spp.) have both direct and indirect transmission by fecal-oral route or through infected prey ingestion. The oocysts somewhat resemble those of whipworms (*Trichuris* spp.) of dogs. *Capillaria* spp. typically inhabits the intestinal tract but may also migrate to other organs. Pathology due to these species is unclear. Diagnosis is made by fecal floatation and treatment is indicated on identification.

Strongyloides spp. have a somewhat complex life cycle with direct transmission by a fecal-oral route or through skin penetration. *Strongyloides* spp. inhabit the gastrointestinal tract and greatly resemble the lungworms *Entomelas* spp. on fecal flotation. Diagnosis for either species is made by fecal floatation and identification of larvae (*Strongyloides* spp.) or embryonated eggs (*Entomelas* spp.). Diarrhea, anorexia, or weight loss may be seen with *Strongyloides* infection. Increased respiratory secretions, pneumonia, anorexia, and weight loss may be seen with *Entomelas* infections.

Treatment of all intestinal and respiratory nematodes consists of fenbendazole (Panacur) at a dose of 50 mg/kg PO once daily for 3 days, then repeat in 3 weeks followed by repeat fecal flotation (Klingenberg 1996). Because the majority of nematode parasites have direct transmission, proper hygiene and sanitation are imperative.

Cestodes

Tapeworms are infrequently encountered in captive lizards. Transmission is indirect typically through an arthropod intermediate host as seen in dogs and cats. Diagnosis is made by observations of proglottids in stool or the identification of oocysts on fecal flotation. Treatment consists of praziquantel (Droncit) 5 to 8 mg/kg PO or IM and treatment is repeated in 2 weeks (Klingenberg 1996).

Treatment of intestinal parasites in lizards is not without potential side effects. Anecdotal reports of sudden deaths in *Chamaeleo* spp. treated with standard single doses of fenbendazole and ivermectin (Stahl 1998) are known and the author has observed this effect on several occasions. Over several years, the author has made similar observations of a dramatic decline in health following the deworming of some individuals of wild-caught *Uromastyx* spp., *Varanus* spp., and *Chlamydosaurus* spp. at a reptile wholesale distribution facility. Some of the affected animals had no apparent compromised health prior to treatment, but were housed with conspecifics in relatively small cages, experienced repeated movement of humans around the enclosures, and may not have been on the optimal plane of nutrition. See color plates 3.9 through 3.20.

EMERGENCIES

Many health disorders of lizards are potential emergencies simply because of the latency in which they are presented or other related or consequential disorders with which they present. A few diseases or presenting complaints, however, are considered critical and death is imminent without immediate medical care. Some critical cases may present moribund or deceased and may require the same level of diagnostic attention to determine the cause of death.

Trauma
Trauma, as with any animal, may be an emergency. Many cases of trauma present ambiguously because the patient is found in a compromised state and the owner did not observe the inciting cause. Trauma should be suspected whenever the onset of clinical

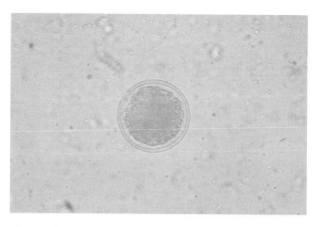

Plate 3.10. Roundworm, original magnification 40×. (Photo courtesy of ZooAtlanta) (See also color plates)

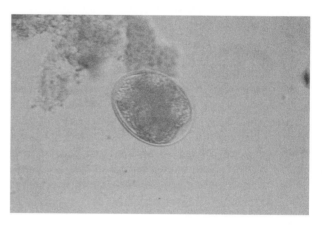

Plate 3.11. Ascarid, original magnification 40×. (Photo courtesy of ZooAtlanta) (See also color plates)

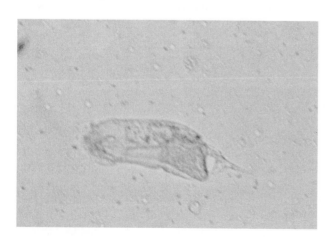

Plate 3.9. Flagellate, original magnification 40×. (Photo courtesy of ZooAtlanta) (See also color plates)

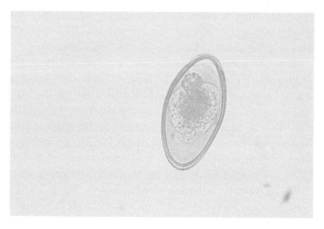

Plate 3.12. Oxyurid, original magnification 40×. (Photo courtesy of ZooAtlanta) (See also color plates)

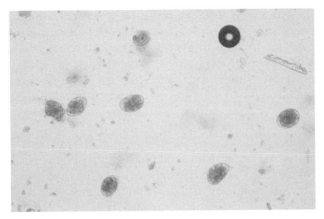

Plate 3.13. *Ascarid, original magnification 10×. (Photo courtesy of ZooAtlanta) (See also color plates)*

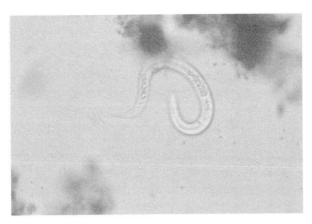

Plate 3.16. *Strongyle larva, original magnification 40×. (Photo courtesy of ZooAtlanta) (See also color plates)*

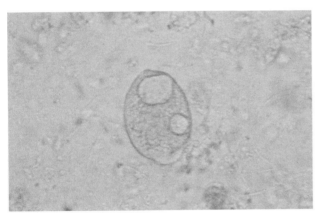

Plate 3.14. *Coccidia, original magnification 40×. (Photo courtesy of ZooAtlanta) (See also color plates)*

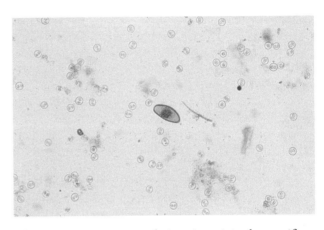

Plate 3.17. *Pinworm and eimeria, original magnification 10×. (Photo courtesy of ZooAtlanta) (See also color plates)*

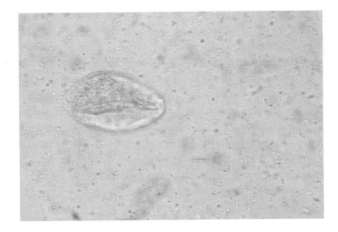

Plate 3.15. *Nyctotherus, original magnification 40×. (Photo courtesy of ZooAtlanta) (See also color plates)*

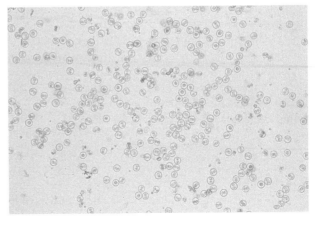

Plate 3.18. *Eimeria, original magnification 10×. (Photo courtesy of ZooAtlanta) (See also color plates)*

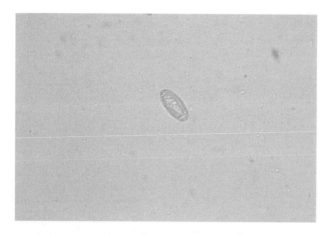

Plate 3.19. Capillaria, original magnification 40×. (Photo courtesy of ZooAtlanta) (See also color plates)

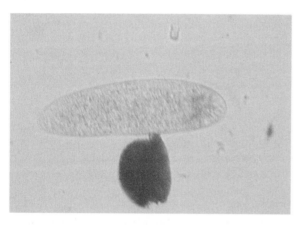

Plate 3.20. Pinworm, original magnification 40×. (Photo courtesy of ZooAtlanta) (See also color plates)

signs is acute; that is, within hours of the patient observed in a normal state and no history of gradual onset of lethargy, anorexia, weight loss, pregnancy, or other abnormal physiology. The presence of a thin or dehydrated animal or any history of anorexia should indicate the presence of another or an additional underlying disease process. Infectious or metabolic diseases rarely show acute clinical signs in lizards.

Diagnosis of trauma may be speculative as no external clinical abnormalities may be apparent. Radiography is the desired diagnostic test to evaluate for abnormal anatomy. Hematocrit and blood profile parameters may be normal, though creatine kinase (CK) values are commonly elevated with skeletal muscle injury. Radiographically suspected intracoelomic fluid may be aspirated for analysis.

With a high degree of suspicion of traumatic injury, empirically derived doses of corticosteroids are indicated in addition to providing proper thermal gradient. Warmed intravenous, intraosseous, or intracoelomic fluids are indicated for hypotension. Stabilization of fractures or luxations is performed following cardiovascular and thermal stabilization.

Toxicity

Unless presented with the known history of chemical toxicity, the veterinary staff must be meticulous at obtaining a history to support this diagnosis. The clinical signs of chemical or pesticide toxicity in reptiles are ambiguous, which leads to a diagnosis by exclusion of other metabolic diseases and delay in appropriate treatment. Generally, chemical toxicities in lizards are relatively acute and have no history of anorexia, paralysis, or weight loss preceding the onset of clinical signs.

The most common exogenous chemical toxicities in lizards are exposure to pesticides containing pyrethrins or organophosphates that are applied to treat mite infestations of the patient or the enclosure. Profound depression, death, or a variety of neurologic abnormalities including muscle postural abnormalities, tremors or fasciculations, seizures, and paralysis may occur.

With reasonable suspicion of pesticide toxicity, treatment is similar to that of mammals including cleaning or removal of the inciting cause, supportive care, and treatment with anticholinergics (see above, "Common Disorders"). Diazepam at 2.5 mg/kg IV or IM is reported for seizures (Rossi 1998a; Schumacher 2002b).

Hypocalcemic Metabolic Bone Disease

This form of MBD is separated from the classic osteopathic MBD. Diagnosis of hypocalcemic MBD should be suspected of any patient presenting with abnormal neurologic signs and no history of trauma or toxin exposure. Physiologically this disease is gradual onset, though the onset of clinical signs may be acute or subtle and unnoticed by the owner. Herbivorous or insectivorous lizards are clinically most affected, but all lizards are susceptible to hypocalcemia. History regarding diet and light exposure may help to confirm suspicion of this disease prior to diagnostic testing.

The most common clinical signs include hindlimb paresis or paralysis, muscle fasciculations or twitching, and depression. It is not uncommon for the only clinical sign to be hindlimb paresis with a normal appetite and no other physical abnormality. The progression of clinical signs from paresis to profound mental depression is usually gradual. Hypocalcemic MBD is a critical emergency when the patient presents substantially depressed or stuporous.

Diagnosis is highly suspected and supported by history in herbivorous lizards fed improper diets, no calcium or vitamin D_3 supplements, or little to no exposure to ultraviolet light. Diagnosis is confirmed with blood chemistry. Radiographs may be helpful in excluding other disorders such as trauma or diminished bone density, but they do not confirm hypocalcemia.

Treatment is supportive with warming, IV, IO, or IC fluids, and calcium gluconate at 100 mg/kg SC, IM, or IC. Treatment is long term and prognosis for recovery is grave for the most critical cases.

Gastrointestinal Obstruction

Signs of gastrointestinal obstruction may be vague, though history supports a gradual onset (days) anorexia, constipation, depression, weight loss, bloating, and rarely regurgitation. All species of lizards are susceptible, but terrestrial lizards are much more likely to ingest foreign materials from their environment. Impaction or constipation may occur in arboreal insectivorous lizards especially if dehydrated. A diagnosis of obstruction may also be supported by the history of feeding improper foods such as processed meat products to herbivores.

Diagnosis is based on history, physical exam, and radiographs. The radiographic presence of a foreign body or generalized gas distention of small and/or large intestine is indicative of obstruction. Because large herbivorous lizards have a relatively large distensible gut and relatively narrow pelvic canal, obstruction may occur much lower in the gastrointestinal tract than is classically seen in dogs and cats. Obstructions at the pelvic inlet exhibit marked abdominal bloating and commonly large and small intestinal gas distention. If these signs are observed radiographically in the absence of a detectable foreign body, retrograde percloacal barium is indicated to identify the obstruction. On rare occasions, repeated enemas administered by the owner or veterinary staff may result in colonic perforation and stricture that may mimic foreign body obstruction. With the degree of gas distention commonly seen in obstruction, ultrasound may be of little value diagnostically.

With high degree of suspicion of obstruction in the depressed patient, supportive care and surgery are indicated. Trocharization to relieve gas is not indicated as the thin gastrointestinal membranes may rupture and spill their contents into the coelomic cavity. Careful advancement of an oral feeding tube may aid in the reduction of bloating presurgically.

Dystocia

Dystocia, also called egg-binding, in oviparous species has varying degrees of presentation in lizards with many similarities to birds. Single or multiple eggs may be retained and the lizard may be in varying degrees of physical health. Those lizards presented with dystocia in a profoundly weakened state must receive immediate supportive care and surgery. Placement of IO catheter and fluid therapy are indicated.

Diagnosis is confirmed with history, physical exam, and radiographs. Ovariosalpingectomy is indicated for lizards with dystocias of more than a few retained eggs as surgery time is greatly extended for multiple salpingotomy incisions that are required for multiple eggs. Lizards will retain reproductive ability when ovariosalpingotomy or unilateral ovariosalpingectomy is performed.

Pneumonia

Though generally a straightforward diagnosis, at first appearance pneumonia may be confused with severe cases of stomatitis with no associated respiratory disease in lizards. History usually indicates a gradual onset of disease with a moderate to prolonged period of anorexia, weight loss, and increased respiratory effort. Oral or nasal exudates may or may not be present. A thorough physical exam including thoracic auscultation and thoracic radiographs is required for definitive diagnosis of pneumonia. Stomatitis may be concurrent or absent. Profound weakness and depression may be the result of profoundly reduced ventilatory capacity or secondary septicemia. Diagnostics and medical treatment are discussed above in "Common Disorders."

Oxygen therapy is generally not indicated due to respiratory suppression (see above, "Anesthesia"). IO fluid therapy and antibiotics are indicated. Nutritional support may be required for prolonged periods. Asphyxiation is a concern as the lizard may be too weakened to expel pulmonary exudates. Passage of a rubber feeding tube and aspiration of tracheal secretions may be performed with caution. Transtracheal wash procedures are performed only in patients that are not critically compromised.

Cloacal Prolapse

Cloacal prolapse is diagnosed by physical examination alone. This disease is an emergency with respect to potential necrosis and loss of tissue from time delay in presentation and treatment.

First aid of cloacal prolapse is cleaning and hydrating prolapsed tissue with isotonic solution. Following diagnosis of the specific nature of the prolapse, hypertonic solutions such as 50% dextrose may be applied to reduce swelling. Sedation or general anesthesia is often indicated to reduce patient struggling and pain. Reduction of viable tissue is first attempted manually when possible and then approached surgically. Systemic antibiotics are indicated despite the method of reduction. Corticosteroids may be administered empirically. The occurrence of reperfusion injury in reptiles is not known.

TECHNIQUES

Intravenous and Intraosseous Catheter Placement

Intravenous (IV) catheter placement is generally limited to the medium to large species of lizards approximately 20 cm or larger in the cephalic vein, though with proper equipment and skill there is no reason not to consider catheterization of smaller lizards (fig. 3.15). Sedation is required for catheterization (Jenkins 1996).

Standard sterile preparation of the catheterization site is performed and a transverse skin incision is made across the dorsal distal aspect of the antebrachium, just dorsal to the carpus. The incision in smaller lizards can be made with the sharp angle of a hypodermic needle or with a scalpel blade in the case of larger lizards. Once the vein is identified, standard catheterization technique is used with an appropriate-sized intravenous catheter. The catheter is secured with tape or suture.

Intraosseous (IO) catheters are indicated in smaller lizards or those with anatomy or disease that prohibits intravenous catheter placement. The bones of choice

for intraosseous catheterization are the femur, tibia, or humerus. Consideration must be given to the location with respect to the ability of the patient to interfere with or manipulate the catheter while hospitalized.

For femoral IO catheterization, standard sterile preparation is performed over the distal femur and a spinal needle of appropriate size is passed through a cutdown in the skin. The needle is advanced through the cortical bone of the distal diaphysis and then directed proximally into the medullary cavity of the bone. The tip of the needle should rest in the medullary cavity approximately one-third the distance from the proximal femur (Jenkins 1996). The catheter is then secured with taping that will also somewhat immobilize the stifle. See fig. 3.16.

If spinal needles are not available, sterile hypodermic needles of appropriate size may be used. The tibia is catheterized with a proximal to distal approach. Intravenous and intraosseous fluid therapy is performed with lactated Ringer's solution (LRS) and LRS + 2.5% dextrose at a rate of 0.5 to 1.0 ml/kg/hr (Jenkins 1996).

Venipuncture

Blood collection in lizards is performed from the caudal tail vein or rarely from the ventral abdominal vein. Small patients are placed in dorsal recumbency and

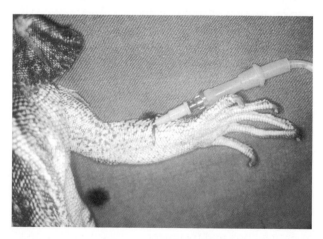

Fig. 3.15. *Cephalic catheter placement. (Photo courtesy of Dr. Stephen J. Hernandez-Divers, University of Georgia)*

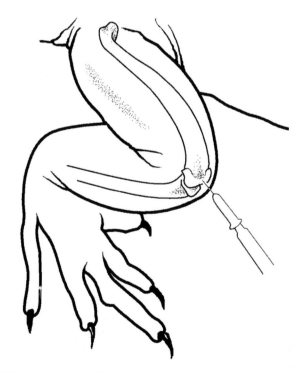

Fig. 3.16. *IO catheter placement. (Drawing by Scott Stark)*

may be wrapped in a towel to ease restraint. Large lizards may remain in ventral recumbency with the tail supported off the edge of a table. Fractious, dangerous, or very small and delicate lizards may require brief anesthesia for blood collection.

A portion of the proximal third of the tail from the vent is selected and aseptically prepared as if for surgery. A needle of appropriate length and gauge is selected for the patient. For lizards greater than 60 cm total length, a 22 gauge 1.0 to 1.5 inch needle on a 3.0 cc syringe is appropriate. For lizards less than 60 cm total length, a 22 to 25 gauge 0.5 to 0.75 inch needle on a 1.0 cc syringe is appropriate. For lizards less than 25 cm total length, a 27 gauge 0.5 inch needle on a 1.0cc or smaller syringe is appropriate. Insulin syringes are commonly used for these smallest patients.

Blood collection is performed in a manner similar to that of venipuncture of the tail vein of a cow. The needle is advanced through the skin along the ventral midline in a perpendicular to slightly cranially directed angle until the tip of the needle contacts the vertebral body. Slight vacuum is applied to the syringe as the needle is slowly withdrawn until blood is seen entering the needle hub. Blood collection is slow and may require 15 to 30 seconds for large lizards and up to 45 seconds for smaller lizards.

Care is taken to slowly expel blood into the collection tube(s) to prevent hemolysis from narrow-gauge needles. Lithium heparin (green top) tubes are the collection tube of choice for reptile biochemistry and complete blood count (CBC). EDTA may lyse reptilian erythrocytes when used for CBC (Mader & Rosenthal 2000). Whenever possible, the needles of 25 gauge or smaller should be removed from the syringe prior to transferring blood. Most labs that perform reptilian blood chemistries are capable of using samples as small as 25 μL (0.25 cc). The CBC may be submitted as a blood smear instead of whole blood when only a small sample is available for serum chemistry.

The ventral abdominal vein may be accessed in very small lizards or in those in which tail autotomy is likely. These patients should be anesthetized. The blood collection site is prepared with the patient in dorsal recumbency and accessed along the ventral midline at a point between the sternum and one-third the distance proximal to the pelvis. The bevel of the needle is directed dorsally and the needle advanced just beneath the skin while applying slight suction (Jenkins 1996). Blood collection may be faster when compared to the ventral tail vein. Cardiocentesis is not recommended for blood collection in lizards because of the risk of trauma and the relative lack of access of the heart in lizards (fig. 3.17).

Transtracheal Wash

Microbiology and cytology specimens may be collected from the lungs in a matter consistent with that of mammals. The glottis is easily visualized in patients that cooperate with opening the mouth. For patients that are reluctant to open the mouth, light sedation may be required. Following a diagnosis of pneumonia, a sterile catheter of appropriate diameter and length is advanced through the glottis and directed into the right or left lung as indicated by radiographs. A sterile wire may be inserted into the catheter and molded (using sterile technique) to aid the direction of the tip into the left or right mainstem bronchus (Murray 1996). At no time should the tube be forced if resistance is encountered. A speculum is employed to keep fingers out of the mouth and aid in visualization during the procedure.

Following placement of the catheter, warmed (to ambient temperature of the patient) sterile saline solution is infused at a dose of 1 to 5 ml/kg body weight and then retrieved into the syringe (Murray 1996). Repeated flushing of the saline, gentle coupage, or gentle rolling of the patient following infusion will increase the return of diagnostic material. Following collection, the patient is carefully monitored for normal respiration and heart rate. Samples should be submitted for appropriate culture and sensitivity and cytology. Portions of the sample may be preserved in EDTA or fixed on a microscopic slide for cytologic analysis.

When a transtracheal wash is contraindicated, bacterial culture and sensitivity may be obtained from pulmonary exudates swabbed from the glottis by culturette. By observing the patient's respiratory cycle, a microtip culturette is carefully inserted into the glottis and then retrieved in a manner not to retrieve oral secretions. This method may not reflect the bacterial population present in the lower respiratory tract.

Cloacal and Colonic Wash and Enema

Techniques for cloacal and colonic wash are applicable for microbiologic and cytologic sample collection, enema, and barium administration for contrast radiography. Colonic wash is performed in the absence of a fresh fecal sample for parasite analysis. Retrograde percloacal colonic catheterization is not as routine and as simple as performed in mammals and improper technique can result in severe health consequences to the patient. Sedation is not commonly required except in fractious patients.

A clean catheter similar to that used for transtracheal wash, a saline-filled syringe, and water-based lubricant are used. Dosage for colonic wash is approximately 10 ml/kg (Schumacher 2002b).

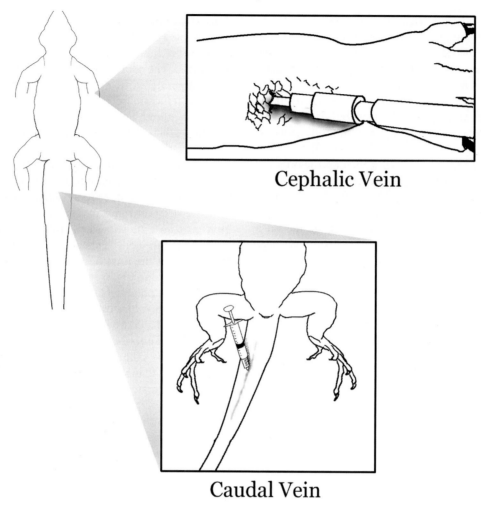

Cephalic Vein

Caudal Vein

Fig. 3.17. Lizard venipuncture sites. (Drawing by Scott Stark)

Copious lubrication of the tube is recommended for all procedures. Careful and slow advancement of the catheter in a retrograde fashion through the cloaca will reach the colon. On occasion the urinary bladder may be accessed accidentally. The urodeum lies ventrally and the coprodeum lies dorsally in the cranial cloaca.

It is imperative not to force the catheter if any resistance is encountered upon advancement. The coelomic tissues may be ruptured easily and the technician or clinician may not perceive a rupture based on the resistance encountered. Occasionally, the slow infusion of fluid upon advancement of the catheter will aid in reducing resistance especially with constipated animals. Once the catheter has reached the lower intestine, saline solution is infused and retrieved several times and gentle massage of the colon may be applied to maximize return of diagnostic material. A swab and floatation may be performed on the retrieved sample.

Administration of saline or stool softeners such as docusate sodium solution is applied in a manner similar to that of other companion animals. Resistance should never be achieved upon the syringe plunger with the administration of any colonic solutions.

In the event of suspected or confirmed iatrogenic colonic or cloacal rupture, surgery is immediately indicated for primary repair of the defect and copious lavage of the coelom. Most cases of iatrogenic ruptures unfortunately go unnoticed until the animal presents with life-threatening coelomitis and sepsis.

Cloacal swabs for bacterial culture and sensitivity may be obtained in a manner similar to that performed in birds. Washing of the external vent is indicated to reduce contamination of the culturette upon insertion and sample retrieval.

Bandaging

Bandage application and wound care for skin defects are consistent with those of other companion animals with the exception that the healing process is prolonged. Except for deep or extensive wounds or those that may become contaminated, wounds on most lizards are best maintained open in a clean environment rather than bandaged. Bandages may be cumbersome to lizards or may be a source of rubbing or other behaviors that attempt to remove the bandage. Tape is contraindicated on all geckos or other lizards with fragile skin.

Bandage application may be indicated for tail autotomy and amputations temporarily after surgery. Application of antibiotic ointments and gauze-packed syringe casings is ideal to allow hemorrhage control and to prevent contamination. Typically these bandages are required for only a few days.

External coaptation of limbs is commonly performed as part of fracture management using materials and techniques applied for other companion animals. The same principles of stabilizing one joint above and below the fracture are followed. A potential splint for larger lizards is their own body. Under sedation, forelimbs are secured to the lateral chest wall, with care not to compress the chest cavity especially in sedated animals. A similar application may be employed with the hind limb to the tail. With this technique, however, proximal humeral and femoral fractures may not receive adequate reduction in motion of the proximal bone fragment resulting in malalignment.

Spica splints are ideal for both fore limb and hind limb unilateral or bilateral fracture management. Under sedation the rigid splint for fore limb humeral fractures is incorporated into the soft bandage ventrally across the sternum and in the hind limb the splint is applied dorsally across the dorsal pelvis. The soft support bandage of the hind limb is wrapped in a figure-eight pattern incorporating both hind limbs dorsally creating abduction of both hind limbs. Similar technique is applied for forelimb soft bandage. This technique allows for the cloaca to remain free of bandage material and to reduce contamination of bandage material (Bennett 1996b). For more distal fractures of limbs, a modified Robert Jones bandage incorporating or encased by a plastic syringe casing and stirrups is ideal.

Carpal, tarsal, and digital fractures may be bandaged with soft bandage material. A ball bandage composed of a cotton ball applied to the palmar or plantar aspect of the affected foot is wrapped by soft bandage (Bennett 1996b). For all bandage applications, lizards should be maintained on clean nonorganic substrate such as paper or carpet including those lizards requiring a higher humidity environment. Strict attention should be given to cage and bandage sanitation and hygiene.

Force-Feeding

One of the most common signs of any disease state in lizards is anorexia. Force feeding or assist feeding is employed when the normal feeding response is diminished or when the animal is physically incapable of normal prehension or swallowing of food or water.

The technique for force feeding may also be applied to gastric oral medication administration and diagnostic gastric lavage. Some species of lizards may require sedation to access the oral cavity (*Uromastyx* spp., *Corucia zebrata*, and occasionally *Iguana* spp. and *Varanus* spp.). These species, especially *Uromastyx* and *Corucia*, are candidates for pharyngostomy tube placement when repeated force feeding or oral medication is required.

Assist feeding of lizards is accomplished in several ways. Voluntary feeding for smaller lizards is applied when the patient's normal feeding response or mobility is compromised, but with a little enticement the patient will readily prehend and swallow food. For large or dangerous lizards, tongs or forceps are used to introduce food. Assist feeding is used for patients that can swallow but are otherwise reluctant to prehend prey items; the mouth may be gently opened and the food item placed into the mouth for the patient to swallow. Prepared foods such as vegetarian gruels may be fed by syringe in this matter. Force-feeding is used for patients that are depressed and will not swallow or are incapable of chewing; food is provided by gastric or pharyngostomy feeding tube.

For insectivorous and carnivorous species that are fed only every other day or every few days in normal health, the normal feeding schedule may remain the same. It is important for all lizards to not over feed, especially if assist feeding normal dietary food items. Constipation or obstruction can result from overzealous feeding in these patients. For those species fed specially prepared gruels either by mouth or through a feeding tube, daily feeding is recommended as it is likely that these diets are more rapidly digested and absorbed when compared to the diet of normal health.

The procedures of tube force-feeding are similar to those applied for neonatal companion animals. The stomach of quadruped lizards is measured to the last few ribs. Anguiform lizards are treated as snakes for tube feeding purposes. Rubber catheters or stainless steel ball-tipped dosing needles are appropriate to use as feeding tubes. Because of the stresses imposed on the patient from restraint and opening the mouth by assist and force feeding, feeding frequency is generally no more than once daily for these patients. Alternatively, placement of a pharyngostomy tube accommodates smaller volume multiple daily feedings (fig. 3.18).

Diets are based on identifying the patient as carnivorous (including juvenile omnivorous) or herbivorous (including adult omnivorous). The amount of feeding is a calculated daily energy need based on standard metabolic rate (SMR) measured in kcal/day. The formula is $SMR = 32 \times BW^{77}$, where BW = body weight in kg. Alert and relatively noncompromised patients receive 75% to 100% of daily energy needs in the first 24 to 48 hours. Weak or debilitated patients receive 40% to 75% of their daily energy needs in the first several days (Donoghue & Landenberg 1996). The amount of feeding of the daily energy requirement is gradually increased to 100% as the patient's health and responsiveness improve. And, because the goal of force-feeding is to bring the patient back to voluntary feeding, the amount and frequency of force-feeding decreases or may abruptly stop pending the patient's recovery.

A variety of enteral diets is available for both human and veterinary use. These include: for omnivores, Ensure (Ross Laboratories, Columbus, OH); for herbivores, Sustacal Enriched (Ross Laboratories, Columbus, OH); and for carnivores, Clinical-Care feline and canine liquids (Pet-Ag, Elgin, IL). The available energy in kcal/ml as well as protein, fat, carbohydrate, and fiber contents are stated on the packaging.

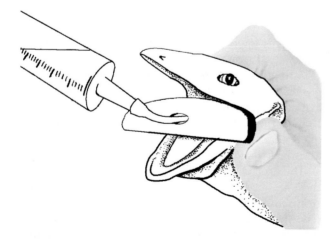

Fig. 3.18. Force-feeding. (Drawing by Scott Stark)

Therapeutic Administration

Treatment of lizard patients with pharmaceuticals is performed in a manner consistent with that of mammals with several exceptions. First, the oral administration is not always the route of choice: (1) Oral access may be difficult or stressful for some patients receiving daily medications; (2) Gastrointestinal transit time and factors affecting absorption of medications varies among species; (3) Inexperience or reluctance of the client in administering oral medications may lead to unnecessary trauma to the patient or noncompliance by the owner. When properly counseled, however, most clients enjoy the opportunity to take an active role in restoring the health of their pets.

Examples of antibiotics commonly administered orally in lizards are enrofloxacin injectable and compounded suspensions (Baytril), griseofulvin suspension (Fulvicin), metronidazole injectable and compounded suspensions, sulfamethazine (Albon), trimethoprim-sulfamethoxazole (Bactrim), and compounded tetracyclines. Additionally, many injectable antibiotics or ophthalmic preparations may be applied directly to oral mucous membranes rather than by injectable method in order to achieve higher drug concentrations at the site of infection. The parasiticides fenbendazole (Panacur) and praziquantel (Droncit) are administered PO. The author does not recommend the application of antibiotics to drinking water or to food items for lizards because of potential drug inactivity and the difficulty in accurate dosing.

Injections are performed using five methods. Subcutaneous (SC) and intramuscular (IM) techniques are most common. Intracoelomic (ICe) technique is used for large volumes of fluids or for drugs that need rapid systemic absorption such as calcium gluconate. Intravenous and intraosseous are typically performed through an indwelling catheter.

It is generally uncommon practice for clients to administer injectable medications to mammalian patients for routine infections. This practice is relatively common for reptile patients, but it must be approached with great attention to both the client's ability and the patient's cooperation. Considerations include:

1. What is the risk of injury to both the client and patient from the proposed procedure?
2. Is the client capable of adequately restraining the patient while administering the medication?
3. Is the client capable of determining if an undesirable side effect has occurred that prohibits further treatment?

4. Is there risk for abuse of the medication dispensed?

When dispensing injectable medication for the client to administer, adhere to the following:

1. Dispense the medication *premeasured* in syringes for each dose and *only* the amount for the specified number of doses. Administration should be only by the SC or IM route for home administration. If long-term treatment is required, dispense a portion of the amount and only refill the medication with a recheck exam or consultation.

   Accurately and fully label drug name, concentration, route, frequency, and duration of administration with no abbreviations.

   Never dispense medications that are potentially dangerous to humans at the prescribed dose (large doses of aminoglycosides, chemotherapeutics, narcotics).
2. Describe, show, and allow the client to practice administration of the medication. Sterile saline may be used for a practice injection.
3. Instruct the client on the appropriate uncapping and capping of needles and handling of the sterile needle.
4. Counsel the client on potential side effects of the drug and potential side effects administration. Describe "what can possibly go wrong" scenarios.
5. Provide the name and number of an employee at the clinic who can be reached at any time if there is a problem.
6. Have the client bring all medical waste products to the hospital or clinic for disposal.

Subcutaneous injections are made in the lateral scapular region. The skin is not drawn or lifted above the body wall as is common practice in mammals. The needle is advanced into the subcuticular space, gentle aspiration is applied to check for incidental venous access, and the injection is administered. Serial injections are alternated between the left and right sides and among different locations within the region. Subcutaneous injections are contraindicated in most *Chamaeleo* spp., all *Phelsuma* spp., and many other Gekkonidae because of skin autotomy, scarring, and skin discoloration caused by the injection. PO administration is indicated in these species.

Intramuscular injections are administered in epaxial muscles or triceps muscles in large lizards. IM injections are generally not possible in smaller lizards. When possible intramuscular injections are preferred for lizards to decrease the risk of skin inflammation.

Intracoelomic injections are administered in the right lower quadrant of the abdomen slightly cranial dorsal to the rear leg (Klingenberg 1996). Drugs administered in this way are sterile fluids, calcium gluconate, potassium penicillin, and some injectable anesthetics.

It is essential to understand not only the intended use of the medication, but also potential undesired or side effects. Side effects may be the result of a single administration, a series of administrations, a route of administration, or a cumulative dose. Individual variation as seen in mammals may also occur in reptiles. Side effects also involve the restraint or manipulation necessary to administer a particular administration. When considering the use of therapeutics, the old adage "do no harm" must be remembered.

EUTHANASIA

Euthanasia of captive lizards may be required for several reasons. The procedures for lizard euthanasia more closely resemble those of domestic laboratory animals than of dogs and cats. The relative inaccessibility of peripheral veins for injection of euthanasia solution necessitates injection of euthanasia solution directly into the heart (Mader 1996b) or occasionally into the occipital sinus or foramen magnum. Intracoelomic injection of euthanasia solution can be performed, but cardiac arrest may be prolonged and detection of death uncertain. The client must be fully prepared for euthanasia techniques prior to performing the procedures.

Humane euthanasia in the veterinary hospital is best performed under heavy sedation with the dissociative agents ketamine or Telazol. Ketamine at a dose of 100 mg/kg IM, or Telazol at a dose of 25 mg/kg IM will assure adequate sedation (Mader 1996b). Euthanasia solution as specified by the manufacturer for mammals is applied to lizards. Injections may be given intracardially with a sternal or lateral percutaneous approach to the heart. If the patient is dehydrated or severely debilitated and the cardiac approach is not possible, injection into the occipital sinus is indicated.

REFERENCES

Balsai, M. 1997. *General Care and Maintenance of Popular Monitors and Tegus*. Escondido: Advanced Vivarium Systems.

Barten, SL. 1996a. "Biology: Lizards." In *Reptile Medicine and Surgery*, edited by Douglas R. Mader, 47–61. Philadelphia: W.B. Saunders Co.

Barten, SL. 1996b. "Differential Diagnosis by Symptoms: Lizards." In *Reptile Medicine and Surgery* edited by Douglas R. Mader, 324–32. Philadelphia: W.B. Saunders Co.

Barten, SL. 1996c. "Specific Diseases and Conditions: Bites from Prey." In *Reptile Medicine and Surgery*, edited by Douglas R. Mader, 353–55. Philadelphia: W.B. Saunders Co.

Barten, SL. 1996d. "Specific Diseases and Conditions: Paraphimosis." In *Reptile Medicine and Surgery*, edited by Douglas R. Mader, 395–96. Philadelphia: W.B. Saunders Co.

Barten, SL. 2002. "Diseases of the Iguana Oral Cavity." In *Proceedings of the North American Veterinary Conference (16).* Gainesville, FL.

Bennett, RA. 1996a. "Special Techniques and Procedures: Anesthesia." In *Reptile Medicine and Surgery*, edited by Douglas R. Mader, 241–47. Philadelphia; W.B. Saunders Co.

Bennett, RA. 1996b. "Special Techniques and Procedures: Fracture Management." In *Reptile Medicine and Surgery*, edited by Douglas R. Mader, 281–87. Philadelphia: W.B. Saunders Co.

Bennett, RA. 1996c. "Specific Diseases and Conditions: Cloacal Prolapse." In *Reptile Medicine and Surgery* edited by Douglas R. Mader, 355–59. Philadelphia: W.B. Saunders Co.

Bennett, RA. 1996d. "Specific Diseases and Conditions: Cryptosporidiosis". In *Reptile Medicine and Surgery*, edited by Douglas R. Mader, 359–63. Philadelphia: W.B. Saunders Co.

Bennett, RA, Mader DR. 1996. "Special Techniques and Procedures: Soft Tissue Surgery." In *Reptile Medicine and Surgery*, edited by Douglas R. Mader, 287–98. Philadelphia: W.B. Saunders Co.

Boyer, TH. 1996. "Specific Diseases and Conditions: Metabolic Bone Disease." In *Reptile Medicine and Surgery*, edited by Douglas R. Mader, 385–92. Philadelphia: W.B. Saunders.

Cranfield, MR, Graczyk, TK. 1996. "Specific Diseases and Conditions: Cryptosporidiosis." In *Reptile Medicine and Surgery*, edited by Douglas R. Mader, 359–63. Philadelphia: W.B. Saunders Co.

Daly, J., et al. 1994. "Dietary Source for Skin Alkaloids of Poison Frogs (Dendrobatidae)" *Journal of Chemical Ecology* 20 (4): 943–98.

DeNardo, D. 1996a. "Special Topics: Reproductive Biology." In *Reptile Medicine and Surgery*, edited by Douglas R. Mader, 212–24. Philadelphia: W.B. Saunders Co.

DeNardo, D. 1996b. "Specific Diseases and Conditions: Dystocias." In *Reptile Medicine and Surgery*, edited by Douglas R. Mader, 370–74. Philadelphia: W.B. Saunders Co.

de Vosjoli P. 1992. *The Green Iguana Manual.* Lakeside, CA: Advanced Vivarium Systems.

de Vosjoli, P. 1993. *The General Care and Maintenance of Prehensile-Tailed Skinks.* Lakeside, CA: Advanced Vivarium Systems.

de Vosjoli, P. 1995. *Basic Care of Uromastyx.* Santee, CA: Advanced Vivarium Systems.

de Vosjoli, P. 1997. *The Lizard Keeper's Handbook.* Santee, CA: Advanced Vivarium Systems.

de Vosjoli, P., Ferguson, G. (eds.). 1995. *Care and Breeding of Panther, Jackson's, Veiled, and Parson's Chameleons.* Santee, CA: Advanced Vivarium Systems.

de Vosjoli, P., et al. 1997. *The Leopard Gecko Manual.* Mission Viejo, CA: Advanced Vivarium Systems.

de Vosjoli, P., et al. 2001. *The Bearded Dragon Manual.* Irvine, CA: Advanced Vivarium Systems.

Donoghue, S, Landenberg, J. 1996. "Special Topics: Nutrition." In *Reptile Medicine and Surgery*, edited by Douglas R. Mader, 148–74. Philadelphia: W.B. Saunders Co.

Frye, FL. 1991. *Biomedical and Surgical Aspects of Captive Reptile Husbandry.* 2d ed., vol. 1&2. Melbourne, FL: Krieger Publishing Co.

Gehrman, WH. 1994. Spectral Characteristics of Lamps Commonly Used in Herpetoculture. *Vivarium* 5(5):16–21.

Glaw, F, Vences, M. 1994. *A Field Guide to the Amphibians and Reptiles of Madagascar.* 2d ed. Bonn, Germany: Koenig.

Goin, CJ, Goin, OB, Zug, GR. 1978. *Introduction to Herpetology.* 3d ed. New York: W.H. Freeman and Co.

Helfman, GS. 1990. "Mode Selection and Mode Switching in Foraging Animals." *Advances in the Study of Behavior* 19: 249.

Innis, CJ. 2000. "Diagnosis and Treatment of Renal Disease in Tortoises." In *Proceedings of the North American Veterinary Conference (14).* Gainesville, FL., 954–55.

Jacobson, ER. 2002. "Chlamydiosis: An Underreported Disease of Reptiles." In *Proceedings of the North American Veterinary Conference (16).* Gainesville, FL., 916–17.

Jenkins, JR. 1996. "Special Techniques and Procedures: Diagnostic and Clinical Techniques." In *Reptile Medicine and Surgery*, edited by Douglas R. Mader, 264–76. Philadelphia: W.B. Saunders Co.

Johnson-Delaney, CA. 1996. "Introduction: Reptile Zoonoses and Threats to Public Health." In *Reptile Medicine and Surgery*, edited by Douglas R. Mader, 185–203. Philadelphia: W.B. Saunders Co.

Klingenberg, RJ. 1993. *Understanding Reptile Parasites.* Lakeside, CA: Advanced Vivarium Systems.

Klingenberg, RJ. 1996. "Special Techniques and Procedures: Therapeutics". In *Reptile Medicine and Surgery*, edited by Douglas R. Mader, 229–321. Philadelphia. W.B. Saunders Co.

Lane, TJ., Mader, DR. 1996. "Reptile Medicine and Surgery. Special Topics: Parasitology." In *Reptile Medicine and Surgery*, edited by Douglas R. Mader, 185–203. Philadelphia: W.B. Saunders Co.

Levell, JP. 1998. *A Field Guide to Reptiles and the Law.* Melbourne, FL: Krieger Publishing Company.

Mader, DR. 1996a. "Specific Diseases and Conditions: Acariasis." In *Reptile Medicine and Surgery*, edited by Douglas R. Mader, 341–46. Philadelphia: W.B. Saunders Co.

Mader, DR. 1996b. "Special Techniques and Procedures: Euthanasia and Necropsy." In *Reptile Medicine and Surgery*, edited by Douglas R. Mader, 277–81. Philadelphia: W.B. Saunders Co.

Mader, DR. 1996c. "Specific Diseases and Conditions: Gout." In *Reptile Medicine and Surgery*, edited by Douglas R. Mader, 374–79. Philadelphia: W.B. Saunders Co.

Mader, DR. 1996d. "Specific Diseases and Conditions: Upper Alimentary Tract Disease." In *Reptile Medicine and Surgery*, edited by Douglas R. Mader, 421–24. Philadelphia: W.B. Saunders Co.

Mader, DR. 2000a. "Reptilian Microbiology and Antibiotic Therapy." In *Proceedings of the North American Veterinary Conference (14).* Gainesville, FL., 961–64.

Mader, DR. 2000b. "Thermal Burns in Reptiles." In *Proceedings of the North American Veterinary Conference (14).* Gainesville, FL., 965–67.

Mader, DR. 2002a. "Metabolic Bone Diseases in the Green Iguana." In *Proceedings of the North American Veterinary Conference (16).* Gainesville, FL., 921–22.

Mader, DR. 2002b. "Ventral Midline Approach for the Lizard Coeliotomy." In *Proceedings of the North American Veterinary Conference (16).* Gainesville, FL.

Mader, DR, Rosenthal, K. 2000. "Proper Collection of Laboratory Samples." *Proceedings of the North American Veterinary Conference (14).* Gainesville, FL., 958–60.

McKeown, S. 1993. *The General Care and Maintenance of Day Geckos.* Lakeside, CA: Advanced Vivarium Systems.

McKeown, S. 1996. "Introduction: General Husbandry and Captive Management." In *Reptile Medicine and Surgery,* edited by Douglas R. Mader, 9–19. Philadelphia: W.B. Saunders Co.

Murray MJ. 1996. "Specific Diseases and Conditions: Pneumonia and Normal Respiratory Function." In *Reptile Medicine and Surgery,* edited by Douglas R. Mader, 396–405. Philadelphia: W.B. Saunders Co.

Obst, FJ, et al. 1988. *The Completely Illustrated Atlas of Reptiles and Amphibians for the Terrarium.* Neptune City, NJ: TFH.

Ritchie, BW. 1992. Class Notes: Exotic Animal Medicine. University of Georgia College of Veterinary Medicine.

Rossi, J. 1998a. "Emergency Medicine of Reptiles." *Proceedings of the North American Veterinary Conference (12).* Gainesville, FL.

Rossi, J. 1998b. *What's Wrong with My Iguana?* Escondido: Advanced Vivarium Systems.

Rossi, JV. 1996. "Special Topics: Dermatology." In *Reptile Medicine and Surgery,* edited by Douglas R. Mader, 104–17. Philadelphia: W.B. Saunders Co.

Schumacher, J. 2002a. "Anesthesia of Reptiles." In *Proceedings of the North American Veterinary Conference (16).* Gainesville, FL: ESVA.

Schumacher, J. 2002b. "Critical and Supportive Care of Reptiles." In *Proceedings of the North American Veterinary Conference (16).* Gainesville, FL.

Silverman, S, Janssen, DL. 1996. "Special Techniques and Procedures: Diagnostic Imaging." In *Reptile Medicine and Surgery,* edited by Douglas R. Mader, 258–64. Philadelphia: W.B. Saunders Co.

Stahl, SJ. 1998. "Common Medical Problems of Old World Chameleons." In *Proceedings of the North American Veterinary Conference (12).* Gainesville, FL., 814–17.

Stahl, SJ. 2000. "Reptile Obstetrics." In *Proceedings of the North American Veterinary Conference.* Gainesville, FL. 971–74.

Williams, DL. 1996. "Special Topics: Ophthalmology." In *Reptile Medicine and Surgery,* edited by Douglas R. Mader, 175–84. Philadelphia: W.B. Saunders Co.

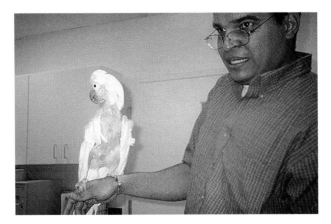

Plate 2.1. *A feather picker. (Photo courtesy of Dr. Sam Rivera)*

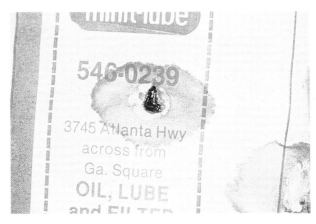

Plate 2.4. *Hematuria and melena. (Photo courtesy of Dr. Sam Rivera)*

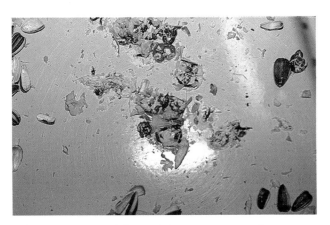

Plate 2.2. *Normal feces. (Photo courtesy of Ryan Cheek)*

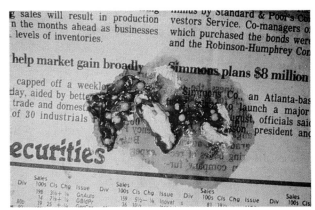

Plate 2.5. *Undigested seeds. (Photo courtesy of Dr. Sam Rivera)*

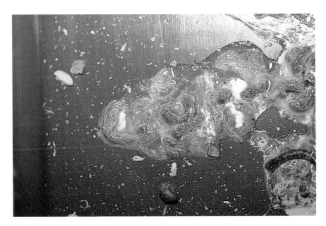

Plate 2.3. *Normal feces. (Photo courtesy of Ryan Cheek)*

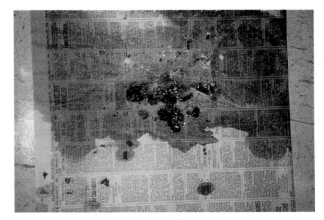

Plate 2.6. *Polyuria. (Photo courtesy of Dr. Sam Rivera)*

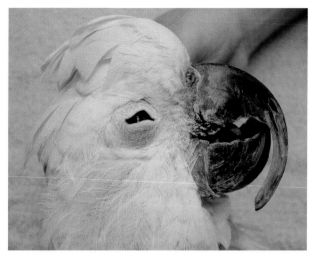

Plate 2.7. *Bird with PBFD. (Photo courtesy of Dr. Stephen J. Hernandez-Divers, University of Georgia)*

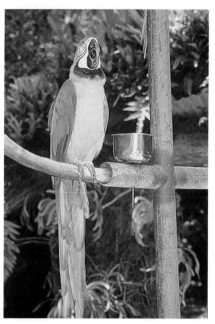

Plate 2.10. *Blue and gold macaw. (Photo courtesy of Cherie Fox)*

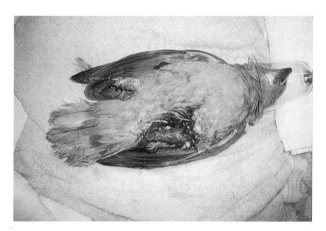

Plate 2.8. *Amazon parrot with trauma from a cat. (Photo courtesy of Dr. Sam Rivera)*

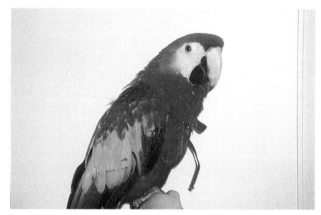

Plate 2.11. *Scarlet macaw. (Photo courtesy of Dr. Sam Rivera)*

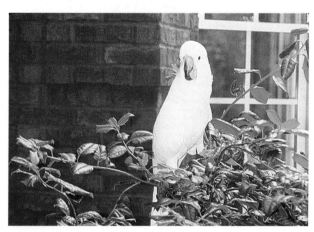

Plate 2.9. *Umbrella cockatoo. (Photo courtesy of Cherie Fox)*

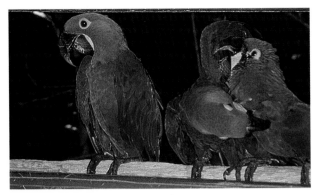

Plate 2.12. Hyacinth macaw. *(Photo courtesy of Cherie Fox)*

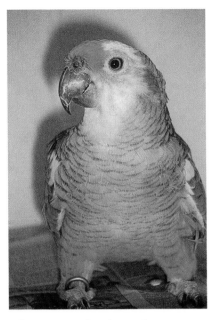

Plate 2.15. *Blue-fronted amazon. (Photo courtesy of Dr. Sam Rivera)*

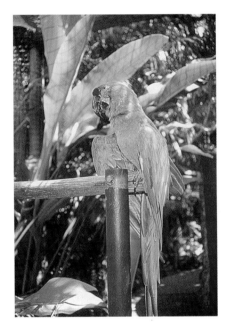

Plate 2.13. *Military macaw. (Photo courtesy of Cherie Fox)*

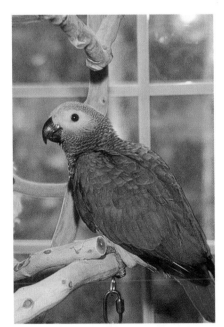

Plate 2.16. Congo African grey. *(Photo courtesy of Cherie Fox)*

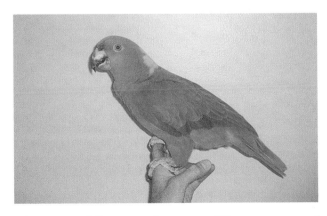

Plate 2.14. *Yellow-naped amazon. (Photo courtesy of Dr. Sam Rivera)*

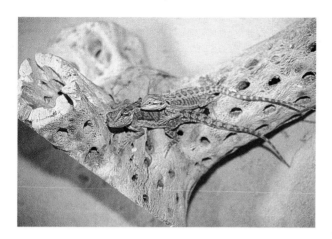

Plate 3.1. *Bearded dragon. (Photo courtesy of Ryan Cheek)*

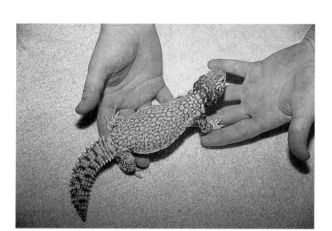

Plate 3.2. *Mali uromastyx. (Photo courtesy of Ryan Cheek)*

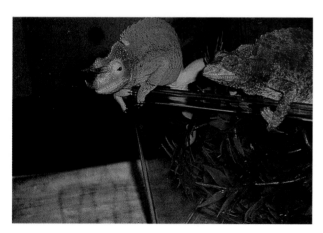

Plate 3.3. *Jackson chameleon. (Photo courtesy of Dr. Sam Rivera)*

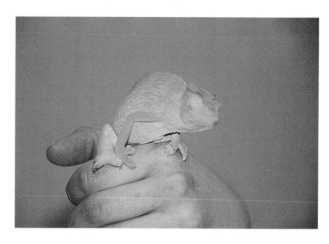

Plate 3.4. *Chameleon. (Photo courtesy of Ryan Cheek)*

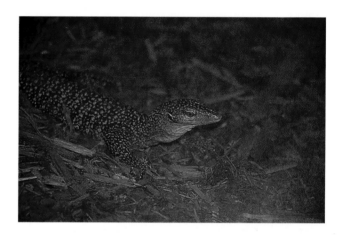

Plate 3.5. *Mangrove monitor. (Photo courtesy of Ryan Cheek)*

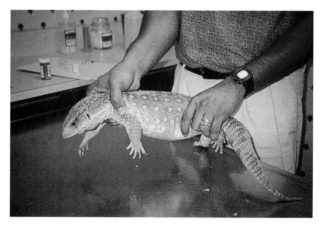

Plate 3.6. *Savannah monitor. (Photo courtesy of Dr. Sam Rivera)*

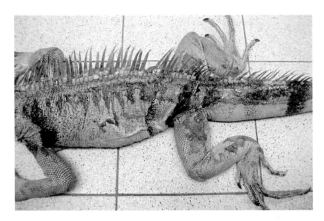

Plate 3.7. *Thermal burns. (Photo courtesy of Dr. Stephen J. Hernandez-Divers, University of Georgia)*

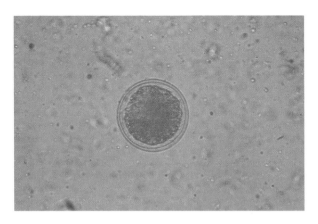

Plate 3.10. *Roundworm, original magnification 40×. (Photo courtesy of ZooAtlanta)*

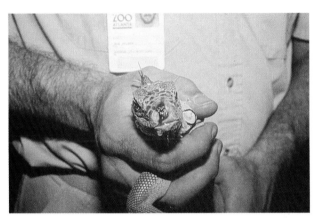

Plate 3.8. *Rostrum abrasion. (Photo courtesy of ZooAtlanta)*

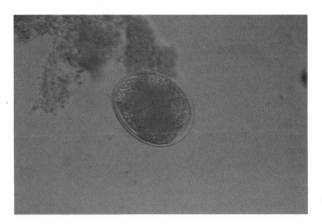

Plate 3.11. *Ascarid, original magnification 40×. (Photo courtesy of ZooAtlanta)*

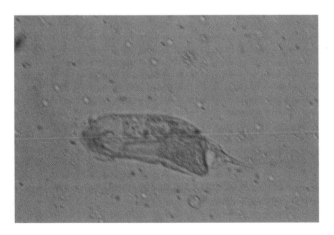

Plate 3.9. *Flagellate, original magnification 40×. (Photo courtesy of ZooAtlanta)*

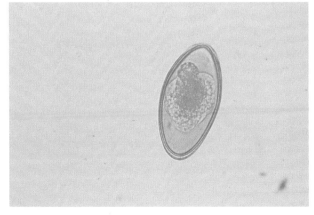

Plate 3.12. *Oxyurid, original magnification 40×.. (Photo courtesy of ZooAtlanta)*

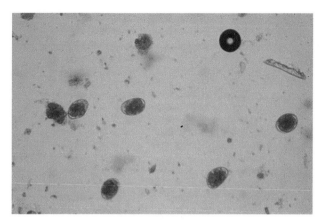

Plate 3.13. *Ascarid, original magnification 10×. (Photo courtesy of ZooAtlanta)*

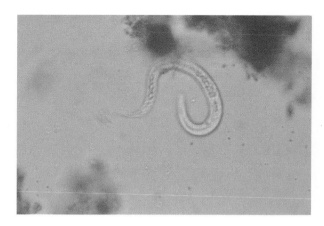

Plate 3.16. *Strongyle larva, original magnification 40×. (Photo courtesy of ZooAtlanta)*

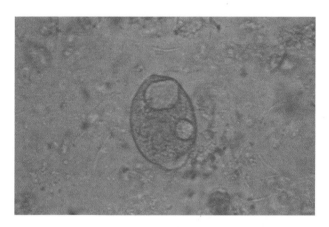

Plate 3.14. *Coccidia, original magnification 40×. (Photo courtesy of ZooAtlanta)*

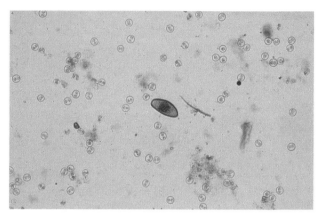

Plate 3.17. *Pinworm and eimeria, original magnification 10×. (Photo courtesy of ZooAtlanta)*

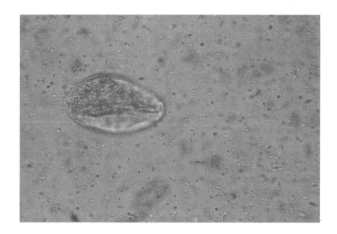

Plate 3.15. *Nyctotherus, original magnification 40×. (Photo courtesy of ZooAtlanta)*

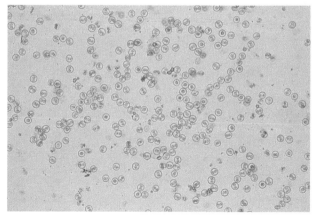

Plate 3.18. *Eimeria, original magnification 10×. (Photo courtesy of ZooAtlanta)*

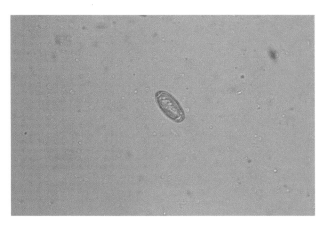

Plate 3.19. *Capillaria, original magnification 40×. (Photo courtesy of ZooAtlanta)*

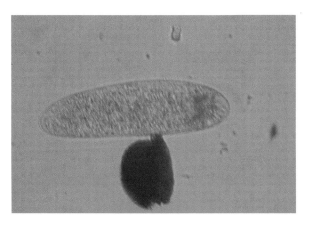

Plate 3.20. *Pinworm, original magnification 40×. (Photo courtesy of ZooAtlanta)*

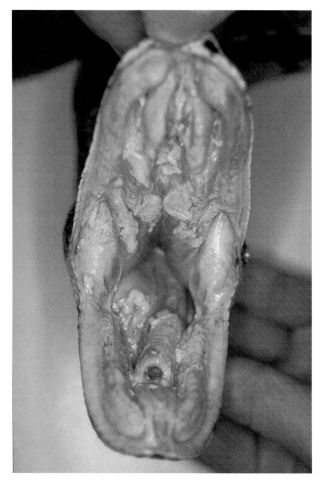

Plate 4.2. *Stomatitis in a snake. (Photo courtesy of Dr. Stephen J. Hernandez-Divers, University of Georgia)*

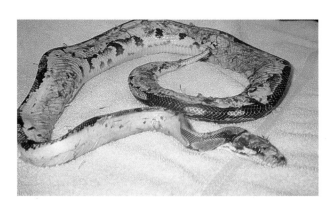

Plate 4.1. *A snake suffering from trauma from a prey item. (Photo courtesy of Dr. Sam Rivera)*

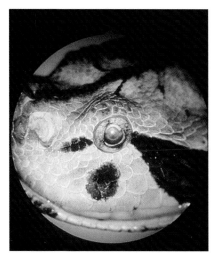

Plate 4.3. *Ocular larva migrans in a snake. (Photo courtesy of ZooAtlanta)*

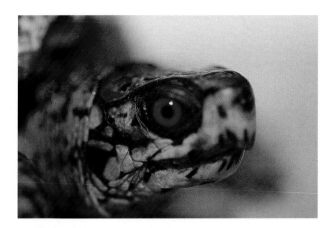

Plate 5.1. Male eastern box turtle showing red eye.

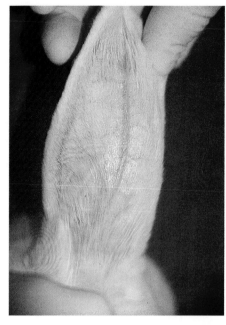

Plate 8.1. Marginal lateral ear vein on the left and the prominent central auricular artery. (Photo courtesy of Ryan Cheek)

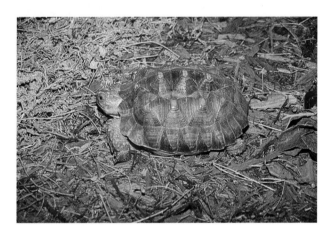

Plate 5.2. Sulcata tortoise.

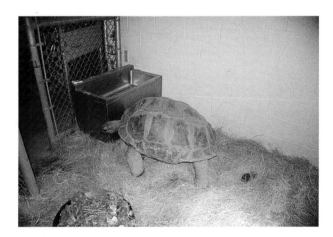

Plate 5.3. Aldabra tortoise.

CHAPTER FOUR

The Snake

Ryan Cheek and Shannon Richards

INTRODUCTION

Keeping snakes in captivity has become increasingly popular over the years. With the increase in captive specimens there has become a large demand for veterinarians and veterinary technicians who are educated in proper husbandry and treatment of reptiles. The veterinary staff must be willing to keep up with current treatment protocols (through continuing education courses or literature) as reptile medicine is ever changing and still evolving. One important tool in the diagnosis of any reptile is a thorough history. This is important because most reptiles in captivity become ill due to improper husbandry. Snakes kept in ideal conditions in captivity can live 10–20 years (depending on the species). This chapter contains general husbandry information on snakes to assist the veterinary staff through the diagnostic process.

CAPTIVE-BRED VERSUS WILD-CAUGHT

It is important to know whether a captive snake has been wild-caught or captive-bred. Wild-caught snakes are those that have been taken from their natural habitats and sold through the pet trade. Unfortunately, this is a common occurrence in the reptile industry. Wild-caught specimens typically have parasites (ticks, mites, and various internal parasites) and can take a long time to adjust to a captive environment, if they do at all. They also can have a host of other illnesses such as respiratory infections that become apparent while in captivity due to stress. Feeding wild-caught snakes can prove to be challenging as well due to their reluctance to eat in captivity. This reluctance to eat is usually due to the difficulties that a wild-caught snake may have adjusting to a captive environment (especially if husbandry guidelines are not being followed) and the snake not being offered the natural diet it is accustomed to. For example, a snake feeding primarily on frogs in its natural environment may not be receptive to the white lab mice that are sold commercially as snake feeders. This is not to say that it will never feed on mice in the future, but it will take some time to adjust and may take some "trickery."

Captive-bred snakes are snakes that have been bred and raised in a captive environment. These are obviously better specimens due to their lack of exposure to the diseases and parasites found in wild-caught specimens. Captive-bred snakes also accept "commercially available" diets better (such as feeder rodents) when offered and are not as finicky about accepting prekilled prey items, which is the recommended method of feeding. Although the temperament of a snake can never be guaranteed, captive-bred snakes tend to be more docile overall and can become more accustomed to handling.

For these reasons, it is important to know whether a snake was wild-caught or captive-bred. One should always recommend the purchase of captive-bred specimens to potential buyers to better ensure the snake's overall health. There are many reputable snake breeders to buy from who can provide a more reliable history on the snake. In a lot of cases, they are less expensive than buying from pet retail stores.

BEHAVIOR

Snakes are solitary animals and should be housed separately unless attempting to breed. Some can exhibit territorial behaviors and be aggressive to other inhabitants. Signs of aggressive behavior toward other snakes include biting, constricting, and "head pinning." The head pinning is a courtship behavior as well. During breeding season, some of these behaviors are observed more often. If these signs of aggression are observed with snakes being housed together, one should be removed immediately. As with any animal, if snakes are fighting, care should be taken if interference is necessary. A person could be bitten while trying to separate the combating snakes. Using hooks or tongs is recommended when human interference is warranted.

Another downside with housing snakes together is that some species (i.e., king snakes) eat other snakes as part of their natural diet. For this reason, all king snakes should be kept separate. Size or gender does not affect the snake's instinctive predatory behavior.

It is also important to know whether the snake is diurnal (active during day hours) or nocturnal (active during night hours). Knowing when the snake is the most active will aid in making several decisions, such as handling and ideal feeding times.

ANATOMY AND PHYSIOLOGY

Integument

As in mammals, the skin of snakes plays several crucial roles. The skin is the cellular protective barrier from the snake's outside environment. By being a protective barrier, it serves to protect the body from microbes and parasites, resists abrasions, and buffers the internal environment from the extremes of the external environment. The skin also holds other tissues and organs in place while being elastic enough to allow for respiration, movement, and growth. The skin also serves other roles such as physiological regulation, sensory detection, respiration, and coloration.

The snake's skin consists of two main layers, the dermis and epidermis. The epidermis is covered completely by keratin. This layer of keratinous cells, stratum corneum, shields the living tissue below. The stratum germinativum, the innermost layer of the epidermis, divides continuously to replace the outer layer of dead keratinous cells. As the cells in the stratum germinativum are pushed outward, they slowly flatten, die, and keratinize to form the stratum corneum. The stratum corneum is composed of three layers, the Oberhautchen layer, the beta-keratin layer, and the alpha-keratin layer, from the surface inward, respectively.

The dermis consists of two layers, the stratum compactum and the stratum spongiosum. The stratum compactum is the innermost layer of the dermis. It consists of densely knit connective tissue. The stratum spongiosum consists of connective tissue, blood vessels, glands, nerve endings, and other cellular structures.

Ecdysis, or shedding of the skin, is a normal occurrence for the duration of the snake's life. Young snakes will shed much more often and begin to have a longer resting period as they reach adult size. Because the top layer of snake skin consists mostly of keratin, which is

dead material, it is incapable of expanding during the snake's growth process. Therefore, it needs to be shed every so often. The cells of the upper stratum germinativum, the outer-generation layer, begin to proliferate and differentiate. The germinative layer begins to divide producing new layers of cells. These new cells form the inner generation layer, which is the precursor to scales, or the outer-generation layer, for the next ecdysis cycle . At this stage the new epidermal layer is ready. The Oberhautchen then fills with lymph and enzymatic action produces a cleavage zone and the old epidermis is shed (Zug et al. 2001, 49).

Before a snake sheds, it secretes a lubricant underneath the outermost layer of skin. This is to assist with the shedding process. This lubricant is most noticeable on the snake's eyes. The eyes become opaque or blue in color due to this lubricant being secreted. Sometime after this optical opacity or dullness in appearance is noticed the snake will begin to shed its skin. It can take a week or two before the entire shedding process is over and should be repeated at regular intervals. The snake may attempt to use any furnishings in the enclosure to assist in removing the dead skin. For this reason, one should make sure all of the furnishings are not so abrasive as to cause injury to the snake. The snake may also attempt to soak in its water bowl to assist in shedding. Water softens the old skin and makes it easier to remove. If the humidity is too low, the snake may have problems shedding. A snake sheds its entire outer layer of skin all at once. All snakes, with the exception of large boids, should shed in one piece. If there are numerous pieces of the snake's shedded skin or some still present on the snake, this is an abnormal shed. Snakes with abnormal shedding may need husbandry changes or may have ectoparasites and should be checked thoroughly. Age, nutrition, species, reproductive status, overall health, and hormonal balance also play a role on frequency of ecdysis.

If some shedding is still present on the snake, soaking or spraying can be tried to assist in the removal of the skin. If skin is allowed to build up and not "slough" off naturally, infections can occur underneath the old skin.

While snakes are in shed, they should not be handled or fed. Their senses are dulled (eyes opaque) and because they feel vulnerable, they can also be very defensive. To avoid potential bites, handling is not recommended during this time. Also it is unlikely the snake will eat, so feeding should not occur until after the snake has shed. If offering live prey items, feeding should not occur while the snake is in shed due to the higher potential for rodent bites.

Snakes are either entirely or partially covered by overlapping scales. The surface of each scale is composed of beta-keratin while the interscalar space, or sutures, is composed of alpha-keratin. This distribution of keratin gives a protective covering while allowing for flexibility and expansion. Certain species of colubrids and viperids are nearly scaleless. These species may only have labial and ventral scales. The remainder of the body is covered in a smooth keratinous epidermis. This anomaly is a recessive homozygous trait.

Snakes have paired scent glands at the base of their tails. These glands open at the outer edge of the cloaca. A large amount of semisolid, malodorous fluid is released for defensive behavior in some species and for courting behavior in other species.

Musculoskeletal System

Snakes possess a very complex cranial skeleton. Snakes have a cartilaginous anterior chondrocranium, the portion of the cranium that covers the brain (Zug et al. 2001, 52). This anterior portion of the chondrocranium consists of continuous internasal and interorbital septa and a pair of nasal conchae (Zug et al. 2001, 50). The chondrocranium calcifies between the eyes and ears and forms the basisphenoid. Farther posteriorly, a pair of exoccipitals, the supraoccipital bones, and the basioccipital form just below and behind the brain. These occipital bones encircle the foramen magnum. The exoccipitals and the basioccipitals form a single occipital condyle and the articular surface of the skull and atlas.

The maxilla is loosely connected to the other cranial bones. The maxilla connects to a special process on the prefrontal bone. They are connected via a movable articulation. The maxilla is also loosely connected to the cranial bones by the ectopyerygoid (Romer 1997, 126). The snout structures, the premaxilla, nasal, septomaxilla, and vomer, are movable as a separate series of bones from the maxilla and are also loosely connected to the cranial bones. This adaptation allows snakes to swallow large prey.

The mandible is highly specialized to allow for a large gape when swallowing large prey items (Romer 2001, 209). The mandible lacks a mandibular symphysis; an intramandibular hinge allows for the mandible to flex in the middle, and an articulated streptostylic quadrate allows the mandible to move sideways.

The vertebral column in snakes is divided into the atlas and axis, 100–300 trunk or precloacal vertebrae, several cloacal vertebrae, and 10–120 caudal vertebrae (Zug et al. 2001, 57). Each precloacal vertebra has a rib attached. The zygapophyses, the intervertebral articular surfaces, possess a posterior and anterior pair on each vertebra. The anterior zygapophyses flare outward and upward while the posterior zygapophyses flare inward and downward. The angle of the zygapophyses gives reptiles their flexibility or rigidity. Snakes are able to have such great flexibility due to these articular surfaces being angled toward the horizontal plane (fig. 4.1).

The muscular system of snakes consists of several hundred multisegmental muscle chains composed of elongated and interconnecting segmental muscles and tendons. Movement is achieved through individual contraction patterns of the muscle chains. There are six types of locomotion divided into two classes (Pough et al. 2001, 272). Lateral undulation and slide-pushing have no static points of contact with the substrate. Rectilinear, concertina, sidewinding, and saltation do have static points with the substrate.

Lateral undulation is the most widely used method of locomotion in snakes. At fixed points in the snake's environment, force is generated by horizontal waves traveling down alternating sides of the body. These fixed points can be a rock, tree, or any other physical object that the snake comes in contact with. At each point the body generates a force that pushes the body posterolaterally.

Slide-pushing is similar to lateral undulation but does not use fixed points in the physical environment. Slide-pushing involves very rapid alternating side body waves that generate sliding friction. This friction propels the snake forward.

Concertina locomotion is very slow and consumes large amounts of energy. This is a very complex system of locomotion. First, the anterior portion of the body will remain still while the posterior portion will draw up in a series of tight curves. The posterior end will then be stationary and the anterior end will extend forward. The sequence then repeats.

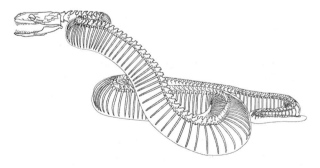

Fig. 4.1. *Snake skeletal anatomy. (Drawing by Scott Stark)*

Concertina locomotion is most effectively used on the ground where static friction is used to prevent rearward slippage.

Sidewinding is most commonly used on shifting soil such as mud or sand. Most snakes appear to have the ability to sidewind. The forces in sidewinding are directed vertically on the substrate. Sections of the body are alternately lifted, moved forward, and then set down. This produces a series of tracts that are parallel producing forward motion.

Saltation involves a very rapid straightening of the body from anterior to posterior lifting the entire body off the ground. This is used only by small species.

Rectilinear motion relies on the lateral muscles to work at the same time. The costocutaneous superior muscles pull the skin forward relative to the ribs. The ventral scales then anchor themselves to the ground. The costocutaneous inferior then pulls the ribs and with them the rest of the body forward relative to the stationary ventral scales. This form of locomotion is used by large body snakes such as boids and vipers.

Cardiovascular System

The Heart

The heart size, shape, structure, and position are all dependent on the species' anatomy, physiology, and behavior. Heart position has a direct correlation with arboreal, terrestrial, and aquatic habits (Vasse 1994, 75). Terrestrial species have a heart that is close to the head and have blood vessels in the distal portion of the body that dilate to receive extra blood. The heart of arboreal species is also located close to the head so that blood can more easily reach the brain when hanging vertically. Marine species have a heart that is found in the middle of the body so the pumping effort is minimal. Marine species do not have blood accumulation in the tail and the low blood pressure is compensated for by the external water pressure (Vasse 1994, 75). The heart consists of three chambers, a right and left atria and a single ventricle. The ventricle is further divided into the cavum arteriosum, cavum venosum, and the cavum pulmonale. Even though the ventricle lacks a septum, the snake can still separate oxygenated and deoxygenated blood and can maintain different systemic and pulmonary pressures because the heart is functionally five chambered (Pough et al. 2001, 206). There is a muscular ridge in the ventricle that separates the cavum pulmonale and the cavum venosum. The cavum arteriosum is located dorsal to the other two compartments and communicates with the cavum venosum through an intraventricular canal. There are two inflow routes, the right and left atria, and three outflow routes, the pulmonary artery, and the left and right aortic arches. The right atrium receives blood from the sinus venosus. The sinus venosus is a large chamber located on the dorsal surface of the atrium. It receives blood from four veins, the right and left precaval vein, the postcaval vein, and the left hepatic vein. The left atrium receives blood from the right and left pulmonary veins.

Blood flow through the heart starts when both atria contract. The atrioventricular valves open and allow blood to flow into the ventricle. When the atria contract, the valve between the right atria and the cavum venosum seals off the intraventricular canal allowing the oxygenated blood from the left atrium to flow into the cavum arteriosum and the deoxygenated blood from the right atrium to flow into the cavum venosum and then to the cavum pulmonale. When the ventricle contracts, the blood pressure inside the heart increases. First, because resistance is lower in the pulmonary circuit, deoxygenated blood is expelled from the cavum pulmonale through the pulmonary artery. When the ventricle shortens, the muscular ridge that separates the cavum venosum and the cavum pulmonale comes into contact with the wall of the ventricle and closes off the passage between the two compartments. The atrioventricular valves are forced shut as the pressure inside the ventricle increases. When the atrioventricular valves are shut, the oxygenated blood from the cavum arteriosum is pushed through the intraventricular canal into the cavum venosum and out the left and right aortic arches. At this point, the pressure inside the cavum venosum is more than twice of that in the cavum pulmonale.

Another remarkable ability that snakes, as well as other squamates and chelonia, have is the ability to perform intracardiac shunting. Intracardiac shunts are classified as left-to-right or right-to-left. In a right-to-left shunt, the deoxygenated blood that should normally be flowing out to the pulmonary circuit is being expelled out to the systemic circuit via the aortic arches. This shunt increases the amount of circulating blood and decreases its oxygen content. Primarily, the right-to-left shunt is used to increase the body temperature and to bypass the lungs during breath-holding. The left-to-right shunt is used to help stabilize the oxygen content of the blood. The direction and degree of intracardiac shunting is dependent on the pressure differences between the pulmonary and systemic circuits and the washout of blood remaining in the cavum venosum.

The renal-portal system exists in all fish, reptiles, and birds. The system collects blood from the caudal portion of the body and carries it to the kidneys. The blood is then filtered and is returned to the heart via the post caval vein. Blood that travels through the renal-portal system only goes through the convoluted tubules and not the glomeruli (Holz 1999, 249).

The location of the heart, being so cranial, has two disadvantages. First, when a snake is holding its head down, blood flow to the tail will be compromised. Second, most important, when the head is up or the entire body is in a vertical position, the blood from the tail has to travel all the way to the heart against gravity. The veins of snakes do not have valves to prevent back flow so snakes have adapted three ways to ensure that the blood continues to flow toward the heart even while being vertical. The contractions of the smooth muscles that line the vessels help push the blood toward the heart. Snakes will undulate or contract their skeletal muscles massaging the blood toward the heart. The tight skin of arboreal species acts as an antigravity suit further assisting the blood in traveling toward the heart.

The lymphatic system in snakes, as well as all reptiles, is an elaborate drainage system. Microvessels collect lymph from all over the body. These microvessels merge into larger vessels that eventually empty into larger lymphatic trunk vessels and then into lymphatic sinuses. All three parts, the trunk, vessels, and sinuses, empty into veins. The lymph can be bidirectional but mostly flows toward the pericardial sinus and into the venous system. Reptiles have a pair of lymph hearts located in the pelvic region but do not possess lymph nodes.

Respiratory System

Snakes have upper respiratory anatomy similar to mammals. Air enters and leaves the trachea through the glottis located in the back of the pharynx. The glottis and other cartilage form the larynx. The trachea of snakes has incomplete cartilaginous rings. The ventral portions of the rings are rigid and the dorsal portion is membranous.

Most snakes only have a single right lung and a small nonfunctioning left lung. The right lung is generally one-half or more of the snake's body length. In most species, the posterior one-third is an air sac. Very few snakes have a right and left functioning lung. In those species that do have a very small functional left lung, it is about 85% smaller than the right. The right bronchi enters the lung and empties into a wall that is lined with faveoli. The faveoli are richly supplied with blood. Most of the gaseous exchange occurs in the faveoli (Zug et al. 2001, 173). Snakes that have only one functioning lung possess a tracheal lung. The tracheal lung is a vascular sac that contains many faveoli

for gas exchange. The tracheal lung extends from the point where the tracheal rings are incomplete dorsally and posteriorly until it is touching the right lung. The air sac, or saccular lung, is not used as a site for gas exchange but as a site for air regulation.

All reptiles breathe using a negative-pressure ventilation (Pough et al. 2001, 200). During inspiration, the intercostal muscles expand the ribs the entire length of the body dropping the pressure inside the lungs to below atmospheric pressure drawing in air. Then the intercostal muscles relax and the glottis closes closing the respiratory tract. The snake then pauses for several seconds to several minutes before exhaling. Terrestrial and arboreal species normally have a period of apnea between respiratory cycles. When snakes are swallowing large prey, the ribs in the anterior portion of the body are not able to expand for proper inspiration. During ingestion of prey, the posterior ribs expand causing the saccular lung to inflate and deflate moving air through the respiratory system. (See table 4.1)

Nervous System

The central nervous system is organized the same in snakes as it is in all reptiles and similar to mammals. The brain of snakes is divided into the forebrain and hindbrain. The forebrain contains the cerebral hemispheres, the thalamic segment, and the optic tectum and is further broken down into the telenchephalon, diencephalon, and mesencephalon. The cerebral hemispheres are pear shaped. They contain olfactory lobes that project anteriorly and end in olfactory bulbs (Zug et al. 2001, 61). The thalamic region is hidden by the cerebral lobes and the optic tectum. The thalamic region is tube shaped with a thick wall. The dorsal portion of the thalamic region has two dorsal projections. The anterior projection is the parietal body and the posterior projection, the epiphysis, is the pineal organ. The pineal organ is glandular in most snakes. The ventral portion contains the hypothalamus. The optic tectum is located on the dorsal part of the posterior portion of the forebrain and the ventral part contains the optic chiasma. The hindbrain contains the cerebellum and medulla and is also broken down into the metencephalon and myelencephalon. Both are small in extant species of reptiles. Reptiles also have 12 pairs of cranial nerves.

The spinal cord runs the entire length of the vertebral column. Each vertebra contains a bilateral pair of spinal nerves. Each spinal nerve contains a sensory and motor root that fuse near their origin. The diameter of the spinal cord is uniform all the way down to the end.

Sense Organs

Cutaneous Sense Organs

Boids, pythonids, and viperids have specialized structures in the dermis and epidermis that contain heat receptors (Zug et al. 2001, 62). These pit organs sense infrared heat and are located in different locations in each taxon. In the boids, the pit organs are scattered on unmodified supralabial and infralabial scales. Boids have intraepidermal and intradermal types. Pythonids have a series of pit organs in the labial scales. The heat receptors lay on the floor of each pit. In viperids, the pit organs are located bilaterally between the eyes and the nares. The opening of each pit is forward facing and is overlapped by other receptors. The heat receptors are contained inside a membrane that stretches across the pit further enhancing its heat-seeking ability.

Ears

The ears of snakes have the same two functions as they do in mammals, hearing and balance. The middle ear in snakes is virtually nonexistent (Platel 1994, 51). It is a very narrow cavity that does not contain a tympanic membrane but does contain one ossicle, the columella, that abuts the quadrate bone for transmission of vibrations. The inner ear of snakes is very similar to the inner ear of mammals. The utricle and saccule make up the semicircular canals that ensure balance. Vibrations are received in the inner ear via the columella and pass through the cochlear canal and onto the basilar papilla. Even with the absence of an outer ear and the virtual absence of a middle ear, snakes are adept at hearing (Platel 1994, 52). Since the columella senses vibrations from the quadrate bone that is located on the upper jaw, snakes will pick up vibrations from the substrate on which their head rests (Funk 1996, 42). It is believed that arboreal snakes can pick up aerial vibrations enabling them to catch avian prey in midflight.

Smell

It is difficult to determine the amount of olfactory sensation snakes have. Snakes have a large number of olfactory nerves, which leaves no doubt that snakes are macrosmatic animals. Their olfactory abilities do not work alone; they are closely associated with the vomeronasal sense as well as sight.

Vomeronasal Sense

The vomeronasal organ, or Jacobson's organ, plays a vital role in predation. It is connected to the oral cavity by the vomeronasal duct. The role of the vomeronasal organ is to detect nonaerial, nonvolatile particulate odors. These odors are picked up by the chemoreceptors on the forked tongue. After picking up a scent, the snake then carries that scent to the vomeronasal organ. The sensory cells inside the vomeronasal organ react with certain molecules that then transfer the scent to the accessory olfactory bulbs, other encephalic centers, and the nucleus globosus. The vomeronasal organ is also used for interspecies relations. Snakes can use the vomeronasal organ to sense a den for hibernating and for reproductive behaviors such as picking up pheromones.

Eyes

The snake has very different eye anatomy than other reptiles. Embryologically, the eyelids of snakes fuse to form a transparent spectacle (Zug et al. 2001, 64). This spectacle has an extensive vascular network that is optically transparent. The anterior layer of the spectacle is shed during each ecdysis cycle. The spectacle is separated from the cornea by an epithelial lined subspectacular space. The globe of the eye is kept moist via secretions made by the harderian glands. The nasolacrimal ducts drain from the medial canthus to the roof of the oral cavity at the base of or just behind the vomeronasal organ. The globe has poorly developed rectus muscles and limited rotational muscles. Snakes lack the scleral ossicles and cartilage that lizards and chelonians have. Snakes possess a soft and pliable lens. They are able to focus by the forward movement of the lens by increased pressure of the vitreous applied by the ciliary muscle. The iris contains striated muscle making dilation and contraction of the pupil voluntary.

The retina, pupil shape, and lens color have gone through evolutionary changes to better fit the species lifestyle (Platel 1994, 54). Diurnal species, most often, have a round pupil, yellow lens, and a retina made of all cones. Crepuscular species have a paler lens and the retina contains both rods and cones. Nocturnal species have a vertical slit-shaped pupil, a colorless lens, and a retina consisting of mostly rods with very few cones. These are just generalized statements with many exceptions. For example, crepuscular or nocturnal pythons have a round pupil and a retina that contains a large quantity of both rods and cones.

Snakes have a very wide range of vision from 125° to 135° for most species. Snakes are also able to perceive depth and distance using binocular vision. The area that both eyes can see is between 30° and 45° (Platel 1994, 55).

Digestive System

The digestive system in snakes is a linear tract (Funk 1996, 40). It starts with the mouth that opens directly into the buccal cavity. The buccal cavity contains rows of teeth on the upper and lower jaw, the vomeronasal organs, the primary palate, the internal nares, and a highly specialized tongue. Aniliids, the false coral snakes, have developed a partial secondary palate. The morphology of the tongue is variable dependent on the feeding behavior of the snake. The buccal cavity contains many glands throughout the entire cavity. Multicellular glands are a component of the epithelial lining of the tongue. These glands produce and secrete mucous that coats the prey making passage down the esophagus smooth. Snakes also have five types of salivary glands: labial, lingual, sublingual, palatine, and dental. Venom glands are modified salivary glands. The pharynx contains a muscular sphincter that controls the opening of the esophagus (fig. 4.2).

The esophagus is a muscular walled tube that connects the buccal cavity to the stomach. In snakes, the esophagus may be one-quarter to one-half of the body length. The stomach is a very large muscular tube that has the primary role of mechanical digestion and starting the chemical digestion process. The stomach lining has numerous glands that produce secretions to aid in digestion. The pyloric valve controls the food bolus that enters into the small intestine. The small intestine is a long, narrow, straight tube. The small intestine also has glands to help with the digestion process. At the junction with the large intestine, there is a marked difference in the size. The large intestine has a diameter several times that of the small intestine. Boidea have a small cecum located at the proximal colon. The large intestine is the weakest and most thin-walled structure in the digestive tract. The large intestine ends at the anus and then leads to the dorsal portion of the cloaca, the coprodaeum.

The primary function of the liver in snakes is the same as in mammals. The liver produces bile that is stored in the gall bladder and then sent to the duodenum via the common bile duct. Bile aids in the digestion of fat. The liver is elongated and spindle shaped. The pancreas produces digestive fluids into the duodenum. The pancreas is usually located in a triad with the spleen and gallbladder, or some species have a splenopancreas (fig. 4.3).

Since the feeding behavior of snakes is not all the same, different physiological and morphological changes occur with different feeding behaviors. Snakes that eat small, frequent meals tend to have a

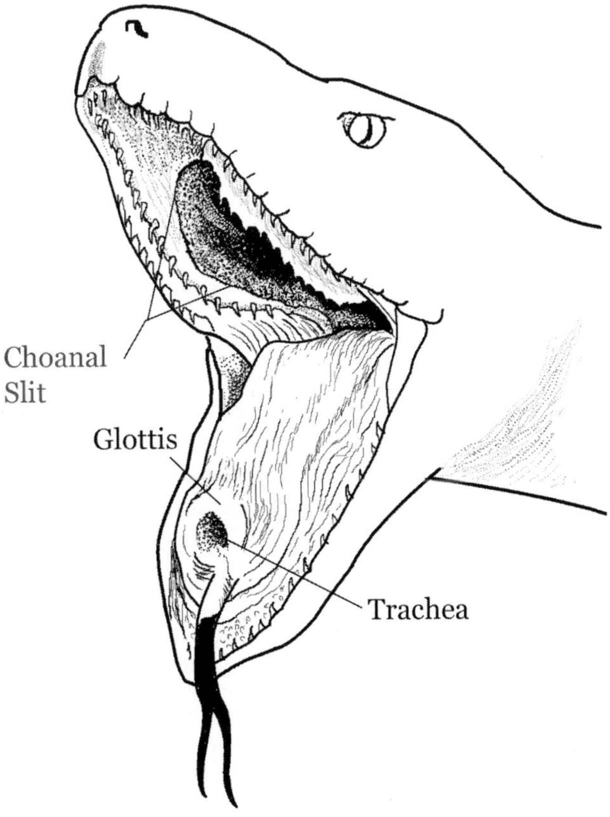

Fig. 4.2. *Oral cavity of a snake. (Drawing by Scott Stark)*

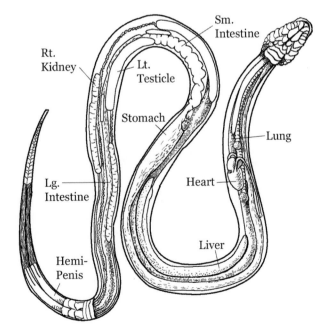

Fig. 4.3. *Visceral anatomy. (Drawing by Scott Stark)*

digestive system that is always in an active state. On the other hand, snakes that eat large, infrequent meals maintain their digestive system in an inactive state until a prey item has been ingested. When the prey is ingested, the gut begins to increase secretions of hydrochloric acid and digestive enzymes. Within one day, the small intestine will double in size and other organs in the digestive, respiratory, and circulatory system will also gain size. When the digestive tract is activated, the metabolic rate will increase as much as 44 times that of the resting metabolic rate. The energy needed to activate the intestinal tract must be received from stored reserves before the digestive process will begin for the new prey. Infrequent feeders usually maintain a metabolic rate half that of frequent feeders.

Urinary System

Snakes have a bilateral pair of lobulated and elongated kidneys. They are located in the dorsal caudal coelomic cavity. The right kidney is located cranial to the left kidney. The kidneys are metanephric in structure and have few nephrons and lack a loop of Henle and a renal pelvis (Divers 2000, 217). The ureters empty into the urodeum in the cloaca. Snakes do not have a urinary bladder.

Snakes excrete nitrogenous waste as uric acid. Uric acid is a purine and is synthesized in several interlocking pathways. Uric acid is very insoluble in water. In the kidney tubule, urine stays dilute. Water is reabsorbed when the urine reaches the cloaca, making the urine solution more concentrated and some of the uric acid precipitates. The precipitation of uric acid reduces the concentration of the uric acid allowing more water to be reabsorbed. Again, this leads to more precipitation of uric acid. This process allows nitrogen to be excreted using very little water. The end product is a white or gray semisolid pasty material containing uric acid.

Endocrine and Exocrine Glands

Pituitary Gland

The pituitary gland is the so-called master gland of the body. It consists of two parts, the neuropophysis and the adenopophysis. The neuropophysis produces hormones that stimulate the adenopophysis or act directly on the target organs. The adenopophysis releases six hormones: adrenocorticotropin, follicle-stimulating hormone, luteinizing hormone, prolactin, somatotropin, and thyrotropin.

Pineal Complex

The pineal complex consists of an epiphysis and a parapineal organ. They act as light receptors and are associated with cyclic activities such as circadian rhythms and seasonal cycles. As a gland, both organs release melatonin. All snakes have a pineal gland that lies on the brain but does not exit the skull as in some iguanids.

Thyroid Gland

The thyroid is located in the throat adjacent to the larynx and trachea and is nearly spherical. Snakes can have either a single or paired thyroid gland. The thyroid is responsible for accumulating iodine and producing and regulating hormones that control growth and development as well as ecdysis.

Parathyroid Gland

The parathyroid is located just cranial to the thyroid. The parathyroid functions as a blood calcium regulator.

Pancreas

The pancreas in snakes, like in mammals, functions as an endocrine and exocrine gland. As an exocrine gland it secretes digestive enzymes, and as an endocrine gland it secretes the hormone insulin via clusters of cells called the islets of Langerhans.

Gonads

The gonads produce the sex hormones. The function of the gonads is closely regulated by the brain and the pituitary. Hypothalamohypophyseal hormones and gonadotropins are produced by the brain and the pituitary, respectively, when the gonads are triggered by a hormonal response. Along with stimulating reproductive structures, the sex hormones also produce secondary sexual characteristics and provide a feedback mechanism to the hypothalamic-pituitary complex.

Adrenal Glands

The adrenal glands are a pair of bilateral glands located anterior to the kidneys. The adrenal glands have many functions. They produce adrenaline and noradrenaline, they affect sodium, potassium, and carbohydrate metabolism, and they affect the androgens and the reproductive process.

Table 4.1. Approximate Organ Location in Snakes

First quarter	Trachea, esophagus, heart
Second quarter	Heart, liver, lung, stomach
Third quarter	Stomach, gallbladder, gonads, small intestine, pancreas, spleen, adrenal glands
Fourth quarter	Colon, kidneys, cloaca
Tail	Hemipenes, musk glands

REPRODUCTIVE BIOLOGY AND HUSBANDRY

The Male Anatomy

All male snakes have a right and left testicle and a pair of hemipenes. The testicles are in the shape of an ovoid mass that consists of seminiferous tubules, interstitial cells, and blood vessels. They are located dorsomedially within the coelomic cavity between the pancreatic triad and the kidneys. The right testis is located just cranial to the left. Snakes do not have an epididymis. The hemipenes are located in the base of the tail and are held in place by a retractor muscle. Sperm is produced in the seminiferous tubules. During copulation, sperm travels to the hemipenis through the Wolffian ducts. The sperm is able to enter the female by means of the sulcus spermaticus located on the outside of the hemipenis. During copulation, only one hemipenis is used. Many snakes, especially boids, have vestigial (pelvic) spurs. These spurs are used in copulation as stimulation and to help position the two cloacae together (fig. 4.4).

The Female Anatomy

The paired ovaries are located similarly to testes. The ovaries consist of epithelial cells, connective tissue, nerves, blood vessels, and germinal cell beds encased in an elastic tunic. An inactive ovary is small and granular. Active ovaries are large, lobular sacs filled with spherical vitellogenic follicles. Snakes do not have a true uterus. The oviducts empty directly into the cloaca and have an albumin-secreting and shell-secreting function.

Fertilization

Prior to egg production, fertilization will occur in the upper portion of the oviducts when the sperm and egg

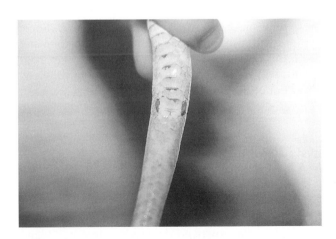

Fig. 4.4. Large pelvic spurs. (Photo courtesy of Ryan Cheek)

unite. In snakes, fertilization is usually delayed for a few hours to years after copulation. The sperm storage structures facilitate storage of sperm for long periods of time. This process of delayed fertilization permits females to mate with other males allowing multiple paternity among the offspring and having a higher fecundity rate, although not all snakes practice this.

Sexual Maturity

Sexual maturity in snakes is dependent on many factors. Husbandry and nutrition are more important factors than age. Ultimately, it is the size of the snake that determines sexual maturity. Due to the large difference in care provided to captive snakes, the age of sexual maturity will consequently be different as well. With proper husbandry and nutrition, snakes will grow quickly and become sexually mature within their first or second year of life.

Follicle Maturation and the Fat Cycle

In the months before the female's reproductive cycle, she will begin to store fat (Ross et al. 1990, 60). This fat plays a major role in the reproductive cycle. Vitellogenesis, the production of yolk, will only occur if enough fat is stored. Also, at the end stages of gestation, snakes may not eat so the fat bodies are used for energy. The follicles mature within the ovaries. When the follicles are mature and palpable, some ova are released into the oviduct while other ova may be released before or after copulation. At this point the snake will find a male and copulate and the female will become gravid. After the proper gestation period, the female will either lay eggs or give live birth. The female is now very thin and weak after using up all of her fat deposits during gestation and/or incubation. Until the fat stores have been built back up, she will not be able to stimulate follicular maturation. She then begins to eat and increases her fat bodies. After a couple to several months, the female snake is back to full weight and can begin the follicular maturation cycle again.

Courtship

It is important to know and observe signs of courtship so proper changes can be made. If communal cages are kept, insubordinate specimens should be separated from the courting pair. Temperature cycling patterns should be started before or right at the first signs of copulation. Specimens should be removed or added if either of the specimens seen courting is inappropriate for breeding.

There are many courtship behaviors observed in snakes. Most behaviors are not species specific.

Following is an explanation of four common courtship behaviors that are seen in many taxa (Ross et al. 1990, 55).

1. The tactile chase behavior is characterized by the male pursuing the female in often jerky and erratic movements. The male may flick his tongue over the female's body and begin to crawl over her dorsum trying to align his body with hers. The female will continue to crawl away if unreceptive to the behavior.
2. In the tail search copulatory attempt the male will rotate his tail under the female's tail in an attempt to bring both cloacae together. A receptive female will then lift her tail or allow her tail to be lifted by the male. The male may use his spurs to stimulate the female to lift her tail.
3. Tactile alignment is characterized by the male aligning his tail with the female's, using his spurs as stimulation and to help align the cloacae.
4. Intromission and coitus occurs when a female raises her tail and everts her cloaca to a male. The male will then align the two cloacae and copulation occurs. This behavior is also known as cloacal gaping.

Oviparous, Ovoviviparous, and Viviparous

Oviparous snakes are snakes that lay eggs that are protected by a hard shell. Around 70% of snakes are oviparous. Some of the more common oviparous species seen in a veterinary practice are king snakes and milk snakes (*Lampropeltis* spp.), rat and corn snakes (*Elaphe* spp.), and all pythons. Oviparous snakes will go to much trouble finding an appropriate place to lay their eggs. Some snakes will lay in a natural cavity, hollow stumps, or small mammals' burrows while others will dig their own burrow or make a nest. Most pythons will incubate their eggs by hugging the eggs and increasing their own body heat through rhythmic contractions of their abdominal musculature.

Ovoviviparous snakes will incubate the eggs inside the oviducts until the eggs hatch. This process ensures proper humidity and temperature levels within the mother's thermoregulative capabilities. Ovoviviparous snakes are found mainly in places where the ground is too cold to incubate eggs (Saint-Girons 1994, 99). There are many disadvantages to ovoviviparous snakes. The gravid female moves very slowly, which opens her up to predation; she is only able to eat very small prey, which are hard to find at times; and she must focus more on thermoregulation. Some examples of ovoviviparous snakes are all boas, all vipers, and garter snakes (*Thamnophis* spp.)

Snakes do not practice true viviparity.

Egg Anatomy

After fertilization, the embryo begins to develop on the dorsal surface of the yolk. The yolk is then covered by the yolk sac and attached to the embryo by the yolk stalk at the umbilicus. Nourishment is provided by the yolk via the blood vessels of the yolk sac. The amnion is a fluid-filled sac that surrounds and protects the embryo. The allantois is a closed sac that collects waste products. The chorion is a membrane that surrounds and protects the embryo and yolk sac. The shell membranes that cover these three membranes provide gas exchange throughout the shell. The blood vessels in the shell membranes and the yolk stalk combine to form the umbilicus. As the egg passes through the oviducts, the shell and shell membranes are gradually applied by the shell glands.

Timing and Frequency of Reproduction

In most species, environmental factors trigger the breeding season. While other species will breed year round, for temperate species, breeding season usually begins in spring after a hibernation period. Most equatorial species will breed year round. There are exceptions to these rules. Some tropical boids reproduce in the cooler part of the year though temperature changes have a greater diurnal change than a seasonal change. Many species that live in areas where there is a rainy season, like the monsoons in Southeast Asia and India, time their reproductive cycle with the rainfall.

It is not common for a snake to reproduce more than once in a single year due to the lengthy gestation periods and having to gain back a large amount of fat deposits. The entire reproductive process starting with follicle maturation and ending with the snake back at full weight could take several months to over a year depending on species.

Maternal Care

Very few snakes show any maternal care. Some pythons will coil around the eggs incubating them and protecting them from predators. Some viviparous species will show maternal care by helping the newborns out of the amniotic sac and consuming the infertile yolk sac.

EGG INCUBATION AND MANAGEMENT

Artificial Incubation

It is recommended that eggs only be artificially incubated only by experienced herpetoculturists. Many herpetoculturists artificially incubate eggs to increase the chance of hatching. In captivity, it is difficult for the female snake to keep the relative humidity high enough to incubate her own eggs. If the decision is made to artificially incubate the eggs, the herpetoculturists must be prepared several days before the female lays the eggs. It is recommended that the incubator be ready several days in advance. The incubator should maintain a constant temperature and humidity that is ideal for the species being incubated. For most species, a temperature range of 86°F to 91°F is ideal. Eggs do not benefit from temperature variations so a constant temperature should be maintained. It is not critical to measure the relative humidity although a high relative humidity should be maintained. As long as condensation appears on the sides of the incubator, the humidity should be high enough.

When the female lays the eggs, the herpetoculturists should move quickly to remove them. Within a few hours after oviposition, the eggs will become adherent. It is preferable that the eggs be laid singly in the incubator so they can be properly monitored. Also, the conditions inside the enclosure may be inadequate for proper incubation, which can be detrimental to the eggs. Eggs can dehydrate within 48–72 hours. Gently remove the eggs and place them in the preheated incubator. The incubator should be checked several times a day for proper temperature and humidity and the eggs should be checked for viability.

Maternal Incubation

There are several reasons why maternal incubation should be performed. The eggs should be maternally incubated if the female is too large or aggressive to safely remove the eggs, if the female unexpectedly laid eggs and an incubator was not ready, or if normal incubation parameters are not known. The humidity in the cage should not fall below 75%. Because of the high humidity that must be maintained, the cage should be kept in a very clean environment with adequate circulation. The temperature in the cage should be constant. The incubating female should not have to thermoregulate. Thermoregulation requires an excessive amount of energy that many incubating females do not have. The cage should be kept at 88°F for most species of python. If maternal incubation was chosen due to the lack of experience of artificial incubation, extensive research on the natural history of the species should be done to determine the proper incubating temperature.

Incubator Design

Incubators can be commercially bought or one can easily be made. The basic requirements of an incubator are: the construction should prevent excessive heat and humidity loss, there must be a constant and reliable heat source, and there must be a thermostat to control the temperature. The actual design of the incubator can vary as long as the above three rules have been met. When constructing an incubator, some general guidelines should be followed. The incubator should be uniformly heated. An easy way to accomplish this is by using heat tape that can be evenly positioned on the bottom of the incubator. Hot water can also be used. An inner container should be installed that is not resting on the bottom of the incubator. This will allow the heat to be evenly distributed throughout the entire incubator. The thermostat should be sensitive enough to control the temperature fluctuation within one degree. The temperature should be monitored from the outside of the incubator. To ensure adequate humidity, spray the incubator and eggs with water every two to three days. The water should be the same temperature as the incubator. The incubator should be lined with Styrofoam to maintain a proper temperature. The best substrates to use are vermiculite, sphagnum moss, potting soil, sand, shredded newspaper, pea gravel, and paper towels.

Determining Egg Viability

A viable clutch should be uniform in size, have a brilliant white color, and be pliable or elastic (Ross et al. 1990, 103). If an egg is smaller, discolored, or hard or rubbery, it usually is not fertilized. Some female snakes will reject an unfertilized egg from the clutch. If an egg does not adhere to the rest of the clutch, it should still be incubated until signs of egg death appear. Wrinkles or depressions at the time of oviposition are not signs of nonviability. A fertilized egg will not show significant change during the incubation period. An unfertilized egg will quickly begin to show signs of decomposition.

It can sometimes be very difficult to determine the viability of an egg. If the viability is uncertain, the egg should be incubated until further signs appear. The rest of the clutch will not be in danger. The texture of an egg or irregular calcification should not be used as an indication of nonviability. Another method for determining egg viability is a technique called candling. This technique involves the use of a high intensity light to transilluminate the egg. A viable egg should have a network of blood vessels and an embryo during the late stages of incubation. The absence of blood vessels indicates a nonviable egg.

Manual Pipping

Sometimes manual pipping is necessary for the embryo to live. An egg should be manually pipped only if most eggs in the clutch have hatched, no eggs have pipped by the estimated due date, or the due date is unknown. Manual pipping is a very delicate procedure that with time and practice can be a very effective method of saving a clutch. All that is needed to perform this technique is a pair of iris scissors and thumb forceps. Using the iris scissors, a small perforation is made in the shell. With the scissors pointing up toward the inner surface of the eggshell, a small incision is then made in the shell. At the site of the puncture, another small incision is made. This should make a "V" shaped incision. The wedge can be elevated using the thumb forceps and removed. If done properly, the shell membranes should all still be intact. During this process, one should avoid cutting large blood vessels—small vessels are impossible to avoid. The embryo should not be visible. With the thumb forceps, the shell membranes should be gently separated from the shell. One should start at the window that was made and begin working outward. More pieces of shell can be removed as the membrane is separated. When a large enough window has been made, the embryo can then be stimulated. To stimulate the embryo, prod it gently with a blunt tip instrument. If it is alive, the embryo will move freely in the egg. The embryo should be intermittently stimulated until the neonate has emerged from the shell. This process usually takes 12 to 24 hours.

HOUSING

When obtaining housing for a snake, a couple of things must be taken into consideration: (1) the size (length) of the snake to be housed, (2) whether it is a terrestrial or an arboreal species, (3) will it be secure (escape proof), (4) does it have proper ventilation, (5)and does it allow for necessary cleaning/disinfecting.

Aquariums are certainly suitable and aesthetically pleasing enclosures for most species of snakes, but can be quite costly to obtain, especially when housing some of the larger species. Ideally the length of the enclosure should be *no* less than half of the length of the snake being housed. When housing arboreal species (i.e., green tree python), the enclosure should have more vertical space than horizontal to allow for placement of perches for the snake. If an aquarium is used, one needs to make sure that a lid can be secured on the tank appropriately. Lids that rest on top of the aquarium without any locking mechanisms are NOT appropriate for snakes as they are escape artists!! Also, if using an aquarium, the lid should allow prop-

er ventilation (i.e., screen lids) if the aquarium itself does not have any ventilation holes (which most do not). One should make sure to choose a lid that does not present a potential fire hazard if using heat lamps above it. Plastic lids will melt (fig. 4.5).

Any aquariums with cracks should be avoided due to the potential for the glass to shatter resulting in injury to the animal. In short, aquariums can make wonderful enclosures and can be easily disinfected if the cost of obtaining an aquarium is not an issue.

Building an enclosure for a snake is usually the preferred method of acquiring housing. It is less expensive in most cases and allows for customizing according to the snake's needs. If one has the time and know-how, this is usually the best way to ensure the snake being housed has adequate room and the caging can be built using secure locking mechanisms. It can be enjoyable customizing an enclosure as long as a couple of guidelines are followed. Obviously, it would not be ideal to construct a cage solely of wood without any way to view the snake. Glass or Plexiglas should be included when constructing a wooden enclosure. Screen can be used on the sides or even the top of the enclosure to ensure proper ventilation. Without proper ventilation, bacteria can accumulate and it will become stagnant inside the enclosure. Having screen incorporated into the top of the enclosure will allow for proper lighting/heat fixtures to be affixed on top of the cage to allow lighting in but not allow the snake to come into contact with it. Heat lamps should not be placed inside the enclosure where the snake can come into contact with them due to the potential to sustain burns. An enclosure should not be constructed solely of screen, however, as it can become too drafty. The wood used should be sanded and free of abrasive sur-

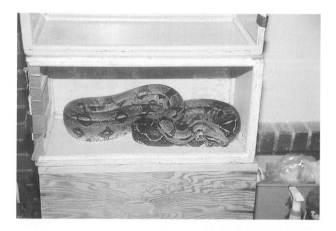

Fig. 4.5. Inappropriate housing for a snake. (Photo courtesy of Ryan Cheek)

faces to prevent potential injuries to the snake. Wood that is used also needs to be treated/painted to allow regular cleaning without damaging the wood. Sealing/painting will also be necessary for cleaning purposes because of the possibility that feces and such may soak into the porous wood. Priming and painting the inside of the enclosure white can assist you in spotting problems such as mites in the caging. The white paint reflects the lighting better as well.

Depending on what is preferred to access the inside of the cage, different locking mechanisms can be chosen. Everything from hinged doors with padlocks to sliding glass doors are suitable for securing the custom enclosure.

There are commercially available enclosures specifically made for keeping reptiles, such as Neodesha and Visions cages. These are perfectly suitable for housing snakes if one does not mind the added expense and as long as an appropriately sized enclosure can be obtained.

Substrate

There are many different types of substrate that are used in snake enclosures (fig. 4.6). There also is a lot of debate on what is appropriate and what can be harmful. It is necessary to read as much literature about the snake as possible to obtain more information about its natural habitat to better assist in making husbandry-related choices.

Below is a brief summary of commonly used substrate items and whether they are appropriate to use.

Cedar/pine shavings are not recommended as substrate for any reptiles. The oils and natural aroma of these shavings can be toxic to snakes and can even lead to respiratory disorders. Although some companies claim that they are great for snakes because they "repel mites and ticks," using any cedar or pine shavings should be avoided. Shavings can also lodge in the snake's oral cavity, which could cause stomatitis (mouth rot).

Aspen shavings can be used for some of the snake species requiring an arid climate. Aspen shavings should not be used for snakes requiring high humidity. There are more suitable substrates for maintaining high humidity. One should make sure the aspen shavings have been treated through a "baking" process, which can help to eliminate any potential for parasites contained in the shavings and to ensure the shavings are free of toxic oils. Aspen shavings can also become lodged in the snake's mouth so as a precaution, the snake should not be fed on aspen shavings.

Indoor/outdoor carpet or Astroturf is commonly used as substrate. It is aesthetically pleasing and does not present any immediate harm to the snake. It can be purchased by the yard at most local hardware stores. Routine cleaning and disinfecting will be more demanding than with other substrates because the carpet costs more and needs to be replaced frequently. When a snake defecates or passes urates, the carpet will absorb some of the matter and will need to be washed or replaced all together. Otherwise the carpet will become pungent and allow bacterial and/or mold growth. Animals with parasite infections should have the carpet changed completely to avoid recontamination.

Aquarium gravel and corncob should *not* be used. Some gravel can be abrasive and they can both cause impactions if ingested in large amounts.

Sand is used often for desert species. There are many contradicting statements regarding the use of sand in any reptile enclosure. However, it is the "natural" substrate of many desert species. There is debate as to whether it causes digestive problems and obstructions.

Any loose substrate ingested in large amounts could potentially cause these problems as well as stomatitis. To reduce the chance of this happening, the snake should not be fed in the enclosure. Some people feed their snakes in plastic tubs or boxes to eliminate the opportunity to ingest substrate while feeding. While some people buy play sand at the hardware store to use, others buy the sand sold at pet stores for reptile substrate. Some of the commercial brands of sand used as substrate for reptiles claim that if ingested the sand is less likely to cause impactions than regular play sand due to its calcium contents and fine grain. However, caution should still be used when feeding any reptile on a sand substrate. Also, large amounts of calcium consumption can be just as harmful as calcium deficiencies. Personal preference determines which one to get if sand is the substrate of choice. One needs to make sure it is not being ingested, or change the type of substrate used.

Cypress mulch is another good substrate especially for species requiring higher humidity. It can make an enclosure look very natural and it is relatively inexpensive. One needs to make sure that it is cypress mulch and not another type of mulch (i.e., eucalyptus) because these can be very aromatic and lead to respiratory problems. The mulch can be mixed with sphagnum moss if the goal is to make a natural appearing environment.

Newspaper is frequently used as substrate, especially when an individual keeps multiple snakes. Newspaper is plentiful, inexpensive, and easily obtained. It is absorbent and easily replaced when

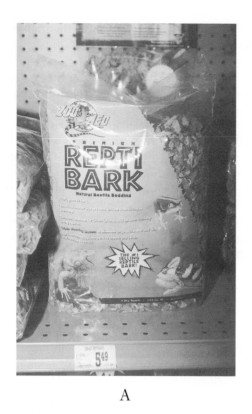

A

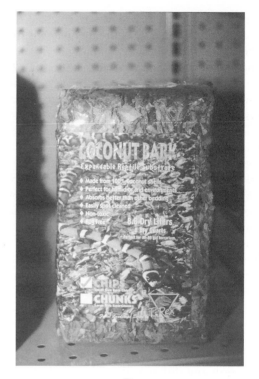

B

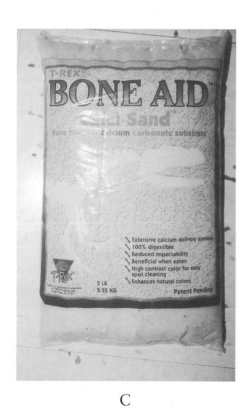

C

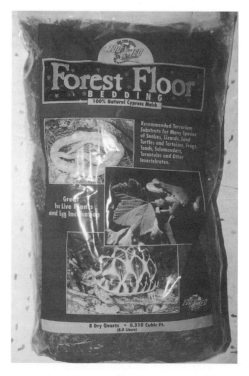

D

Fig. 4.6. *Various common commercially available substrates.* **A.** *Repti Bark (fir bark).* **B.** *Ground coconut shell.* **C.** *Calcium carbonate granules.* **D.** *Cypress mulch. (Photos courtesy of Ryan Cheek)*

doing routine cleanings. It is especially good to use for animals in quarantine and the substrate best suited for feeding as the chances of it being ingested are not as great as "loose" substrate. Although not as aesthetically pleasing as some forms of substrate, it is definitely easier to maintain.

Potting soil should be used with caution. Most potting soils have fertilizers and other chemicals that could be toxic to snakes. If top soil is used, one should make sure that it is organic and free of chemicals. Otherwise, top soil can be a good substrate to use for snakes requiring high humidity because of its ability to retain moisture. This can be used for terrestrial and burrowing species.

Caution should be used if any tree limbs, substrate, or any other objects are collected from outside. They can contaminate the enclosure with parasites, molds/fungus, and so on. Sterilization can be attempted with these objects via boiling/baking or disinfecting with a diluted bleach solution to minimize contamination. Tree limbs taken from outside should not have any "sticky" substances such as sap on them.

Good judgment must be used when choosing an appropriate substrate. Knowing the geographic range of the particular snake housed will aid in making husbandry decisions.

Heating and Lighting

Snakes are ectothermic, meaning they rely on their surroundings to regulate their body temperature. Unlike mammals, they are unable to do this on their own. Because of this, snakes kept in captivity require heating/lighting supplementation (see table 4.2). Failure to maintain appropriate temperatures for the particular snake can lead to respiratory disorders, food regurgitation, anorexia due to lethargy, and even death.

There are many species of snakes kept in captivity today and sold commercially. Whether the snake is a desert-dwelling or tropical snake, it is necessary to maintain an enclosure that mimics its natural surroundings and climate zone. Ideally, snakes need a warm basking area to maintain good health and also a cooler area to retreat to in case they get too warm. To ensure that necessary temperatures are being met, thermometers must be purchased. These can be bought at most pet stores and have adhesives so they can be easily placed into the enclosure. Ideally, one thermometer should be affixed in the enclosure where the hottest temperature is achieved and one should also be affixed in the "cool zone." If the snake is a terrestrial species, the thermometer should be placed close to the bottom. With arboreal species, the thermometers should be placed near the areas where the snake can perch (fig. 4.7).

Heat rocks are sold commercially for reptiles as an artificial heat source. These are not reliable heat sources and can in fact can injure the snake. The heating element is not on a thermostat and can get extremely hot. If the snake is allowed direct contact with the rock, the snake can sustain serious burns. Other times the rock can be cool to the touch providing no supplemental heat at all. Heat rocks are not recommended by the author, however, if used they should be buried under the substrate so the snake does not have direct contact with them. If heat rocks are used, they should not be the only source of heat provided.

Heating tape/pads/under tank heaters are good sources of heat for snakes. These products are also sold commercially in the pet trade and if used correctly, are safer than heat rocks. The pads and tape can be placed on the outside of the enclosure underneath the tank where the snake can not have direct contact with the units but still benefit from the heat being emitted. These heating mechanisms distribute the heat more evenly and in some cases cover the entire length of the enclosure. If a heating pad is used that has a temperature setting control, the setting should be kept on low. If the enclosure is made of thick wood or if there is a thick layer of substrate, one can place the pad on medium if the low setting is not producing enough heat to benefit the snake. The bottom of the enclosure should always be tested (via touch or thermometers) thoroughly to ensure it does not get too hot. A high setting should never be used. One should not trust that the snake will move if the heating element gets too hot. Thermal burns are easily prevented if caution is used and regular checks are performed on the heating elements.

Heat lamps are acceptable primary heat sources and also provide the snake with necessary day and night cycles if actual lights are used. These can be used in conjunction with under the tank heaters for snakes requiring high temperatures. Clamp light fixtures are relatively inexpensive and can be purchased from a local hardware store (fig. 4.8). These can be placed on top of the enclosure (on a screen, not plastic or flammable material) or clamped to a surface allowing the light to be directed into the enclosure. Bulbs should be selected based on the snake's temperature needs and the design of the enclosure itself. Incandescent bulbs, ceramic heat emitters, or flood lamps can be used for heating purposes. It depends on the dimensions of the enclosure and the snake's temperature needs as to what wattage bulb should be used. In most cases, a 50–75 watt bulb is sufficient. Extremely high wattage bulbs or bulbs used for food warming purposes should not be used as these get extremely hot. The heat-emitting bulbs should be of sufficient distance from the

Table 4.2. Husbandry Data for Selected Species of Snakes

Common name	Scientific name	Average length*	Ambient temperature in Fahrenheit (day)**	Humidity	Geographic range
Boas					
Common boa	*Boa constrictor*	~6'–10'	80–85	50–70%	Central America and South America
Brazilian rainbow boa	*Epicrates cenchria cenchria*	5'–7'	80–85	75–90%	Brazil
Emerald tree boa	*Corallus caninus*	4'–6'	75–82	85–90%	Amazon Basin
Rosy boa	*Lichanura trivirgata*	2'–3'	80–85	20–30%	Southern CA, AZ, Mexico
Pythons					
Ball python	*Python requis*	3'–5'	80–85	60–65%	Central Africa, Western Africa, Borneo
Blood python	*Python curtus*	3'–6'	80–85	70–75%	Borneo Islands, Malaysia, Sumatra
Burmese python	*Python molurus bivittatus*	12'–20'	80 –85	70–80%	S.E. Asia
Green tree python	*Morelia chondropython viridis*	4'–6'	75–85	85–90%	Australia, New Guinea
Carpet python	*Morelia spilota*	6'–10'	80–85	60–70%	Australia
Reticulated python	*Python reticulatus*	10'–25'	80–85	65–70%	Thailand, Indonesia, Philippines (S.E. Asia)
African rock python	*Python sebae*	12'–20'	80–85	65–70%	Africa
Colubrids					
Common king snakes	*Lampropeltis getula*	4'–5'	75–85	30–50%	North & South America
Corn snakes	*Elaphe guttata*	4'–5'	75–85	50–60%	Easter United States, Midwest United States
Rat snake	*Elaphe obsoleta*	5'–7'	75–85	50–60%	North America
Milk snake	*Lampropeltis triangulum*	2'–5'	75–85	50–60%	North & South America
Gopher/Bull/Pinesnake	*Pituophis* spp.	4'–7'	75–85	30–50%	United States & Mexico
Garter/Ribbon snakes	*Thamnophis* spp.	2'–4'	75–80	60–75%	United States

*Lengths refer to average adult lengths (in feet) not absolute min./ max. lengths.

**Temperatures given are average ambient temperatures; basking spots should be 5–10°F higher with a night time drop of 5–10°F.

snake that burns do not occur. The snake should not have direct access to the bulbs. Burns can be sustained from *any* heat source including bulbs if the snake is allowed direct access to them or if they are not placed at a safe distance from the snake being housed.

By placing the lamp on one end of the enclosure, the snake is allowed a good basking area. One end of

the enclosure should be free of any heat sources to provide a cooler zone to retreat to (fig. 4.9).

When using lights as heat sources, they should not be kept on all the time. Timers can be purchased that will control what times the light comes on and off. This will assist in maintaining natural photoperiods or day/night cycles. Ideally, the snake should have

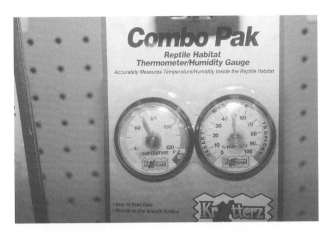

Fig. 4.7. Thermometer and hygrometer. (Photo courtesy of Ryan Cheek)

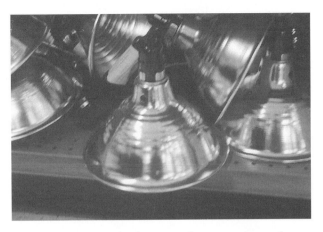

Fig. 4.8. Clamp light fixture. (Photo courtesy of Ryan Cheek)

around 12–13 hours a day of "daylight" followed by 11–12 hours of darkness to mimic "nighttime." The timers can be set to mimic the different seasonal day/night cycles by synchronizing them with the different day/night cycles that change slightly from season to season. For example, in the summer there are longer daylight hours than in winter. Therefore, daylight should be provided for approximately 13 hours where as in winter 11 hours of daylight is typical. The photoperiod in snakes is particularly important to follow if breeding the snake is considered. Some snakes are only receptive to breeding during certain seasons so these seasonal changes must be recreated in captivity for successful breeding activity. However, if bulbs are the only source of heat being used, it may be necessary to purchase "night bulbs" to ensure the snake does not get too cool during the night hours. A slight drop in temperature at night is a natural occurrence but too much can lead to illness. Night bulbs emit heat yet allow darkness. Red, blue, black light, ceramic bulbs or commercially available "night" bulbs can be purchased to achieve this. Reading the temperature gauges in the enclosure will assist you in making the appropriate decision on whether night bulbs will be necessary. Keeping the enclosure in a temperature-controlled room and away from drafty areas (i.e., windows) will aid in preventing drastic temperature changes at night when the heat lamps go off.

UV lighting or natural sunlight certainly could be beneficial to the snake, but if not provided, it is not detrimental to the snake's overall health as with diurnal lizards (fig. 4.10). It should be clear though that there is not any bulb available that can replace natural sunlight. During the warmer months, if it is decided to keep a snake outside, which is not recommended, special precautions need to be taken. Glass or

Plexiglas enclosures should *not* be used at all outside as they can get extremely hot with the direct sunlight and prove to be fatal to the snake. The inside of the enclosure can become hot much like in a car with the windows rolled up and no air flow. With other enclosures used outside there should always be a shaded area provided for the animal. They must be able to retreat to an area that is not receiving direct sunlight when they are finished basking. They will become overheated if this is not done.

It is beneficial to wire the heating device (bulbs or pads) to a thermostat. This can assist in more accurately maintaining temperatures and decrease the chance of thermal burns. This is not to say that thermostats are always accurate or 100% dependable but it certainly helps. Frequent temperature checks should be performed when synchronizing thermostats.

Water and Humidity

Depending on the geographic range the snake derives from, it may be necessary to supplement humidity as well as heat. Tropical species (i.e., emerald tree boas) need relatively high humidity and require some form of supplementation. In some cases, it may be necessary to make husbandry choices to prevent high humidity as with desert species requiring arid environments.

Hygrometers (humidity gauges) can be purchased with thermometers and placed inside the enclosure to provide humidity readings. This will provide information as to when humidity needs to be increased or decreased so any changes necessary can be made for ideal conditions.

High humidity can be maintained by misting the entire enclosure and even the snake. The mist should be fine and not extremely cold or hot water. It may be necessary to mist multiple times a day for tropical

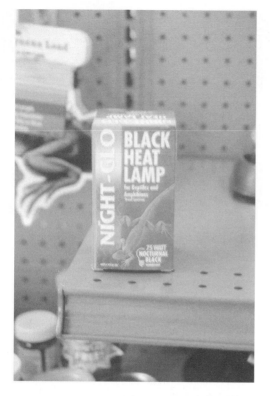

A

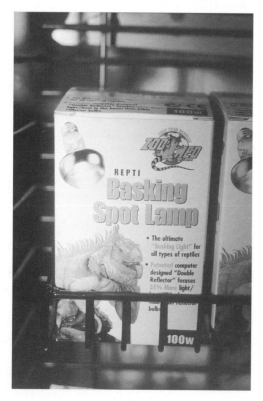

B

C

Fig. 4.9. *Various commercially incandescent heat lamps.* **A.** *Night light.* **B.** *Basking day light.* **C.** *Incandescent heat light. (Photos courtesy of Ryan Cheek)*

species. Some people even set up misting systems on timers to provide constant and consistent humidity (see fig. 4.7).

One should remember that humidity is the presence of moisture in the atmosphere itself. If the enclosure does not allow humidity to stay contained, than it needs to be modified or a different enclosure should be used. Using enclosures made of screen exclusively for snakes requiring high humidity is not ideal due to the inability to keep moisture within the enclosure. The moisture will escape. Aquariums are good for maintaining humidity however an appropriate lid needs to be made or purchased. One should ensure that it does have some sort of ventilation however because the air and substrate can become stagnant. Typically, if water is added to supplement humidity (via misting, etc.), it should be evaporated at least within 24 hours. If it does not evaporate, then the enclosure is lacking appropriate ventilation. It may take some trial and

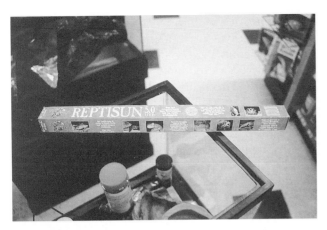

Fig. 4.10. UV lightbulb. (Photo courtesy of Ryan Cheek)

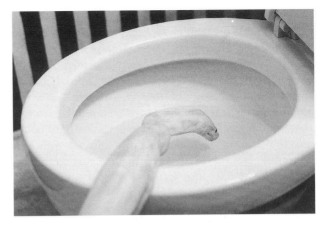

Fig. 4.11. This is not an appropriate method of providing water to a snake. (Photo courtesy of Stacy Bailey)

error to get the humidity right. If one is obtaining tropical species requiring humid environments, appropriate methods should be established before placing the snake in the enclosure. However, most species may not require any supplementation if appropriate enclosures and substrates are used.

A water supply is essential for all snakes and can assist in maintaining humidity as well. All snakes need an appropriately sized water container in the enclosure. Some enjoy soaking in the water prior to shedding, so the snake's size should be taken under consideration when choosing an appropriate bowl. Small ceramic bowls work well for smaller snakes (they can not be tipped as easily as light-weight bowls) and plastic tubs work well for larger snakes. One needs to be careful not to overfill as the snake can cause large amounts of water to spill over when submerging. The water should be changed if it becomes soiled or stagnant. It should be changed no less than once a week otherwise. If the water container is placed over the heating element (heating pad or tape) it will create some humidity and will evaporate quickly so the water levels should be watched closely. If the species requires low humidity, obviously the water should not be placed near the heating elements (fig. 4.11).

Substrate can play a vital role in maintaining high humidity. Substrate materials such as topsoil, moss (sphagnum or peat), and mulch are great substrate choices for species requiring high humidity. They absorb and hold moisture well unless too much water is added. Regular mistings in conjunction with appropriate substrate are keys in maintaining high humidity. Items such as newspaper, shavings, or rock gravel allow "pooling" and are not ideal for humid terrestrial environments.

Other Cage Furnishings

Hide boxes are easily constructed structures and really make a difference in the snake's overall demeanor. If the snake has a place to go where it feels secure, it will be less stressed in its captive environment. This has also been known to assist in the feeding response in some snakes (i.e., ball python). Hide boxes can be constructed out of everything from boxes, plastic pots, Tupperware (not clear), or logs. They also may be purchased from reptile supply stores/dealers. No matter how elaborate or simple they are, hide boxes serve the same purpose and should be provided.

Tree branches or some sort of perching material should be provided with arboreal species. PVC pipe can be used for this purpose as well. The perch should not be any bigger in diameter than the largest part of the snake's body. Any bigger than this will make perching difficult. One needs to make sure all perching materials are secured properly and free of abrasive surfaces.

Decorative rocks are nice additions to an enclosure but can also injure the snake if there are sharp edges. Snakes often use cage furnishings to assist them when shedding by rubbing against them. Anything with rough texture should not be placed in the enclosure.

QUARANTINE

All reptiles brought into a home or facility should undergo a quarantine period. This is especially necessary in environments where numerous reptiles are housed. There are some diseases in reptiles that can wipe out whole collections if proper quarantine procedures are not used (i.e., inclusive body disease).

A room should be set aside for quarantine purposes and should be absent of other animals especially other reptiles. During the quarantine period, physical exams and fecal exams should be performed to check for internal/external parasites. Ideally, a fecal culture for *Salmonella* should be performed as well. *Salmonella* is transmissible to other reptiles and is zoonotic as well. The quarantine period should be no less than 30 days. Some facilities have a 6-month quarantine period for all reptiles. The quarantine period should be extended if the snake becomes ill and continue until the snake is healthy.

Proper cleaning and disinfecting is very important during this time. The enclosures should be set up to meet the snake's individual requirements but also should allow for frequent cleaning. Newspaper is a good substrate to use for quarantined animals due to the ease of cleaning. It is easily changed and is cheap to replace. When the snake defecates or passes urates, the substrate should be changed completely. A dilute bleach solution (½ cup bleach to 1 gallon of water) should be used to clean surfaces in the enclosure. One needs to make sure it is dry before placing the snake back in the enclosure. Gloves should be worn when cleaning soiled cages to prevent contamination. Any cage furnishings should be properly disinfected or replaced.

NUTRITION

All snakes are carnivores that feed on whole prey items. Their digestive system is made to digest whole prey and they "cast out" or defecate the parts of the prey that are not digested such as fur. Eating whole carcasses provides them with added nutrients such as calcium from bone so that no further supplementation is needed. Feeding packaged meat and poultry products is not an appropriate, balanced diet for snakes. Feeding in this manner may be convenient for some, but it is not as nutritionally beneficial as whole prey items are. It should be remembered that just because a snake eats something readily does not mean it is nutritionally sound. It is the responsibility of the person who cares for the captive snake to make sure its nutritional needs are properly met.

Although some commonly kept species feed on invertebrates, most will readily feed using commercially bred mice and rats. What to feed the snake depends on multiple factors: (1) availability of prey item, (2) natural diet, (3) whether the snake was captive-bred or wild-caught, and (4) size of the snake.

Prey Items

With the increase in popularity of keeping snakes in captivity, there is a larger and more diverse market for buying varieties of food items. At one point, the most accessible food items involved buying "pet rodents" at pet stores. Not only was this costly, but the pet rodent's nutritional needs were probably not as closely monitored as they are when sold as food items. It is essential that any prey item is fed a nutritionally sound diet. Prey items that were starved, fed inappropriately, or otherwise neglected are going to be of little nutritional benefit to the snake that eats them. Just going through the motions of feeding the snake does not ensure nutritional requirements are being met. Remember, "you are what you eat."

Today, there are many companies that breed insects and rodents specifically for food items. Every growth stage of rats and mice can be purchased from these companies. Commercially available snake food includes various stages of mice, rats, gerbils, rabbits, guinea pigs, chickens (and other birds such as guinea chicks). For smaller snakes (i.e., garter and ribbon snakes) that feed primarily on invertebrates, there are crickets, various worms, and even small fish available for feeding purposes. In some cases, other reptile and/or amphibian species, such as anoles or frogs, may be used to encourage finicky eaters to feed in captivity. However, most of the commonly kept species will feed on rodents. Below are some of the terms used when specifying the stage of feeder rodent desired if standard adult size is not ideal:

Pinkies—baby mice, no fur present yet
Fuzzies—baby mice that have just gotten fur
Hoppers—juvenile mice that have fur and all adult characteristics but not as large as adult mice
Pups—usually unweaned/nursing baby rats
Weanlings— baby rats that are no longer nursing
Otherwise (for rats)—small, medium, large, or jumbo is used to obtain desired size.

Choosing an appropriately sized meal can be done by offering a prey item that is no larger than the biggest part of the snake's body. Some people try to gauge prey size by the size of the snake's head. This can be deceiving because the snake will dislocate its jaw for feeding; therefore it can feed on prey items that are much larger than that of its head. Gauging by the actual body itself will help to ensure the snake is being fed a large enough prey item and yet not one too big that could cause an uncomfortable, large bulging appearance.

Another benefit of commercial rodent breeders being accessible is the ability to purchase rodents prekilled and/or frozen. Some people find it disheartening and difficult to feed live rodents to snakes. In the wild, the snake will feed on live prey, but with the availability of prekilled prey on the market, there is no need for this in captivity. Captive-bred specimens will readily feed off prekilled or previously frozen prey items. Offering live prey to snakes causes unnecessary suffering to the rodent, and the snake can endure rodent bites as a result. Significant rodent bites can cause many dermatological problems; some even warrant systemic antibiotics and/or topical treatments of a dilute betadine or chlorhexidine solution. Scars from bite wounds are usually apparent in snakes that are offered live prey items. See color plate 4.1.

Offering previously frozen prey rather than live prey has many other benefits. It is usually cheaper to buy them in this fashion and they may be purchased in bulk rates if freezer space is available. Another benefit is that a frozen rodent will certainly be less likely to introduce parasites to the snake and/or enclosure. Rodents are one of the main sources of parasitic contamination in captive snakes. They can harbor mites, for instance. If a frozen prey item had parasites (endoparasite or ectoparasite), the parasites will most likely be dead due to the freezing process. This is not to say, however, that it is acceptable to knowingly offer parasite infested animals as food just because they were frozen. Buying snake food from a reputable company will assist in making sure the snake's nutritional needs are being met.

One should not attempt to feed a frozen rodent to the snake. It must first be thawed out. Putting it in a ziplock bag and submerging it in hot water is an easy way to do it. Some people even place the rodent on a warm surface (under a heat lamp, on a heat pad, etc.) to ensure the rodent is properly thawed. Microwaves are not an option for thawing rodents.

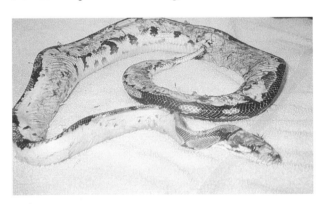

Plate 4.1. A snake suffering from trauma from a prey item. (Photo courtesy of Dr. Sam Rivera) (See also color plates)

Feedings only need to occur about once a week to every 14 days for adult snakes due to their slow digestive process. For juveniles, it may be necessary to feed twice a week to ensure that proper nutritional requirements are being met during the growth process. If a snake refuses one meal, do not panic. This occurs occasionally and the snake will not starve in one week's time. If several consecutive meals are skipped, then the snake's inappetence needs to be addressed.

Why Won't My Snake Eat?

Some people claim that their snake will not take previously frozen prey and will only accept live prey items. Some people have snakes that are reluctant eaters in general. Below are some feeding guidelines and tips to follow for all reluctant eaters.

Some snakes, such as Boidae and pit vipers, have heat-seeking pits that they rely on for locating their warm-blooded prey. Some people confuse these "pits" for "nostrils." These bilateral openings are located on the skin of the upper lip usually under the nares. If they confront a cold prey item (previously frozen), they are unlikely to show any interest. One should make sure that the prey item is warm before offering it to the snake, using the warming techniques described above.

Besides warmth, motion also can trigger a snake to feed. However, tongs should always be used when placing a prekilled rodent into the enclosure. This is especially true when one "entices" the snake by moving the prey item around. Many snakebites occur during feedings and can be easily avoided if using tongs (not hands) when feeding and keeping a safe distance from the snake.

If the snake was wild-caught and is not feeding in captivity, there are several things to check for. Wild-caught specimens are frequently reluctant to eat in captive environments. It should be remembered that they have been taken from their natural habitat and placed in a cage. Not only that but in most cases they are being offered prey they would have never encountered in their natural habitat. For example, a green tree python will feed primarily on birds, frogs, and occasional small mammals in its natural habitat. Once in captivity, it is offered white mice. This an unnatural prey item and small mammals are not a large part of the natural diet to begin with. This is not to say that it will never accept commercially bred rodents in captivity, but adjusting to a new captive environment is tough. One should at least try to offer a natural diet initially. One can try feeding colored rodents rather than the typical white feeder rodents, if the snake is reluctant to eat white rodents. Although more expensive than mice and rats, gerbils are another option to be used for prey. This sometimes helps with wild-caught snakes that are reluctant to eat because gerbils look more like a natural source of prey than white rodents. Wild-caught specimens will most likely be reluctant to take prekilled prey initially. They are accustomed to live prey items. So attempting to feed prekilled or frozen prey items to newly acquired wild-caught snakes will most likely be unsuccessful and will take time. Besides the moral issues with keeping wild-caught snakes, this is another reason why they should be avoided as purchases.

Some people attempt to speed up the process of getting a wild-caught snake to accept commercially bred rodents by "scenting" them. This does work occasionally. This is achieved by taking the rodent and rubbing a natural prey item on it to leave a scent. This works mostly for hobbyists that keep multiple species of reptiles and amphibians. For example, if trying to feed a mouse to a snake that will mostly feed on lizards and frogs naturally, a person can rub the feeder rodent on a lizard or frog that is kept in their collection. This will leave the scent of that animal on the rodent, and possibly "trick" the snake into eating it.

Another common reason a snake may refuse food is inadequate heat being provided. If a snake is cold, it will most likely refuse food. A snake needs to be warm to properly digest food. Regurgitation occurs frequently in snakes kept too cold. If it is cold then it will spend most of its time in a heat-preserving posture and will not be interested in feeding at all. One should make sure all heat requirements are being met when dealing with a reluctant eater.

As a rule, when a snake refuses prey, one needs to check to make sure all husbandry requirements are being met properly. Even something as simple as absence of a hide box (a secure place) will cause a snake to refuse prey.

If a snake is about to shed, it will most likely refuse food. Food items should not even be offered until the snake has fully shed to avoid excess stress.

Snakes that are ailing from respiratory disorders or other illnesses will most likely stop feeding as well. The onset of illness will affect their appetites just like any other animal. It is extremely important for the snake's owner to read as much literature as possible on the snake being kept. Once again, knowing the natural geographic range of the snake will help in making husbandry decisions, which may be the root of many problems. All too often, snakes are impulse buys and the buyer does not bother with reading up on the requirements and responsibilities involved with that particular snake.

DISEASES AND CLINICAL CONDITIONS

Diseases Affecting the Reproductive Tract

Cloacal prolapse is a common problem seen in snakes. The prolapse can be the colon, hemipenes, uterus, or oviduct. It is usually caused by excessive straining or during copulation. It is important to determine which organ has prolapsed before initiating treatment. The hemipenes are solid and do not have a lumen. The colon is smooth and has a lumen. Feces will normally be seen if it is the colon that prolapsed. The oviduct or shell gland will have longitudinal striations with a lumen. There will not be any feces present if it is the oviduct or shell gland.

Hemipenile prolapse, or paraphimosis, can be caused by several things. Infections from bacteria, fungus, or parasites, swelling secondary to forced probing, forced separation during copulation, constipation, or neurologic dysfunction in the hemipenes retractor apparatus, cloacal vent, or anal sphincter muscles can all cause hemipenile prolapse. Treatment should start as soon as the diagnosis is made. The prolapsed hemipenis should be cleaned, lubed, and replaced. If replacement is unsuccessful or the hemipenis is necrotic, the hemipenis should be amputated. Since snakes have two hemipenes, their reproductive ability will not be affected.

A *prolapsed colon* is caused by excessive straining, usually from constipation. The tissue must be moistened and replaced. Most colon prolapses can be replaced through the cloaca, but occasionally surgery is required. When the tissue is replaced it must also be inverted. If replaced properly a purse string suture is not required. Since this condition is not the primary problem, both conditions must be treated.

Oviductal or shell gland prolapses are most commonly seen during normal oviposition or parturition. They are treated much the same as a colon prolapse. The prolapsed tissue must be kept moist and replaced through the cloaca. If a large amount of the oviduct is prolapsed or if the tissue is necrotic, resection is recommended.

Dystocia is another common reproductive disorder. There are two types of dystocia in reptiles, obstructive and nonobstructive (Lock 2000, 734). An obstructive dystocia is caused by an anatomic inability to deliver the eggs or live young or by a complication during oviposition. The anatomic defect may be fetal or maternal. Some common maternal anatomic defects including misshapen pelvis, oviductal stricture, nonoviductal masses, oviduct scarring from previous infection, or retained eggs or fetuses from previous pregnancy. Fetal defects including an egg that is too large or eggs that have adhered. Diagnosis is made through a physical exam, history, and radiographs or ultrasound. Treatment includes the surgical removal of the eggs or fetuses.

Nonobstructive dystocias are mostly caused by poor husbandry, infection, or poor physical condition (Lock 2000, 735). Improper temperature, humidity, diet, and nesting site can all cause a dystocia. Oviposition requires great strength. Most captive-raised snakes do not have the muscle mass that wild snakes have, which makes it very difficult to deliver eggs or live young. Treatments include massaging the eggs down, percutaneous ovocentesis, posterior pituitary hormones, and, as a last resort, surgery. When massaging, care must be taken to not trap a portion of the oviduct posterior to the egg or live young. If this happens, one should massage the egg or embryo back to its original position and start over (Ross et al. 1990, 79). Percutaneous ovocentesis can be performed in oviparous snakes. A needle is inserted into the egg through the ventrum and the contents aspirated. It is important that the coelomic cavity is not contaminated with egg contents. The egg should pass within 48 hours naturally. Posterior pituitary hormones such as oxytocin can be used to assist with the oviposition. If all attempts have been made and the eggs or embryos are still retained, then surgery must be performed. Successful incubation of eggs after a dystocia is rare. Live fetuses have been raised after a salpingotomy, but it is not common. The prognosis for the female is good following a dystocia. The future reproductive status is also good as long as there were no complications and at least one of the reproductive tracts was left in tact. The female is more likely to retain eggs and live young again.

Disorders of the Integument

The most common disorder affecting the integument is dysecdysis, or difficulty in shedding. Causes of dysecdysis are numerous but are mostly associated with poor husbandry. Some common husbandry problems associated with dysecdysis are too high temperature, too low humidity, no shedding implement such as a rock or log, and malnutrition. Other causes of dysecdysis include systemic disorders, metabolic disorders, stress from excessive handling, loud noises, vibrations, and overcrowding, or anything that limits the snake's movements. Treatment includes soaking the snake in tepid water for 1 to 8 hours a day and treating the underlying problem.

Increased ecdysis frequencies can occur in snakes. Hyperthyroidism and dermatitis are the main causes of this condition. After a severe trauma, the natural function of healing is frequent ecdysis.

There are many clinical signs of dermatosis. Abscesses, abrasions, blisters, bullae, discoloration, and nodules are all signs of a diseased integument (Rossi 1996, 106). Abscesses are the most common dermatologic condition seen in captive reptiles. They are commonly caused by bites from prey or cage mates. Most abscesses are filled with a solid exudate. Treatment for abscesses include surgically removing the abscess and irrigating the area and using antibiotics pending a culture and sensitivity.

Bacterial dermatoses are also a very common condition. The most common bacterial infection is caused by *Pseudomonas* spp. Other common bacterial pathogens include *Salmonella* spp., staphylococcus, and streptococcus, as well as many other possible bacterial pathogens.

Fungal dermatoses are commonly seen in snakes that live in humid environments. The clinical signs are much the same as in bacterial infections. Clinical signs of both fungal and bacterial infections include a brown to greenish yellow discoloration, blisters, ulcers, nodules, crust, and granulomas.

Vesicular dermatitis, commonly known as blister disease, is common in snakes kept in dirty, very humid enclosures (Rossi 1996, 114). Fluid-filled blisters will appear all over the body. These blisters will get contaminated with bacteria and septicemia and death quickly follows without treatment.

Another bacterial infection caused by poor cage hygiene is ventral dermal necrosis (Lawton 1991, 254). Snakes kept in dirty enclosures can develop infections underneath their ventral scales. The signs include petechiation, echymosis, and eventual necrosis of the ventral scales. Fluid therapy is often needed due to the fluid loss from the damaged skin.

Contact dermatitis occurs when the snake is exposed to harsh chemicals such as pesticides, cleaners, and harsh aromatic compounds.

The diagnosis for all dermatosis includes a physical examination and history, culture (aerobic, anaerobic, and fungal), and cytology (Rossi 1996, 114). Treatment usually involves topical or systemic antimicrobials and husbandry and nutritional changes. During the treatment of any of these dermatoses the snake should be housed on clean paper. The paper should be changed daily and the cage should be disinfected daily as well until the condition has resolved.

Disorders of the Cardiovascular System

Cardiovascular disorders are not commonly seen in snakes. The clinical signs are nonspecific ranging from weight loss to a change in skin color. Nutritional disorders such as hypocalcemia, hypovitaminosis E, and hypercalcemia with hypervitaminosis D_3 have been associated with cardiovascular disease. Infectious diseases affecting the cardiovascular system are usually secondary to a systemic illness. There is potential for endocarditis with any gram-negative bacterial pathogen. If bacterial sepsis is suspected, a blood culture should be taken. There have been reported cases of congested heart failure associated with infectious disease and with cardiomyopathy diagnosed.

Conditions of the Nervous System

Spinal osteopathy has been observed in all species of snakes (Bennett 1996b, 145). The exact etiology is unknown. This condition has not been observed in wild populations. There are several possible causes to this disorder. It is suspected that a virus found in mice or a virus of snakes that is spread by mice may be a causative agent. Septicemia is suspected because bacteria are often cultured from the spinal lesions. An immune-mediated disease secondary to septicemia is also suspected. Finally, chronic trauma from excessive handling is thought to be a cause of this disease. Clinical signs include focal or multifocal swelling along the dorsum, pressure inducing a pain response, hyperflexic cranial to the lesion, motor deficits, trembling, and spinal deformities. The diagnosis is made via clinical signs and radiographs. In the early stages of this disease, the snake is still able to function on its own. As the disease progresses, the snake will no longer be able to move, constrict, or swallow prey. Treatment includes blood and local aspirate cultures, antibiotics, and surgical debridement.

Organophosphate and carbamate toxicity have been reported in snakes. Treatment is similar to that of mammals. The snakes should be given atropine and fluid therapy to maintain hydration and renal function. Its temperature should be decreased to slow conduction velocity of nerves to control seizures.

Conditions of the Respiratory Tract

The most common illnesses in snakes are respiratory infections. Respiratory infections can be caused by bacterial, viral, fungal, or parasitic pathogens (Driggers 2000, 524). Bacterial pneumonia is the most common cause of respiratory illness. Gram-negative pathogens are the most common. Viral infections are underdiagnosed due to the lack of diagnostic assays. Fungal infections are rare but have been reported. Common clinical signs of pneumonia include cyanosis, bubbles coming from the nares or glottis, wheezing or crackles heard during auscultation, and petechiae of the oral cavity. Stomatitis is commonly seen in snakes with pneumonia (Driggers 2000, 524). The diagnostic plan should include culture and sensitivity, cytology, and radiographs. A transtracheal wash should be performed to obtain samples for the culture and cytology. Antibiotics should be started and changed pending the results of the culture and sensitivity. Fluid therapy should be initiated with dehydrated snakes. The most common cause of pneumonia in snakes is husbandry related. It is crucial to keep the snake within its POTZ and keep proper humidity levels. Also, the cage needs to be kept clean at all times.

Other causes of respiratory disease include masses, trauma, aspiration of substrate, and dehydration. Dysecdysis can also compromise the respiratory tract causing disease (Driggers 2000, 528).

Disorders of the Urinary System

Unfortunately, early detection of renal dysfunction has not been observed in reptiles. Renal diseases are among the most common problems in older snakes.

Gout, not as common in snakes as it is in other families of reptiles, does occur. Gout is the result of excessive protein metabolism or catabolism. In this case uric acid production is greater than uric acid excretion. All diseases that lead to renal failure can cause gout (Miller 1998, 96). Gout is found in two forms. In the first form, urates are deposited on mesothelial surfaces. Urate deposits commonly occur on the pericardial sac, the peritoneum, the capsule of the liver, and within the parenchyma of the kidneys. In the other form of gout, urate deposits are made in joints, tendon sheaths, ligaments, and periosteum. Both forms of gout can occur simultaneously. Treatment for gout involves diuresis and diet change to a low-purine diet. The prognosis is poor.

Bacterial nephritis is a common disease associated with the urinary system. It is often secondary to other bacterial infections or an immunosuppressive event (Miller 1998, 98). The primary cause should be detected and treated accordingly.

Disorders of the Eye

Retained spectacles are a common reason snakes are brought into the veterinary clinic. Spectacles are retained when dysecdysis occurs. To remove the retained spectacle, place the snake in a very damp environment for 24 hours. After that time, wipe the eye with a gauze sponge or damp tissue. The retained spectacle usually will come off easily. If the retained spectacle does not come off easily, the snake should be kept in a warm damp environment until the next ecdysis cycle and proper ecdysis occurs.

Surgical intervention should be a last resort. This is a delicate procedure and should be done carefully so the eye is not damaged. Sterile lubricant should be applied to the eye and the spectacle gently removed with forceps. If the old spectacle is still attached firmly, force should not be used to remove it. It may take several days of soaking and/or applying lubricant to fully remove the retained spectacle or any retained piece of shed.

Intraspectacular dermatitis will occur as a localized dermatitis or as part of a more generalized dermatitis. The majority of these cases is caused by retained spectacles. Often, enucleation is the treatment.

Bullous spectaculopathy is caused by obstruction of the nasolacrimal duct (Williams 1996, 181). The obstruction is usually secondary to either infectious stomatitis or a congenital obstruction. The lacrimal fluid is not able to drain from the eye, which causes the distended subspectacular space. Long-term treatment involves surgically removing a 30° wedge of the ventral spectacle allowing for drainage.

Subspectacular abscesses are usually the result of an ascending infection in the oral cavity (Williams 1996, 181). Treatment for these abscesses involves a wedge resection of the spectacle and flushing. The debris should be cultured and the snake should be started on appropriate antibiotics.

Infectious Stomatitis

Infectious stomatitis is a disease that is caused by poor husbandry and nutrition, stress, poor feeding techniques, or trauma. It is crucial that the snake be kept in its POTZ and proper humidity be maintained. When proper husbandry is not met, the snake's immune system is weakened allowing for opportunistic bacteria to reproduce. Stress from being in overcrowded cages, excessive handling, or loud noises can also weaken the immune system. Snakes that are fed live prey will commonly have small abrasions in their oral cavity that can lead to an infectious stomatitis. Finally, snakes that rub on the sides of the cage will have rostral abrasions that lead to an infectious stomatitis. See color plate 4.2.

Vomiting and Regurgitation

Vomiting can occur for many reasons. Stress can make a snake vomit. If disturbed after a meal, a snake may get nervous and vomit its meal. Also, feeding a prey that is too large, feeding a prey that is partially autolyzed, and keeping the snake below its POTZ are all common causes of vomiting. Infectious diseases such as parasitic infections, inclusion body disease, and bacterial infections can also cause vomiting in snakes. Regurgitation is usually associated with lesions in the esophagus, oral cavity, or pharynx.

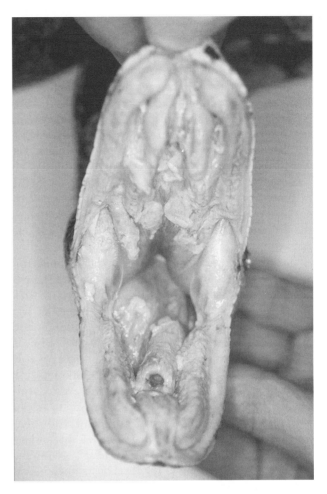

Plate 4.2. Stomatitis in a snake. (Photo courtesy of Dr. Stephen J. Hernandez-Divers, University of Georgia) (See also color plates)

Diagnosing Lumps and Bumps

Lumps and bumps are a common finding in snakes. These lumps and bumps occur on the outside as well as on the inside. When a lump or bump is found on the surface of the snake a fine needle aspirate should be performed. Cytology, culture, and sensitivity should be performed on the sample. If the lump or bump is palpated in the coelomic cavity, a radiograph or ultrasound should be performed to determine the origin. A sample should be obtained and cytology performed. Causes of lumps and bumps in snakes range from parasites to abscesses to neoplasia. Once the diagnosis is made, treatment should begin accordingly.

Viral Diseases

Paramoxyvirus is mainly found in viperids but has been isolated in most taxa of snakes (Schumacher 1996, 229). It is transmitted through secretions of the respiratory tract. Clinical signs are characterized by severe respiratory disease. Occasionally neurologic signs such as trembling are seen. A diagnosis of paramoxyvirus should be made when the pneumonia is unresponsive to antibiotics. A hemagglutination test has been developed and can be used to measure antibodies against ophidian paramoxyvirus. A diagnosis can also be made by histological examination of postmortem lung samples. There is no treatment for paramoxyvirus. Supportive care and antibiotics to treat secondary bacterial infections should be in the treatment plan. Prognosis is poor. If an outbreak of paramoxyvirus occurs in a collection, all sick snakes should immediately be quarantined and strict hygiene procedures must be followed.

Inclusion body disease (IBD) is another serious viral infection that is only found in boids (fig. 4.12). It is believed that this disease is caused by a retrovirus. Species of boa constrictors have been found to harbor species of retroviruses that do not cause disease (Marschang 2001, 37). The route of transmission is unknown. It is suspected that arthropods play a role in the transmission. In boas, the most common first clinical sign seen is regurgitation. In pythons, regurgitation is not seen. The disease slowly progresses to more neurologic signs such as head tremors, disorientation, and the loss of the righting reflex. Secondary bacterial infections are common. Eventually the snake will become anorectic and die. Pythons show clinical signs much more rapidly than boas. In boas, a diagnosis can be made by taking a sample of the liver and performing a histologic exam. There are no diagnostic tests for pythons. There are no treatments for retrovirus infections except for supportive care and treating secondary bacterial infections. The snake will eventually die from this virus. Prevention of this disease involves strict quarantine procedures when introducing new boids to a collection. If there are affected snakes in the collection, euthanasia is recommended to prevent more specimens from being infected with the virus.

Zoonotic Diseases

Snakes possess very few zoonotic diseases (Glynn 2001, 9; table 4.3). There are two ways in which zoonotic diseases are passed (Siemering 1986, 64). One, is by direct contact with the infected animal. The other is by indirect contact, which can be from contaminated feces, urine, secretions, blood, soil, fomites, and aerosols. Zoonotic diseases, for the most part, are easily avoided by following a few simple rules. One should not use the bathtub, sink, or shower as a place to soak a snake. One should not kiss a snake and

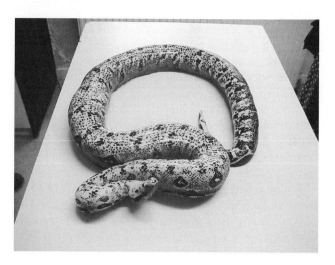

Fig. 4.12. *Inclusion body disease: note absence of righting reflex. (Photo courtesy of Dr. Stephen J. Hernandez-Divers, University of Georgia)*

hands should be washed after handling. A physician should be consulted if one is bitten by a snake and the area should be washed thoroughly. Finally, one should never clean any of the cage furnishings where human food is kept or prepared.

The most talked about zoonotic disease associated with reptiles is salmonellosis. It is believed that most reptiles carry *Salmonella* organisms in their intestinal tract and sporadically shed the organisms in their feces. An estimated 93,000 cases of reptile associated human salmonellosis is diagnosed each year (Glynn 2001, 9). All clients that either own a reptile or are considering owning a reptile for a pet should be educated about *salmonella*. By simply following the guidelines above, salmonellosis is easily preventable.

TAKING A HISTORY

Being able to take a complete history of a snake patient is the first crucial step in diagnosing and treating a sick snake. Such things as signalment, presenting complaint, husbandry and nutrition information, and any previous medical history are keys to proper diagnosis and treatment.

Signalment

Signalment includes the common and scientific names (ball python, *Python regius*), age, amount of time in owner's possession, whether it was captive-bred or wild-caught, and whether it is kept as a pet or as a breeder.

Table 4.3. Common Zoonotic Diseases in Reptiles

Pathogen	Threat to humans	Mode of transmission
Salmonella spp.	Gastrointestinal	Fecal oral contact
Campylobacter spp.	Diarrhea and acute gastroenteritis	Fecal oral contact
Klebsiella spp.	Diarrhea and genitourinary infections	Direct contact
Enterobacter spp.	Diarrhea and genitourinary infections	Direct contact
Yersinia enterocolitica	Gastroenteritis and severe abdominal pain	Environmental contact
Pseudomonas spp.	Cutaneous, respiratory, and digestive	Ingestion, inhalation, or scratches or bites
Mycobacterium spp.	Cutaneous and subcutaneous nodule	Fecal oral contact, inhalation of oral or respiratory mucosa, or bites or scratches
Coxiella burnetii	Q-fever	Inhalation or direct contact

It is important that the common and scientific names of the snake are acquired when the appointment is made. With approximately 2,400 extant species of snake, it would be impossible for a single person to know the natural history, husbandry, and nutritional needs of every species. Therefore, it is important that the medical staff be prepared ahead of time to ensure that the owner meets proper husbandry and nutritional needs. Many species of snake also have two or more common names, which can make identification very difficult. For example, most Americans refer to *Python regius* as a ball python, where as most Europeans refer to *Python regius* as the royal python. By knowing the scientific name of the snake, proper identification can be made, and therefore proper husbandry and nutritional needs can be met.

Another key component to signalment is the age of the snake. If the actual age of the snake is unknown, then the amount of time that the owners have had possession of it is important information. The average life span of captive snakes is very short. However, snakes are capable of living to a very geriatric age, with some species known to live more than 30 years. The reason for such short life spans is mostly associated with poor husbandry.

At this point, the origin of the snake should be noted. Wild-caught snakes are often imported in very substandard conditions and arrive at the pet store with a subclinical disease. Most commonly seen with imported specimens are internal and external parasites and respiratory infections. Captive-bred specimens, generally speaking, are much tamer, are disease and parasite free, and live longer than wild-caught specimens. It is also important to urge owners to buy captive-bred specimens due to the depletion of wild populations caused from the collection of wild animals for the pet trade.

It also needs to be noted if the snake is kept as a pet or as a breeder. Snakes kept solely as pets usually do not need to be hibernated, photoperiods do not need to change throughout the year, and nutritional needs usually do not change throughout the year. Snakes kept for breeding do have nutritional and husbandry changes throughout the year. Temperate species should be hibernated, which takes several weeks of preparation. If hibernation is not done properly, the snake can become very sick and possibly die while hibernating. With regard to nutrition, many female snakes will not eat while gravid. The females will normally start eating again when the clutch is laid, the clutch hatches, or the live babies are born. Special nutritional needs must be met before the breeding season starts and when she starts eating again. Also, to ensure a successful breeding season, the photoperiod must be changed to simulate the natural photoperiod.

All snakes that are large enough should be sexed. It is a very simple procedure that should be included in the initial exam.

Presenting Complaint

The presenting complaint is the reason the owner brought the snake to be examined. Some common presenting complaints include wheezing, dysecdysis, anorexia, and lethargy. One should approach the presenting complaint as if it were a dog or cat. The owner should be asked when the problem started, were there any husbandry/ nutritional changes, have the owners noticed any other problems, and so on. The medical staff is like a team of detectives that must gather as much evidence as possible to come up with a diagnosis and treatment plan. It is important to get as much information from the owners as possible.

Husbandry and Nutritional Information

The single leading cause of death in captive snakes is poor husbandry and/or nutrition. It is up to the veterinary technician to find out every detail of the husbandry practices and advise the owner if corrections need to be made. This part of the history will take 15 to 20 minutes. It is crucial to take time and record every detail. Following is a list of questions that should be asked at the initial exam:

- What is the day and night temperature range?
- What is the day/night cycle?
- What light sources are available?
- What are the primary and secondary heat sources available?
- What is the humidity in the enclosure?
- What humidity devices and methods are used?
- How big is the cage?
- Where is the cage located?
- What is the cage made of?
- Is the cage designed for an arboreal or terrestrial species?
- What substrate is used?
- How often is the cage cleaned and disinfected?
- What type of disinfectant is used?
- What cage furnishings are available (rocks, branches, hide box, etc.)?
- How is water offered (drip system, misting, bowl, etc.)?
- What food items are being offered and what time of day are they offered?
- Is the snake fed live, frozen thawed, or fresh-killed prey items?
- How is the prey offered (feeding tongs, set in the • bottom of the cage, in a separate cage, etc.)?
- What is the feeding schedule?
- How are the prey items stored?
- Where were the prey items acquired?
- What is the ecdysis/defecation schedule?
- Are there other reptiles or other animals in the same air system?
- Are any of these animals sick or have any died within the past 3 months?
- Is proper quarantine performed on new and sick specimens?

Previous Medical History

Any previous medical condition or diagnostic tests should be noted in the record. The owner's fecal check and deworming schedule should also be noted in the record.

PREPARING FOR THE PHYSICAL EXAM

The exam room must be prepared ahead of time to ensure a quick and complete physical exam. The exam room needs to be "snake proof." The doors must be sealed so the snake can not escape under the door, large drains in the sink should be covered, air vents should be covered with mesh to not allow the snake to craw in, and any other holes or cracks that the snake can get into should be covered or sealed to keep the snake from escaping or getting stuck. Appropriate-sized sex probes with lubrication for sexing and a spatula or credit card for oral examination should be in the exam room. Restraining devices such as snake hooks, clear plastic restraining tubes, and capture tongs should be readily accessible for aggressive or venomous species. Large snakes could need two or more people for proper restraint. It may be necessary to have other technicians or assistants close by in the event that more help is needed. Other essential instruments that are needed for a physical exam are a good light source, ophthalmic scope, stethoscope, fecal collection system, and a magnifying glass to check for external parasites.

RESTRAINT

As stated previously, snakes can be very unpredictable and should be treated as such to avoid being bitten. Even the most docile of snakes will bite if it feels threatened or cornered. One should watch for warning signs, such as hissing or an S-shaped striking posture before attempting to handle a snake (fig. 4.13).

Whether restraining or simply holding the snake it is important to do so properly. If not held properly, not only can one get bitten, but the snake can sustain injuries, too. The body should always be supported as much as possible. With larger snakes, it will take more than one person to hold and offer necessary support.

When manually restraining the snake, one should ensure that someone has control of the head. This should be the first part of the body restrained. The head should be held right at the base and without applying too much pressure around the neck area. This could obstruct the trachea causing a strangling effect and the snake could suffocate. In addition, the snake could panic making it very difficult to manage. The rest of the body can be held with a free hand or by assistants when handling large or aggressive snakes. Do not place a snake (especially large snakes and/or constrictors) around your neck. This is commonly done and can be dangerous. If the snake feels threatened and insecure it will begin to constrict around the neck.

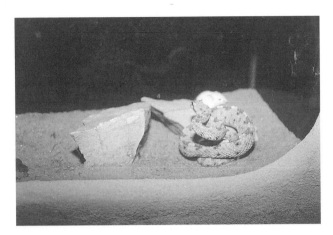

Fig. 4.13. A snake in a striking pose. (Photo courtesy of Ryan Cheek)

Different tools can be used to move snakes or assist in immobilization, including hooks, tubes, and tongs. They are discussed below.

Snake hooks allow a person to move a snake without having to touch the animal or having to get too close. This is advantageous when handling aggressive snakes. It can be used to get a snake out of an enclosure, as a guide, or as a pinning device. For example, to remove a snake from an enclosure, the hook is used to "hook" the snake one-third of the way down its body and then gently lift it. The hook can then be used to pin the head to take control of it but extreme caution must be used as any thrashing on the part of the snake can cause severe spinal cord injury. Only handlers experienced with the hook should use the pinning technique. If the snake is hooked too close to the head or tail, the snake will usually slide right off. It may be necessary to use more than one hook for larger snakes (fig. 4.14).

Snake hooks are also used when coercing a snake into a snake tube for physical exam or immobilization. Hooks can be purchased at most reptile supply shops (figs. 4.15 and 4.16).

Snake tubes are open-ended, clear, hard plastic or acrylic tubes that are used to hold a snake and view it safely during examination. The tube's diameter must be just large enough for the snake's head to fit into, but not allow the snake to turn around in. One end of the tube should be aimed toward the snake's head and a snake hook used to entice the snake into the tube. Once one-third to one-half of the snake's body is in the tube, the handler should grasp the snake and the base of the tube so it can not back out. A face mask can be placed on the other end of the tube to administer gas anesthesia and immobilize the snake com-

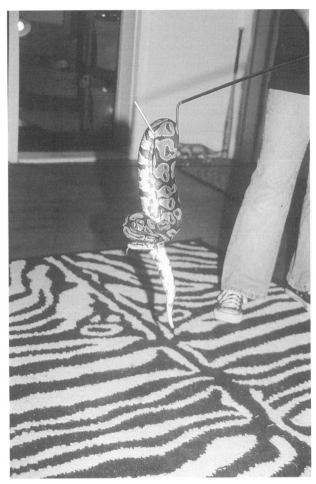

Fig. 4.14. Proper use of a snake hook. (Photo courtesy of Ryan Cheek)

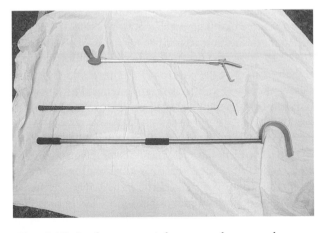

Fig. 4.15. Snake tongs at the top and two snake hooks below. (Photo courtesy of Ryan Cheek)

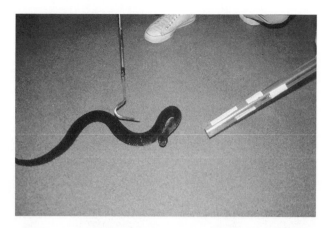

Fig. 4.16. *Using a hook to coax a snake into a plastic tube. (Photo courtesy of ZooAtlanta)*

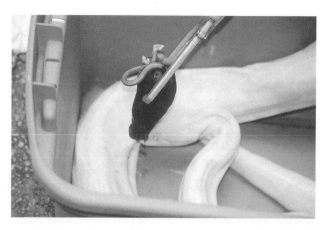

Fig. 4.17. *Feeding a python with tongs. (Photo courtesy of Ryan Cheek)*

pletely, if necessary. This is the safest way to manage aggressive snakes and venomous species. Most of these tubes are purchased from reptile supply stores or hardware stores (if appropriate materials are found) and come in various sizes.

Another method of capturing an aggressive snake is to place a clear shield over its head. Once the shield is in place, the handler can grasp right behind its head taking control of it.

Snake tongs can be used for many purposes. The most common use is for feeding (fig. 4.17). Offering food items via tongs is obviously safer than using one's hands to offer prey. Tongs allow the feeder to have distance from the snake and the prey item. Although some people use tongs to assist in restraining snakes, this method is not recommended. Grabbing the snake with tongs can apply too much pressure and, depending on what part of the body is grasped, the snake can be injured. Snakes can also easily free themselves from tongs if not grasped properly. Tongs can be used to assist in tubing the snake but not as a *primary* handling mechanism.

An undesirable method of restraint is to allow a snake to partially swallow prey. This will allow the handler time to take control of the head and the body before the snake can strike. However, often the snake will regurgitate the prey making this technique undesirable.

To avoid bites, some reptile hobbyists believe that snakes should not be fed inside their primary enclosure, especially when the only time the enclosure is opened is when the snake is being fed. This creates a feeding response and makes bites more likely to occur. Feeding outside the primary enclosure would be a safer practice and also could help to ensure that any loose substrate located inside the primary enclosure is not ingested during feeding.

THE PHYSICAL EXAM

After a very thorough history has been taken and the exam room is prepared, a complete physical exam should be performed. The physical exam should begin as soon as the owner brings the snake into the exam room. The snake should be observed as it moves around its environment. Body/muscle tone, proprioception, and mobility should also be observed. Any abnormalities should be noted. An accurate weight in grams or kilograms as well as the snout to vent length (SVL) should be measured to determine organ location and monitor growth in juvenile snakes. The cloacal temperature should be recorded to help determine the thermal environment in which the snake lives.

There are several approaches to performing a physical exam. Some clinicians prefer a head to tail evaluation while others have a specific order of body systems that are examined. It is important to do the same routine with every physical exam so nothing is left out or overlooked.

Integument
The skin should be checked for parasites, thermal burns, trauma, skin tenting or ridges to assess hydration, dysecdysis, and bacterial or fungal infections. If ecdysis is currently in process, the stage of ecdysis should be recorfded.

Respiratory System
The upper and lower airways should be auscultated for any crackles or increased respiratory sounds. It must be kept in mind that most snakes only have a right lung with the exception of the boids, which have a right lung and a small left lung. The nostrils should be clear of debris and any discharge. The glottis can

easily be observed for proper function and for any inflammation. When the glottis opens during respiration, one should look down the trachea for any swelling, mucous, or foreign material.

Cardiovascular System

Auscultation of the snake's heart can sometimes prove to be difficult. It is crucial that the exam room be silent. Using a damp cloth or gauze sponge can help enhance the heart sounds. The heart is generally around 25% down the body from the snout. A heart rate should be obtained during auscultation. Peripheral pulses should be assessed via the use of a Doppler flow detector. The Doppler can be placed on the ventral tail vein or just cranial to the heart at the base of the glottis.

Neurologic Examination

Neurologic exams are very simple to perform on snakes (Bennett 1996b, 142). The exam starts with the initial presentation of the snake. One needs to watch for any jerking motions, absent or slow righting reflex, or the inability to strike at prey. The site of a spinal cord injury can be found by using the righting reflex. Snakes will right themselves up to the point of the injury. A hypodermic needle may be used to stimulate the panniculus reflex. A neurologically normal snake's skin will twitch up to the point of spinal injury. A cranial nerve exam should be performed if a neurologic disorder is suspected. Following are methods to use to examine the 12 cranial nerves in snakes.

CN I—A snake with a properly functioning olfactory nerve will recoil from the smell of noxious odors. Alcohol can be placed in front of the snake's nose to see if it reacts to the smell.

CN II—Since reptiles have an iris that is composed of skeletal muscle, pupilary light reflex can not be used to determine the function of the optic nerve. Carefully watch the eye movements of the snake to assess the function of the optic nerve.

CN III, CN IV, CN VI—This group of cranial nerves is extremely hard to assess in snakes. They are responsible for eye movement coordination.

CN V—Snakes with a malfunctioning trigeminal nerve will have abnormal jaw function and a loss of feeling around its face. It will not be able to thermoregulate or find prey.

CN VIII—The acoustic nerve is difficult to assess. Snakes may show signs of nystagmus, head tilt, rolling, and abnormal righting reflex.

CN IX, CN XI, CN XII—Dysphagia and abnormal tongue movements can be seen in a snake if one or more of these cranial nerves is damaged or malfunctioning.

CN VII and CN X—The facial and vagus nerves are impossible to assess in snakes.

Palpations

The entire length of the snake should be palpated for any abnormalities such as enlarged organs, internal masses, lumps, and bumps. In breeding females, eggs and preovulatory follicles can be felt on palpation. Digital palpation of the cloaca can reveal several abnormalities and should be performed on all snakes that are large enough. An otoscope or endoscope can be used as well.

Ophthalmic Exam

As discussed in the anatomy section, snakes have a transparent spectacle that covers the cornea. The eyes should be clear and smooth. Any retained sheds can easily be seen and removed. Any other abnormalities should be further examined with an ophthalmic scope.

Fecal Exam

All snakes that come in for a physical exam should have a fecal examination performed. This exam should include a fecal floatation and two direct fecal smears, one prepared with a normal saline solution and the other prepared with a Lugol's iodine solution.

Oral Exam

Because most snakes become distressed during the oral exam, it is often best to perform the oral examination last. Gently open the mouth using a spatula or plastic card. Determining the proper mucosa color can be difficult. Most species have a pale mucosa color while others may have a more pink or bluish color. It is important to know the normal color for that species before the physical exam is performed. With all species the oral cavity should be moist without any stringy or tenacious mucus. The clinician should look for any caseous exudates, hemorrhage, and necrosis.

RADIOLOGY

Creating a Technique Chart

A separate technique chart should be made for snakes. A variable kVp or variable mAs technique chart can be made although a variable mAs technique chart is preferable. The technique chart should start at 2 cm and go to at least 20 cm. Describing the proper method of creating a technique chart is out of the scope of this text. There are numerous texts that describe in detail this process. It is an easy but time-consuming task that if performed correctly will save much time when a radiograph is needed.

Positioning

As with all other animals, two views should be taken, a lateral and dorsoventral (DV). Snakes should not be radiographed in the coiled position as this can distort internal organs and decrease detail. The snake should be stretched out over the cassette. If properly collimated, two or more regions of the body can be radiographed on one film. If possible, radiograph both views of the same region on one film to make interpretation much easier. If multiple films are required, the films should be labeled to match the region taken. There are several methods of doing this. The method that this author uses is based on the number of films required to radiograph the snake. If four films are needed, the first film is labeled 1/4, the second film is labeled 2/4, and so on.

Restraint

With the exception of very sick snakes, most snakes will not be still enough to radiograph without proper restraint. For docile snakes, manually holding them on the table will be sufficient enough restraint for proper technique. For less-docile snakes, placing them in clear plastic tubes will allow for proper positioning and technique. If this method is used, the kVp or mAs, depending on the technique chart used, may need to be slightly increased to compensate for the plastic. As a last resort, chemical restraint can be used. Either injectable or inhalant anesthesia can be used. If injectable anesthesia is used, a short acting drug or one that is reversible is preferred. Some injectable anesthetics can last for hours or even days in reptiles.

ANESTHESIA

Anatomy and Physiology Considerations

The lungs of reptiles are very fragile. When performing intermittent positive pressure ventilation (IPPV) always stay under 20 cm water to avoid pulmonary rupture (Bennett 1996a, 30). Since reptiles do not have a diaphragm, respiration is accomplished through other muscles throughout the thoracic and abdominal areas. Some of the muscles are paralyzed when the reptile reaches a surgical plane of anesthesia making IPPV necessary. One should keep in mind also that many snakes can breath hold and convert to anaerobic metabolism. Many species can live for

hours without oxygen. This adaptation makes induction difficult to impossible in some species if inducing with inhalant anesthesia.

Preanesthetic Examination and Considerations

Before placing a snake under anesthesia a very thorough physical examination should be performed. Also, a minimal amount of diagnostics including a packed cell volume and total solids should be recorded to help determine the health status of the snake. More diagnostics may be needed such as a biochemical profile, complete blood count, fecal analysis, radiographs, or cultures if infection is suspected. Any abnormalities on the physical examination or diagnostic testing should be treated or stabilized before the anesthetic episode. The snake should be fasted for 1 to 2 weeks for any elective procedures or nonemergency anesthetic procedures. The cardiopulmonary function can be compromised if a large prey is still being digested in the stomach.

Intravenous fluid therapy is needed for any debilitated snake or during long procedures (Bennett 1997, 32). If the snake is dehydrated, rehydration should occur before beginning the anesthetic episode. Any of the crystalloids are appropriate for use in reptiles (Lawton 2001, 788). There is a lot of debate over the use of any fluids containing lactate (Wright 1999, 817). Lactate in reptiles builds to high levels after muscle fatigue and can only be metabolized by the liver. There has been no research performed on this issue as of the date of publication of this text. Until further research has been conducted, it is recommended that fluids containing lactate not be used on a long-term basis in reptile patients. If lactated Ringer's solution is chosen for fluid therapy, potassium chloride must be added to prevent hypokalemia. If fluids are needed interoperatively, an intravenous catheter must be placed in either the jugular vein or directly into the heart. The interoperative fluid rate should be 5 to 10 ml/kg/hr.

Preanesthetic Medications

Preanesthetics are not routinely used in reptiles. Preanesthetics will provide much smoother induction and recovery afnd will improve muscle relaxation.

Anticholinergics

Anticholinergics such as atropine sulfate and glycopyrrolate for the most part are unnecessary as a preanesthetic medication. Glycopyrrolate has been shown to help prevent bradycardia, however, bradycardia is usually not a concern in reptile anesthesia.

Tranquilizers

As a preanesthetic, tranquilizers will help decrease the amount of induction and maintenance needed. Tranquilizers also help keep the induction and recovery smooth by reducing the excitatory phase of anesthesia. Acepromazine given 1 hour before induction has been shown to smooth the induction process and reduce the amount of induction needed.

Injectable Anesthetics

The use of injectable anesthetics in reptiles is very unpredictable. The same dose given to two individuals of the same species can yield completely different levels of sedation (Bennett 1996a, 243). Once the injection is given, the depth of anesthesia cannot be controlled. Since reptiles have a very slow metabolism, recovery time can take from a couple of hours to a week with some anesthetics. Reptiles require a very high dose of narcotics to produce any sedative effects, making narcotics not recommended in reptiles.

Barbiturates have a questionable use in reptiles. It is unknown how reptiles eliminate barbiturates from their body. It is believed that reptiles rely on metabolism for eliminating barbiturates instead of redistribution to nonnervous tissue (Bennett 1996a, 244). Thiobarbiturates have a recovery time of several days. This recovery time can be quickened by increasing the ambient temperature in the cage. The ultrashort barbiturates work well in reptiles with a relatively short recovery time of only a few hours. As with all injectables, there is a significant variation in response.

Ketamine is frequently used in snakes for sedation and induction at a dose of 22 to 44 mg/kg. Ketamine can also be used as a surgical anesthetic at a dose of 55 to 88 mg/kg. Due to metabolic scaling, larger species require the lower end of the recommended dose (Bennett 1997, 34). Ketamine can be given every 30 minutes during a procedure at a dose of 10 mg/kg to maintain a proper level of anesthesia. Ketamine should not be used on debilitated patients. Recovery time is usually greater than 24 hours.

Medetomidine has been used with great success in snakes. When given, it greatly reduces the amount of induction needed and also at higher doses gives enough sedation for quick procedures. Medetomidine is reversible with atipamezole. Medetomidine when given with ketamine shows better anesthetic effects than when given alone.

Telazol is recommended as a tranquilizer or induction agent and not the sole anesthetic. At a dose of 4 to 5 mg/kg, Telazol will sedate the snake enough for diagnostic procedures or for intubation. Even at high levels, snakes will still respond to stimuli.

Propofol is a very short acting nonbarbiturate that can be used as an induction agent or for short surgical or diagnostic procedures. The only disadvantage of Propofol is that it must be given intravenously, which can be very difficult in some snakes (Schumacher 2002a, 946). The advantages of Propofol is that it produces very rapid induction and recovery times, it has minimal accumulation with repeated doses, and it produces very little hangover effect after recovery.

Several neuromuscular blocking agents have been used in snakes. Since these drugs do not produce unconsciousness or analgesia, the use of neuromuscular blockers should be limited to nonpainful diagnostic procedures. Since respiratory paralysis is likely, intubation with IPPV is necessary.

Inhalant Anesthetics

Inhalant anesthetics have become the standard of practice for reptiles (Bennett 1997, 36). There are many advantages of inhalant anesthetics versus injectable anesthetics. First, the level of anesthesia is much more precisely controlled. Another large advantage is that the patient is intubated and receiving supplemental oxygen. The recovery time of inhalant anesthetics is much quicker than with injectable anesthetics. Usually the patients are recovered in less than one hour after the anesthetic episode. A nonrebreathing system is recommended for patients weighing less than 5 kg and an oxygen flow rate of 300 to 500 ml/kg/min is recommended. Patients weighing more than 5 kg can use a rebreathing system at an oxygen flow rate of 1 to 2 L/min. IPPV is recommended in all anesthetized reptiles at a rate of two to four breaths per minute.

Methoxyflurane has been used successfully in snakes. The disadvantage of this inhalant is that it produces slow induction and recovery times, and 50% of the drug is metabolized by the liver making it inappropriate in patients with any liver problems. Elapids and some pythons have shown sensitivity to methoxyflurane.

Halothane produces a quicker induction and recovery than methoxyflurane. Also, only 12% of halothane is metabolized by the liver making this drug a better choice for patients with liver problems. When inducing with halothane, start with a low concentration and slowly increase to prevent irritation. This process can induce breath holding. Venomous species seem to require a higher concentration of halothane, with viperids requiring more than elapids.

Isoflurane is the inhalant anesthetic of choice of this author. It is completely eliminated by the lungs so it causes no metabolic compromise, and can safely be used on debilitated or compromised patients.

Induction is quick taking five to ten minutes with recovery taking less than 30 minutes on most patients.

The newest inhalant anesthetic on the market is *sevoflurane*. Sevoflurane gained popularity in the human and veterinary market because of the low blood-gas solubility. This low blood-gas solubility allows for very fast induction and recovery times and improving the control of anesthetic depth (Schumacher 2002b, 950). In humans, cardiovascular stability is better maintained with sevoflurane than with isoflurane. Sevoflurane is also completely eliminated by the lungs. There has been very little research conducted on the effects of sevoflurane in reptiles. Clinical experience shows that species and individuals respond differently to sevoflurane with some being much more resistant than others (Schumacher 2002b, 950).

Analgesics

It was once believed that reptiles do not feel pain. Reptiles have the neurologic components, antinociceptive mechanisms, and behavioral responses to pain that other animals have (Bradley 2001, 45). Reptiles can and do feel pain and therefore analgesics should be provided. Since pain is easier to prevent than treat, analgesics should be given before an anticipated painful procedure. Snakes also share many of the same signs of pain as domestic species. Commonly, snakes will shows signs of avoidance of handling, withdrawal, restlessness, agitation, being easily startled, or anorexia when they are in pain. Some more obvious signs of pain are holding the body less coiled at the site of pain, stinting on palpation, and being tucked up and writhing in the affected area.

Recovery

Recovering patients should be placed in an environment that is quiet and within the species POTZ. Close attention should be paid to the respirations since all anesthetics compromise the respiratory system. Also observe the patient for any pain or discomfort and treat with analgesics accordingly. If the patient was receiving fluids during the procedure, the fluids should be continued until the patient is fully recovered.

Anesthetic Monitoring

The depth of anesthesia in snakes is very difficult to assess. As snakes become anesthetized, relaxation begins cranial and goes caudal and is reversed when recovering. One of the first reflexes a snake loses is the righting reflex. Other reflexes to check are the cloacal reflex and the tail pinch to help determine the depth of anesthesia. At a surgical plane, snakes should still have

a tongue withdraw, and will lose it if the snake is beyond the surgical plane. Each anesthetized snake should be connected to an electrocardiogram as well as a Doppler flow device since the cardiovascular system is very difficult to assess. The heart rate and respiratory rate should be monitored continuously starting when the patient is induced and ending after the patient is fully recovered. Pulse oximetry is only useful in reptiles to monitor trends in arterial oxygen saturation.

SURGERY

The basic principles of surgery are universal. Aseptic techniques should always be used. To prepare the patient for surgery, induce with anesthesia, intubate, and place on maintenance inhalant anesthesia. Tracheal intubation is easy on snakes (figs. 4.18 and 4.19). The trachea sits at the base of their tongue and is easily visible when the mouth is open. One should perform an initial scrub with an approved surgical scrub such as chlorhexidine or betadine to remove any dirt or debris from the substrate. When the patient is stable under anesthesia, the patient can then be moved into the surgical suite. Once inside the surgical suite, all assistants should put on a cap and mask to maintain asepsis. The patient should be properly positioned and taped down to secure it to the table. Snakes can be positioned either in sternal, dorsal, or left or right recumbency. Once the patient is secured to the table, a sterile surgical scrub should be performed. The fluids used to prep the patient should be warmed to prevent cooling the patient. The patient should also be kept at its POTZ during the entire procedure and through recovery. This can be achieved by using a circulating hot water pad or hot water bottles.

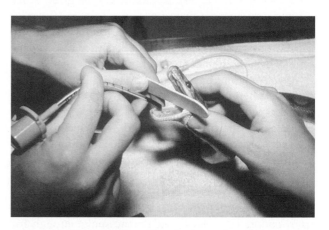

Fig. 4.18. *Endotracheal intubation of a snake. (Photo courtesy of ZooAtlanta)*

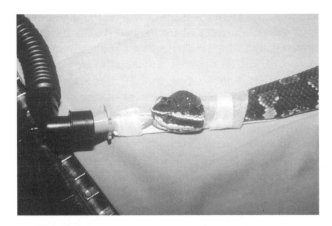

Fig. 4.19. Stabilizing the endotracheal tube with a tongue depressor. (Photo courtesy of ZooAtlanta)

Wound Healing

Wound healing has been studied extensively in snakes (Bennett & Lock 2000, 718). When a wound forms, proteinaceous fluid and fibrin fills the space to form a scab. A single layer of epithelial cells grows under the scab and then proliferates to restore the full thickness of the epithelium. Underneath this layer of epithelial cells, macrophages and heterophils move in to clean up any pathogens. Fibroblasts migrate to the area forming a fibrous scar. Heterophils are present until maturation has occurred. Ecdysis seems to help with the wound healing process (Bennett 1997, 38). It has also been observed that incisions that have a cranial to caudal orientation heal faster than a transverse incision. Also staying in the upper end of the species POTZ promotes good wound healing (Bennett & Lock 2000, 719).

The incised skin of reptiles has a tendency to heal inverted. The skin should be closed using an everted suture pattern such as mattress pattern. Skin staples can also be used for skin closure. The sutures should be removed in four to six weeks and preferably after the next ecdysis cycle.

Common Surgical Procedures

Celiotomies are routinely performed on snakes. The incision for a celiotomy should be made between the first two rows of scales dorsolateral to the large ventral scales (Bennett & Lock 2000, 721). This approach is performed to avoid the large midabdominal vein. A zigzag incision is made between the scales in the softer skin. Celiotomies are commonly performed for foreign body removal and exploratory surgery.

The most common surgery of the respiratory tract is removal of granulomas from the trachea. The approach is the same as for a celiotomy. The granuloma is found and removed. The two ends of the trachea are then anastomosed and the incision is closed. The snakes are usually back to breathing normally immediately.

Gastrointestinal surgeries are routinely done to repair abnormalities. These abnormalities may include foreign body removal or resection and anastomosis.

Surgery on the reproductive tract is usually not performed to prevent a reproductive problem (Lock 2000, 737). The most common female reproductive surgical procedure is dystocia and ovariectomy or ovariosalpingohysterectomy. The last two procedures are performed to prevent another dystocia, to remove cysts or tumors, or to prevent another prolapse. The most common surgical procedure on the male reproductive tract is penile amputation. The hemipenis will prolapse and become inflamed and will not be able to be retracted. Oftentimes the hemipenis can be replaced, but occasionally the hemipenis will become necrotic and have to be amputated (fig. 4.20).

PARASITOLOGY

Diagnosing Parasites

Parasitic infections are relatively easy to diagnose. A fresh stool sample should be obtained being careful not to collect any urates. When an appointment is made for a snake, the client should be asked to bring in a fresh stool sample. The client can put the stool sample in a plastic sandwich bag and kept it in the refrigerator for up to three days. It is not recommended that the stool sample be stored in a refrigerator that

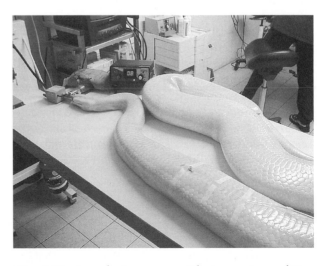

Fig. 4.20. A snake in surgery. (Photo courtesy of Dr. Stephen J. Hernandez-Divers, University of Georgia)

also stores food for human consumption. A double or even triple bag system can be used if the sample is stored with food for human consumption. If a fresh sample is not available, a colonic wash can be performed to obtain a sample. Three diagnostic tests should be performed: a flotation, centrifugation, and saline prepared direct smear. The fecal flotation is used to diagnose nematode ova. The centrifuge will help diagnose protozoan cysts. The direct smear is used to diagnose moving or live parasites. The techniques used to perform these diagnostics are the same techniques used for diagnosing parasites in small animals. Some parasites, like *Cryptosporidium*, require specialized diagnostic testing.

COMMON PARASITES OF SNAKES

External Parasites

Ticks
Ticks are a common finding on snakes. Ticks can be very difficult to find on snakes, especially if the snake has dark skin. Rarely are ticks in such a high number on snakes to cause anemia, but ticks can transmit blood parasites and viruses. All ticks should be removed with extra care to remove all the mouthparts from the skin.

Mites
Ophionyssus natricis, the snake mite, is a common finding in pet snakes. The mites are small and appear red, gray, or black. Snakes that are infected may spend long periods of time soaking in water or appear to rub or twist their bodies. Visualizing the mite is the only diagnostic method. If mites are suspected, a clean white paper towel or hand towel can be rubbed down the entire length of the snake's body. Often, the mites will come off onto the towel making for easier visualization. Treatment includes cleaning and disinfecting the cage and ivermectin. Ivermectin can be made into a spray or used as an injection. It is also recommended that all wood and porous cage furnishings be removed and paper be used as a substrate until the mites have been eradicated from the area.

Internal Parasites

Protozoa

Amoebiasis: Of the many species of amoebae that are found in snakes, *Entamoeba invadens* is the most pathogenic (Lane & Mader 1996, 190). This amoeba causes a very high mortality and morbidity rate in snakes. This species is transmitted via the ingestion of infected reptile feces. This parasite has a direct life cycle leading to great difficulty in eradicating it from snakes. Clinical signs of amoebiasis are anorexia, dehydration, and wasting away. Later stages of the disease will show clinical signs of ulcerative gastritis and colitis. This organism can spread to other tissues causing renal and hepatic necrosis and abscesses. A diagnosis is made through a positive culture. Treatment of this disease includes a broad-spectrum antibiotic, an amoebicide, and supportive care. The snakes can also be kept at a temperature of 95°F.

Coccidia: Coccidiosis is a common finding in captive snakes. In wild snakes, coccidiosis is a self-limiting infection, but in captivity, coccidia can cause severe illness and in young or small species can cause death. Coccidia does have a direct life cycle. Sulfonamides are the preferred treatment.

Cryptosporidium is becoming a serious coccidial infection in snakes. The exact source of infection is unknown but it is believed that snakes contract the parasite by either contact with shedding reptiles or from mammalian prey items. Clinical signs for the disease includes midbody swelling, weight loss, and regurgitation. The midbody swelling is a result of chronic gastric hypertrophy caused by the parasite. Cryptosporidiosis is diagnosed by visualization of oocysts on a microscopic exam. A dimethyl sulfoxide (DMSO) acid-fast fecal exam should be performed for proper diagnosis. *Cryptosporidium* spp. oocysts are difficult to find due to their small size of less than 4 microns. The oocysts contain no sporocysts and four sporozoites. There are no safe and effective treatments for cryptosporidiosis. Trimethoprim sulfa, spiramycin, and paromomycin have been shown to reduce clinical signs and reduce or eliminate oocyte shedding. These drugs were given in conjunction with supportive care including fluids, high environmental temperatures, and tube feeding. It is not known if there is a zoonotic potential with this disease, so proper precautions should be taken.

Flagellated Protozoa: There are many genera of flagellates found in snakes. Most are nonpathogenic although there is the potential of *Giardia* spp. to cause disease. Clinical signs include anorexia and weight loss (Barnard 1996, 71). Metronidazole is the treatment of choice for flagellates.

Cestodes
The life cycle of cestodes involves many intermediate hosts. Snakes that are susceptible to cestode infections are those that are fed amphibians, fish, or crustaceans.

Nematodes

Several species of nematodes affect snakes. The life cycle involves one or several intermediate hosts. Nematode infections usually appear subclinical but signs can appear with severe infections. The only species of great concern are the *Rhabdias* spp. and *Strongyloides* spp. (Barnard 1996, 73). *Rhabdias* spp. are known as the lungworm in snakes. These nematodes migrate to the lungs. There are few clinical signs with minimal inflammatory response. Severe infections will show signs of dyspnea and mouth gaping. The diagnosis of lungworms can be made by discovering eggs and free-stage larvae in the oral secretions or in the feces. Strongyles are nematodes that feed on the blood of the host. Clinical signs include anorexia, weight loss, hemorrhagic ulceration, and gastrointestinal obstruction. A fecal exam is performed for diagnosis. Treatment for all nematodes includes any of several anthelmintics and supportive care. See color plates 3.9 through 3.20 and 4.3.

Blood Parasites

Extracellular and intracytoplastic blood parasites are commonly seen in snakes. These parasites rarely cause disease and are normally found on routine blood smears. Extreme cases can cause hemolytic anemia. If anemia is found, an antimalarial medication is indicated.

Preventing Parasites

With parasites, like most other diseases, the prevention is easier than the cure. A few simple guidelines should be followed. The enclosures should be kept clean and be disinfected often. New specimens should follow proper quarantine procedures. Do not feed wild prey items. Feed only frozen prey to the snakes. If live prey must be fed, start a breeding colony at home with a parasite free male and female. Varying the prey offered can help to break any parasite life cycle (Lane & Mader 1996, 202).

EMERGENCY AND CRITICAL CARE

As more and more snakes are kept as pets, the need for proper emergency and critical care is increasing. The basics of emergency and critical care in snakes are the same as in any other animal. The patient is assessed and diagnostics and treatments are quickly started. An emergency is defined as a sudden generally unexpected occurrence, or set of circumstances, demanding urgent action. Unfortunately, the need for urgent care is in the eye of the owner and not trained medical professionals. Many owners wait to seek medical attention days to months after first noticing a problem with their snake, so that the initial problem turns into an emergency situation.

Phone Calls

Many owners will call the veterinary hospital seeking advice on their pet snake to determine if emergency medical treatment is necessary. Many problems with snakes that are reported after hours can wait until the morning when the regular veterinarian is available. Most diseases have been developing for weeks to months and initiating treatment can wait another several hours. It is important that the technician screening the phone calls be familiar with snakes. Some clinical signs in dogs could be very serious while in a snake it is very normal. A common phone call that is not an emergency is an owner worried that his or her ball python (*Python regius*), or any other species, has not eaten in a week or sometimes several months. Obviously, for a snake this is not an emergency. Some of the more common emergencies that do need to be seen immediately are trauma, bite wounds, burns, hypothermia, hyperthermia, dyspnea, and cloacal prolapse. Common nonemergency clinical signs in snakes are lethargy, anorexia, dystocia, and constipation.

Initial Presentation and History

As soon as the patient comes into the veterinary hospital, a veterinary technician should make a quick assessment to determine the urgency of care. If the patient is stable, a thorough history should be obtained. If the patient is critical and needs immediate care, the patient should be taken to the attending veterinarian and a quick history should be obtained. This history should include such questions as:

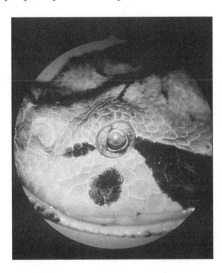

Plate 4.3. *Ocular larva migrans in a snake. (Photo courtesy of ZooAtlanta) (See also color plates)*

What is the ambient temperature in the enclosure?
Is the snake eating and drinking normally?
Do you feed live or dead prey?
What heat sources are used?
Has your snake been lethargic?
Have you seen any coughing, wheezing, or nasal discharge?
Has your snake regurgitated any food?
Have there been any other medical problems in the past?

A more complete history can be obtained after the patient is stable and more time can be focused away from the patient. More questions may need to be asked pending the results of the physical examination.

Diagnostics
After the physical examination has been performed, the clinician will have a diagnostic plan. This plan may include a fecal analysis, biochemical profile, complete blood count, packed cell volume, total protein, or radiographs.

Treatment
After the diagnosis is made the treatment should begin. For dehydrated or severely ill snakes, fluid therapy should be initiated. Intravenous fluid therapy is preferable but other methods of fluid therapy will suffice. The fluids should be warmed to the preferred body temperature for the species being treated. The snake should be placed in a cage that is heated to the species POTZ. A full-spectrum UV light should also be provided. Analgesics should be administered to patients that are in pain. Finally, other therapeutics should be started to treat the clinical signs and disease. Nutritional support should be started only after the patient is stable.

EMERGENCY CONDITIONS

Trauma
Trauma of any kind should be treated as an emergency. Bite wounds are common in snakes. Bites normally occur from cage mates and live prey items left in the cage unattended. Lacerations are not as commonly seen in snakes. Most commonly lacerations occur from exposed ends of wire mesh used on cages. Large snakes can easily break through glass cages causing severe lacerations. Bite wounds and lacerations are treated by either primary closure or secondary intention healing. If the wound is left open, antibiotic ointments rubbed on the wound work well as a barrier.

Also, systemic antibiotics should be used on all bite wounds or lacerations. Analgesics should also be used.

Hypothermia
Occasionally snakes will escape from their enclosure and be found in a place that is excessively cold causing metabolism to cease. Frostbite may be seen on the tip of the snake's tail. If not necrotic, some pigment will be lost. Hypothermic snakes are not able to digest food and will often regurgitate prey. It is common to see respiratory disease several days to weeks after an episode of hypothermia. Snakes should be warmed up slowly over several hours and supportive care should be started.

Hyperthermia
Hyperthermia often occurs when the owner lets the snake outside in a glass or plastic enclosure in direct sunlight. Radiant heat quickly warms the snake and the snake is not able to get into a cooler environment. Treatment for hyperthermia includes subcutaneous or intracoelomic fluids and a quick cool water bath to decrease the core body temperature. Steroids may also be indicated.

Dyspnea
Snakes do not normally open-mouth breathe. If acute dyspnea occurs the snake should be seen immediately. Dyspnea can be caused by several pathogens or disease processes, but it is most commonly associated with pneumonia.

Thermal Burns
Thermal burns are one of the most common emergencies seen in practice. Often, snakes will not show clinical signs of a burn for several days making them difficult to treat. Thermal burns are most commonly caused by a malfunctioning heat source or improper use of a heat source. The two most common causes of thermal burns in snakes are hot rocks (or what this author refers to as "death rocks") and heat lights that snakes will coil around.

Burns are classified as superficial, partial, or full thickness. A superficial burn involves only the epidermis. The snake may appear to be in pain and have some discoloration on its scales. In severe superficial burns some scales may be singed. Snakes with a superficial burn have a good prognosis. Antibiotic therapy should be initiated if any infection is noted. The snake should be housed in its POTZ and should heal by the next ecdysis. Little or no scarring is seen with superficial burns.

Partial-thickness burns involve complete destruction of the epidermis and extend into the underlying layers of skin. These burns appear red, ooze plasma, and will blister. Partial-thickness burns are also very painful. Treatment for partial-thickness burns can take several months to completely heal. Since these burns are very painful, analgesics should be administered immediately. The burn should be flushed thoroughly and supportive care should be started. It is not uncommon for these patients to be in shock. After cleansing the burns, a burn cream such as 1% silver sulfadiazine should be applied and a sterile nonstick bandage should be placed. Wet to dry bandages can also be used. The bandages should be replaced every day. The snake should be housed in a glass or Plexiglas container with no substrate until the wound is completely healed. The cage should also be disinfected daily. Antibiotics should be started to prevent infections that are common in burn victims.

Full-thickness burns are characterized by a black eschar. Full-thickness burns are not painful due to all of the nerves in the skin being destroyed. Full-thickness burns have a poor to grave prognosis and require very intensive treatment. The wound initially should be treated with a thorough cleansing and fluid therapy to treat for shock. The burn should be debrided to promote healing and a bandage should be placed. Antibiotics should also be started. Daily bandage changes and debridement are necessary for successful treatment. As the skin heals, the wound will become very painful. Analgesics should be started as soon as the patient feels pain. It can take months to a year for full granulation to occur. The owners must be told of the poor prognosis, long-term care, and financial expense of treating a full-thickness burn before treatment begins.

CRITICAL CARE MONITORING

The same principles apply to monitoring a critically ill snake as apply to monitoring a critically ill dog or cat. Neurologic, respiratory, and cardiovascular function all must be monitored and assessed.

The cardiovascular system should be monitored by using a Doppler and electrocardiogram. A heart rate should be obtained from both the Doppler and ECG and recorded in the record (figs. 4.21 and 4.22). Auscultation should be performed to monitor the respiratory system. The breath sounds should be clear without any wheezing or crackles. A respiratory rate should be obtained and recorded in the record. The patient should also be observed for dyspnea. A neurologic exam should be performed daily. The snake should also be housed in its POTZ.

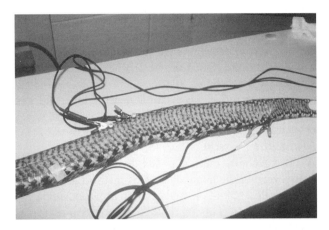

Fig. 4.21. ECG lead placement on a snake. The head is to the right. (Photo courtesy of ZooAtlanta)

SEX DETERMINATION

Since snakes do not possess external genitalia, determining the sex can sometimes be challenging. There are several acceptable methods used to determine the sex of snakes. Of the methods available, there are various degrees of simplicity and accuracy. It is important to choose a method that best suits the particular snake. For a snake that is kept as a pet, it is best to stick with a more simple method of sex determination. Snakes kept for breeding should be sexed using the most accurate method for that species.

Secondary Sexual Characteristics
With the exception of the boids, most snakes do not show any secondary sexual characteristics. Male boids will sometimes have larger cloacal spurs than females. Only technicians that are very familiar with boids will

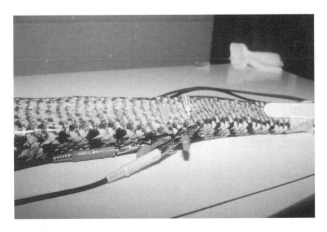

Fig. 4.22. ECG lead placement close-up to show detail. (Photo courtesy of ZooAtlanta)

be able to accurately determine the sex by using this method. Another secondary sexual characteristic that can be used to determine the sex is looking for a small bulge in the tail. Since the hemipenes are kept inside the tail, a small bulge may be seen. Using secondary sexual characteristics is a simple method but produces the least amount of accuracy.

Manual Eversion

A more accurate method of sex determination is manually everting the hemipenes. This method is best used in juvenile snakes or snakes that are too small for other methods. This method of sex determination is often referred to as popping. For this process, firmly roll one thumb up the base of the tail starting distal and working proximal to the cloaca. If it is a male, the hemipenes will "pop" out. Care must be taken not to apply too much pressure or the hemipenes can be damaged. This method is unreliable in large snakes and some colubrids where manual eversion of the hemipenes is not possible.

Cloacal Probing

This is the preferred method of sex determination. It is very simple and accurate if done properly. The probe used can be anything that is straight and has a blunt end. Commercial sex probes are available in sets of various diameters. Insert the lubricated probe into the cloaca and angle it caudally. Position the probe just lateral to the midline. Then gently slide the probe caudally into the base of the tail. If the snake is male, the probe will enter the inverted hemipenis and slide down several millimeters. If the snake is a female, the probe will either not be able to enter the tail base or will go only a couple of millimeters. Female snakes have blind diverticula that are smaller in diameter and shorter in depth than the hemipenes. A major cause of error in sexing is using a probe that is too small. A very small probe can enter the diverticula in females giving a false diagnosis. The technician must also be careful not to be forceful with the probe. The probe should slide smoothly with very little force needed. Generally, the distance the probe enters the base of the tail is measured in either millimeters or number of subcaudal scales. This number should be recorded in the file with the sex diagnosis (figs. 4.23 and 4.24).

Hydrostatic Eversion

Hydrostatic eversion is the most accurate yet difficult method of sex determination. This method involves injecting isotonic saline into the base of the tail just caudal to where the hemipenes would be located. Keep injecting the saline until the hemipenes are everted or resistance is felt on the syringe. A possible dan-

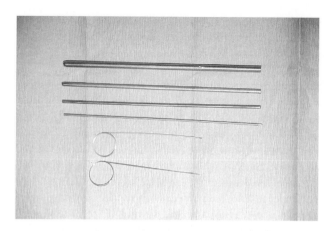

Fig. 4.23. Probes used for sexing snakes. (Photo courtesy of Ryan Cheek)

ger of this procedure is injecting the saline into the hemipenes instead of caudal. For very large snakes, anesthesia is required to perform this procedure. This method is very accurate because the hemipenes are everted in males, and if the snake is female, the swelling around the cloaca allows for visualization of the oviductal papillae.

CLINICAL TECHNIQUES

Administration of Medications

Intravenous (IV)
Intravenous injections can be given in the tail vein or directly into the heart. Use the same technique used for venipuncture to give the injection. Another vein that can be used for IV injections is the palatine vein. This vein is located in the oral cavity and is best suited for very experienced phlebotomists due to its small size. The palatine vein should only be used in snakes with a healthy oral cavity and no signs of stomatitis.

Subcutaneous (SC)
Subcutaneous injections can easily be given when the snake is coiled. When a snake is coiled, skin folds will appear. The needle should be placed between the scales on the lateral coelomic body wall, aspiration applied to the syringe to ensure a blood vessel has not been entered, and then the injection given. If the snake is not coiled, a small piece of skin can be lifted and the injection given.

Intramuscular (IM)
Intramuscular injections can be given in the epaxial and lateral muscle groups. The needle is placed

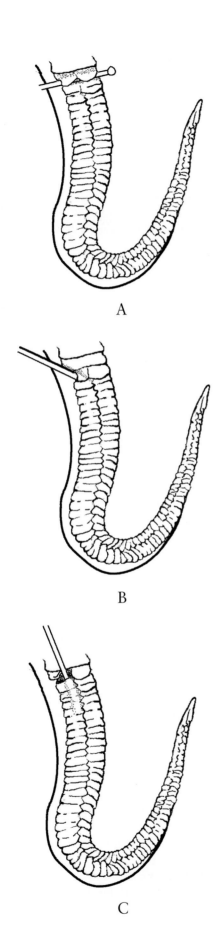

A

B

C

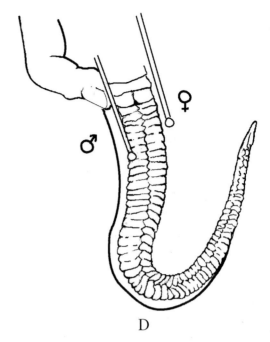

D

Fig. 4.24. *Sexing a snake. A. Appropriate placement of probe prior to insertion. B. Initial insertion of the probe. C. Advancing the probe. D. In males the probe advances farther than in females. (Drawings by Scott Stark)*

between the scales, aspiration applied to the syringe to ensure a blood vessel has not been entered, and then the injection given.

Intracoelomic (ICe)

The snake should be restrained in dorsal or lateral recumbency. The needle is placed between scales in the lower quadrant of the coelomic cavity being careful to be far enough caudal to avoid the lung. It is very important to aspirate back on the syringe before injecting. If any blood or other questionable fluid is aspirated, the needle should be removed and a new syringe and medication should be prepared. If giving ICe fluids, the fluids should be warmed up to the snake's POTZ before administering.

Oral (PO)

Oral medications are very easy to give to snakes. The medication is drawn up into a syringe and then a red rubber catheter is attached to the end. To prevent the red rubber catheter from passing into the trachea, a catheter should be chosen that is too large to fit into the trachea. One should also open the mouth to ensure that the catheter has gone down the esophagus. After checking for correct placement, administration of the medication can begin. With another syringe filled with water, the medication should be flushed down to ensure that no medicine is left in the catheter. This method can also be used to force-feed snakes.

Venipuncture

Tail Vein

The snake can be placed in either dorsal or ventral recumbency (fig. 4.25). With the bevel of the needle facing cranial, the needle is inserted exactly on midline at a 45° angle. While maintaining gentle suction, the needle is advanced until a flash of blood is seen. Occasionally the coccygeal vertebrae will be hit first and the flash of blood will be seen as the needle is withdrawn. The needle should be inserted caudal to the hemipenes and scent glands. With smaller snakes, a gentle suction and release may be done to receive enough blood to perform diagnostic testing.

Cardiocentesis

Locate the heart by either manually palpation or by Doppler. One should apply pressure just caudal and cranial to the heart to stabilize it. After the heart has been stabilized, the needle is inserted at a 45–60° angle. The needle is advanced until a slight pop is felt and the needle has entered the heart. One should then aspirate back until enough sample has been taken. Occasionally, pericardial fluid may be aspirated. If this happens, the needle should be withdrawn and the procedure started over with a fresh needle and syringe (fig. 4.26).

Palatine Vein

As stated previously, the palatine vein is only recommended in a snake with a clean oral cavity and no signs of stomatitis. This technique will only work on very docile or anesthetized snakes. One should

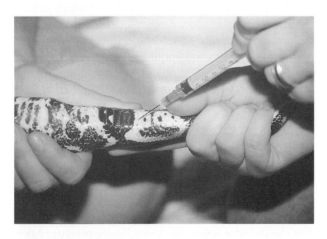

Fig. 4.25. *Venipuncture using the tail vein. (Photo courtesy of Ryan Cheek)*

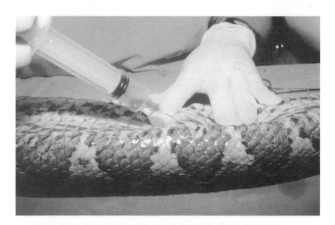

Fig. 4.26. *Cardiocentesis. (Photo courtesy of ZooAtlanta)*

restrain the snake with its mouth open. A 25–27-gauge needle should be advanced into the vein. One should then aspirate gently to prevent the vein from collapsing. Due to the chance of contamination from the saliva, this vein is best used only for IV injections.

Intravenous Catheter Placement

Jugular Vein

A cut down incision is required for this procedure. The skin should be surgically prepped. The incision should be made at the junction of the ventral scutes and lateral scales just cranial to the heart, about four to seven scutes. It will be necessary to bluntly dissect to expose the vein. After the vein has been exposed, the catheter is inserted until a flash is seen in the hub. The catheter is then advanced into the vein. The skin is closed using sutures and with the catheter sutured to the skin. A bandage can be placed to keep the catheter site clean.

Heart

In an extreme emergency, a catheter can be placed in the heart for a short time. The technique used for venipuncture can be used to place the catheter. Once the catheter is placed, it should be secured with suture or tape.

Force-Feeding

One should properly restrain the snake with its mouth open. An appropriate-sized prey item is grasped with large hemostats and a large amount of lubrication is applied to the entire body of the prey. The prey is inserted into the snake's mouth gently forcing it down. Once the prey is completely inserted, one should milk the prey down the esophagus until it reaches the stomach. One should be very careful that the prey does not scratch the esophagus with its incisors or claws. An easy way to prevent this is to trim the claws and teeth before force-feeding.

Snakes can also be force-fed by using the same technique for giving oral medications (figs. 4.27 and 4.28). Liquefied whole prey or artificially prepared foods can be used. For neonates or smaller snakes a device called a pinkie press can be used.

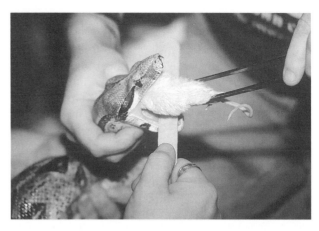

A

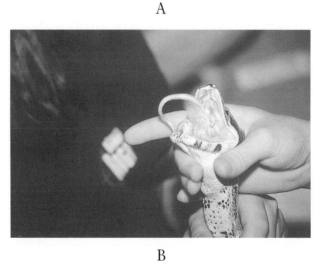

B

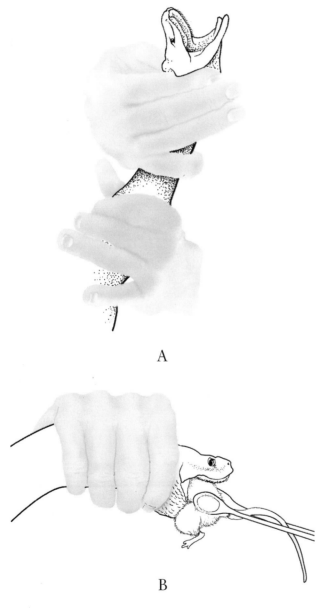

A

B

Fig. 4.27. Feeding a snake. A. Restraint with the mouth open for insertion of prey. A tongue depressor may be used to open the mouth. B. Using a pair of large hemostats, the prey is gently pushed down into the esophagus. (Drawings by Scott Stark)

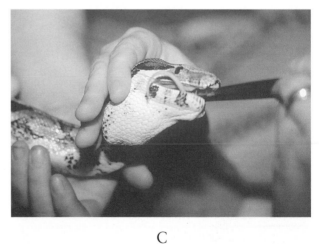

C

Fig. 4.28. Force-feeding a snake. A. The snake is properly restrained and a tongue depressor is used to open the mouth. The prey is then inserted into the oral cavity. B. The prey is almost completely into the oral cavity. C. Then the prey is gently pushed down the esophagus. (Photos courtesy of Ryan Cheek)

Tracheal and Lung Wash

Restrain the snake with its mouth open. Pass a sterile red rubber catheter into the trachea. Once the catheter is in place, infuse sterile saline into the trachea and lung. Do not place more than 5 ml/kg into the lung. After the sterile saline has been administered, aspirate back as much of the saline as possible. The saline can be injected and aspirated as many times as needed to receive a proper amount of sample (figs. 4.29 and 4.30).

Colonic Wash and Enema

With a well-lubricated red rubber catheter, one should insert the catheter into the colon. To enter the colon, the cloaca should be entered and the catheter aimed ventrally. With a syringe filled with saline, one should then begin flushing the saline into the colon and aspirating it back. This step should be repeated several times to get an adequate sample. This process also helps soften stools in constipated snakes. After aspiration, the sample can then be analyzed for parasites, cytologic examination, and culture (fig. 4.31).

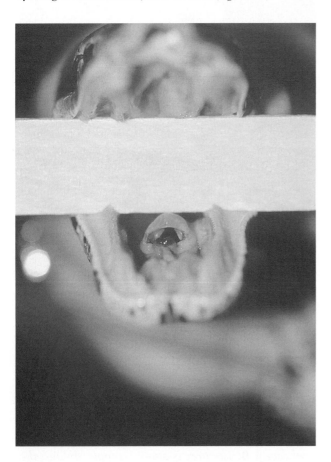

Fig. 4.29. View of the glottis. (Photo courtesy of Ryan Cheek)

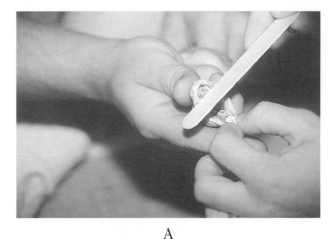

A

B

C

*Fig. 4.30. Tracheal wash. **A.** With the snake properly restrained the mouth is opened. **B.** A tongue depressor is used as a mouth gag, and the red rubber catheter is inserted into the trachea. **C.** 0.9% sodium chloride is then gently flushed into the trachea and then aspirated back. (Photos courtesy of Ryan Cheek)*

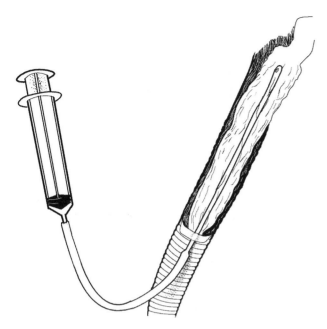

Fig. 4.31. Colonic wash. (Drawing by Scott Stark)

TRANSPORTATION

When it becomes necessary to transport a snake, there are several ways to do it. The most common item used to transport snakes are "snake bags." Snake bags can be burlap sacks, pillow cases, laundry bags, or other linens as long as it is a "breathable" fabric and can be secured. When using bags, the snake should be placed in the sack and a knot tied at the open end. One should remember that when transporting the snake in the bag, the bag should be grabbed above the knot, as a bite can still occur through a bag. (The bag should be moved using tongs if the snake is venomous). Venomous snakes should be transported in something more durable to safeguard against bites.

Plastic tubs or clean paint buckets with lids can be used as well. This works well for larger species if a large enough bag cannot be obtained. One should ensure that the lid snaps down or can be secured properly in case the snake pushes on it. Breathing holes need to be cut in the plastic if tubs or buckets are used. One should make sure not to create abrasive or sharp edges that the snake could come into contact with when adding breathing holes in plastic containers.

VENOMOUS SNAKES

It is not recommended to keep venomous snakes in private collections, especially by novice hobbyists. In some cases, it may be illegal to keep venomous snakes without proper permits. For this reason, it is rare that one would be brought into private practice for medical care. If this occurs, however, proper protocols need to be implemented. Whether a veterinary practice is even equipped for safe handling of venomous snakes needs to be addressed. At the very least, snake tongs, hooks, and tubes are needed for safer handling. Also, someone trained in handling venomous snakes is needed. Although one can practice tubing and handling techniques on nonvenomous snakes, there is obviously more risk involved in dealing with the venomous ones and one could be putting others at risk as well.

Most procedures on venomous snakes should be done while the snake is under anesthesia. This involves either tubing or placing the snake in an immobilization chamber. One should not attempt to manually restrain the head of a venomous snake. Those who milk snakes for venom have to do so but it is not a safe method of restraint. Some fangs are long enough to still penetrate a hand while restraining the head.

An envenomation protocol also needs to be in place at the facility. Most human hospitals (if they carry antivenin at all) only have those of indigenous species. So imported species are of higher risk to handle due to the lack of accessible antivenin. Most facilities that handle venomous snakes keep the different types of antivenin in stock, not necessarily for self-administration should a bite occur, but to bring to the nearest hospital if the hospital does not have any on hand. This is difficult though, due to both the expenses involved and the lack of accessibility. Expiration dates on the antivenin have to be closely monitored as well.

One should make sure to have a line of communication established with local hospitals to see who is able to handle a venomous snakebite. Contacting the local poison control facility to establish a protocol would be helpful as well. Once again, these are all things that need to be addressed before venomous snakes are managed at the facility. Minutes count should a venomous snakebite occur. One cannot afford to waste time calling hospitals to see if they can handle that particular bite. If this seems like too much of a hassle, then handling/treating venomous snakes should not be performed at that facility at all.

EUTHANASIA

Unfortunately, not all patients can be saved. Fortunately, veterinary medicine has the privilege of being able to humanely euthanize suffering animals with terminal illnesses. Euthanizing snakes can prove to be a difficult task. There are several humane methods of euthanasia that are acceptable in snakes. Only the methods that this author feels are humane will be discussed here.

This author's favorite method of euthanasia in snakes starts with an injection of Telazol or ketamine HCl. If injectable anesthetics are not available, inhalant anesthesia can be used. Due to the ability of snakes to hold their breath for long periods of time this can be a very lengthy process. After the snake is anesthetized, a cardiac stick is performed and an overdose of a barbiturate is injected. In very small species or very dehydrated snakes, a cardiac stick can be difficult. In that case, a simple ICe injection of a barbiturate can be performed. It can take several minutes to several hours before the snake is finally deceased using this method.

The toughest part of euthanizing snakes is determining death. There is not a good answer to the question. Is the snake deceased? An electrocardiograph, auscultation of the heart, or a Doppler can all be used to determine if the snake is deceased. Due to the fact that reptile hearts can still beat for several hours postmortem or can even beat once or twice per minute postmortem, these three tests can prove to be inaccurate. Many reptile clinicians have heard stories of the snake coming back to life 24 hours after the euthanasia. This can be easily avoided if the snake is left in the hospital overnight for observation.

BEING A RESPONSIBLE SNAKE OWNER

As a part of the veterinary team, the technician is responsible to properly inform and educate clients of the needs of particular animals. It is also important to offer guidance when purchases are being considered. Knowing what is involved in snake care and knowing specifics about different species of snakes will aid in giving advice to those considering purchasing a snake as a pet. Offering consultations to clients before purchases will help to eliminate a lot of the problems that arise after a snake is purchased. Snakes, in general, do not make good "pets." This should be kept in mind when offering advice to potential buyers. Buying a snake that will reach lengths of 20 feet or more is obviously not a choice that should be made by most people either. These snakes usually become neglected and the owners sometimes begin to fear them due to their size and sometimes their predisposition, which may become aggressive.

More and more people are beginning to devise ways to "get rid of" their snakes when it is no longer convenient to own them. All too often these snakes are impulse buys that are thought of as disposable belongings. The most appalling of these occurrences is when people let them go in their backyards when they "don't want to deal with them anymore." Most captive specimens are not even indigenous to the country where their "owners" set them free. Not only will it most likely kill the animal, but it can upset the natural balance of that particular ecosystem. Some even choose to freeze the snake as their way of "humanely euthanizing" the animal so they will no longer be burdened. There is nothing humane about freezing a live animal. It is in fact a slow, painful death.

If it is decided that a snake is no longer wanted, then attempts should be made to place it in a home or facility ready and able to meet its needs. Most of the time, this occurs with the larger species of snakes. They can reach astounding lengths and girths and can be extremely dangerous—not to mention the size of the enclosure needed to properly house them. These are obviously not for novice keepers and should be discouraged when an inexperienced individual inquires about obtaining one.

Another point to be made about being a responsible snake owner is understanding that a lot of people fear them. Taking them out to public places to "show them off" is not doing the public any good and especially not the snake. It can scare the snake being around a lot of commotion and can cause the people to panic as well. This in turn, is doing more injustice to the snake than one would think. The public, as a whole, has a terrible phobia of snakes and forcing the issue by bringing snakes into public places makes it worse. If individuals want to display their snakes, they should offer educational exhibits and lectures. That way they can create a learning environment and the people have the choice whether to participate or not. A phobia (no matter how silly one thinks it is) is a phobia, and it is not something that can be a forced change.

BIBLIOGRAPHY

Barnard, SM. 1996. *Reptile Keepers Handbook*. Florida: Krieger Publishing Company.

Bennett, R. 1998. "Urinary Diseases in Reptiles: Pathophysiology and Diagnosis." In *Seminars in Avian and Exotic Pet Medicine*, edited by Allen M. Fudge. Philadelphia: W.B. Saunders Co.

Bennett, RA. 1997. "Reptilian Surgery, Parts 1 and 2." In *Practical Exotic Animal Medicine*, edited by Karen L. Rosenthal. New Jersey: Veterinary Learning Systems.

Bennett, RA. 1996a. "Anesthesia." In *Reptile Medicine and Surgery*, edited by Douglas R. Mader. Philadelphia: W.B. Saunders Co.

Bennett, RA. 1996b. "Neurology." In *Reptile Medicine and Surgery*, edited by Douglas R. Mader. Philadelphia: W.B. Saunders Co.

Bennett, RA, & Lock, BA. 2000. "Nonreproductive Surgery in Reptiles." In *Veterinary Clinics of North America: Exotic Animal Practice*. Phildadelpia: W.B. Saunders Co.

Bradley, T. 2001. "Pain Management Considerations and Pain-Associated Behaviors in Reptiles and Amphibians." In *Proceedings of the Association of Reptilian and Amphibian Veterinarians*. Eastern State Vet Ass.

Divers, SJ. 2000. "Reptilian Renal and Reproductive Disease and Diagnosis." In *Laboratory Medicine: Avian and Exotic Pets*, edited by Allen M. Fudge. Philadelphia: W.B. Saunders Co.

Driggers, T. May 2000. "Respiratory Diseases, Diagnostics, and Therapy in Snakes." In the *Veterinary Clinics of North America: Exotic Animal Medicine*. Philadelphia: W.B. Saunders Co.

Funk, RS. 1996. "Snakes." In *Reptile Medicine and Surgery*, edited by Douglas R. Mader. Philadelphia: W.B. Saunders Co.

Glynn, MK, et al. 2001. "Knowledge and Practices of California Veterinarians Concerning the Human Health Threat of Reptile-Associated Salmonellosis." *Journal of Herpetological Medicine and Surgery* 11(2): 9–13.

Holz, PH. 1999. "The Reptilian Renal-Portal System: Influence on Therapy." In *Zoo and Wild Animal Medicine: Current Therapy*. 4th ed., edited by Murray E. Fowler and R. Eric Miller. Philadelphia: W.B. Saunders Co.

Lane, TJ, & Mader, DR. 1996. "Parasitology." In *Reptile Medicine and Surgery*, edited by Douglas R. Mader. Philadelphia: W.B. Saunders Co.

Lawton, MP. 2001. "Fluid Therapy in Reptiles." In *Proceedings of the North American Veterinary Conference*. Eastern States Vet Ass.

Lawton, MP. 1991. "Lizards and Snakes." In *Manual of Exotic Pets*, edited by Peter H. Beymon et al. Ames: Iowa State University Press.

Lock, BA. May 2000. "Reproductive Surgery in Reptiles." In *Veterinary Clinics of North America: Exotic Animal Practice*. Philadelphia: W.B. Saunders Co.

Marschang, RE. 2001. "Isolation of Viruses from Boa Constrictors, *Boa constrictor* spp., with Inclusion Body Disease." In *Proceedings of the Association of Reptilian and Amphibian Veterinarians*. Eastern States Vet Ass.

Miller, HA. April 1998. "Urinary Diseases of Reptiles: Pathophysiology and Diagnosis." In *Seminars in Avian and Exotic Pet Medicine*, edited by Allen M. Fudge. Philadelphia: W.B. Saunders Co.

Platel, R. 1994. "Nervous System and Sensory Organs." In *Snakes: A Natural History*, edited by Roland Bauchot. New York: Sterling Publishing.

Pough, FH, et al. 2001. *Herpetology*. 2d ed. New Jersey: Prentice-Hall Inc.

Romer, AS. 1997. *Osteology of the Reptiles*. Reprint. Malabar, FL: Krieger Publishing.

Ross, RA, et al. 1990. *The Reproductive Husbandry of Pythons and Boas*. The Institute for Herpetological Research, Stanford, CA.

Rossi, JV. 1996. "Dermatology." In *Reptile Medicine and Surgery*, edited by Douglas R. Mader. Philadelphia: W.B. Saunders Co.

Saint-Girons, H. 1994. "Growth and Reproduction." In *Snakes: A Natural History*, edited by Roland Bauchot. New York: Sterling Publishing.

Schumacher, J. 2002a. "Anesthesia in Reptiles." In *Proceedings of the North American Veterinary Conference*. Eastern States Vet Ass.

Schumacher, J. 2002b. "Sevoflurane in Reptiles." In *Proceedings of the North American Veterinary Conference*. Eastern States Vet Ass.

Schumacher, J. 1996. "Viral Diseases." In *Reptile Medicine and Surgery*, edited by Douglas R. Mader. Philadelphia: W.B. Saunders Co.

Siemering, H. 1986. "Zoonoses." In *Zoo and Wild Animal Medicine*, 2d ed., edited by Murray E. Fowler. Philadelphia: W.B. Saunders Co.

Vasse, Y. 1994. "A Cardiovascular System Working Against the Forces of Gravity." In *Snakes: A Natural History*, edited by Roland Bauchot. New York: Sterling Publishing.

Williams, DL. 1996. "Ophthalmology." In *Reptile Medicine and Surgery*, edited by Douglas R. Mader. Philadelphia: W.B. Saunders Co.

Wright, K. 1999. "Fluid Therapy for Reptiles." In *Proceedings of the North American Veterinary Conference*. Eastern States Vet Ass.

Zug, GR, et al. 2001. *Herpetology: An Introductory Biology of Amphibians and Reptiles*. 2d ed. New York: Academic Press.

CHAPTER FIVE

The Chelonians

Samuel Rivera

INTRODUCTION

Turtles belong in the class Reptilia. This class is divided into four orders, Chelonia (all turtles), Crocodylia (crocodilians), Squamata (snakes and lizards), and Rhynchocephalia (tuatara). There are approximately 270 species in the order Chelonia. This order contains a primitive group of animals that evolved into a shelled form millions of years ago and is considered the most primitive group of living reptiles. Chelonians include turtles, tortoises, and terrapins. The terms "turtle," "tortoise," and "terrapin" are sometimes confusing because they have different meanings in different parts of the world. In the United States, tortoise refers to terrestrial chelonians; turtles often refer to aquatic or semiaquatic chelonians with the exception of the box turtle, which is terrestrial; and terrapins are semiaquatic, hard-shelled chelonians. Because of the confusion in terminology, chelonians are often listed by their binomial scientific name, which is uniform around the world. There are hundreds of species of chelonians kept in captivity. See color plates 5.1, 5.2, 5.3. Unfortunately, many of the diseases seen in captive chelonians are related to improper husbandry and/or inadequate diet. Accurate identification of chelonian species will aid in the evaluation of husbandry and nutritional management. The goal of this chapter is to provide a basic understanding of chelonian husbandry, nutrition, biology, basic clinical techniques, and common health problems.

ANATOMY AND PHYSIOLOGY

Musculoskeletal System

In this section, the North American eastern box turtle (*Terrapene carolina carolina*) will be described. The most remarkable feature of turtles is their shell, which is divided in two parts. The dorsal part is the carapace and the ventral part is the plastron. The carapace normally consists of approximately 50 bones. The nuchal bone is the most cranial along the dorsal midline. It is followed by 7 neural, 1 suprapygal, and a pygal bone, consecutively. The neural bones are attached to the vertebrae. The costal bones are located on either side of the neural bones. The peripheral bones are located on the lateral aspect of the costal bones and extend from the nuchal to the pygal bones on both sides of the carapace (fig. 5.1).

The plastron consists of nine bones. The cranial part of the plastron is composed of the entoplastral bone, which is surrounded by the epiplastral bones cranially and two hypoplastral bones caudally. The hypoplastral bones are followed caudally by a second pair of hypoplastral bones, and a pair of xiphiplastral bones, consecutively. The bones of a turtle shell articulate with each other by a suture. Box turtles have a movable hinge located transversely between the two pairs of hypoplastral bones.

The bones of the shell are covered with structures made of keratinized epithelium called scutes. The most cranial scute along the dorsal midline is the cervical. The cervical scute is followed caudally by five vertebral scutes. The scutes adjacent to the vertebrals are the pleurals. The scutes outlining the periphery of

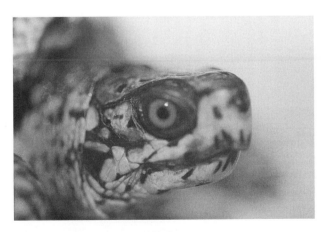

***Plate 5.1.** Male eastern box turtle showing red eye. (See also color plates)*

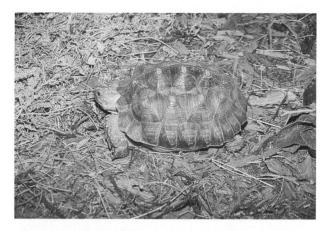

Plate 5.2. Sulcata tortoise. (See also color plates)

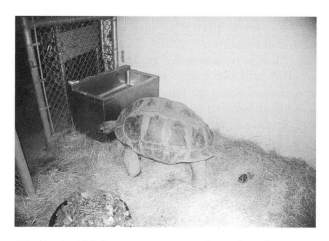

Plate 5.3. Aldabra tortoise. (See also color plates)

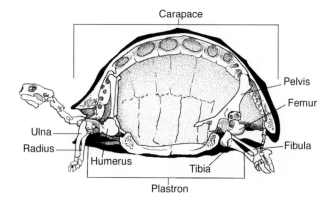

Fig. 5.1. Skeletal anatomy. (Drawing by Scott Stark)

the plastron are the peripherals. The plastron has six pairs of scutes. The cranial pair is the gular, followed by the humeral, pectoral, abdominal, femoral, and anal scutes, consecutively. The movable hinge is located between the pectoral and abdominal scutes. This hinge allows the plastron to be folded up to enclose the head and forelimbs within the shell. The pelvic and pectoral girdles are contained within the rib cage that is fused to the carapace.

The bones of the limbs of most chelonians are similar to those of other vertebrates.

Respiratory System

Turtles breathe through a pair of nostrils located at the dorsocranial aspect of the premaxilla. The glottis is located at the base of the tongue. The trachea is relatively short and bifurcates into two mainstream bronchi that open into the dorsal aspect of the paired lungs. The lungs are large, compartmentalized structures with a reticular surface containing bands of smooth muscle and connective tissue. The lungs attach dorsally to the ventral aspect of the carapace and ventrally to a membrane that is attached to the stomach, liver, and intestinal tract. Turtles do not have a diaphragm. Respiration is achieved by the contraction of the proximal muscle mass of the pectoral and pelvic limbs (Wood & Lenfant 1976). Aquatic turtles can exchange oxygen through the mucosal surface of the oral cavity and cloaca. Soft-shelled turtles can exchange oxygen through their skin (Girgis 1961).

Gastrointestinal System

The tongue of turtles is large and unable to distend from the oral cavity. They have salivary glands that produce mucus but not digestive enzymes. The esophagus courses along the neck. The stomach lies on the left cranioventral side of the coelomic cavity and has a gastroesophageal and a gastroduodenal valve. The small intestine is relatively short. The pancreas is pale pink and can be located near the spleen or in the mesentery along the duodenum. The liver is large, saddle-shaped, and located ventrally under the lungs. The liver has two lobes and it envelops the gall bladder. It also has indentations for the heart and stomach. The small intestine joins the large intestine at the ileocolic valve. The cecum is not well developed. The large intestine is the primary site of microbial fermentation in herbivorous turtles. The digestive tract empties into the cloaca (fig. 5.2).

Genitourinary System

The paired kidneys are located on the ventrocaudal aspect of the carapace, cranial to the acetabulum. The

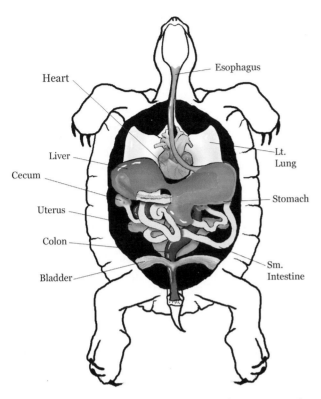

Fig. 5.2. Visceral anatomy. (Drawing by Scott Stark)

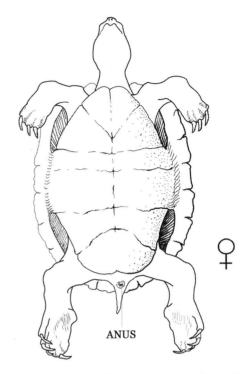

Fig. 5.3. Female reproductive anatomy. (Drawing by Scott Stark)

paired gonads are located cranial to the kidneys. The urogenital ducts empty into the neck of the urinary bladder. The urinary bladder is bilobed with a thin membranous wall. Male turtles have a single, large, dark-colored penis. It is located in the floor of the cloaca and it is not used for urination.

Many turtles are sexually dimorphic. The male tortoise has a concave plastron. The males of aquatic turtle species have long nails on their front feet. Generally, the tail is relatively larger in males than in females (fig. 5.3 and 5.4; see also color plate 5.1).

Circulatory System

Chelonians have a three-chambered heart consisting of two atria and one ventricle. Like other reptiles, turtles have a renoportal circulation system. Its function is to provide an alternate blood supply to the renal tubular cells, and prevent ischemic necrosis, when the arterial blood supply to the glomerulus is compromised (Holz 1999).

HUSBANDRY AND NUTRITION

There are hundreds of species of turtles seen in the pet trade. It is beyond the scope of this chapter to cover turtles by species. A brief overview on the husbandry of aquatic and terrestrial turtles will be discussed. The general public often seeks advice from veterinarians and their support staff in regard to the care and feeding of their newly purchased turtle. It is essential that one have a basic understanding of the husbandry and feeding practices of chelonians. Whenever possible, the turtle should be identified so accurate information on its husbandry and eating habits can be obtained.

Aquatic Turtles

Aquatic turtles are one of the most labor intensive reptiles to maintain. Inadequate husbandry often results in health problems. The housing requirements depend on the size and the number of turtles kept. As a rule of thumb, the combined surface area of all the turtles' carapaces should not exceed 25% of the tank's floor surface area (Anonymous 1990). The water should be as deep as the width of the turtle's shell, so that if overturned it will be able to right itself. The simpler the setup, the easier to clean. Clean water is essential to the health of turtles. The best way to keep the water clean is by doing full water changes. The larger the volume, the less the frequency of water changes. The number of animals, the feeding frequency, and the type of food offered will also determine the frequency of cleaning. Avoid drastic temperature changes when replacing the

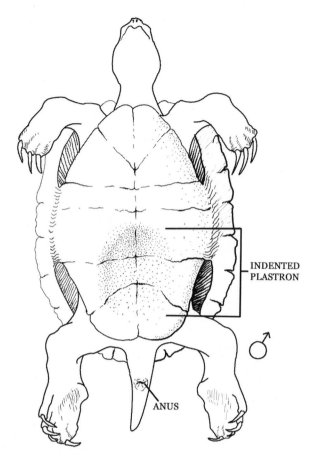

Fig. 5.4. *Male reproductive anatomy. (Drawing by Scott Stark)*

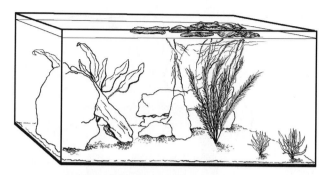

Fig. 5.5. *Aquatic habitat. (Drawing by Scott Stark)*

water as this can be detrimental to the turtle's health. A filtration system will minimize but not eliminate the need for complete water changes (fig. 5.5).

Adequate environmental and water temperature are important for good health. Turtles are ectothermic: they rely on the environmental temperature to regulate their body temperature. Turtles have a preferred optimal temperature zone (POTZ), which is the temperature at which they are the most comfortable. The POTZ also allows for normal physiologic functions to occur, such as digestion and fighting disease. Most aquatic turtles have a preferred optimum water temperature of 24 to 29°C (75 to 82°F). A dry area should be available so the turtle can dry off and bask. Basking is a process by which turtles can regulate their body temperature. An incandescent 50 to 150 watt lightbulb with a reflector directed toward the basking area will create a hot spot for basking. Place the basking light approximately 12–18 inches away from the basking area.

An adequate diet is essential for good health. Aquatic turtles are omnivorous with a few exceptions. Younger rapidly growing animals tend to eat a larger

percentage of meat but will switch to eating more vegetable matter as they get older (Frye 1991). A varied diet is the key to a healthy turtle. Too much of one food item can often lead to nutritional imbalances. Fish (goldfish, guppies, and bait minnows) is accepted by many turtles. Chopped, skinned adult mice are a good source of vitamins and minerals. Earthworms and a variety of insects can also be fed. Many adult turtles can be fed dark green leafy vegetables and a small amount of fruits. Most pet turtle owners will feed a commercial pelleted diet. Turtle owners that feed strictly pelleted food should always be encouraged to supplement the diet with other food items in order to provide the most balanced nutrition possible. Adult turtles can be fed two to three times per week. Young turtles should be fed daily or every other day. Aquatic turtles eat in the water and can be quite messy. Some turtles can be trained to eat in a separate container. This will minimize but not eliminate the need for frequent water changes.

There are some species of chelonians that spend the majority of their time in the water but spend some time on land. For these chelonians, a variation of the aquatic environment is the semiaquatic one. This setup involves all the same features of an aquatic setup but includes a land portion for basking (fig. 5.6).

Terrestrial Turtles
Land turtles can be kept in a variety of enclosures, depending on the size and number of animals kept. Where weather permits, tortoises should be kept outside. This allows the animals plenty of room to exercise and graze. Healthy tortoises can be placed outdoors when the temperature is above 18°C (65°F), and the midday temperature reaches 24°C (75°F) or above (Boyer & Boyer 1996). The outdoor enclosure should have a hiding place and a shaded area. The sides of the outdoor enclosure should be made of wood or any solid material that can provide a visual barrier. Wire fencing is not recommended because tortoises can injure them-

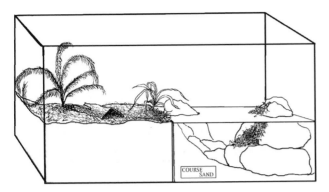

Fig. 5.6. Semiaquatic habitat. (Drawing by Scott Stark)

selves while trying to climb or push through the fence. The walls should be at least three times the height of the largest tortoise. Some tortoise species like to dig; therefore wire can be buried around the perimeter, at least 10 to 12 inches, to prevent escape.

Tortoises can be kept indoors. Generally they require more space than most reptiles of similar size. As a general rule, the combined size of all the tortoises' carapaces should not exceed 25% of the enclosure's floor (Anonymous 1990). Aquariums, or a wide variety of plastic containers, can be used for small tortoises. Larger species can be kept in enclosures made of wood or cement. A garage or spare room can serve as a holding area for tortoises. The room temperature should be between 24° and 32°C (75° and 90°F). A thermal gradient between 75° and 90°F is ideal to allow for thermoregulation. This gradient can be created by placing a basking light at one end of the enclosure. The basking light should be placed 18–24 inches away from the animals. At night, supplemental heat can be provided with heating pads placed under the enclosure, ceramic heaters with a reflector, or night heat lights. Acceptable substrates include cyprus mulch, large conifer bark nuggets, alfalfa pellets, newspaper, and indoor-outdoor carpeting, among others. Inappropriate substrates include sand, fine gravel, cat litter, crushed corncob, or walnut shells because these can lead to gastrointestinal impactions. Pine and cedar shavings are not recommended because of the presence of oils that can adversely affect the respiratory tract. The cage should be cleaned several times per week. The substrate can be changed as needed. If the tortoises are kept indoors all year, a source of UV light needs to be provided. There is a wide variety of UV lights and the manufacturer's instructions must be followed closely. Two points to keep in mind are that most UV bulbs must be kept at a minimum distance from the animals to be effective, and the lifespan of

the bulbs is limited and must be replaced on a regular basis. Natural light is ideal and must be provided whenever possible (fig. 5.7).

Tortoises are mainly herbivores. In the wild, tortoises eat a variety of leaves, stems, flowers, and fruits, additionally some will eat snails, earthworms, and other invertebrates. The ideal diet should be made of 85% vegetables (dark leafy greens, grasses), 10% fruits, and 5% high-protein foods (Boyer & Boyer 1994). The high-protein foods can be provided once or twice weekly. Alternatively, commercially made pelleted diet can be provided and supplemented with high-fiber food items. Adult animals can be fed two to three times per week, whereas juveniles can be fed daily or every other day.

COMMON DISEASES

Metabolic Bone Disease
This disease is caused by an improper calcium and phosphorus ratio in the diet and/or a vitamin D_3 deficiency. Turtles fed liver, heart, or muscle meat will often develop metabolic bone disease. The resulting calcium deficiency often leads to a depletion of calcium from bone resulting in fibrous osteodystrophy. Clinical signs include anorexia, soft and or deformed shell, and abnormal scute growth. The treatment involves diet correction and proper vitamin D_3 supplementation.

Vitamin A Deficiency
This is a common presentation in aquatic and terrestrial turtles. It is caused by feeding a diet deficient in vitamin A. The clinical signs include conjunctivitis, blepharitis, swollen eyelids, nasal discharge, dyspnea,

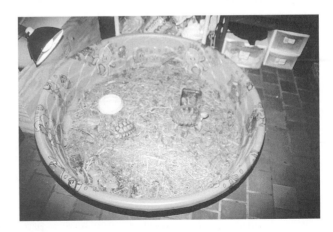

Fig. 5.7. Setup for a small tortoise. (Photo courtesy of Ryan Cheek)

and ear abscesses. This condition is treated with parenteral vitamin A and diet correction.

Vitamin A Toxicity

This can be caused by excessive supplementation or administration of parenteral vitamin A. The clinical signs include dry flaky skin, or sloughing of the skin with secondary bacterial infection. Treatment requires systemic antibiotics if secondary bacterial infection is present, and discontinuation of parenteral vitamin A or any source of oversupplementation.

Diseases of the Shell

"Shell rot" is a term used to describe infections of the shell involving loss of scutes. The terms "wet" and "dry" shell rot are used to describe the appearance of the lesions. The wet form is usually associated with a hemorrhagic discharge between the scutes. This form is often associated with bacterial infections. The dry form has a dry appearance and is often associated with fungal or bacterial infections. In some mild cases of shell rot, the lesions can be treated topically. Aquatic turtles need to be kept dry for 30–60 minutes after topical treatment. Septicemic cutaneous ulcerative disease (SCUD) is a common disease seen in aquatic turtles. The clinical signs include cutaneous ulcerations, anorexia, and lethargy. Treatment of any shell lesion involves debridement and topical antimicrobial treatment. In some cases, systemic antibiotics may be indicated.

Traumatic injuries to the shell are relatively common, especially in wild chelonia. In many cases, radiographs can help determine the extent of the damage. The prognosis is poor if the spinal cord is damaged. Once the animal is relatively stable, the wounds must be cleaned, debrided, and flushed with sterile saline and diluted disinfectant (i.e., chlorhexidine). Be careful when cleaning full-thickness fractures with exposed coelomic cavity. Turtles with full-thickness fractures or severe soft-tissue trauma need systemic antibiotic treatment (fig. 5.8).

Repair of Shell

Superficial cracks on the shell can be repaired using sterile fiberglass cloth impregnated with polymerizing epoxy resin. Contact with the soft tissue should be avoided. Dental acrylic can also be used. Full thickness fractures where the coelomic cavity has been exposed require surgical repair. In addition to shell repair, these animals require fluid and nutritional support and antibiotic therapy. They often have a prolonged recovery and adequate treatment is needed until the turtle is eating on its own and is free of infection.

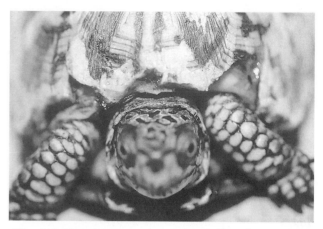

Fig. 5.8. Traumatic injury to the shell. (Photo courtesy of Ryan Cheek)

Overgrown Beak

Some turtles will develop an overgrown beak in captivity. This has been associated with an inadequate diet. The overgrown beak needs to be trimmed on a regular basis. For the most part this can be done without sedation. A dremmel tool works well (fig. 5.9 and 5.10).

Respiratory Disease

This is one of the most common presentations in clinical practice. Turtles do not have a diaphragm and as a result they cannot clear discharge in their lungs by coughing. Some predisposing factors to respiratory disease include improper diet, inadequate temperature and humidity, unhygienic conditions, and/or inappropriate substrate. Clinical signs of respiratory disease include a mucopurulent nasal discharge, ocular discharge, dyspnea, open-mouth breathing, anorexia, weight loss, and lethargy. Aquatic turtles may show

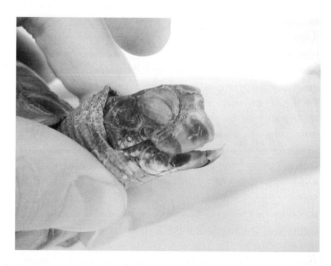

Fig. 5.9. Overgrown beak. (Photo courtesy of Dr. Stephen J. Hernandez-Divers, University of Georgia)

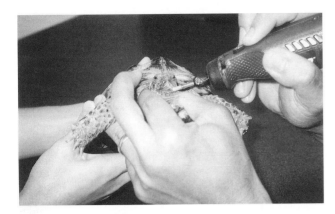

Fig. 5.10. Trimming an overgrown beak with a Dremmel tool. (Photo courtesy of Stephen J. Hernandez-Divers, University of Georgia)

inability to swim normally as they lose control of buoyancy. Pneumonia can be caused by bacteria, viruses, mycoplasma, and certain parasites. The diagnosis is based on the clinical signs, radiographs, transtracheal wash, and culture and sensitivity results. Treatment includes bactericidal antibiotics, nebulization, warmth, fluid therapy, and nutritional support.

Gout

Gout is a condition that involves the deposition of uric acid in the visceral organs and/or joints. It can be caused by kidney disease, dehydration, and diets high in protein. Clinical signs include lethargy, anorexia, lameness, and swollen joints. The diagnosis can be made by measuring serum/plasma uric acid levels, radiographs, and cytological evaluation of the material in the affected joints. The treatment involves the correction of the primary problem, but it is often unrewarding.

Gastrointestinal Tract Disease

There is a wide range of diseases that affect the gastrointestinal tract of chelonians. Stomatitis, parasites, foreign bodies, bacteria and fungal enteritis, and amoebic enterohepatitis are some of the most common conditions encountered in private practice. The clinical signs of gastrointestinal disease include anorexia, vomiting, weight loss, lethargy, dehydration, and abnormal stools. The diagnosis is based on a complete blood count, plasma biochemistries, fecal examinations, radiographs, endoscopy, and in some cases ultrasonography. The treatment is based on the disease present. Fluids and nutritional support are an important part of the therapy.

Reproductive Disorders

Dystocia is one of the most common reproductive problems seen in chelonians. The clinical signs include anorexia, lethargy, straining, and sometimes bloody discharge from the cloaca. The diagnosis of dystocia is based on radiographs. The predisposing factors include poor environmental conditions, metabolic disease, and improper husbandry. Cloacal prolapse in females during parturition and penile prolapse in males during copulation are common presentations in chelonians. This can be caused by trauma, infection, or cloacal impaction. Severe cases of penile prolapse often require amputation (fig. 5.11 and 5.12).

Aural Abscesses

While relatively common to see, the pathogenesis of aural abscesses isn't completely known. Improper husbandry and malnutrition may be predisposing factors. Treatment involves surgical intervention. The tympanic membrane is incised and exudate removed, followed by debridement and lavage of the wound. An antibiotic ointment may then be applied to the wound. The wound will be left open and lavaged daily, followed by ointment application until the wound heals by second intention (fig. 5.13; Murray 1996).

ZOONOSES

The greater number of zoonotic diseases associated with keeping turtles involve bacterial pathogens. The most widely recognized disease is salmonellosis. Children, immunosuppressed individuals, and the elderly are at greater risk of contracting salmonellosis. In the 1960s and 1970s, there was a large number of human cases of salmonellosis linked to pet turtles as the source of infection. In 1975, laws went into effect banning the sale of baby turtles with a carapace length of 4 inches or less. In 1999, the Centers for Disease Control estimated that of the millions of cases of

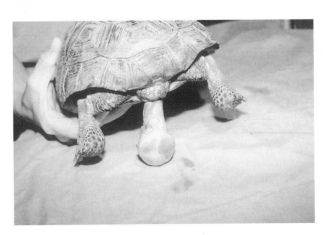

Fig. 5.11. Penile prolapse. (Photo courtesy of ZooAtlanta)

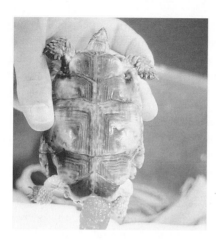

Fig. 5.12. Cloacal prolapse. (Photo courtesy of ZooAtlanta)

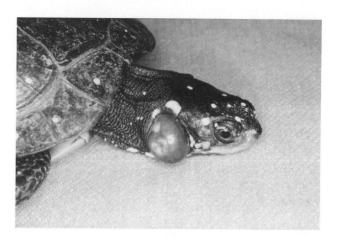

Fig. 5.13. Aural abscess. (Photo courtesy of Dr. Stephen J. Hernandez-Divers, University of Georgia)

human salmonellosis reported between 1996 and 1998, only 7% per year was associated with reptile or amphibian contact (CDC 1999). The vast majority of human salmonellosis (approximately 80%) cases was associated with eating contaminated food. The genus *Salmonella* contains many species with thousands of different serotypes. Many of theses serotypes have been isolated from healthy turtles and have been associated with human salmonellosis. The symptoms in humans include abdominal pain, diarrhea, nausea, vomiting, and fever. Owners should be made aware of the potential health hazard when keeping turtles as pets. Proper sanitation is essential to decrease the risk of exposure. There is no effective or practical way to eliminate the bacteria from the intestinal flora of positive animals. The bacterial burden in the environment will greatly increase when the feces are allowed to build up in the enclosure. This will cause contamination of the turtle's environment and body surface increasing the risk of transmission to humans. That is why it is so important to practice strict hygiene when keeping turtles. By cleaning frequently, the bacterial contamination in the enclosure will be greatly reduced. Perhaps the decline in percentage of human cases of salmonellosis associated with pet turtles has been due to the increased awareness and practice of adequate hygiene.

Aeromona, *Campylobacter*, and *Pseudomonas* of reptile origin have been associated with illness in humans.

Reptiles can also be affected by several species of *Mycobacterium* that are known to cause disease in humans. *Mycobacterium* can cause a variety of lesions in reptiles. The route of transmission for humans is through direct contact or inhalation of contaminated particles.

The hallmark of disease prevention and decreased risk of exposure to potential zoonoses is adequate hygiene. This goes for both the pet owner and the health care provider. When sick turtles are hospitalized, it is imperative that they be kept in a clean environment and be handled carefully to prevent contamination of the hospital environment.

OBTAINING A HISTORY AND PERFORMING A PHYSICAL EXAMINATION

A thorough history is one of the most important aspects of the clinical evaluation. Improper diet, enclosure, temperature, and humidity are often major contributors to illness. One should always ask about previous illness. Any change in appetite, behavior, weight, and defecation (consistency and frequency) should be recorded. The origin of the animal (wild caught versus captive bred, bought from a pet store versus a private breeder) must be ascertained. Also inquire about other animals in the collection, whether there are other types of turtles and/or other reptiles in the household. Were any animals bought recently? Was the animal quarantined? All these questions will help to formulate a picture of the animal's husbandry and potential exposure to pathogens. As part of an initial evaluation, one should do a visual exam. Assess motor function if the animal is willing to walk. Check the plastron and carapace for any evidence of trauma or infection. Look at the skin of the legs and nails. Evaluate the head, eyes, nares, oral cavity, and tympanic membrane. Note any discharge, redness, or swelling. The lungs of chelonians can be auscultated by placing a wet hand towel between the carapace and the stethoscope to enhance the surface contact.

Restraint

The neck of most turtles has an S-shaped curve that allows the animal to withdraw the head within the shell. In most turtles the head can be extended by applying gentle pressure with your thumb and index finger behind the mandibles. In many cases the head can be grabbed by reaching from underneath. Turtles will quickly withdraw the head when approached from the top. Once you have a hold behind the temporomandibular joints, apply gentle traction to overcome the turtle's resistance; be careful not to be too forceful. It is important to avoid dorsoventral pressure with your fingers as this can cause damage to the soft tissue of the neck and trachea. This technique is limited by the size, physical condition, and disposition of the turtle. The head of box turtles can be a little harder to exteriorize. A box turtle can move the cranial part of the plastron upward, making the shell an almost impenetrable fort. In this case a tongue depressor or smooth stainless steel speculum can be used to pry the shell open. Insert your tool between the carapace and plastron and apply gentle pressure downward. Once exposed, a limb can be grabbed and one can attempt to restrain the head as described above. A more gentle approach is to place the turtle in a small amount of warm water. Most turtles will attempt to get out of the water and when it does, you can attempt to restrain a limb or the head. If the first attempt to restrain the turtle fails, the animal should be placed in its holding container and tried later. Patience is your best ally. In aquatic species, with long nails, a towel can be used to wrap the animal and hold the legs within the shell. Nails can inflict painful scratches to the handler. The towel can also be used to keep the head inside the shell in aggressive species. Remember that turtles, like other animals, will stress easily when handled excessively (fig. 5.14).

RADIOLOGY

Radiographs are an important diagnostic tool in the assessment of the musculoskeletal, respiratory, gastrointestinal, and reproductive systems. The dorsoventral (DV), lateral, and anterior-posterior views are recommended. The DV radiograph can be easily taken by placing the turtle on the table. Most often it will stay still long enough for you to take the radiograph. For the lateral and anterior-posterior views, a horizontal beam is desired. Elevate the turtle by using a round container that will fit under the plastron. Make sure the feet do not come in contact with the container. It is desirable to keep the patient in the sternal position. Tilting the turtle on its side is not recommended as this will often cause distortion of the lungs and visceral and reproductive organs. (see fig. 5.15)

ANESTHESIA

The overall health of the patient animal should be established in order to assess the anesthetic risk. Turtles should be well hydrated prior to anesthesia. The environmental temperature is also important. When anesthetized, turtles should be kept at their POTZ. Keeping them slightly warmer during recovery is recommended.

There are several techniques for anesthetizing chelonians. The preferred method is the use of parenteral drugs. Chelonians can be anesthetized using inhalation agents via mask or chamber induction but they can hold their breath for a long time making this technique time-consuming. If you are using gas induction, the uptake of the anesthetic agent can be increased by

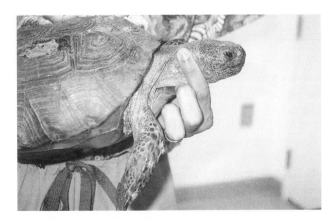

Fig. 5.14. Proper restraint. (Photo courtesy of Dr. Sam Rivera)

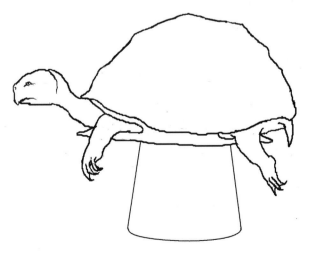

Fig. 5.15. Restraint for radiographs. (Drawing by Scott Stark)

manipulating the limbs in and out. This will enhance ventilation of the lungs. The IM and IV routes are frequently used for the administration of induction agents. Once the turtle is anesthetized it can be maintained using isoflurane or sevoflurane. The animal can be intubated using a proper size endotracheal tube. Alternatively, small red rubber catheters can be modified to serve as endotracheal tubes. In small patients, large-bore intravenous catheters can be used. The laryngeal opening is located near the based of the tongue. A cotton tip applicator can be used to gently move the tongue cranially while inserting the endotracheal tube. It is recommended to use a speculum to keep the mouth open and prevent the animal from biting the endotracheal tube. One should keep in mind that large chelonians have a strong jaw tone even if slightly sedated and can cause serious damage to fingers.

Monitoring anesthesia in chelonians can prove challenging. An EKG is ideal to monitor the cardiac function. An ultrasonic Doppler can be used to monitor the peripheral pulse in the limbs. The withdrawal and palpebral reflexes are sometimes helpful but not always reliable. A pulse oximeter with a cloacal probe can often be used to monitor oxygen saturation. It is recommended to use intermittent partial pressure ventilation in chelonians (four to eight breaths per minute). This will help ventilate the lungs and keep an adequate flow of oxygen and anesthetic agent in the lungs.

PARASITOLOGY

Turtles can be affected by a wide range of parasites. It is important to collect a fresh fecal sample. Dry feces are not recommended for use as many protozoan organisms die as the feces dry. You can advise the client to collect the feces at home, place the sample in multiple sealable plastic bags, and keep it refrigerated. Reiterate to the client the dangers of keeping reptile feces where food for human consumption is kept. If the sample is to be kept refrigerated, extreme hygiene is important to prevent cross contamination. The sample can be refrigerated overnight, but longer refrigeration is not recommended. The fecal exams must be done using fecal material and not urates. If a fresh sample is not available, a cloacal wash (see below) can be done to obtain a sample.

Direct fecal exam. Using a small wooden stick, place a small amount of feces on a microscope slide. Place a cover slip on top and examine immediately. The longer the sample sits the more likely motile protozoans will die. Do not use a cotton tip applicator as the cotton can absorb a substantial amount of your sample. Certain cysts can be difficult to identify. You can stain the sample by adding one drop of Lugol's solution. It is ideal to prepare two direct smears, one stained and one unstained. The Lugol's solution will kill motile protozoans. Some of the protozoans commonly encountered are hexamita, balantidium, nyctotherus, and coccidia.

Flotation. The flotation technique is done in the same manner as that for small animals. Use as much fecal sample as possible to increase the chances of finding parasite ova.

Cloacal wash. Using a soft rubber catheter, instill a small amount of saline solution in the cloaca. Collect the fluid for examination. This sample can be used for direct exam and flotation.

Turtles can be subclinical carriers of pathogenic amoeba species. *Entamoeba invadens* is an example of an amoeba that causes low morbidity in turtles but can cause severe illness and death in snakes and lizards. Nematodes, trematodes, and cestodes are common in turtles, particularly wild caught animals. It is important to keep in mind that chelonians are also affected by ectoparasites. Ticks, leeches, and cuterebra larvae can be found in turtles. See color plates 3.10 through 3.20.

EMERGENCY AND CRITICAL CARE

The most common emergency seen in private practice is trauma. Wild turtles hit by cars are unfortunately seen too often. The initial stabilization of the patient requires proper assessment of the injuries, antimicrobial therapy, fluid support, and adequate environmental temperature. When a turtle with severe trauma is presented, the shell as well as the limbs, head, and neck must be evaluated for the presence of blood. Once the wounds are identified, they must be cleaned thoroughly using sterile saline and a disinfectant. Antibiotics may be required to avoid infection of the wounds, which can lead to fatal septicemia. Turtles with massive trauma can become dehydrated quickly. Adequate fluid support is essential for a full recovery. Fluids can be given subcutaneously or in the intracoelomic cavity. Once the patient is stabilized, it should be kept at its preferred optimal temperature zone. This will allow for the immune system and other physiologic functions needed for healing to work efficiently. It is also important to provide nutritional support to the patient as soon as possible. Wild chelonians will not eat on their own initially and need to be force-fed. Adequate nutrition is important for a full recovery.

Chelonians with severe trauma take a long time to heal, but if they are handled properly from the time of initial presentation the recovery time can be reduced significantly.

CLINICAL TECHNIQUES

Blood Collection

The sites for blood collection in chelonians are the jugular, brachial, subcarapacial, tail(ventral and dorsal), and femoral veins, as well as the occipital sinus and the heart. Chelonians can prove challenging for blood collection. It is always a good idea to familiarize yourself with multiple venipuncture sites. The supplies needed depend on the size of the animal. Prior to blood collection, slides, hematocrit tubes, small-volume (0.5 ml) heparinized tubes, alcohol swabs,

needles (22–27 gauge), and syringes (0.5–3 ml) should be prepared. In patients smaller than 300 g, use a 25 to 27 gauge needle in a 0.5–1 cc syringe. In patients greater than 300 g, one can use a 22 gauge needle in a 3 cc syringe. Larger needles (20 g) can be used in turtles weighing over 5 kg (fig. 5.16).

Jugular Vein

The jugular vein is relatively superficial and located dorsally on the neck. Some turtles may need sedation for jugular venipuncture. In most turtles blood can be collected from this location as long as the head can be exteriorized. The neck should be held in the extended position. In some patients the vein can be visualized by applying digital pressure at the base of the neck, however this is not always the case. Once the vein is located, the needle should be inserted at a 30° angle and negative pressure applied as the needle is advanced.

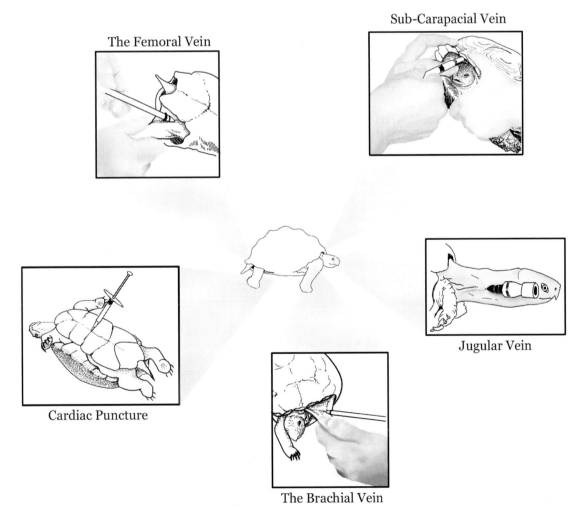

The Femoral Vein

Sub-Carapacial Vein

Cardiac Puncture

Jugular Vein

The Brachial Vein

Fig. 5.16. *Venipuncture sites. (Drawing by Scott Stark)*

The syringe will fill with blood as soon as the vein is entered. In some cases, the flow is slow. Once blood fills the hub of the needle, stop advancing and release suction on the plunger. Sometimes the vein will collapse. One should reapply gentle suction until the desired amount of blood is obtained.

Brachial Vein

The animal should be placed in sternal recumbency. One should then gently pull either forelimb to expose the brachial-antibrachial joint. The brachial vein is located deep to the triceps tendon. This tendon can be palpated on the caudal aspect of the extended leg. The needle should be inserted perpendicular to the skin, in the groove located ventral to the distal end of the tendon. Once the skin is entered, negative pressure should be applied and the needle advanced. Redirecting the needle may be needed to find the vein. Once the vein is entered, the vein blood will flow into the syringe.

Subcarapacial Vein

This vessel is located on the ventral aspect of the carapace along the dorsal midline. The animal should be restrained in sternal recumbency with the front end elevated at a 45° angle. With one hand, the head should be held inside the carapace. With the index finger of the other hand, the first vertebrae that is fused to the carapace along the dorsal midline should be palpated. The needle is inserted in the midline position and slowly directed to the space between the carapace and the vertebrae. Negative pressure should be applied as the needle is advanced. Blood will fill the syringe as the vein is entered.

Ventral Tail Vein

The turtle is restrained vertically with the plastron facing the phlebotomist or in dorsal recumbency. One should keep in mind that placing the animal in dorsal recumbency is stressful, therefore this should be done for the shortest amount of time possible. The tail should be extended and held as straight as possible. One should then insert the needle in the ventral midline, distal to the vent. It should be kept in mind that the further distal one goes, the smaller the diameter of the vein. The needle is then inserted at a 60° angle with the hub directed cranially. The needle should be advanced until the vertebral body is hit. One should then apply negative pressure and gently move the needle out (1–2 mm) until blood flows. This site is generally not productive as only a small volume can be obtained. Larger turtles in good physical condition can hold the tail close to the body making the tail very difficult to exteriorize.

Dorsal Tail Vein

The animal should be restrained in sternal recumbency. The tail should be held as straight as possible and the needle inserted in the dorsal tail midline. One should insert the needle, at a 30–45° angle, proximally near the junction between the tail and the caudal margin of the carapace. The needle is then advanced until the vertebral bodies are encountered. Negative pressure should be applied and the needle moved gently out (1–2 mm) until blood flows. If the tail cannot be exteriorized, the needle should be inserted in the proximal aspect of the tail midline and the steps followed as described above.

Femoral Vein

The turtle should be restrained vertically with the plastron facing the phlebotomist or in dorsal recumbency. It should be kept in mind that placing the animal in dorsal recumbency is stressful, therefore this should be done for the shortest amount of time possible. The femoral vein courses through the femoral triangle (the space through which the femoral vessels run to and from the hind limb), which is located at the most proximal end of the medial aspect of the hind limb. With one hand, the hind leg should be extended, and the other hand should be used to withdraw the blood sample. This, like many of the other techniques, is a blind stick. The needle should be inserted at a 45° angle and suction applied as the needle is advanced. Blood will fill the syringe as the vein is entered. Repositioning the needle should be minimized as damage can be done to nerves and other vessels located in this area.

Occipital Venous Sinus

The animal should be restrained in sternal recumbency and the head extended. The caudal aspect of the skull is then palpated. The sinus is located in the dorsal midline near the cranial cervical region. The needle should be inserted at a 60° angle. Negative pressure should be applied once the skin is penetrated as the needle is advanced. The syringe will fill with blood as the sinus is entered. Sometimes the needle can be repositioned to either side of the midline as the sinus can extend laterally. One should be careful not to go too deep.

Heart

This technique is relatively invasive as it requires drilling a hole through the plastron. A sterile drill or intramedullary pin can be used to perforate the plastron. The site of entry is where the ventral midline suture intersects the caudal suture of the pectoral scutes. The needle is then inserted perpendicularly as suction is applied. The correct location of the needle can sometimes be corroborated by the slight movement of the syringe caused by the heartbeat. Once blood is collected, the hole must be repaired using dental acrylic or epoxy resin. This is the author's least desirable site for blood collection and is used rarely.

Administration of Medications

Routes of Administration

Intramuscular Route: Antimicrobial agents and certain anesthesia induction agents are often given intramuscularly. Intramuscular injections are given in the muscle mass of the front legs. Chelonians have a renoportal circulation system. It is believed that medications injected in the caudal half of the body are filtered by the kidneys before entering the general circulation. However, this concept has been challenged in recent studies (Holz 1999). Until more is known about the role the renoportal circulation plays in filtering parenteral drugs, these medications should be given in the front half of the body—particularly drugs with potential nephrotoxic side effects.

Subcutaneous Route: Subcutaneous injections can be given in the inguinal and ventral neck skin folds. Fluid replacement can be given at a rate of 20 ml/kg every 24–48 hours.

Intravenous Route: The jugular vein can be used for the administration of fluids. This and the subcarapacial vein can be used for the administration of intravenous anesthetics.

Intracoelomic Route: The coelomic cavity can be accessed through the prefemoral fossa. The prefemoral fossa is the space just cranial to the pelvic limb into which the limb is retracted when the animal feels threatened. The intracoelomic route is most commonly used for the administration of fluids. Restrain the turtle in lateral recumbency; this will cause the viscera and reproductive organs to shift away from the injection site. Insert the needle parallel to the plastron and directed cranially in the ventral aspect of the fossa. If the needle is directed dorsally, there is a risk of injecting the fluids in the lungs. If the needle is directed medially, the fluids can go in the bladder. If the turtle urinates, you may be in the bladder; pull and reposition the needle. When injecting fluids into the coelomic cavity, keep in mind that the needle does not have to be inserted very deep. The fluids can be given at a rate of 20 ml/kg every 24–48 hours.

Oral Route: The supplies needed to administer oral medications or force-feeding are round-tip stainless steel tubes or red rubber catheters, speculums, and syringes of various sizes. Many sick turtles are anorexic. Nutritional support is essential for a full recovery. The most challenging part in many cases is opening the mouth. Some turtles will open their mouths when restrained. You can take advantage of this and insert a speculum or feeding tube quickly. If this fails, you must pry the mouth open. The upper beak in turtles hangs slightly over the lower beak. A blunt tool can be inserted under the upper beak and inserted in the mouth. Once in the oral cavity, twist the tool to pry the mouth open. Once the mouth is opened, the feeding tube or speculum can be inserted. The tube feeding volume is 1–2% of the body weight every 24–48 hours. Hold the head fully extended; measure the distance from the mouth to the mid plastron. Insert the feeding tube to the desired length and administer the feeding formula.

Intraosseous Route: This route is not frequently used but is available when needed. The two most commonly used sites are the tibia and the plastrocarapace bridge that connects the plastron and carapace on the lateral aspect of the body. An intraosseous needle with a stylet is desirable. A 22–20 gauge needle with a 25 gauge needle inside to serve as a stylet can be used which keeps the primary needle from becoming clogged (fig. 5.17).

Cloacal Route: Fluids and deworming medications can be administered via the cloaca. A lubricated red

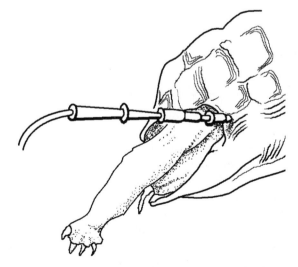

Fig. 5.17. Intraosseous catheter. (Drawing by Scott Stark)

rubber catheter or ball-tipped stainless steel tube can be placed in the cloaca and the desired medication delivered. It is recommended to hold the turtle at an angle, with the cloaca elevated above the turtle's head to improve the absorption rate (Bonner 2000).

Nebulization: One of the most common problems seen in clinical practice is respiratory disease. Nebulization is a relatively stress-free method to deliver medications into the respiratory system. Turtles have lower respiratory rates than mammals and birds, therefore the nebulization time must be extended. In many cases, turtles have to be nebulized for an hour or longer to ensure that an adequate amount of medication is administered.

Catheter Placement (IV)

Jugular catheterization is reserved for patients that are extremely weak and in a very critical condition (fig. 5.18). Patients that are relatively stable will make it difficult to maintain and clean the catheter site. The procedure for IV catheter placement in a jugular vein is as follows:

1. Scrub the area of the jugular vein in the anesthetized patient.
2. Make a full thickness incision on the skin.
3. Identify the jugular vein using blunt dissection
4. Insert the IV catheter of adequate size depending on the size of the turtle.
5. Place a butterfly tape over the catheter and cap and suture to the skin.

IV bolus fluids can be given at a rate of 1–2 ml/kg over a 15 to 30 minute period.

EUTHANASIA

In some cases, euthanasia is the most humane course of action. Ill animals with a poor to grave prognosis or severely injured animals may require humane euthanasia. The hardest part of euthanizing turtles is knowing whether or not they are dead. This can be a tricky question to answer. Some of the signs that help determine if the patient is dead include absence of a heartbeat, no response to pain (i.e., corneal reflex), rigor mortis, cyanotic mucous membranes, and sunken flat eyes. An EKG or ultrasound can be used to assess the heartbeat; however, keep in mind that in turtles the heart can continue to beat several hours after euthanasia. The author's preferred method of

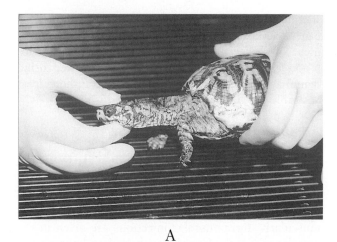

A

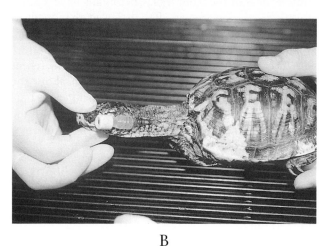

B

Fig. 5.18. *Jugular catheter placement.* **A.** *Proper restraint for jugular catheterization.* **B.** *Placement of jugular catheter. (Photos courtesy of Ryan Cheek)*

euthanasia in turtles is lethal injection. The euthanasia solution can be given intravenously or intracoelomically. In some cases, it is recommended that the turtle be kept in the clinic overnight to ensure the animal is dead. Several sources have referred to freezing as an alternative method for euthanasia but this is considered inhumane.

REFERENCES

Anonymous. 1990. "Guideline for the housing of turtles and tortoises: Minimum standard housing guidelines for pet shops, wholesale animal dealers, and other commercial establishments." *New York Turtle and Tortoise Society Newsletter* 19(5).
Bonner, BB. 2000. "Chelonian therapeutics." *The Veterinary Clinics of North America, Exotic Animal Practice.* Ed Fronefield, SA. 3(7): 257–332.

Boyer, TH, Boyer, DM. 1994. "Tortoise care." *Bull Assoc Reptil Amphi Vet* 4(1): 16–27.

Boyer, TH, Boyer, DM. 1996. "Turtles, tortoises, and terrapins." In *Reptile Medicine and Surgery*, edited by Douglas R. Mader. Philadelphia: W.B. Saunders Co.

Centers for Disease Control and Prevention. 1999. "Reptile-associated salmonellosis—selected states 1996–1998." MMWR 48, 1009.

Frye, FL. 1991. *A practical guide for feeding captive reptiles.* Melbourne: Krieger Publishing

Girgis, S. 1961. "Aquatic respiration in the common Nile turtle, *Trionyx triunguis*." *Comp Biochem Physiol* 3: 206.

Holz, PH. 1999. The reptilian renal portal system—a review. *Bull Assoc Reptil Amphi Vet* 9(1): 4.

Murray, M. 1996. "Aural abscesses." In *Reptile Medicine and Surgery*, edited by Douglas R. Mader. Philadelphia: W.B. Saunders Co.

Wood, SC, Lenfant, CJM. 1976. "Respiration: Mechanics, control, and gas exchange." In *Biology of Reptilians*, vol 5, edited by C. Gans, 225–274. San Diego: Academic Press.

CHAPTER SIX

The Amphibians

Brad Wilson

INTRODUCTION, TAXONOMY, AND NATURAL HISTORY

A fascination with amphibians has gripped humans since the first recorded history and continues today through scientific discoveries of remarkable healing and disease resistance properties of amphibian tissues, the discovery of potential therapeutic compounds in amphibian skin, and the understanding of potential human and animal health consequences resulting from environmental alteration. Interest in captive amphibians over the last decade has increased tremendously and the knowledge gained regarding the husbandry, physiology, and breeding habits of many species has likely exceeded that of any other exotic pet group during this time period.

Similarly, the demand for veterinary care for these species has exceeded the capabilities of the veterinary profession and has far exceeded the provisions of formal veterinary education. The recent publication of Wright and Whitaker (2001) is the first major step in educating the profession in the health care of amphibians. In general, scientific literature regarding amphibian medicine has been restricted to symposia presentations, society journals (American Association of Zoo Veterinarians), and several hobbyist books and publications. Awareness of the demand for health care in these animals and the willingness of many clients to treat these pets has stimulated and necessitated a demand for more education by veterinarians and veterinary technicians.

Taxonomy

The biological saying "ontogeny recapitulates phylogeny" is most appropriately applied to the natural history of amphibians. The life cycle of the amphibian from egg to adult (ontogeny) is the abridged version of the monumental evolutionary adaptations of amphibians (phylogeny) that enabled the vertebrates to leave water and colonize the land 350 million years ago (Wright 2001e; Goin, Goin, & Zug 1978). Modern amphib-

ians comprise over four thousand species (Wright 2001g) that are classified into three orders based on anatomic characteristics. The orders are listed with the modern accepted nomenclature followed by commonly used traditional nomenclature in parentheses: the caecilians, Gymnophiona (Apoda); the sirens, salamanders, and newts, Caudata (Meantes and Urodela); and the frogs and toads, Anura (Salientia). See table 6.1 for species commonly kept in captivity.

Amphibians of the order Gymnophiona, caecilians, are uncommonly kept as pets and even less commonly observed clinically. Originating in the eastern and western tropics, caecilians may be terrestrial (yellow-striped caecilian, *Ichthyophis kohtoaensis*) or totally aquatic (*Typhlonectes compressicauda*) as adults. To many, caecilians resemble snakes or oversized earthworms. All known species are limbless with greatly reduced eyes. Some species are oviparous (egg-laying) and some are viviparous (live-bearing). All known species are carnivorous and consume various arthropods, annelids, or gastropods. Because of their secretive nature, it is likely that many species remain undiscovered. Longevity of captive caecilians is reported at 9 years (Goin et al. 1978).

The order Caudata, tailed amphibians, consists of salamanders, newts, sirens, and amphiumas. Sirens were once classified in a separate order, Meantes (Trachystomata). The majority of species inhabits North America with one species in Africa, and no species in Australia or Antarctica (Goin et al. 1978; Duellman & Trueb 1994). Many species of all suborders are maintained as pets, though few are commercially available. Few species venture far from water or moist environs and most species require water for some portion of reproduction or development. Some species are fully aquatic, some facultatively aquatic, some terrestrial; and some American newts (*Notophthalmus viridescens*) are aquatic as larvae, terrestrial as juveniles, and aquatic again as adults. Salamanders are carnivorous as both larvae and adults and consume various arthropods, gastropods,

Table 6.1. Amphibians Commonly Kept in Captivity

Common name/species name	Origin	Habitat	Size (cm)[1]	T/H[2]	Repro[3]	Feed[4]	Care[5]	Handling concerns[6]
Gymnophiona								
Yellow-striped, *Ichthyophis kohtoaensis*[7,13]	SE Asia	fossorial, tropical	50	25/mod	oviparous	an,ar	mod; large	docile, sturdy; escape
Aquatic caecilian, *Typhlonectes* spp.[7,13]	S America	aquatic, tropical	to 50	25	viviparous	an,ar	easy; medium	docile, sturdy; escape
Caudata								
Cryptobranchidae (Giant salamanders)								
Hellbender, *Cryptobranchus alleganiensis*[7]	N America	aquatic, temperate	to 75	15	oviparous	cr,ar,v	diff+; large+#	occas aggressive, sturdy
Sirenidae (Sirens)								
Greater siren, *Siren lacertina*[7]	e N America	aquatic, temperate	80	20	oviparous	ar,cr,v	mod; large+	occas aggressive, sturdy
Amphiumidae (Amphiumas)								
Amphiuma, *Amphiuma means*[7]	e N America	aquatic, temperate	to 100	20	oviparous	ar,cr,v	mod; large+	aggressive, sturdy
Proteidae (Neotenic salamanders)								
Mudpuppy, *Necturus maculosus*[7]	e N America	aquatic, temperate	40	15	oviparous	ar,cr,v,g	diff; large#	docile, sturdy
Ambystomatidae (Mole salamanders)								
Axolotl, *Ambystoma mexicanum*[7]	C America	aquatic, tropical	20	20	oviparous	ar,cr,v	easy; medium	aggressive, sturdy
Tiger salamander, *Ambystoma tigrinum*[7]	N America	terrestrial, fossorial	25	22/mod	oviparous	ar,an,v	easy; small	aggressive, sturdy
Waterdog, *Ambystoma tigrinum*[9]	N America	temporary aquatic; terrestrial	20	20	n/a	an,ar, cr,v	easy; small	aggressive, sturdy
Plethodontidae (Lungless salamanders)								
Arboreal salamander, *Aniedes lugubris*[10,11]	w N America	terr/arbor, temperate forest	10	14 to 17/ mod	oviparous	ar	mod; small	occas. aggressive, sturdy
Palm salamander, *Bolitoglossa* spp.[13]	C,S America	terr/arbor, tropical forest	8 to 14	14 to 20/ high	oviparous	t,ar	diff+; medium	docile, fragile

Species	Distribution	Habitat	Size	Temp/humidity	Reproduction	Zones	Care	Temperament
Ensatina, *Ensatina* spp. [10,11]	w N America	terrestrial, temperate forest	7	14 to 17/ mod	oviparous	ar	mod; small	docile, sturdy
Red salamanders, *Pseudotriton* spp. [11]	N America	semiaquatic, streams, forests	15	20/mod	oviparous	an,ar	mod; small	docile, sturdy
Anura								
Pipidae (Clawed frogs)								
Dwarf frog, *Hymenochirus curtipes* [8,13]	Africa	aquatic, tropical	4	25	oviparous	an,ar	easy; small	docile, sturdy
Surinam toad, *Pipa pipa* [8,13]	S America	aquatic, tropical	20	25	oviparous	v,an,ar	mod; large+	docile, sturdy
African clawed frog, *Xenopus laevis* [8,13]	Africa	aquatic, tropical	12	25	oviparous	v,an,ar	easy; medium	docile, sturdy
Pelobatidae (Spadefoot toads)								
Asian leaf frogs, *Megophrys* spp. [13]	SE Asia	terrestrial, tropical	to 15	20–22/ mod	oviparous	ar,v	mod; medium	docile, sturdy
Bufonidae (True toads)								
Harlequin toads, *Atelopus* spp. [9]	C,S America	terrestrial, montane tropical	to 5	15–20/ high	oviparous	ar,t	diff+; medium	docile, fragile
American toad, *Bufo americanus* [13]	N America	terrestrial, temperate	to 10	20/low	oviparous	ar,g,v	easy; medium	docile, sturdy
Marine toad, *Bufo marinus* [13]	C,S America	terrestrial, temp/ tropical	23	22/low	oviparous	ar,g,v	easy; large	occas. aggressive, sturdy
Asian tree toads, *Pedostibes* spp. [13]	SE Asia	terrestrial, tropical	to 10	25 to 27/ high	oviparous	t	diff; large	docile, fragile to sturdy
Microhylidae (Narrow mouth toads)								
Tomato frogs, *Dyscophus* spp. [8,13]	Madagascar	semiaquatic, tropical	to 10	25/mod	oviparous	ar	easy; medium	docile, sturdy
Malaysian toad, *Kaloula pulchra* [8,13]	SE Asia	terrestrial/fossorial, tropical	7	25/high	oviparous	ar,t	easy; medium	docile, sturdy
Dendrobatidae (Poison dart frogs)								
Dendrobates, *Phyllobates*, *Epipedobates* spp. [12,13]	C,S America	terrestrial, tropical	1.5 to 5	22 to 30/ high	oviparous	ar,t	easy to diff; varies	occas. aggressive - see below
Hylidae (Tree frogs)								
Red-eyed treefrog, *Agalychnis callidryas* [14]	C America	arboreal, tropical	7	25/high	oviparous	ar	easy; medium	docile, sturdy

(Table 6.1 continued)

Table 6.1. continued

Common name/species name	Origin	Habitat	Size (cm)[1]	T/H[2]	Repro[3]	Feed[4]	Care[5]	Handling concerns[6]
Green treefrog, *Hyla cinerea*[13]	N America	arboreal, temperate	6	25/mod	oviparous	ar	easy; medium	docile, sturdy
Monkey frogs, *Phyllomedusa* spp.[14]	C, S America	arboreal, tropical	to 10	25/low to mod	oviparous	ar	mod; med to lg	docile, sturdy
White's treefrog, *Litoria caerulea*[7,14]	Australia	arboreal, desert/forest	10	25/low to mod	oviparous	ar	easy; medium	docile, sturdy
Ranidae (True frogs)								
Mantellas, *Mantella* spp.[13]	Madagascar	terrestrial, tropical	3	18 to 22/high	oviparous	ar,t	easy; small+	docile, fragile to sturdy
American bullfrog, *Rana catesbeiana*[13]	N America	semiaquatic, temperate	to 20	22/mod	oviparous	v,ar	easy; large+	aggressive, sturdy
African pyxie frog, *Pyxicephalus adspersus*[13]	Africa	semiaquatic, temperate	to 20	25/mod	oviparous	v,ar	easy; large+	aggressive, sturdy
Eyelash frog, *Ceratobatrachus guentheri*[13]	Solomon Islands	terrestrial, tropical	8	25/mod	oviparous	ar	mod; medium	docile, sturdy
Leptodactylidae (Tropical frogs)								
Surinam horned frog, *Ceratophrys cornuta*[13]	S America	terrestrial, tropical	20	25/mod	oviparous	v,ar	diff; medium	aggressive, sturdy
Ornate horned frog, *Ceratophrys ornata*[13]	S America	terrestrial, tropical	12	25/mod	oviparous	v,ar	easy; medium	aggressive, sturdy

[1] Average maximum adult size.

[2] Average day temperature/relative humidity for adults of species or typical of genus in captivity.

[3] Oviparous (ovi-) = egg laying; viviparous (vivi-) = live birth.

[4] Diet of the adult amphibian *in nature* listed in order of importance for each species: *an* = annelids; *ar* = arthropods; *cr* = crustaceans; *g* = gastropods; *t* = termites and ants; *v* = vertebrates. Many animals will adapt to domestically raised food items.

[5] Difficulty for captive maintenance of wild-caught and some captive-born animals. (Generally, captive-born animals adapt well with proper conditions.) Second value is minimum terrarium size. *Easy* = adapts well to terrarium; *moderate* = specialized feeding, temperature, housing required; *difficult* = only most experienced keepers; *difficult +* = should only be attempted by zoological parks. *Small* = 10 gallon terrarium; *medium* = 15 to 20 gallon terrarium; *large* = 30 gallon terrarium; *large+* = 55 gallon or specially constructed; # = may require chilled water.

[6] Typical response of patient to handling (all animals will resist handling): *Docile* = will not attempt to bite, no special defenses. All caecilians may escape; terrarium must be well sealed. *Occasionally aggressive* = may attempt to bite, but generally will not cause injury to handler. Can bite and seriously damage or kill cage mates. Avoid skin or direct/indirect mucous membrane contact with wild-caught dart frogs and all marine toads. *Aggressive* = species that will routinely bite as defense (Amphiuma) or conditioned feeding response (mole salamanders) *or* will attempt to eat any cage mates (frogs, mole salamanders). Amphiumas, pyxie frogs, and horned frogs must be approached and handled with caution; bites from adult animals may cut skin and may be painful. *Fragile* = amphibians that may be easily stressed, damaged, or killed by handling. *Sturdy* = amphibians that are not likely damaged from responsible handling.

[7] Wright (2001g, 3–14).

[8] Mattison (1987).

[9] Lotters (1996).

[10] Stebbins (1985).

[11] Petranka (1998).

[12] Walls (1994).

[13] Obst et al. (1988).

[14] de Vosjoli (1996).

arachnids, annelids, crustaceans, and other vertebrates including mammals. Longevity of salamanders is known to be up to 55 years for the Japanese giant salamander (*Adrias japonicus*) (Goin et al. 1978). Generally, the larger species have a longer lifespan than smaller species.

The order Anura, tailless amphibians, consists of frogs and toads. This order represents the great majority of all species of modern amphibians and the majority of captive amphibians. A great number of species is available in the pet trade as captive-born animals. Frogs are to amphibians as lizards are to reptiles. Frogs have managed to adapt to and to populate many terrestrial, arboreal, and aquatic (and even one flying!) habitats on earth. Adaptation and specialization of skin, diet, and reproductive strategy have made this expansion possible. All adult frogs are carnivorous and the majority of their larvae, tadpoles, are herbivorous. Some tadpoles are omnivorous and some are carnivorous. Adult frogs feed on many insects, crustaceans, annelids, and other vertebrates, and some species are specialized to feed primarily on other frogs (*Ceratophrys* spp., *Hemiphractus* spp.). Known longevity for some species is up to 36 years (Goin et al. 1978).

Amphibians begin development as fertilized eggs, and with most species the eggs hatch into free-swimming gilled larvae, which, in turn, metamorphose into adults. The posthatching larvae are dependent upon a moist environment such as open water, inside a gelatinous terrestrial egg (some species undergo direct development and metamorphose to adults inside the eggs), inside a brooding adaptation of the parent, or inside a uteruslike oviduct (some amphibians are live bearing, or viviparous). Not all amphibian larvae require standing water to complete development. Similarly, all adult amphibians are not dependent on standing water to reproduce, though traditionally most amphibians do return to water both to mate and to disperse eggs. Some amphibians are entirely aquatic and cannot survive out of water for any extended periods of time, whereas others inhabit deserts or may aestivate for extended periods (years) with no exogenous water. Completely aquatic amphibians are represented in all three families. Some salamanders are neotenic, in which metamorphosis to the typical adult form never occurs yet the larvae develop gonads internally and the larvae are capable of reproduction.

Though most numerous in temperate to tropical environments, amphibians are distributed worldwide. Frogs are found among nearly every habitat on earth except the open ocean and Antarctica. Particularly interesting among the frogs is their colonization of harsh deserts. Adaptation for desert environments is most widespread among the frogs of Australia as seen in both terrestrial (*Arenophryne rotunda*) (Mattison 1987) and arboreal (*Litoria* spp.) species and among the South African terrestrial species (*Breviceps* spp.). Several South American species (*Atelopus* spp.) are adapted to cool elevations well over ten thousand feet (Lotters 1996) and some species of North American frogs (*Rana sylvatica*) are known to freeze solid during hibernation and then thaw following winter to resume normal physiology (Duellman & Trueb 1994; Mattison 1987; Stebbins 1985).

The veterinary technician should be familiar with herpetological scientific nomenclature and common terminology. It is not uncommon that scientific order, family, or group names of both plants and animals may be modified for use in general conversation or popular and scientific publications. For instance, when speaking of the three orders of amphibians, frogs and toads (Anura) are commonly called anurans. Salamanders (Caudata) are called caudates. With the salamanders and frogs, the family names are commonly modified when discussing several of the larger families: the mole salamanders (Ambystomatidae) are ambystomatids; the lungless salamanders (Plethodontidae) are plethodontids; the poison dart frogs (Dendrobatidae) are dendrobatids; the tree frogs (Hylidae) are hylids; the true toads (Bufonidae) are bufonids; and so on.

Much of this chapter will focus on frogs. This is due to the fact that frogs are, by far, the most popular and widespread amphibian group in the pet industry. Much of the medicine, anesthesia, and surgery techniques applied to frogs are extrapolated to all amphibians. The general discussion of amphibian medicine will focus on metamorphosed juvenile and adult amphibians with a separate general discussion of larvae. The husbandry and disorders of larvae can differ significantly from the adults of some species.

ANATOMY AND PHYSIOLOGY

General anatomy is similar across all three orders of amphibians and is discussed as it applies to all amphibians. Anatomical specializations and clinically significant differences in anatomy are described for the three orders. Physiology varies tremendously even among genera and species of the same order and clinically significant differences are noted in the following discussion.

Integument
The evolutionary development of amphibian skin is one of the greatest adaptations that enabled verte-

brates to leave the water and exist on land. The epidermal layer of amphibian skin is shed routinely (ecdysis) in a manner consistent with lizards and snakes. Ecdysis may occur piecemeal or entirely, and some caecilians, frogs, and salamanders consume the shed skin; a process called keratophagy or dermatophagy. The dermis layers of skin serve a respiratory function and are highly vascularized. Some caecilians possess small scales that are imbedded in the skin (Goin et al. 1978; Duellman & Trueb 1994).

The respiratory function of amphibian skin is particularly important for larvae, adult caecilians, most adult salamanders, and many frogs. Several species of amphibians and one family of salamanders (Plethodontidae) have absent or greatly reduced lungs and rely on cutaneous respiration for the majority of oxygen and carbon dioxide exchange. The hellbenders (Cryptobranchus spp.) and giant Asian salamanders (Adrias spp.), both of which are aquatic, have well-developed lateral skin folds, which increase surface area for cutaneous gas exchange. An interesting behavior exhibited by Cryptobranchus spp. is a rocking motion in which the salamander sways the body from side to side in slow moving or poorly oxygenated water presumably to "ventilate" the skin (Duellman & Trueb 1994; Petranka 1998).

The amphibian epidermis is rich with glands. Some epidermal glands produce secretions that moisten the skin to facilitate cutaneous respiration and some frogs (Phyllomedusa spp.) secrete waxy substances that protect against dehydration and desiccation (Wright 2001b). Poison glands are present in all salamanders and frogs. These are most notable among the poison dart frogs (Dendrobatidae) of Central and South America and toads worldwide. Of all amphibians, the skin secretions of Phyllobates terribilis, the golden dart frog of Colombia, are the most toxic (Walls 1994). The Chaco Indians of Colombia use skin secretions of three species of Phyllobates to coat blow darts used to hunt monkeys, hence the common family name of these frogs. Of the 170 species of Dendrobatidae, only P. terribilis is considered lethal to humans from simply touching the toxin. Interestingly, wild-caught dart frogs of all species fed domestic diets in captivity and frogs born in captivity lose the majority of their skin toxins (Daly et al. 1994).

Several species of toads and salamanders possess large parotid glands dorsally on the head, just caudal to the skull. These glands are elliptical and commonly the site of profuse toxin excretion. Skin toxins from many frogs and toads are dangerous to domestic animals such as dogs and cats. The author has observed a 20 kg Labrador retriever suffer violent vomiting,

diarrhea, and convulsions following the accidental ingestion of a Cuban tree frog (Osteopilus septentrionalis). Anecdotal reports exist of deaths in dogs and cats following exposure to or ingestion of toxic secretions of marine toads (Bufo marinus). In general, all terrestrial frogs and toads should be considered potentially dangerous to dogs and cats. Other captive amphibians that should be considered toxic include the European salamander (Salamandra salamandra), the American newt (Notophthalmus viridescens), and some mole salamanders (Ambystoma spp.).

Many of the more toxic amphibians exhibit aposematic coloration and are conspicuous or active by day. Animals that exhibit aposematic or warning colors rely on a learned response of the potential predator to avoid interaction with the particular animal or suffer distasteful or noxious stimuli. Some of the commonly observed aposematically colored amphibians include the European salamander (Salamandra salamandra), the red eft phase of the American newt (Notophthalmus viridescens), red salamanders (Pseudotriton spp.), some poison dart frogs (Dendrobatidae), some harlequin frogs (Atelopus spp.), the golden mantella (Mantella aurantiaca), and the semiaquatic fire-bellied toads (Bombina spp.). As with some insects and snakes, mimicry in coloration occurs in several "nontoxic" species that co-occur with more toxic species.

Several species of frogs possess unique skin adaptations for raising young. The aquatic female Surinam toad (Pipa pipa) carries eggs on her back over several months during which time the eggs invaginate into the skin and undergo direct development into juvenile frogs. Upon hatching, the juvenile frogs swim out of the holes in the skin ending parental care. Another female South American frog, the marsupial frog (Gastrotheca spp.), possesses a pouch on the dorsum in which eggs hatch into tadpoles (or undergo direct development in some species) and are then released into a suitable aquatic habitat.

Skeletal System

The skeleton of amphibians is composed of both an endoskeleton and exoskeleton that is ossified. The exoskeleton is bone formed in the dermis that fuses with underlying endoskeleton and is most notable in the skull of amphibians, particularly in frogs and toads. The amphibian skeletal system has three functions: protection, locomotion, and support for terrestrial existence. A major adaptation for locomotion on land is the development of pelvic and pectoral girdles. These are absent in caecilians, but well developed in most salamanders and all frogs (Goin et al. 1978).

Great variation of the appendicular skeleton exists among species of frogs and toads. In most frogs and some salamanders, the hyoid bones are modified to eject the tongue for prehension of prey (figs. 6.1 and 6.2).

Digestive System

All adult amphibians are carnivorous and have a digestive tract that is similar to higher carnivorous vertebrates and also similar among the three orders of amphibians. The oral cavity of salamanders and frogs is spacious and generally designed for capturing and swallowing whole prey items. A fleshy tongue is present in most species. Aquatic salamanders have a primary fishlike tongue and aquatic frogs (Pipidae) have no tongue (Goin et al. 1978). Amphibian teeth are replaced throughout life when lost (Goin et al. 1978; Duellman & Trueb 1994).

Prehension of prey may occur by one of several modalities in amphibians: suction, hellbender (*Cryptobranchus* spp.) and Surinam toad (*Pipa pipa*); ambush or direct pounce and capture, mole salamanders (*Ambystoma* spp.) and toads (*Bufo* spp.); luring and capture, horned frogs (*Ceratophrys* spp.); foraging and prehension with tongue, palm salamanders (*Bolitoglossa* spp.) and dart frogs (*Dendrobates* spp.); and scavenging, *Amphiuma* spp., *Siren* spp., and aquatic caecilians (*Typhlonectes* spp.) (Helfman 1990).

The esophagus, stomach, small intestine, and large intestine are similar to that of higher vertebrates (fig. 6.3). The cloaca is homologous to that of reptiles. The pancreas and gall bladder are present and aid in digestion. The liver serves to convert ammonia into nitrogenous waste products, primarily urea. In at least two frog species, the Australian gastric brooding frogs, *Rheobatrachus* spp., the female ingests the fertilized eggs into the stomach where the eggs hatch into tadpoles and then metamorphose into juvenile frogs. During the brooding period all digestive secretions are stopped in these species (Duellman & Trueb 1994).

Respiratory System

Amphibians exhibit four modalities of respiration: branchial, buccopharyngeal, cutaneous, and pulmonic (Wright 2001c). Adult salamanders use the four modes

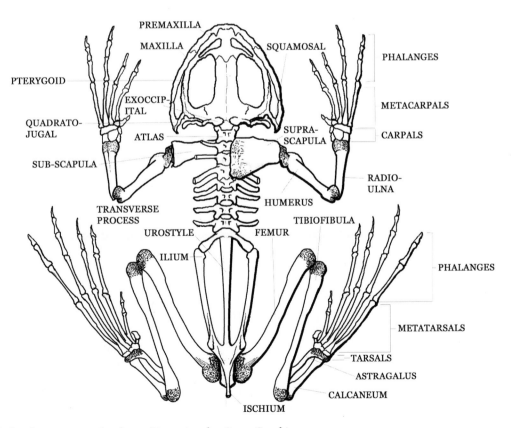

Fig. 6.1. Skeletal anatomy of a frog. (Drawing by Scott Stark)

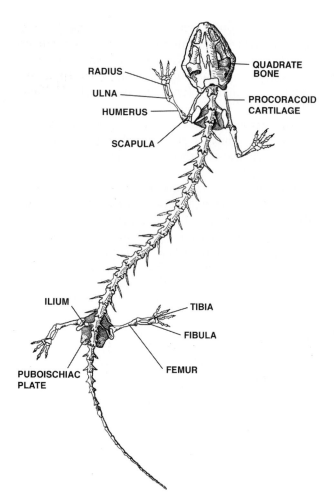

Fig. 6.2. *Salamander skeletal anatomy. (Drawing by Scott Stark)*

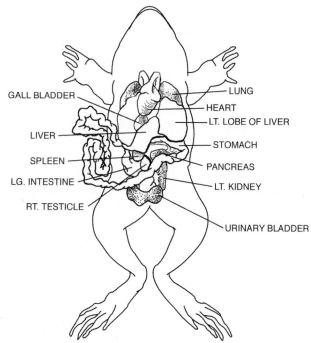

Fig. 6.3. *Visceral anatomy of a frog. (Drawing by Scott Stark)*

of respiration and adult caecilians and frogs do not use the branchial mode. In most amphibians, left and right lungs are of equal size. Some caecilians have a greatly reduced or absent left lung as observed in snakes.

Branchial or gill respiration is present in free-swimming larvae of all amphibians and in neotenic or aquatic salamanders. Those species with external gills may exhibit varying degrees of gill development dependent upon environmental conditions such as dissolved oxygen. In more stagnant oxygen-deprived environments, the gills are larger to increase oxygen-absorbing surface area. In well-oxygenated water, the gills are typically smaller. Some aquatic species (Sirenidae, Proteidae, Pipidae) may rely more on buccopharyngeal and pulmonic respiration by gulping air when oxygen content is critically low. Cutaneous respiration is discussed above in the integument system.

Buccopharyngeal respiration is primarily driven by air gulping in aquatic species and gular or buccal pumping in terrestrial species. Atmospheric air is pulled in through the nostrils to the nasopharynx and oral cavity by negative pressure during buccal expansion and then driven out by the collapse of the gular skin. Oxygen exchange occurs through the thin-walled buccopharyngeal capillaries. This pumping action also drives both inspiratory and expiratory pulmonic respiration in terrestrial amphibians. Buccopharyngeal gas exchange in amphibians is analogous to that of some freshwater air-gulping fishes such as the electric eel (*Electrophorus electricus*) and the lungfishes (*Protopterus* spp. and *Lepidosiren* spp.).

All terrestrial amphibians except salamanders of Plethodontidae, which do not have lungs, utilize pulmonic respiration. Amphibian lungs are saclike with alveoli most well developed in the Anurans. The lungs of some aquatic amphibians serve as hydrostatic or buoyancy organs in addition to the respiratory function (Wright 2001c).

Vocalization is most well developed in frogs, but is also observed in caecilians and salamanders of various species. Frogs are the only order of amphibians in which anatomic vocal structures are well developed and in which vocalization is known to serve as communication for mating, territorial defense, and escape from predators (Duellman & Trueb 1994). Vocalization is unique for every species and is also present in aquatic species. Males are the most vocal of the sexes, but females of some species have "distress calls," which are used when escaping predators, or "release calls" to signal males when the female is unreceptive during opportunistic breeding congregations.

Excretory System

The kidney of amphibians is mesonephric and empties into a urinary bladder. The urinary bladder of some amphibians may be bilobate. As in reptiles, urine is collected by the Wolffian duct (mesonephric duct in amphibians, metanephric duct in reptiles) and then routed to the cloaca and not the urinary bladder. Urine passes retrograde from the cloaca into the urinary bladder (Goin et al. 1978).

Nitrogenous wastes of primarily aquatic amphibians are excreted as ammonia whereas many terrestrial amphibians secrete urinary wastes as urea or uric acid. This conversion of ammonia to urea and uric acid conserves water for terrestrial amphibians and reduces the toxicity of ammonia in the blood. Frogs of the genus *Phyllomedusa* are uricotelic, being able to convert urea to uric acid for excretion (Wright 2001c).

Reproductive System

Amphibians have paired internal gonads that are hormonally regulated. Collecting ducts (oviducts in female) transport gametes to the cloaca where they are expelled from the body. Viviparous species are present in all three orders and the larvae undergo metamorphosis in the oviduct of the female and are born as fully functional juveniles. Fat bodies are located adjacent to the gonads of all amphibians and are presumed to provide nutrient stores for developing gametes. These bodies enlarge during nonbreeding season and are greatly diminished at the end of breeding season.

The testes of frogs are a collection of seminiferous tubules connected to the mesonephric ducts by collecting ducts. Frogs exhibit the greatest organizational structure of seminiferous tubules among the amphibians. The testes (and ovaries) enlarge dramatically in response to the breeding season. Copulation is observed in all caecilians and only one species of frog and fertilization is internal in these species. Fertilization for all other frogs is external. Interestingly, fertilization for all but two families of salamanders (Hynobiidae and Cryptobranchidae) is internal with no copulation. Male salamanders secrete a jellylike substance in the cloaca that encases the sperm, the spermatophore, and expel this structure during breeding. The female salamander collects the spermatophore in the cloaca and fertilization occurs

internally. Fertilization is internal in only a few frog species.

The amphibian ovaries are located in proximity to the kidneys as seen in higher vertebrates. Following ovulation ova are contained within a thin membrane, the ovisac, which ruptures and releases eggs into the coelom. Eggs are funneled into the ostium of the oviduct by cilia lining the coelomic mesentery and then passed to the cloaca to be expelled into the environment. The lining of the oviduct of viviparous caecilians is consumed by developing larvae as nourishment during development. In oviparous species the oviducts serve to store or hold eggs until spawning occurs. In salamanders a diverticulum of the dorsal wall of the cloaca forms the spermatheca, which stores collected sperm to fertilize eggs upon spawning.

Amphibians, especially frogs, exhibit tremendous adaptation in parental care of developing eggs and larvae. These adaptations are discussed throughout the various sections.

Cardiovascular System

The cardiovascular system is composed of a three-chambered heart, arteries, veins, and lymphatics. The heart of *Siren intermedia* and *Necturus maculosus* contains an interventricular septum making a four-chambered heart (Goin et al. 1978). As with reptiles, oxygenated and deoxygenated blood mixes minimally in the common ventricle.

The three orders of amphibians exhibit great variation in the development of aortic arch vasculature. A prominent ventral abdominal vein is present in amphibians as in reptiles. This is the vein of choice for blood collection in large frogs or toads. In salamanders not capable of tail autotomy (release of the tail when stressed), blood can be sampled from the ventral tail vein as described for snakes and lizards. Many frogs can also be sampled from the ventral lingual plexus in the mouth (see below, "Techniques").

Lymphatics and lymphatic circulation is well developed in amphibians. All blood cells and proteins except erythrocytes are found in amphibian lymph. Lymph hearts that beat synchronously and independently of the cardia control lymph circulation. In various locations of the body are lymph sacs from which diagnostic samples may be retrieved. Most notable of these are paired lymphatic sacs in the skin dorsal and caudal to the pelvis in frogs.

Amphibian blood and tissue fluids have a lower osmolality (200 to 250 mOsm) than mammals (300 mOsm) (Wright 2001c). Thus, isotonic fluids used for mammals are hypertonic to amphibians and will result in dehydration of the amphibian patient with long-term exposure. Mammalian saline is 0.9% NaCl. A 0.6% NaCl solution is most appropriate for use with amphibians.

Nervous System

The amphibian nervous system is modified from that of fishes with the enlargement of the cerebral hemispheres and the development of more complex neural networks in the spinal cord for the innervation of pectoral and pelvic limbs. A withdrawal response is observed in amphibians as a result of trauma such as damage to limbs and toes.

Sense Organs

Amphibian eyes, though not as highly adapted as those of reptiles for complete terrestrial existence, are greatly modified from the eyes of most fishes. Movable eyelids and lacrimal glands to moisten the eye are among the most notable adaptations. The eyelids are not present in amphibian larvae, most aquatic amphibians, and the neotenic axolotl. A third eyelid or nictitating membrane is present in many terrestrial frogs. It is similar to the same membrane of dogs and cats and its closure is passive, being achieved by contraction of the retractor bulbi muscle followed by withdrawal of the eye into the eye socket. A portion of the levator bulbi muscle actively controls retraction of the third eyelid back to its resting position.

The amphibian auditory system, while anatomically and physiologically interesting, has relatively little clinical significance. Jacobson's organ, the vomeronasal organ, is present in amphibians, but much less developed than in snakes and lizards. This sense organ is suspected to function in food recognition and in plethodontid salamanders (and possibly other genera) is thought to function for pheromone detection during courtship and mating.

HUSBANDRY

Knowledge of basic amphibian natural history and husbandry is sparse in the veterinary community. A basic understanding of the life history requirements of the species in question (or extrapolated from a closely related species) is needed to gain a thorough history and develop a diagnostic and treatment plan for amphibians. Even among different related species of amphibians, however, there may be dramatic diversity within a single genus. These differences are particularly evident among the genera of Dendrobatidae (*Dendrobates*, *Phyllobates*, *Epipedobates*), and the genera *Atelopus* and *Mantella*. The Dendrobatids are a diverse and geographically widespread group occurring from sea level to 2,600 m elevation; some species are terrestrial, some are entirely arboreal; some are 1.5 cm as adults, some are over 5 cm (Walls 1994). Similarly, the Atelopids have species groups that are termed highland (2,600–4,500 m) or lowland (< 1,000 m) (Lotters 1996). If a highland species is maintained as a lowland species or vice versa, the frog will fail to thrive and typically perish within days. Similar though less-extreme environmental diversity is seen among *Mantella* spp. (Staniszewski 1997).

Many of the natural history-related criteria for evaluating lizards (see chapter 3) apply to amphibians. The following list highlights the more pertinent information with which the technician and clinician should be familiar for a given species:

1. *Origin of the captive patient.*
   Is the patient captive-born or wild-caught? For the more common species in captivity, know which of these are more likely caught in the wild or propagated in captivity (see table 6.1).
2. *Preferred microhabitat.*
   Is the patient fossorial, terrestrial, arboreal, aquatic, or semiaquatic?
   What is the preferred air and/or water temperature of the patient?
   What is the preferred humidity of the patient?
3. *Behavior.*
   At what time of day is the patient active in normal health?
   Does the patient exhibit seasonal behavioral patterns such as hibernation?
   Does the patient exhibit certain defensive postures or behaviors when stressed or threatened?
4. *Diet.*
   What is the patient's preferred food in nature and what food items is it known to consume in captivity?
   What is the preferred size of food item?
   Is the patient an aggressive feeder that may attack or consume cage mates?
   At what time of day or night does the patient feed in habitat?
   What is the normal feeding behavior of the species in question?
5. *Anatomy and physiology.*
   What is the anatomy of the normal healthy patient including size or coloration differences between sexes of a given species?
   Are certain physical characteristics seasonally variable?
   Is the patient potentially toxic to cage mates?

The diversity of species' environmental adaptations necessitates this knowledge of amphibians even more than among the lizards, snakes, tortoises, and terrapins. Unfortunately, the majority of amphibian diseases progress rapidly or have a narrow window of treatment making the speed of diagnosis and treatment critical.

The greatest progress in successfully maintaining amphibians in captivity, particularly with the frogs, may be attributed to an understanding of the captive environment for each species. As with many reptiles, success with captive maintenance and breeding of amphibians has improved dramatically in the last 10 to 15 years through the research and experimentation of zookeepers and private hobbyists.

Enclosures and Environment

The four basic generalized amphibian cage designs are arboreal, terrestrial, semiaquatic, and aquatic. On occasion a mix of these designs is appropriate for some animals and each design may be slightly modified to house a particular species. With each of these habitats, there may be dramatic variation between species with regard to temperature and humidity in any given environment. With many species in their permanent enclosure, an effort is made to somewhat reproduce the natural environment to reduce stress and increase adaptability. Once again, having fundamental natural history knowledge of the patient is essential.

The health of the captive amphibian is directly proportional to the "health" of the terrarium. Certain characteristics apply to all amphibian enclosures. These include security from escape, visual and noise security, refuges for hiding, live plants, substrate, and the environmental parameters of lighting, temperature, humidity, ventilation, and water quality.

Security to prevent escape is of primary importance. The most elaborate climate-controlled naturalistic enclosure is of no help to the dried out carcass of an amphibian on the floor of a room. The evolutionary development of legs has greatly improved the ability for escape by amphibians when compared to fishes; some of the most escape-prone amphibians, however, are the legless caecilians and the sirens and amphiumas both of which have reduced limbs. Many fish enthusiasts can attest to similar escapes with eels, ropefish, lungfish, and other anguiform fish species. Though many aquatic and semiaquatic amphibians will perish in the dry environment of a climate controlled room, some, if they find suitable moist habitat elsewhere in the room, can survive quite well outside their intended enclosure. Barnett mentions the placement of "moist oasis" along the walls of such rooms to prevent desiccation in case an escape occurs (Barnett et al. 2001). These may be plastic containers lined with moistened moss and an adequate opening for entry.

Security from visual, noise, and vibration disturbance is essential for many species. With the exception of the most dominant or aggressive species (*Ceratophrys* spp., *Pyxicephalus* spp., large *Bufo* spp., large Ranidae spp., some *Ambystoma* spp., *Amphiuma* spp.), many amphibians rely on camouflage or escape as the first defense. Thus, when threatened, many frogs will attempt escape by jumping. Most enclosures are not of adequate size to prevent collision with the cage walls and the collisions may stimulate further escape behavior. Similar evasion may be seen with some salamanders and many aquatic amphibians though salamanders typically seek retreats or subterranean refuge. Physical trauma, however, may not be as significant as the stress created and the resultant maladaptation to a captive environment without adequate cover.

Visual security is provided by both internal and external cage design. Painting the external surfaces of the terrarium or applying other external visual barriers is helpful to prevent incessant escape attempts through the cage walls and to reduce sudden visual stimulation from movements outside the enclosure. Certain cage ornaments, accessories, and artificial or live plants are applied inside the cage for refuge and visual security. Clean plastic pots, sections of PVC pipe, the bases of plastic soda bottles, cork bark, sticks or logs, and rocks are all valuable as refuges. Though less naturalistic, the benefit of plastic refuges is that they are easily cleaned or sterilized for reuse. Cork bark may be autoclaved (if an autoclave is available) though it is not recommended to use detergents, ammonia, or bleach on any natural or porous cage accessories for amphibians. Thorough rinsing or detoxifying (from the cleaning agents) of these materials is almost impossible, and leaching into the enclosure is likely in a moist humid environment. Dried hardwood leaves are an excellent renewable refuge for salamanders and smaller frogs.

Understanding the behavior of a species in nature is helpful to proper cage design. Many arboreal frogs, for example, will not utilize substrate-interfaced or many horizontally oriented refuges but instead require vertically suspended flat leaves (*Agalychnis* spp., *Hyla* spp.) or horizontal branches (*Phyllomedusa* spp.) for resting. Similarly, terrestrial salamanders typically do not benefit from vertically spacious heavily planted terrariums, though the terrestrial cover provided by such plantings may be beneficial for reducing ground lighting. Larger terrestrial amphibians such as marine toads and mole salamanders seem particularly fond of artificial refuges in a terrarium and will regularly return to these areas when inactive. Aquatic caudates such as *Cryptobranchus* spp. and *Necturus* spp. occur in fast-moving coldwater streams and require large rocks, logs, or other submerged refuges to escape the currents. Often these animals also forage for food in these microhabitats as many food items similarly utilize the refuges to avoid strong currents.

Certain plants provide ideal refuges for some caudates and anurans. Bromeliads are an ideal tropical enclosure plants for smaller hylids, some dendrobatids, and the tropical *Bolitoglossa* spp. Some bromeliads, however, may have sharp defensive spines that can prove perilous to many amphibians and their owners! Many smaller aroids (peace lilies, *Spathiphyllum* spp.) are ideal for tree frogs (Gagliardo, personal communication). Large terrestrial amphibians are best maintained in terrariums that are sparsely planted or contain large sturdy plants. Marine toads, horned frogs, tiger salamanders, and large ranids are quite capable of trampling and eventually killing all but the sturdiest plants in a terrarium. In similar fashion, larger aquatic amphibians (all aquatics except dwarf aquatic frogs and newts) will uproot or damage planted aquatic terrariums in a matter of minutes to hours, though these species typically benefit from copious floating or suspended aquatic vegetation.

Plants for the terrarium are selected based on utility and aesthetic quality. Consideration must be given to the possibility for introduction of harmful pesticides, fertilizers, detergents, and potential pathogens. All plants, regardless of their origin, should be cleaned of all soil and thoroughly washed before planting. Also, plants from one established amphibian enclosure should never be moved to another amphibian enclosure to reduce the risk of parasite or other disease transmission to uninfected or otherwise unexposed animals. This must be strictly observed for plants originating from any enclosures containing wild-caught amphibians. Avoid using plants that originate in regions where there are known frog populations inhabiting or contacting the plants.

Basic requirements of an ideal soil-type substrate are a slowly degradable, well-drained, well-aerated, slightly moisture-retentive soil that is free of pesticides, fertilizers, or other potentially toxic chemicals. These soils, though all organic, contain many nontraditional components, which include horticultural grade charcoal, orchid bark, tree fern or palm trunk fiber, milled sphagnum, and some peat. Generally this substrate is adapted from epiphytic orchid or tropical pitcher plant (*Nepenthes* spp.) soil mixes that are designed to be well drained and aerated (Gagliardo, personal communication). The author has maintained several larger well-planted terrariums of dart frogs with these soil mixes for over 3 years with no soil changing. This soil type is best used for dart frogs, harlequin toads, mantellas, hylids, and other arboreal species requiring a well-planted enclosure.

The major benefit derived of this soil type is for the maintenance of plants in the enclosure. An invariable outcome of most peat-based or ready-made houseplant soil mixes in terrariums is rapid decomposition, compaction, and inadequate aeration. As this process progresses, the roots of plants die and the plants fail to thrive. Eventually the health of the entire terrarium deteriorates and animals fail to thrive. The bark/charcoal/peat mix requires a longer time period (2–3 years) for decomposition and rarely, if ever, compacts in the terrarium. A disadvantage to the "*Nepenthes* mix," however, is that it cannot be used for burrowing species of amphibians. The bark, charcoal, and tree fern are all potentially abrasive to amphibian skin. This does not appear to create a problem for most small (<5 cm) terrestrial frogs or toads, but can be irritating to larger frogs and some salamanders.

Another soil suitable for substrate is composted leaf litter that is free of fertilizers, pesticides, or other chemicals. This is particularly useful for salamanders and burrowing frogs. Commercially available topsoil preparations must be used with caution as they may contain chemical additives.

Proper lighting of a terrarium raises many questions regarding the light needs of amphibians. Generally, the specific requirements of ultraviolet light (UV-A and UV-B) are unknown for amphibians (Barnett 1996). Certainly, questions arise regarding the requirements of nocturnal, fossorial, or fully aquatic amphibians. For terrariums containing live plants, attempts are made to simulate natural sunlight so that the plants will thrive. The incidental effects of this lighting scheme on amphibians may be beneficial. As with most terrestrial vertebrates, some light is required for vision and photoperiodic behavior.

The amphibian owner should attempt to recreate the lighting scheme of the amphibian in nature. In general, most terrestrial salamanders and nocturnal frogs do not require bright lighting and may avoid it altogether. A naturalistic method to reduce lighting on the cage floor is a well-planted terrarium with full spectrum lighting. It is not unusual for some nocturnal hylids to rest on leaves or branches that are exposed to full sun during some part of the day (White's tree frog, *Litoria caerulea*; green tree frog, *Hyla cinerea*). Therefore, suitable basking sites should be provided for these species. Light fixtures are suitably placed above the enclosure, preferably within 46 cm (18 in) off the cage floor (Barnett et al. 2001). It is important to note that ultraviolet radiation does not penetrate plastic and glass, thus any lids that may shield the light should be replaced with screen. Also, when a full aquarium hood is used as lid and light source for the enclosure, a tight fit is essential to prevent escape of the inhabitants.

Commercially available full-spectrum lights for terrariums are available as fluorescent tube lights. Most, if not all, of the incandescent lights available for aquariums and terrariums do not produce adequate UV-A or UV-B radiation. Additionally, because most incandescent bulbs produce copious heat, they should be used with caution for amphibian enclosures. Many brands of full-spectrum lights are available for both plants and animals, each with their own claims of benefits.

Temperature, humidity, and ventilation for the terrarium are all interrelated and their control and management often dictates cage design more than any other environmental parameter. As many fish hobbyists can attest, the larger the aquarium the easier it is to manage temperature. The same is true for terrariums. This is particularly true for humidity and ventilation. Surprising to many, amphibians as a group inhabit a wide variety of climates from the equator to the Arctic Circle. Caecilians and salamanders are somewhat less adapted to extreme climates than are frogs. Thus, discussion of the more extreme temperature and humidity requirements primarily pertain to certain species of anurans. Some species of amphibians require seasonal cooling to stimulate ovulation and spermatogenesis for breeding. Knowledge of the specific patient's natural history with regard to environmental parameters is essential.

Enclosure temperature for many amphibian patients will be controlled by room temperature. The great majority of amphibians can adapt to normal household room temperature of 25–30°C (75–85°F), though there are some exceptions. Most highland tropical frogs (*Atelopus* spp. and some *Mantella* spp.) as well as most North American salamanders will fail to thrive for extended periods at temperatures above 21–24°C (70–75°F) (Lotters 1996; Staniszewski 1997; Obst et al. 1988). The Pacific giant salamander (*Dicamptodon ensatus*), the hellbender (*Cryptobranchus alleganiensis*), and the mudpuppy (*Necturus maculosus*) may all require refrigerated water or air conditioning throughout the year. Aquatic species such as the Surinam toad (*Pipa pipa*) and the African dwarf frog (*Hymenochirus* spp.) require heated water with protected submersible aquarium heaters.

Supplemental heating of the terrestrial amphibian enclosure is generally not required, though some species of frogs and toads benefit from basking lights or heat sources such as incandescent lights or ceramic heaters. These species include some toads, monkey frogs (*Phyllomedusa* spp.), and White's tree frogs (*Litoria* spp.). Most diurnal frogs (dendrobatids, atelopids, mantellids) typically do not require basking areas in the terrarium. Avoid heating enclosures with hot rocks or heating elements with which amphibians can make direct contact to prevent desiccation and thermal burns.

Enclosure humidity and ventilation are somewhat inversely proportional. Though other factors such as temperature and amount of water in the enclosure contribute to humidity, ventilation has the greatest and most rapid effect on increasing or decreasing humidity. Ideally the amphibian enclosure should be well ventilated with appropriate humidity. A partial or full-screen terrarium lid or cover is ideal for allowing evaporation and creating ventilation. Partially occluding the screen lid will increase or decrease ventilation and inversely raise or lower humidity. For large or tall terrariums, small ventilation holes may be drilled in the cage wall and covered with screen to allow ventilation of the otherwise stagnant lower reaches of the enclosure. A small fan may be placed outside the roof of the enclosure to create cross ventilation from these lower air intake ports.

Most terrestrial amphibians benefit from a humidity gradient in the terrarium. This gradient is created by shelters in the terrarium, additional ventilation to portions of the terrarium, and basking sites as described with lighting. Small depressions, pools, or streams of water may be created in the terrarium with pond liner or plant watering trays. For small frogs, particularly for dendrobatids and mantellids, it is imperative that even the smallest water reservoir have multiple escape routes. Many small frogs are incapable of swimming and will drown in even one centimeter of water. Many salamanders are capable of semiaquatic life and generally can withstand submersion for longer periods. Placement of limbs, plants, raised gravel, or other cage accessories within or around the water can ensure the ability for escape. Similarly, the sides of water enclosures for terrestrial amphibians should have tapered ramps in all directions for small amphibians to escape the water.

Moving water in the enclosure is also helpful to increase both humidity and to a lesser extent ventilation. Small waterfalls, humidifiers, or vaporizers may be used for this purpose. Transfer of vaporized air is achieved by connecting an appropriate sized PVC pipe from the vaporizer outflow into the enclosure at the desired location. Connecting the vaporizer to an automatic timer is helpful to create several periodic mistings per day. The misting effect in the terrarium can be quite dramatic. Humidifiers and vaporizers must be cleaned weekly to prevent the growth of potential pathogenic organisms in the water reservoir. Soaking with a dilute bleach solution (1 fl oz or 30 ml in 1 qt or 946 ml water) for 15 minutes and then thorough rinsing is sufficient for disinfecting (Barnett et al. 2001).

Water for the amphibian enclosure should be free of potential pathogens and all treatment chemicals. Aged tap water (allowed to ventilate in a container for 24 hours) in most cases is the best water for the terrarium (Barnett et al. 2001). Alternatively, carbon-filtered water may be used, though this water treatment may result in developmental abnormalities of tadpoles. Water moving in the terrarium over soil, gravel, or charcoal will generally be filtered biologically. Water that is stationary in containers should be changed as often as possible. Many terrestrial amphibians will defecate in these water bowls and bacterial or fungal growth in these containers may be rapid. Cleaning of the water bowls in a dilute bleach solution as described for vaporizer reservoirs is recommended at least weekly.

Enclosure Design

The Terrestrial Enclosure

By employing the general principles of security and environmental parameters, design of the amphibian enclosure, based on the species, is relatively straightforward and dictated by practicality. With the exception of temporary housing or quarantine, the smallest recommended amphibian enclosure is a 10 gallon aquarium. Though there is no maximum size limit of a terrarium, access for cleaning, visualization, and environmental control must all be considered.

An appropriate substrate is most important for establishing a well-balanced naturalistic arboreal, terrestrial, or semiaquatic terrarium and the soil composition is quite variable depending upon the species of amphibians and plants contained within. The type of soil or gravel, however, is only one part of establishing a suitable amphibian substrate. Proper design of the cage floor-substrate interface is crucial for maintaining a long-lasting planted or naturalistic terrarium. Ideally the soil mix should be elevated above the cage floor to allow for water and airflow through the soil and the development of a moisture gradient within the soil and terrarium.

Elevation of the soil above the cage floor is achieved by one of several methods. Wright (2001) uses a standard cage design at National Aquarium in Baltimore (NAIB) by creating a raised platform or false floor of overhead fluorescent light panels (egg crate) that were cut to fit the tank floor and then raised 2 cm above the true cage floor by pilings cut from PVC pipe (Barnett et al. 2001). This false floor is then overlaid with window screen or horticultural shade cloth and covered by 1 to 2 cm of gravel and the sheet moss directly above the gravel. In one corner of the enclosure a 2.5 cm diameter clear plastic tube is placed vertically through the false floor extending to just below the roof of the cage. This tube allows siphoning of the cage floor with a separate smaller siphon tube passed to the bottom of the cage. An optional but highly recommended bulkhead and spigot may be placed through a drilled hole in the cage floor to allow drainage and replace the siphon tube.

The author has used a modified version of this design developed by Ron Gagliardo at Atlanta Botanical Garden with great success. The egg crate false floor is typically inexpensive, but when using standard fish aquariums, prefabricated undergravel filters (the economy models) are made to fit the size of the tank and come complete with siphon tubes. One or more of these siphon tubes may be utilized as access for siphon drainage of the cage floor. Additionally, an alternative to the use of aquarium gravel between the filter plate and the soil is to use washed large or medium horticultural grade charcoal that is commonly available for orchids or other special planting mixes. The benefits of the charcoal are lighter weight (especially for large enclosures) and the gradual filtration of organic and inorganic compounds from the water and soil. The benefit of gravel is the large surface area for biologic filtration that likely also occurs with the charcoal. Charcoal has been used as both an enclosure base layer and as a component of custom mixed terrarium soils by the Atlanta Botanical Garden for over 6 years with no known adverse effects on various species of frogs.

For a planted terrarium, a soil depth of at least 5 cm is recommended. Over time some settling of the soil will occur. Plants are added bare root (no soil on the roots) to the soil mix and lightly watered to settle the surrounding soil. Generally, plants smaller than the eventual desired size are planted and allowed to grow in the terrarium. Plants in an amphibian terrarium should never be fertilized! Theoretically, soil decomposition, animal feces, and microbes will provide all the nutrients necessary for the growth of terrarium plants. It is common that many suitable plants will soon outgrow the enclosure and require routine trimming.

The water level of the terrestrial terrarium is maintained to achieve desired humidity and to fill pools or streams contained within. Plumbing for water accessories may be achieved through drilled holes or siphon tubes through the lid of the terrarium. Water pumps, moving part mechanical devices, and electrical cords should never be inside the terrarium proper. These may be routed through sealed conduits or contained outside the terrarium entirely. Similarly, outflow siphon hoses must be fully protected from cage inhabitants and preferably are located beneath the false floor of the enclosure.

The Aquatic Enclosure

The aquatic enclosure for many obligate aquatic or facultative aquatic amphibians is somewhat similar to the basic tropical fish or goldfish aquarium. Large aquatic amphibians such as *Amphiuma* spp., large sirens, and *Cryptobranchus* spp. are best housed in a 55-gallon or larger aquarium. *Cryptobranchus* and *Necturus* spp. both require chilled water with very high filtration. These animals should not be kept in captivity without properly providing for exact water quality conditions. One requirement for aquatic amphibians is sufficient access to the water surface to breath air. Because a majority of aquatic amphibians are relatively large and somewhat active, all refuges and ornaments must be secure in their placement. Aquarium heaters (if required) should be contained within a shroud such as PVC or other durable plastic into which numerous holes or slits are drilled to allow water movement over the element and proper heat dissipation. This is to prevent the accidental breaking of glass or ceramic heating elements. The lid must be tight fitting and preferably latched to prevent escape. With a swimming start, many larger aquatic amphibians are capable of opening lids to a standard aquarium hood.

Some form of water flow is desired for most aquatic amphibians, though frogs such as *Pipa* spp., *Xenopus* spp., and *Hymenochirus* spp. adapt well to still water. Cleanliness of the terrarium is essential and necessitates some type of filtration system. Undergravel filtration as provided for a fish aquarium is ideal for most aquatic amphibians. Those species requiring high water flow typically require a canister filter or other high flow rate external water pump and/or filter. Most temperate aquatic amphibians require no supplemental heating and adapt well to

room temperatures during the entire year. Tropical species are likely to require some supplemental heating if room temperatures fall below 72–75°F.

Amphibian-Environment Interaction

Several common problems can be avoided in captive amphibians with a practical approach to cage design. First the substrate and cage accessories should be appropriate to not physically injure the animal. This includes even "natural" elements such as plants. Sharp spines on certain bromeliads or other plants can be lethal to frogs! Certain plants are toxic to amphibians. The toxicity is not necessarily from direct contact, but occurs secondary to ingestion by food items such as crickets or other insects. This is mostly a concern with the introduction of field-collected insects. For example, some plant-sucking insects such as aphids can feed on toxic plants (such as milkweeds, *Asclepias* spp.) and not become distasteful to the smaller amphibians. In the case of milkweeds, the toxicity usually results in death of the animal.

Substrate ingestion is a major problem for captive amphibians. The substrate should be either too large to ingest or small enough that ingested particles are passed through the digestive tract. This may require modifying the substrate in a particular enclosure as the amphibian pet grows.

Almost paradoxically, water in the terrestrial enclosure can result in fatalities of some amphibians. Small terrestrial frogs (mantellids, dendrobatids, and atelopids) are incapable of swimming or will exhaust very easily in water. If a water enclosure is located in the corner of a terrestrial terrarium with no escape possibility against the glass, death of some cage inhabitants from drowning is a certainty. To adequately maintain these species in captivity standing water is optional or can be provided in the form of a petri dish or other shallow container. Unfortunately, to successfully breed both *Mantella* and *Atelopus* spp., some form of moving or standing water is usually required in the enclosure.

Assume that any opening to the outside of the cage will be utilized for escape. The lid or covering for the enclosure must be tight fitting or completely sealed. Even strictly terrestrial frogs are capable of limited climbing and jumping to reach the top of the cage. Some salamanders are also capable of climbing glass or plastic.

Amphibian-Amphibian Interaction

A common question of many amphibian enthusiasts is "Can different species be housed together?" The safe answer to the question is "No." Nevertheless, with experience and thorough knowledge of the species in question, many species that co-occur in nature may be housed communally with proper cage design.

The ultimate rule of housing multiple species (or even the same species from different sources) is that wild-caught individuals from different sources should never, ever be housed together. Clinically, amphibians (particularly frogs) appear to be more commonly parasitized than reptiles, even among captive-born individuals. Exposure of naïve animals to certain parasites or bacteria and fungi can result in disaster for an entire collection. A recent concern for terrestrial amphibian owners is the chytrid fungus (chytridiomycosis). This pathogenic fungus is suspected to be at least one of the causes of worldwide mortality among wild populations of amphibians and it has been identified to be widespread and easily transmitted among captive amphibians (see below, "Common Disorders") (Berger et al. 1998; Daszak et al. 2000; Morell 1999).

Aside from contagious disease is the question of compatibility. For the average amphibian owner, large frogs and salamanders (*Ceratophrys*, *Pyxicephalus*, large *Rana*, large *Bufo*, and *Ambystoma*) are best housed singly in an enclosure. All large amphibians are typically conditioned to feed on anything that is small enough to fit in their mouth. Ambystomatids in captivity are particularly conditioned to bite anything that touches the flanks, even animals larger than they are. The author has witnessed numerous leg amputations and lacerations of frogs and other salamanders that were temporarily housed with a tiger salamander of equal size. Frogs such as *Ceratobatrachus guentheri*, *Ceratophrys*, *Hemiphractus*, *Megophrys*, and *Pyxicephalus* spp. prey on other frog species and other vertebrates as a substantial part of their diet and therefore are generally unsuited for cohabitation with any other amphibians.

Toxicity between different species of amphibians is also a concern even within the same family of frogs. Many anecdotal reports exist and the author has witnessed that other amphibians (and other *Rana* spp.) enclosed with wood frogs (*Rana sylvatica*) will die rapidly leaving only the wood frogs alive (Duellman & Trueb 1994; Mattison 1987). The exact nature of this suspected toxicity is not fully known. It is possible that similar toxicity exists between different species of wild-collected dart frogs, though there is no observed toxicity among captive individuals.

QUARANTINE

The role of quarantine for new amphibians in a collection cannot be overemphasized. Segregation of new arrivals is most important for those animals that will be introduced into multispecies displays. The quarantine procedure for amphibians, however, is more designed to protect the individual animal from occult disease that may manifest itself some time after arrival into the new enclosure.

The quarantine enclosure is quite basic. A 10 gallon glass aquarium or plastic sweater box with ventilation holes is ideal for quarantine of most terrestrial amphibians. Larger aquatic amphibians should be maintained in an appropriately sized enclosure. For terrestrial amphibians, the cage substrate should be nonbleached paper towel and possibly a hide box or other disposable cage ornament to provide security. The quarantine enclosure should be located in a low traffic area of the room where the inhabitants may be monitored for activity from a distance. If necessary the sides of the enclosure may be painted or covered with paper to provide visual security. If possible a feeding station should be provided in the form of a petri dish or shallow dish so that the feeding response can be monitored. Arboreal frogs and salamanders can be quarantined similarly with the addition of horizontal branches for perching. If forced to remain on the cage floor, arboreal frogs may become stressed and fail to acclimate.

A fundamental purpose of quarantine is the collection of fecal material for analysis. This should be performed as soon as the first sample is available. Subsequent fecal samples should be examined every 3 to 5 days depending on availability and then rechecked every 2 weeks following a negative or "clean" sample. A final recheck 2 months after a negative sample is also advised (Wright & Whitaker 2001c).

The quarantine period should be at least 30 days following a negative fecal sample for apparently healthy individuals (Wright & Whitaker 2001c). Wild-collected amphibians, despite the status of fecal testing, should be quarantined for 60 days. Under no circumstances should wild-collected amphibians be introduced into an enclosure with any other animals! Despite antiparasite, antibiotic, and antifungal treatment, it is possible for these individuals to carry undetected infectious diseases and later transmit them to other naïve animals.

It is not uncommon to prophylactically treat new amphibian arrivals for gastrointestinal parasites and some cutaneous fungi. Though this practice is no substitute for fecal examination, it can be effective in eliminating or reducing the burden of some infectious diseases. Unfortunately, a risk of adverse side effects exists with this practice. The author has observed the death of long-term captive imported frogs following deworming with fenbendazole at recommended doses. The animals were four green and black poison dart frogs, *Dendrobates auratus*, which were confirmed infected with various nematodes including great numbers of lungworms, *Rhabdias* spp. None of the animals had exhibited clinical disease and were breeding in captivity. Following a single oral treatment with fenbendazole at 100 mg/kg two of the four frogs immediately stopped eating and subsequently died within 5 days. A third stopped feeding and then resumed feeding and survived. The fourth frog was not adversely affected. Both surviving frogs continued to shed *Rhabdias* spp. larvae in the feces following treatment, yet the numbers of larvae were reduced. The author has not observed this phenomenon in other similarly infected *Dendrobates* spp. or *Mantella* spp.

A common prophylactic antiparasite regimen includes administering fenbendazole orally at 100 mg/kg followed by ivermectin topically at 0.2 mg/kg (Wright & Whitaker 2001b). Repeating the treatment in 3 weeks is recommended including rechecking a fecal sample prior to treatment. For diagnosed infections, treatments are generally continued with increased frequency until negative fecal tests are achieved.

Record keeping of feeding and treatments is essential. The client should record all observations of activity, feeding response, food items consumed, and other pertinent behaviors. Weekly weights are also beneficial for healthy individuals when this can be performed accurately and in a stress-free manner.

NUTRITION

If the nutritional needs for amphibians were as simple as tossing a few crickets into the enclosure from time to time, they would all be more popular pets. The nutritional maintenance for many captive amphibians is as labor intensive (or more so) as that of insectivorous lizards and the nutritional requirements of amphibians are more a consequence of the animals being such generalists rather than being specialists on one food item. The variety of food items consumed in the wild likely results in a tremendously varied vitamin, mineral, amino acid, and fatty acid intake that is not duplicated with captive diets. Very little scientific data exist regarding the exact diet and its nutritional composition for amphibians in the wild. Unfortunately much is learned about the proper or improper nutrition of amphibians through histopathology.

There is great variability in the feeding preferences of different life stages of metamorphosed amphibians and this variability has been observed in those animals that have been successfully bred over several generations. For instance, froglets of the golden mantella (*Mantella aurantiaca*) are no more than 8 mm in length at metamorphosis (Staniszewski 1997). To a frog this small, even the smallest of domestic fruit flies is too large to eat. These froglets must be raised for several weeks on small insects called springtails (order Collembola) until they may be fed small fruit flies. Adult mantellas, however, are quite ravenous and will eat crickets that are nearly 20% of their body size.

The feeding method of amphibians is also somewhat important when selecting food items. All frogs should be considered food gulpers—after capturing the prey item, they swallow it whole with little to no chewing. In contrast, large salamanders and especially aquatic amphibians (*Necturus, Amphiuma, Siren,* and *Cryptobranchus* spp.) all exhibit some chewing motions when feeding. This is especially seen in sirens and amphiumas that may repeatedly move food items in and out of the mouth while crushing them (personal observation). Choosing appropriate food items or more importantly avoiding improper food items for certain species is important.

Another important point to remember regarding most terrestrial amphibians is that they are sight feeders. Generally, moving food is preferred over stationary food. Some larger frogs, toads, and salamanders may be conditioned to feed on stationary prekilled or frozen and thawed food items, but this is more the exception than the rule. Thus, when approaching the dilemma of a nonfeeding amphibian, always consider the type and size of food offered.

Perhaps the most important consideration when feeding amphibians is the timing of feeding. The client should be fully informed of the feeding habits of the species in question. Nearly all terrestrial salamanders and many tree frogs are nocturnal and will only feed at night. Many of the larger nocturnal frogs and toads, being opportunists, will feed any time in captivity. The tiger salamander, *Ambystoma tigrinum*, though nocturnal in its native habitat, will readily adapt to daylight feeding. Night feeding may make the monitoring of food consumption difficult with some amphibians. For newly established pets, encourage the client to observe the feeding habits with a flashlight or red light illumination if necessary.

To compensate for the known vitamin and mineral imbalances in food items and for suspected deficiencies in amino acids, many hobbyists apply several commercially available vitamin/mineral powders (called dusting) to the food items prior to feeding. The process of dusting food items is discussed in "Nutrition" in chapter 3. Additionally, food products specifically for the prey items to consume are designed to enrich the prey item prior to feeding it to the amphibian pet. This process is called "gut-loading."

Based on known dietary disorders, several basic provisions must be made for captive amphibians. Calcium and phosphorus (Ca:P) should be provided in a ratio of 1:1 to 2:1 to prevent several nutritional diseases (Wright 2001d; Wright & Whitaker 2001a; Donoghue & Langenberg 1996). Additionally, vitamin D_3 is supplemented in the diet or produced endogenously by the amphibian when exposed to appropriate quality and quantity of ultraviolet light. A ratio that is too low in calcium or too high in phosphorus may result in metabolic bone disease (MBD). A ratio too high in calcium or vitamin D_3 may contribute to hypervitaminosis D and secondary renal failure (Wright & Whitaker 2001b). Powdered supplements are available from Rep-Cal (Los Gatos, CA; www.repcal.com) and Nekton (Clearwater, FL; www.nekton.de).

Neonatal and young amphibians appear to be most affected by MBD because of increased calcium demand by growing bones. The frequency for calcium supplementation of these animals is increased compared to that of adults. Neonatal or young growing amphibians may receive calcium and vitamin D_3 supplementation twice weekly when fed daily, and most adult amphibians should receive calcium supplemented food items once weekly or less often. Larger amphibians fed whole-animal vertebrate diets such as thawed frozen rats or mice likely do not require supplemental calcium in the diet.

Aquatic or semiaquatic amphibians fed diets composed solely of fish may develop a thiamine (vitamin B_1) deficiency (Wright & Whitaker 2001b; Donoghue & Langenberg 1996). This disorder is the result of high levels of thiaminase in the food items that inactivates dietary and endogenously produced thiamine in the amphibian. Several susceptible species are aquatic salamanders, aquatic caecilians, horned frogs (*Ceratophrys* spp.), African bullfrogs (*Pyxicephalus* spp.), and other semiaquatic frogs.

Food Items

Most clients who maintain breeding colonies or large colonies of amphibians are required to raise their own food items as the expense of purchasing food items can be excessive. The simplest factor dictating the feeding of captive amphibians is the size of the animal and the size of the food item. The standard diet for most larger salamanders and frogs is crickets and the diet of choice for smaller amphibians is fruit flies. Some wild collected insects such as termites may be

available seasonally or throughout the year in warmer climates.

Domestic or gray crickets (*Acheta domestica*) of various sizes are the standard diet for most medium to large terrestrial amphibians. Crickets are commercially available in sizes ranging from $\frac{1}{16}$ inch (pinheads) in length to 1 inch (adults) from pet shops and mail order from a variety of sources. The Ca:P for crickets is 0.2:2.6 (Donoghue & Langenberg 1996). Periodic dusting of crickets with calcium and vitamin D_3 powders is recommended for all amphibians.

A variety of specialized cricket diets is available to enrich crickets with nutrients. The efficacy of these products is debatable. Generations of frogs that have been fed crickets raised on fresh vegetables and fruits such as squash, greens, and oranges have reproduced and lived for 5 or more years with no apparent health abnormalities for themselves or offspring (personal observation).

Another cultured food item for medium to large amphibians is mealworms. The mealworm is actually larvae of the beetle, *Tenebrio molitor*, which may be cultured easily in one of several different grain meals supplemented with cut pieces of apple or vegetable for moisture. Because the adult beetles are required to reproduce for new mealworms, a tight-fitting ventilated lid is required to maintain the culture. Mealworms are generally a poor food choice for amphibians because of the hard exoskeleton. Though the softer-bodied, newly molted larvae are acceptable, the author has witnessed the unexplained deaths of several frogs and lizards following the feeding of mealworms. Necropsy on several lizards has revealed peritoneal abscessation that was attributed to gastrointestinal perforation from the hard body parts or possibly chewing of the larvae. Because mealworms do not provide an improved Ca:P ratio (0.1:1.2) (Donoghue & Langenberg 1996) as compared to crickets, their use as a primary food item for most amphibians is not recommended.

Similarly, most beetles and other large insects with hard exoskeletons are not a good food source for amphibians. An exception might be made for large frogs and especially toads, which may be observed to nearly consume their weight in beetles while feeding in habitats during summer months. Large terrestrial salamanders and aquatic amphiumas and sirens are generally capable of crushing these insects and crustaceans following capture and therefore may adequately digest these insects and have minimal risk of gastrointestinal injury.

A smaller beetle is available that can safely be fed to small frogs. This is the flour beetle, *Trilobium* spp., which is a relative of the larger *Tenebrio* spp. These beetles are approximately 5 mm in length as adults with comparable small larvae. They are raised and harvested similar to *Tenebrio* spp., though the adult beetle is fed as commonly as the larvae.

Wingless or flightless fruit flies are the standard diet for smaller frogs and salamanders, particularly for poison dart frogs, mantellas, harlequin frogs, and neonatal amphibians. Two species of flies, *Drosophila melanogaster* (the small vestigial or wingless fruit fly) and *Drosophila hydei* (the larger flightless fruit fly), are commercially available. Fruit flies are easily cultured by the client and may be the sole food source for many captive amphibians. These are cultured in reusable canning jars or disposable plastic cups both of which are sealed with a permeable (but escape-proof) ventilated lid. Fruit fly growing media is available from Carolina Biological Supply Co. (Burlington, NC; www.carolina.com) or can be made from instant potato flakes, brewer's yeast, and a mold inhibitor. Fruit flies are typically dusted with powdered supplements as with crickets.

Another small food item that is relished by nearly all amphibians is the termite. In warmer climates, such as the southeastern U.S. coastal plain, termites can be collected any time of year. There are methods of "culturing" termites in the wild by burying coffee cans punctured with drain holes in the ground and filling them with rolled cardboard. Unfortunately the risk of infestation to homes and other wooden structures is great, so this practice should not be recommended to clients. Nevertheless, wild-collected termites do not appear to cause harm to captive amphibians and certain nutrients not otherwise available to these animals may be provided. Similarly, parasites or other toxins ingested by the termites could put captive animals at risk for disease.

An important but often overlooked food item for small frogs is springtails or leafhoppers, of the insect order Collembola. These very small (<1 mm) white to gray insects are commonly seen in most terrariums containing soil. They feed on detritus and decaying plant material and can be easily cultured to feed neonatal or very small frogs and salamanders. A plastic container such as a margarine container or plastic shoebox filled with approximately 1 to 2 inches of potting soil is ideal. The soil is slightly moistened and a few pinches of fish food flakes are sprinkled on the surface of the soil. The springtails may be introduced from a decaying leaf from outdoors or from a previously existing culture. A method for easily removing the springtails is to place a small block (10 cm × 5 cm × 5 cm) of horticultural tree fern fiber on the soil surface, then remove and gently tap the block to remove springtails when feeding is desired.

The only acceptable vertebrate food sources for captive amphibians are fish and thawed frozen pink mice or rats. Large frogs, toads, and salamanders with conditioned feeding responses will usually accept these items when offered by forceps or in the case of fish when offered in a shallow dish. These larger amphibians will generally accept other vertebrate prey such as other amphibians, reptiles, large beetles, and grasshoppers. The client should carefully consider the health risk to the amphibian before feeding such items. The risk of parasitism with endoparasites, bacterial, or fungal infections is great. Of paramount concern must be the chytridiomycosis fungus when offering any amphibians. This disease is extremely serious for amphibians and should be viewed on the level of the immunodeficiency viruses that affect cats and humans when considering the vigilance for prevention.

Aquatic amphibians consume a wide variety of food items. Earthworms and fish are the standard diets with other arthropods and some frozen foods occasionally accepted. Ideally, the food should be cultured or purchased as cultured rather than collected from the wild. This reduces the risk of introducing infectious diseases into the enclosure. Certain amphibians, particularly several frog species, are specialists in their feeding choices and may be difficult to feed in captivity. The bizarre casque-headed tree frogs, *Hemiphractus* spp., of South America and several species of horned frogs, *Ceratophrys* spp., are known frog-eating specialists (Mattison 1987; Obst et al. 1988). It may be necessary to feed live frogs to these species while trying to train them to eat various invertebrate or vertebrate prey items. Another finicky large frog (8–10 cm) is the climbing toad, *Pedostibes hosei*, of southeast Asia. This frog is known to specialize on ants and termites and may not accept crickets or other large invertebrates in captivity (Obst et al. 1988). By feeding smaller size crickets or beetles, this frog may be transitioned to a cricket-only diet. Among aquatic amphibians the hellbenders, *Cryptobranchus* spp., as adults typically feed only on crayfish and must be coaxed to accept other aquatic food items if captive.

Finally, many clients may be misinformed regarding the feeding of manufactured pelleted diets. It is unreasonable to expect any terrestrial amphibians to eat nonmoving prepared foods. It is more likely, though not common, that aquatic amphibians will readily accept these diets. Salamanders and newts more than frogs will adapt to these diets, but they are rarely substitutes for live foods. Clients should be informed regarding this fact prior to purchasing amphibian pets. For some the cost of live foods or the time to culture them may not meet their expectations for proper maintenance of amphibian pets. One exception of note is the fact that marine toads (*Bufo marinus*) have been observed and videotape recorded eating dry dog food from outdoor food bowls in south Florida. So, one can never underestimate the resourcefulness of these animals when it comes to adaptation!

COMMON DISORDERS

Amphibian health disorders arise from infectious bacterial, fungal, and parasitic etiologies, trauma, nutritional, and toxic diseases. Several diseases, such as metabolic bone disease (MBD) and cutaneous bacterial infection (red leg), are well documented in veterinary scientific and popular literature. Many specific infectious and metabolic diseases, however, are relatively unknown.

Integument

As with snakes and lizards, a very common skin disorder seen in frogs is rostral abrasion. This is particularly common in wild-collected animals, but is just as likely to occur in any species transported in small containers. The common etiology is trauma from escape attempts through clear plastic lids, screens, or glass enclosures. Prevention of this disorder is enhanced with opaque transport containers and packing of the amphibian with moss or another soft substrate to reduce movement within the container.

The primary concern with rostral abrasions is secondary infections from opportunistic or pathogenic bacteria and fungus. If the abrasion is clean and shows no signs of erosion, then no treatment is indicated. For chronic or more extensive abrasions where active erosion of the skin or exposure of underlying bone is present, treatment with topical antibiotics is indicated. Topical application of ophthalmic solutions is indicated. Gentamicin or triple antibiotic solutions are applied once or twice daily. Silver sulfadiazine cream is also efficacious to treat fungal elements in addition to bacteria.

Active lesions associated with erosive dermatitis or osteolysis require aggressive diagnostic and therapeutic intervention. Bacterial culture and sensitivity and cytology from an impression smear or tissue sample in formalin may be submitted. In addition to topical therapy, systemic antibiotics are indicated. Enrofloxacin at a dose of 5 to 10 mg/kg PO or TO every 24 hours for 7 days (Taylor 2001) is recommended pending culture results. The client must be vigilant of the patient with

regard to healing of these lesions. Amphibians with substantial rostral abrasions should be maintained in a quarantine enclosure for cleanliness and close observation.

Traumatic injuries to limbs are similar to rostral abrasions. Trauma may occur secondary to accidents with enclosure lids closing on legs, though bite wounds from cage mates are possible with some species. These wounds typically require aggressive antibiotic therapy initially rather than just observation. If severe trauma to underlying bone is suspected, amputation is recommended early in treatment to prevent the development of systemic disease.

Bacterial skin infections are common in amphibians and may present as discolorations, erosions, abscesses, and ulcerations. Bacterial dermatitis may be difficult to diagnose on visual inspection alone. Many infections are the result of immunosuppression from a number of factors including improper husbandry, inadequate diet, or the stress of shipping. The resultant infectious agent may arise from the patient's environment or from an apparently unaffected cage mate.

The diagnostic test of choice for any cutaneous lesion is bacterial culture and sensitivity followed by histopathology of affected tissue if possible. Pending the response to empiric antibiotic therapy, biopsy may be required. Unfortunately, the risk of septicemia from a number of bacterial etiologic agents necessitates the initiation of treatment prior to receiving test results. The commonly referenced "red-leg disease" of frogs is actually the result of hyperemia secondary to septicemia rather than simply cutaneous disease. If not treated rapidly and appropriately, this syndrome carries a poor prognosis for recovery.

For the nonsepticemic cutaneous disease systemic enrofloxacin is initiated for 7 days. For the septicemic patient, a water bath of 0.6% saline to achieve hydration is initial therapy (Taylor 2001). Antibiotic baths with tetracyclines, semisynthetic penicillins (SSP), and aminoglycosides may be indicated.

Many bacteria are implicated in amphibian skin disease and septicemia. A large number of these are gram-negative rods including the widely reported and well known *Aeromonas* spp. and *Pseudomonas* spp. *Mycobacterium* spp. are also implicated in various disease syndromes in amphibians, particularly skin disease. Diagnosis is very difficult premortem as the bacteria are difficult to culture. Because there is no known treatment for *Mycobacterium* infection, isolation and neutralization of affected individuals is recommended.

Fungal infections are a concern for amphibians. Most notable among these is chytridiomycosis caused by *Batrachochytrium dendrobatidis* (Taylor 2001).The initial clinical sign of this fungal dermatitis is an increased rate of skin shedding with possible associated dermal lesions such as pale skin. It is not known how many different species of amphibians are susceptible to this fungus, but suspicion is growing that it may be worldwide (Berger et al. 1998; Daszak et al. 2000; Morell 1999; Taylor 2001).

Patients are diagnosed with chytridiomycosis by the presence of the organism in shed skin or in formalin-fixed skin. Diagnosed cases or prophylactic treatment of suspected infected animals is performed with a bath of itraconazole. A 1% itraconazole stock solution in methylcellulose is diluted to 0.01% in 0.6% NaCl. Treatment consists of a 5 minute bath once daily for 10 days (Taylor 2001). Resolution of clinical signs is rapid if treatment is initiated early.

Ectoparasites are uncommon among amphibians and are clinically most prevalent among toads. Treatment consists of ivermectin at 0.4 mg/kg PO or TO given once weekly for at least 4 weeks (Poynton & Whitaker 2001). Some amphibian species have shown sensitivity to higher doses of ivermectin (2 mg/kg) (Poynton & Whitaker 2001; Klingenberg 1993).

Finally, a multisystemic disease most notable in the skin is bloating or edema syndrome. This disease process has several possible etiologies, the most notable of which is osmotic imbalance secondary to sepsis or toxemia. Other possible causes include renal disease or failure, heart disease, metabolic bone disease, and environmental factors. Cases in which an individual animal is affected may be challenging to diagnose. For cases in which multiple animals in an enclosure are affected, environmental causes and infectious disease are most likely. With a diagnosis and rapid treatment, prognosis may be fair. Often, the inciting cause has remained unnoticed for some time prior to the onset of clinical signs and the underlying disease has progressed beyond possibility of recovery.

Skeletal System

Though not as common as seen in lizards, metabolic bone disease (MBD) follows the same clinical course as in reptiles. Juvenile or rapidly growing individuals are most susceptible. The pathophysiology of MBD is discussed in chapter 3, "The Lizard." An unknown factor regarding MBD in amphibians is the role of ultraviolet light (UV-B) in the development of clinical disease. Because most amphibians are either nocturnal, fossorial, or otherwise found in shaded forests it is possible that oral cholecalciferol (vitamin D_3) plays more of a role in calcium absorption and metabolism than does that of endogenous vitamin D.

It is also possible that another mechanism of calcium metabolism is at work.

An occasional clinical sign of MBD in amphibians is gastrointestinal bloating. If this sign is observed and there is suspicion of MBD based on history or other physical exam findings, a radiographic study should be initiated to confirm the presence of the disease syndrome. The demonstration of decreased bone density is diagnostic for MBD, though in severe cases, especially among young growing animals, soft pliable bones are highly suggestive of MBD. Blood calcium testing is not a reliable method for diagnosing MBD as the blood will remain normocalcemic until the body stores of calcium are depleted.

Treatment of MBD in amphibians is supportive. Oral calcium glubionate at a dose of 1.0 ml/kg/day (Wright & Whitaker 2001b) and dietary correction is essential. Oral vitamin D_3 is recommended to enhance the absorption of calcium from the gastrointestinal tract (Wright & Whitaker 2001b; Donoghue & Langenberg 1996). Patients with neurologic disease secondary to MBD may require calcium gluconate 10% at 100 mg /kg ICe every 4 to 6 hours until signs resolve. Prognosis for the hypocalcemic state of MBD in amphibians as seen in lizards is poor.

A mysterious disease of newly metamorphosed frogs is called spindly leg disease or syndrome. With this abnormality, tadpoles develop normal or nearly normal hind legs but the forelimbs either fail to erupt from the skin or are extremely thin and weak, almost as if there were only skin and bone with no muscle. This syndrome has been reported extensively among dendrobatid frogs. This high rate of occurrence may be due to the fact that these frogs are bred in captivity in such great numbers and therefore the chance for occurrence is greater. Frogs that do metamorphose and leave the water usually fail to eat and die within days.

The potential causes for this syndrome are diet of the tadpole or parents, improper environmental conditions (temperature, lighting, etc.), genetics, toxins, and possibly chytridiomycosis. Presently a dietary cause is most likely as several anecdotal reports exist that dietary variation in clutches of tadpoles from the same parents raised on different foods may exhibit the disease. There is no treatment for this disease process.

Respiratory System

Clinical respiratory disease is uncommon among amphibians. It is more likely that respiratory infections in amphibians are underdiagnosed rather than less frequent than those seen in reptiles. A common respiratory pathogen is lungworms (*Rhabdias* spp.). Though this nematode is diagnosed with moderate frequency among terrestrial frogs, clinical disease associated with the organism is infrequent. It is likely that the migration of larvae through host tissues and secondary invasion of bacteria with or without septicemia contribute greatly to debilitation of the patient.

Rhabdias spp. infection is diagnosed by demonstrating larvae on direct fecal examination or floatation or by cytology of tracheal wash. Patients exhibiting apparent respiratory distress in association with *Rhabdias* spp. infection are best treated with anthelmintics concurrent with antibiotics such as enrofloxacin for secondary bacterial infection. Those patients that exhibit no active clinical disease are treated only with anthelmintics such as fenbendazole 100 mg/kg PO every 14 days for 3 treatments or ivermectin at 0.2 to 0.4 mg/kg PO or TO at the same rate of administration (Poynton & Whitaker 2001). Because the life cycle of this infection (as well as other amphibian nematodal infections) is direct, isolation and strict hygiene is essential to reducing parasite burdens.

Though not an infectious disease, drowning is a common fatal respiratory disease of captive amphibians. It is mentioned only because it is a disease of prevention as described above in the section on husbandry. This avoidable disease results in the deaths of many valuable amphibian pets.

Digestive System

Another rather common though avoidable noninfectious disease in amphibians is foreign body obstruction. Typically the result of inappropriate substrate or feeding practices, this problem often goes unnoticed for some time. The primary presenting complaint is anorexia or occasionally regurgitation. Gravel, soil particles, or rarely invertebrate exoskeleton may cause obstruction. Diagnosis may be presumptive based on history and husbandry practices or definitive with abdominal palpation and radiographic study.

The degree of obstruction, size of patient, and nature of the foreign body dictate treatment. For organic foreign materials, oral laxatives such as psyllium and mineral oil may aid in passage of the obstruction. For larger amphibians, surgery may be indicated.

Intestinal parasitism is clinically widespread among terrestrial amphibians and somewhat less common among arboreal species. Amphibians are infected with a wide variety of protozoa and metazoa parasites. It is common that routine fecal exams of amphibians reveal these organisms in otherwise healthy patients. Some protozoans may not be pathogenic and may not require treatment. Some protozoan and many metazoan (nematodes, trematodes, cestodes) parasites may inhabit amphibian tissues and remain in "balance" with the host with a competent immune system.

The onset of stress and subsequent immunosuppression that results from transport, poor diet, or inappropriate husbandry can rapidly lead to accelerated reproduction, migration, and infestation of these parasites. Similarly, the direct life cycle of many parasites only compounds the reinfection rate when the patient is subject to confinement in a terrarium. This is the likely cause for the apparent higher clinical prevalence of these parasites in terrestrial rather than arboreal species as there is greater likelihood for contact with the infective oocysts or larvae.

When diagnosed, intestinal parasites are best treated. Nevertheless, the client must be educated regarding the potential side effects of treatment. More commonly there is greater risk of death or debilitation from the host's immune response to sudden parasite death than from side effects of appropriate dose medications. For very valuable animals, treatment of apparently healthy animals should be carefully weighed against the potential loss of the patient. When groups of animals are to be medicated, treatment of a few animals in the group is preferable to medicating the entire group at once.

The most important factor to breaking the life cycle of direct parasites is maintenance of the patient in an immaculately clean, well-maintained enclosure. Removal of all feces immediately after passage is imperative. Feeding of the patient should only be performed in an enclosure with no fecal contamination as food items may browse on contaminated surfaces and reinfect the host. Prophylactic treatment for intestinal parasites is discussed above in "Quarantine."

Protozoan parasites present both a diagnostic and treatment challenge. For suspected pathogenic *Trichomonas* spp. and *Entamoeba* spp. infections, metronidazole is indicated. Dose ranges for adults vary from 10 mg/kg PO every 24 hours for 7 to 10 days for *Trichomonas* to 100 mg/kg PO every 14 days for *Entamoeba* (Poynton & Whitaker 2001). Metronidazole baths at 250 mg to 500 mg/L fresh water for 6 to 8 hours once weekly are indicated for larval amphibians (Poynton & Whitaker 2001).

Coccidiosis is not uncommon in amphibians, yet its diagnosis is complicated by the fact that oocysts are intermittently shed in the feces. Thus, repeated fecal exams over protracted periods are required in some cases for definitive diagnosis. As seen in mammals, coccidiosis is primarily a clinical disease to the very young, very old, or immunosuppressed animal. Nevertheless, treatment is indicated on diagnosis and consists of trimethoprim-sulfamethoxazole at 15 mg/kg PO daily for 14 days (Poynton & Whitaker 2001). The dosage of TMS in exotic animals is based on the combined concentration of both the trimethoprim and sulfa medications.

Nematodes are treated as described for lungworms (*Rhabdias* spp.) above in the section on the respiratory system and in the section on quarantine for prophylactic treatment. It may be difficult to specifically diagnose each species of nematode parasite on fecal exam, though the treatment for each is similar.

Trematodes and cestodes have indirect life cycles in amphibians and interruption of the vector for reinfection is essential for treatment. Treatment consists of praziquantel at 8 to 14 mg/kg PO every 14 days for 3 or more treatments (Poynton & Whitaker 2001).

Excretory System

There are no significant renal diseases of amphibians that are not observed in reptiles, birds, or mammals. Renal disease secondary to toxicosis (medications or environmental), mineral imbalances, or gout is possible.

Reproductive System

Failure to lay eggs, or "egg binding," is the most common reproductive disorder of amphibians. Potential causes are categorized as environmental in which a suitable oviposition site is not available, unsuitable mate, or other stress prevents the release of eggs. Other causes include physical inability to lay eggs that may result from environmental factors. If an egg or eggs becomes lodged in the ostium of the oviduct or within the oviduct proper, all retrograde eggs will be retained. Some cases may require surgery when possible.

Ophthalmology

Superficial ocular disease in amphibians is commonly associated with skin disease or arises from a common etiology such as bacterial, fungal, protozoal, or viral disease. Cataracts, corneal lipidosis, and glaucoma have all been diagnosed. Systemic disease or sepsis such as red-leg syndrome may account for uveitis in amphibians as does similar systemic disease in other animals. Diagnosis and treatment of ophthalmic diseases in amphibians are approached as in other animals.

Toxicity

Amphibians are quite sensitive to environmental contamination from both naturally occurring and synthetic toxins. These include ammonia, nitrites, nitrates, excessive salts, chlorine, organophosphates, pyrethrins and pyrethroids, and many solvents used in glues and sealants. It is imperative that any cleaning compounds used to disinfect enclosures or enclosure accessories be thoroughly rinsed, soaked, and dried prior to reintroduction into the enclosure. Diana et al. (2001) reports toxicosis among dendrobatid frogs within enclosures that were misted by a newly constructed system composed of PVC pipes. Organic solvents from the pipe cement were found to be the cause of toxicosis. Similar attention must be observed with aquarium glass sealants.

Zoonoses

Amphibians are known to carry several bacteria that are potentially pathogenic to humans and other animals. Though not infectious, certain amphibian toxins are potentially dangerous to humans and domestic animals.

Bacteria such as *Listeria monocytogenes*, *Salmonella* spp., and *Yersinia enterocolitica* are all reported as isolated from the feces or digestive tracts of some amphibians (Taylor 2001). There is no link to clinical disease in humans from these bacteria arising from amphibians. Care and common sense, however, must be exercised when handling amphibians regarding zoonotic potential. Human carelessness is often a contributing factor to zoonoses when related to exotic animals.

It is the responsibility of the veterinary clinician and technician to educate the client regarding proper handling of the amphibian pet to reduce the risk of potential exposure.

Several guidelines are:

1. Do not handle amphibians unless absolutely necessary. Most (if not all) amphibians show no apparent health or quality of life benefit from human contact. In fact, stress may be increased as well as tissue trauma that may lead to an increased incidence of disease to the animal.
2. Never handle or clean amphibians, amphibian foods or food containers, or amphibian enclosures near a human food preparation area or human sanitation area such as a kitchen sink, kitchen table or countertop, bathroom sink, or bathtub.
3. Never allow children to handle amphibians without direct adult supervision and make sure that hands are washed immediately after handling.
4. Do not allow amphibians to remain loose or uncontained in a building intended for human occupation, sanitation, or food preparation.

Unfortunately, the above suggestions may seem to be common sense, but the breakthroughs in common sense are always reported in the popular press by relatively uneducated media professionals implicating exotic animals in zoonotic disease. Without the responsible education of pet owners, there is great risk of continued legislation prohibiting private possession of these animals.

Larval Amphibians

Tadpoles and larval salamanders face a variety of disorders that, for the most part, are never diagnosed or treated. Under controlled conditions with captive breeding, the incidence of disease is relatively low, yet many may be susceptible to disease when stressed with substandard environmental conditions. There tremendous variability in natural and cultural conditions of larval amphibians and some species demand exacting environmental parameters, while other are adapted to what might be considered nearly unsurvivable conditions.

For practical purposes, all larval caecilians and salamanders are carnivorous. Some caecilians are viviparous and consume oviductal secretions while developing in the adult female and are then born as juveniles. For salamanders, carnivory leads to cannibalism in crowded conditions, particularly as metamorphosis approaches. It is possible that the survival of some communal pond-breeding salamanders depends on this strategy for a few animals to survive. In contrast, most frog larvae, tadpoles, are herbivorous. There are, however, a few notable exceptions. Though not commonly bred by hobbyists in captivity, horned frogs (*Ceratophrys* spp. and some other *Leptodactylidae*) have carnivorous, or more reputedly cannibalistic, tadpoles. Successful rearing of these tadpoles and larvae of other carnivorous species necessitates isolation into individual enclosures for each larva.

The most critical husbandry issue for larval amphibians is water quality. Understanding the natural history and reproductive strategy for a particular species is important for proper care of the tadpoles. Most dart frogs, for example, lay eggs out of water on leaves, in leaf axils, or on flat surfaces near the ground. After hatching, the tadpoles are then transferred to a suitable water area that is generally a small plant with water supplied only from rain. For these species in captivity, elaborate filtration and moving or constantly filtered water is not essential for survival and metamorphosis. Aged tap water or spring water changed periodically generally yields success.

Species that lay eggs above streams or have tadpoles that inhabit moving water usually require some water oxygenation or filtration for survival. Some of these species, such as many larger Central and South American hylids feed on particulates suspended in the water and require the water movement to supply a constant source of food. Many of these species will rapidly perish if maintained in still or stagnant water.

Feeding of larval amphibians, particularly tadpoles, is not difficult in most cases. An exceptional food for larval herbivorous dendrobatids is spirulina powder (Earthrise Co., Petaluma, CA), which is available from most health food stores. The author has raised many generations of various species of dendrobatids and *Mantella* spp. tadpoles on this diet with absolutely no developmental abnormalities. Overfeeding must be avoided, however. Water quality deteriorates rapidly without filtration and death will be rapid. Many dendrobatids and possibly other frog species give parental care to tadpoles in the form of "feeder eggs." Information on these species is available in many hobbyist texts.

Larval salamanders can be problematic in that many species in early development require live foods. Daphnia, gammarus (fairy shrimp), and other small crustaceans must be cultured or readily available. Wild collection of these food items is not recommended, as this is commonly a source for infection with the trematode *Gyrodactylus* spp., the body fluke. These microscopic parasites can be rapidly fatal to larvae, and may be the inciting cause of cutaneous ulcers on adults. Treatment may be accomplished with dilute salt or formaldehyde baths (1.5 ml of 10% formalin in 1.0 liter water for 10 minutes) and survivability is good with early diagnosis. The amphibians undergoing treatment must be watched very closely and removed to freshwater at the first sign of distress in formalin. Dipping the infected animals into the treatment solution within a net is the most practical method for rapid removal.

Larva amphibians are subject to bacterial and fungal infections as adults. Treatment is made with medicated baths rather than by individual dosing. Diagnosis of a specific infection is usually obtained by sacrificing one or more larvae from a group for bacteriologic or microscopic analysis

OBTAINING A HISTORY, RESTRAINT, AND PHYSICAL EXAM

History

A complete and accurate history of the amphibian patient may be the most important procedure in developing a diagnosis of disease (or health). Unfortunately, amphibian patients are commonly presented moribund or altered from the original onset of clinical signs, making it difficult to diagnose the underlying etiology based on physical exam. Similarly, the clinician may be presented with a deceased patient from a group of animals and a diagnosis may be required to develop a treatment plan for the remaining group of apparently healthy individuals. Additionally, when gaining new clients who own amphibians (and reptiles), much time is spent in phone conversations with clients who are reluctant to bring the patient into the clinic. It is important to be very patient when speaking with potential first-time clients.

The first step in obtaining an accurate history is identification of the correct scientific name of the patient to *at least* the genus (and preferably to species) level. It may be difficult to obtain natural history information based on common or colloquial names. Identification to the subspecies level (many salamanders) or the variety level (many Dendrobatidae) is not important for developing a history and diagnosis.

Establish the origin of the patient. Is the patient captive-born or wild-caught and imported? This information is particularly important for amphibians as the likelihood of acclimation to a captive environment and the potential pathogens in wild-caught animals must be considered. The client may not know this history, particularly if the animal was purchased at a pet store or reptile and amphibian trade show or swap meet. A juvenile or relatively young amphibian is likely captive-born rather than wild-caught. Imported animals are usually adults as they are more frequently captured in the wild and more likely to survive shipping. Today there are certain species of frogs that are almost exclusively captive-born. Many salamanders and most caecilians are wild-caught (see table 6.1).

A particularly important question for the client is the medical history of the patient. Has the patient been treated at home prior to or following the client's possession of the patient? Also, has the patient received treatment from another veterinarian? Home treatment of exotic pets, particularly reptiles and amphibians, is common. Occasionally, results are favorable with home treatment, but more commonly the clinical condition fails to respond or deteriorates.

All husbandry parameters should be fully investigated. Descriptions of the enclosure, substrate, accessories, cage mates, feeding schedule, and environmental conditions both of the enclosure and the room housing the enclosure are important. In cases where multiple individuals or species of amphibians are housed together, the client should be questioned regarding the health of these animals as well as any quarantine procedures that were performed.

The exact nutrition (which food items are consumed) of the captive amphibian is generally not as much of a clinical concern as whether or not the patient is actually eating. With respect to food items offered, particularly insects, it is important to learn what size of insect is fed and the timing of the feedings. Also, ask the client if the patient is observed to actually eat the food items or if the food simply disappears from the cage. Many times insects may escape or hide beneath cage ornaments leading the client to believe that the insects were consumed. This is particularly true of nocturnal amphibians. Question the client regarding food supplements such as vitamin-mineral powders and how often these are applied. For aquatic amphibians it is important to know the exact food items offered (live or processed). Many captive amphibians will refuse prepared diets such as pellets initially and must be fed live food.

Restraint

The primary consideration when restraining an amphibian is stress on the patient and the potential health consequences of handling: the patient should be touched or restrained only when absolutely necessary. All diagnostic tests or treatments should be prepared prior to handling to consolidate procedures into the fewest episodes of physical manipulation of the patient. Consideration must also be given to safety of the handler. Some species are capable of producing toxic skin secretions that are irritating, noxious, but rarely lethal to humans.

The following species when known to be wild collected should be handled with extreme caution: golden poison frog (*Phyllobates terribilis*), black-legged poison frog (*Phyllobates bicolor*), Colorado River toad (*Bufo alvarius*), and the marine toad (*Bufo marinus*). It is unlikely that either of the poison frogs listed will ever be seen in practice as wild-caught individuals because they are relatively inaccessible for collection and exportation from Colombia, and both species are now widely available as captive-born juveniles and adults. Captive-born dart frogs have greatly reduced skin toxins and are generally not toxic to humans (Daly et al. 1994). Nevertheless, an imported *Phyllobates terribilis* should be considered lethal to humans. The toxins of *P. bicolor* are only ⅟₅₀ the strength of *P. terribilis*, yet a wild-caught frog should be considered dangerous (Walls 1994).

The *Bufo* spp. are a concern not as much for their degree of toxicity, which is significant, but for the manner in which the toxin may be secreted. Both species are capable of ejecting copious amounts of toxin from the parotid glands. Reports exist of this toxin spraying 6 feet or more from the animal (Wright & Whitaker 2001d). Entry of the toxin into an unprotected eye can be serious not just from the standpoint of direct physical irritation, but also from absorption and systemic effects. All larger *Bufo* spp. and all wild-caught dart frogs are best handled with powder-free latex gloves. Additionally, protective eyewear is recommended when handling or manipulating larger toad species.

Amphibians are best observed in a clear enclosure such as a plastic shoebox, deli cup, plastic bag, or other small enclosure. Handling for all amphibians is performed with a powder-free exam glove that has been cleaned, rinsed, or moistened with distilled water. Small frogs are best restrained with the hind legs extended and held securely between the thumb and index finger. This frees the head, body, and front legs for examination or treatment, yet adequately prevents jumping or escape attempt. Larger frogs and toads may require support by two hands to the body between the front and hind legs. Medium to large salamanders are restrained with a delicate grip of the fist allowing the head to protrude between thumb and index finger and the tail to exit at the little finger. As in lizards, tail autotomy is possible for many species of salamanders. Most adult anguiform amphibians (caecilians, amphiumas, sirens) are nearly impossible to restrain manually and are best examined in an aquarium or chemically restrained (see below, "Anesthesia").

Physical Examination

As with all exotic animals, the most important physical observations of the patient are made without handling. With the exception of some frogs, the posture of amphibians is not as significant in revealing clinical disease. This is due to the fact that many species are nocturnal and cryptic preferring to remain inactive or burrowed during the day. Species in which posture is generally significant are the dendrobatids, atelopids, mantellids, perching hylids, such as *Phyllomedusa* spp., and most newts.

Activity of the patient may be significant for some species. During a daytime examination all the previously mentioned species (with the exception of hylids) should be bright, alert, and responsive. In contrast, nocturnal species such as hylids, some toads, ranids, and salamanders will generally be inactive. A common indication of poor health in hylids, typically nocturnal, is activity during daylight hours. Red-eyed tree frogs, for example, generally are resting on the sides of the enclosure with eyelids shut in daylight. Aquatic amphibians, though generally nocturnal, are generally active in the enclosure on presentation. Exceptions may include some aquatic or large semiaquatic frogs that, by nature, typically are not very active foragers and prefer to wait and ambush prey.

Observing the feeding response of diurnally active amphibians is a practical method to assess overall health. A failure to respond to the proper food item is generally a sign of illness or stress. Nocturnal or shy animals, however, will rarely feed upon observation in daylight hours.

With a basic understanding of normal anatomy and body condition of the species in question, the visual exam should first focus on body condition. Is the patient normal weight, underweight, overweight, or bloated? It is important to remember that some frogs will inflate with air as a defense mechanism and may appear bloated, but suffer from no abnormal physiology. Air inflation is not a physiologic adaptation of salamanders and caecilians. As with other animals, emaciation does not occur in hours or days, but in weeks or months. Even the smallest frogs have distinct muscle groups that reveal weight loss. Poison dart frogs, for example, will exhibit emaciation particularly on the back, scapulas, and pelvis.

Observe the cloaca for prolapse. This abnormality may remain unnoticed by the client. Also observe a fresh stool sample. For most terrestrial amphibians, the feces are ejected as a pellet and should be somewhat moist and dark brown in color. Abnormalities in color and consistency may be significant. A microscopic fecal exam is essential for all captive-born and imported amphibians.

Abnormalities in respiratory effort can be difficult to detect in terrestrial amphibians. Normal respiration is driven primarily by buccal or gular pumping rather than by diaphragmatic or intercostal muscle contraction. There is rarely noticeable variation in this rhythmic pumping motion even in diseased animals. Bubbling from the mouth or nostrils in terrestrial amphibians, however, is abnormal and a possible clinical sign of respiratory disease.

Abnormalities of the integument is one of the more common abnormal physical findings and a common presenting complaint for diseased amphibians. Understanding the natural history and normal characteristics of the integument for a given species is essential. Most toads, terrestrial newts, and some tree frogs have relatively dry skin. Many larger tree frogs such as *Phyllomedusa* spp. and *Litoria* spp. can produce waxy secretions to prevent desiccation. Amphibians slough skin, ecdysis, throughout their life and this process should not be confused with disease. Coloration varies widely, particularly in frogs, and with many this coloration is bilaterally symmetric. Even cryptic amphibians exhibit some color and pattern symmetry; therefore, observe closely for abnormalities in symmetry of color, texture, and morphology. Amphibians typically do not exhibit color-changing ability as seen in some lizards, though variation will occur from day to night in many hylids. Ulcers, erosions, plaques, and crusts are not normal. Newly acquired or recently imported frogs are susceptible to rostral abrasions that may rapidly progress into necrotizing ulcerations.

Most salamanders and terrestrial frogs have closable eyelids and frogs possess a nictitating membrane that is semitransparent. When awake and alert, the amphibian eye should have eyelids open and clear cornea. Iris coloration is variable among amphibians, but is always bilaterally symmetric. As with mammals, unilateral ocular changes are most suggestive of trauma or focal disease, and bilateral ophthalmic abnormalities are more suggestive of systemic disease. Iris vasculature may be apparent in the normal amphibian eye. There is great variation in pupil structure from circular to horizontally and vertically elliptic. An ophthalmoscope illuminator or slit lamp is helpful for examination of the eye. Commonly used mammalian mydriatics such as atropine and proparacaine are not effective in dilating the amphibian eye. Wright recommends the combination of D-tubocurarine and benzalkonium chloride applied topically for mydriasis (Whitaker 2001).

Oral exam requires physical or chemical restraint in most species. Some species of frog, *Ceratophrys* and *Hemiphractus* spp., are known to gape as a defensive tactic making oral examination possible without restraint on occasion. Similarly, some larger terrestrial salamanders (*Ambystoma* spp., *Dicamptodon* spp.), particularly those maintained long term in captivity, may exhibit a conditioned feeding response and can be coaxed into biting a soft speculum to examine the mouth. Though it is not recommended as normal practice, these animals when routinely handfed will bite fingers waved in front of the face. It is unlikely that any injury will result to a human from the bite of ambystomatid salamanders. Large frogs (*Ceratophrys* spp., *Pyxicephalus* spp.) and large aquatic salamanders (*Amphiuma*, *Siren*, and *Cryptobranchus* spp.) are capable of painful bites to humans. These species generally require chemical restraint for both physical restraint and oral examination.

The clinician and technician should be aware that mandibular bones of many small amphibians are easily fractured with improper or forceful techniques to open the mouth. When properly restrained, the mouth of many smaller amphibians may be opened with a variety of apparatus such as plastic cards, laminated paper, coverslips, and small rubber spatulas. Nearly all amphibians will resist the oral exam if not sedated. Observe for uniformity and symmetry in shape and coloration of the oral mucosa and the tongue. Occasionally parasites such as flukes and leeches may be observed attached to the oral mucosa.

Palpation is easily accomplished for larger amphibians, but should generally be avoided in smaller species to prevent iatrogenic trauma. Internal organs of the smallest species may be evaluated by transillumination of the patient through a clear plastic container. This process is ineffective for large or dark-pigmented patients. The heart, liver, spleen, gonads, and some vasculature may be observed in this manner. Palpation of larger species may reveal abnormalities, such as foreign bodies and calculi, though normal structures may be difficult to assess or identify.

The heartbeat may be visible as pulsations of the skin in the region of the xiphoid on the ventral thorax in some amphibians. Similarly, in some frogs, pulsation of the lymphatic hearts is occasionally observed lateral to the urostyle. Cardiac auscultation is possible in larger amphibians, though the clinical significance of this procedure during wellness exams is questionable.

RADIOLOGY

As with reptiles, radiology is valuable in the diagnosis of some amphibian disease. This imaging is particularly useful for the diagnosis of skeletal disorders, urinary tract calculi, tissue mineralization, pulmonary disease, gastrointestinal foreign bodies, and other gastrointestinal disease with the aid of contrast materials. Unless abnormality is present, it is generally not possible to clearly differentiate coelomic cavity structures radiographically in amphibians.

Techniques for radiographic exposure are as follows (similar to those described for reptiles). Because of the small size of most amphibians, a tabletop exposure with detail cassettes yields the best quality image. Generally, an exposure setting consistent with the lowest mammalian extremity setting is sufficient, though with smaller patients overexposure is still possible. For technician safety the use of a collimator to achieve the smallest exposure field is essential. With this technique, multiple exposures are possible on a single cassette.

Restraint of the amphibian patient during radiology is a hands-off affair. Many frogs will sit briefly directly on the cassette for exposure. For those that are reluctant to remain still, placement of the patient in a plastic bag will facilitate restraint and manipulation for proper exposure (Stetter 2001a). When possible, a lateral and dorsoventral exposure should be made of every patient imaged. This typically requires the movement of the radiographic beam into a horizontal beam projection as the patient sits on the tabletop or platform.

Contrast studies are easily performed in amphibians. Barium sulfate is the contrast medium of choice and is given orally via a rubber catheter or feeding tube. The dosage varies greatly based on the size of the amphibian. A range of 10 to 15 ml/kg PO is generally sufficient, although the technician should approximate the volume of the calculated dose to the patient's body size and adjust accordingly. Percloacal barium administration is also performed for suspected colonic foreign bodies, strictures, or other disease. Great care must be used when manipulating catheters with these tissues to prevent iatrogenic trauma.

ANESTHESIA AND SURGERY

Anesthesia

Anesthesia for amphibians is useful for physical examination of aggressive or reluctantly restrained patients, certain diagnostic and therapeutic procedures, and surgery. Reports exist for the use of injectable anesthetics in amphibians, though current consensus regards these medications impractical and ineffective for safe chemical restraint. The anesthetic of choice for amphibians is tricaine methanesulfonate (MS-222, tricaine, FINQUEL, Argent Chemical Laboratories, Redmond, WA) (Wright 2001f), which is a white crystalline powder that may be mixed with water to anesthetize fish and amphibians. Amphibians are immersed in a bath of tricaine methanesulfonate until anesthesia is achieved and then maintained in fresh water for the particular procedure to be performed. For longer procedures, the patient may be immersed in a 50% dilution of the original induction solution or intubated and maintained on isoflurane.

Preparation of tricaine solution requires dissolving the powder into clean distilled water. The standard solution is 0.1% concentration: 1.0 gram MS-222 in 1.0 liter distilled water. Because tricaine is quite acidic, the solution must be buffered to a pH of 7.0 to 7.4, which is the physiologic range of amphibian tissue. This is accomplished with either sodium biphosphate (Na_2HPO_4) or sodium bicarbonate (Na_2CO_3). Wright (2001f) reports the use of 34 to 50 ml of a 0.5M Na_2HPO_4 solution to the 1.0 liter stock solution of MS-222. Stetter (2001b) applies Na_2CO_3 powder (common baking soda) to the stock solution until no more dissolves yielding the preferred pH range. Ideally, pH should be tested with a pH meter.

Tricaine is not stable in water when exposed to light. Therefore, unless multiple anesthesia episodes are planned, it should be mixed only in the quantity desired for a single anesthetic episode. Generally, a 1.0 L solution is adequate. All dissolved tricaine should be discarded after use and not reused for other patients.

Amphibians are induced in a bath of 1.0 g/L tricaine methanesulfonate in a suitable induction chamber that may be a plastic bag or other sealable plastic container. Induction time may vary, but usually 30 minutes exposure achieves surgical anesthesia (Wright 2001f; Stetter 2001b). Loss of the righting reflex and lack of voluntary movement are indications of adequate induction. Loss of the withdrawal or deep pain reflex indicates surgical anesthesia.

The heart rate is then transferred out of the induction chamber onto a treatment pan or receptacle and then maintained in clean fresh distilled water, or a 50% dilution of tricaine (0.05%) for the duration of the procedure (Wright 2001f). The patient's nostrils and mouth must be maintained above the water level to prevent aspiration. At this time, for longer surgical procedures large amphibians may be intubated and maintained on oxygen (with or without isoflurane) with intermittent positive pressure ventilation (IPPV). Continued exposure to the 0.05% tricaine bath will maintain adequate anesthesia in the absence of isoflurane.

The heart rate should be monitored throughout the anesthetic procedure. Respiration is reduced or nearly absent and oxygenation of the tricaine bath with oxygen is recommended to enhance oxygen absorption through the skin. The patient is recovered from tricaine anesthesia in clean distilled water making sure that the nostrils and mouth are not under water to prevent aspiration. The recovery period may range from 30 to 60 minutes.

An additional anesthetic protocol is the topical application of liquid isoflurane. A mixture of 3.0 ml liquid isoflurane with 1.5 ml water and 3.5 ml KY Jelly is made in a 10.0 ml syringe and shaken. The resulting liquid is then applied to the back of the patient at a dose of 0.025 ml to 0.035 ml/g body weight (Stetter 2001b). The lower dose is applied to frogs and salamanders and the higher dose for toads. The patient is induced in a sealed container over 5 to 15 minutes. Following induction, the remaining gel is wiped from the skin and anesthesia will last for 45 to 80 minutes.

Surgery

Though surgical procedures on amphibians are not routine, several pathologic conditions may require surgical treatment. Celiotomy, mass removal, and limb amputation are the most commonly performed procedures. Other procedures include enucleation and orthopedic surgery. All invasive surgical procedures are performed with general anesthesia using tricaine or isoflurane. Pre- and postsurgical administration of antibiotics are recommended for invasive procedures.

The amphibian skin is prepped using 0.2% chlorhexidine (Wright 2001f) or 0.2% chloroxylenol diluted to 0.75% with water. Isopropyl alcohol and iodine compounds are potentially toxic to amphibians and should be avoided. The surgical prep should have as long a contact time as possible prior to surgery, preferably 10 minutes. The surgical site should be moistened with saline prior to draping and surgery. Depending on the procedure, draping may not be performed. For celiotomy, sterile clear plastic drape is applied. Peripheral to the plastic drape a sterile cloth drape may be used to maintain a sterile field for surgical instruments.

As with lizards, a paramedian ventral midline incision is recommended to avoid the large ventral abdominal vein that lies on the ventral serosal surface of the coelomic cavity. Closure of surgical incisions is accomplished with nonabsorbable monofilament sutures of appropriate size.

TECHNIQUES

Venipuncture

Blood collection in amphibians can be a challenge, yet in some species, with proper technique and anatomical knowledge, the task is routine. Prior to sampling, the skin should be prepped with diluted 2% chlorhexidine or at a 1:40 dilution (Wright 2001f). The author uses diluted 2% chloroxylenol. Alcohol should not be used because of irritation and desiccation to the patient. Sampling from salamanders is performed from the ventral tail vein as described for snakes and lizards. A 1.0 cc or smaller syringe with a 25 or 27 gauge needle is ideal for most amphibians and the sample is preserved in lithium heparin.

Phlebotomy in frogs and toads is performed from a variety of locations (figs. 6.4 and 6.5). In larger frogs and toads the ventral abdominal vein is the best choice for both quality and quantity of the blood sample. Sampling from this vein is performed in the same manner as described for lizards. Because the lymphatic system of amphibians courses parallel to the blood vessels, it is not uncommon to collect lymphatic fluids with peripheral blood. Other sites of blood collection that are generally accessible in large frogs include the femoral vein and the lingual vein located on the ventral surface of the tongue. The volume of blood collected should be no more than 1% of the patient's body weight or 0.5% from a debilitated patient (Wright 2001f).

Celiocentesis

This technique is performed to analyze fluid retained in the coelomic cavity of amphibians. This technique may be both diagnostic and therapeutic. Fluid may accumulate in the coelom secondary to cardiac, renal, hepatic, or other osmotic imbalances. Similar to phlebotomy, a 25 or 27 gauge needle on a 1.0 to 3.0 cc syringe is ideal. The sample site is prepped with a 1:40 dilution of 2% chlorhexidine or chloroxylenol. The preferred collection site is from the mid lateral flank or mid ventral coelomic cavity. The syringe should fill with fluid on gentle aspiration and forceful aspiration should be avoided to prevent damage to delicate internal organs. Fluid may be smeared immediately or submitted in lithium heparin for cellular and chemical analysis.

Fecal Examination

Fecal exam is one diagnostic test that can be performed in all terrestrial amphibians and nearly all aquatic amphibians with relative ease. Collection of feces is facilitated particularly well during quarantine. The amphibian is maintained on a paper towel in a clean cage such as a plastic shoebox or storage container that is adequately ventilated and a sample is collected.

The sample should be examined directly in 0.9% saline and by fecal floatation with standard commercially available fecal floatation solutions. Common parasite ova include nematodes, trematodes, coccidia, various protozoans, and lungworm larvae (see above, "Common Disorders").

Cloacal Wash

Cloacal wash is performed in larger amphibians (>5.0 cm) to collect fecal material for microscopic analysis when a fresh stool sample is unavailable for analysis. A lubricated semirigid plastic or rubber catheter attached to a 1.0 ml syringe is gently inserted into the cloaca and isotonic saline (0.6%) is infused from and retrieved into the syringe. The fluid volume may be between 0.5 and 1.0 ml and not all fluid will be retrieved. A portion of the sample is then viewed with a microscope for pathogens. For smaller amphibians (<5.0 cm) cloacal wash is generally too traumatic to attempt. Examination of fresh fecal samples is recommended for these species rather than performing cloacal wash.

Transtracheal Wash

The techniques for tracheal wash are identical to those in other vertebrates. The patient must be anesthetized (see above, "Surgery and Anesthesia") and delicate handling of the tissues and apparatus must be performed. A sterile tomcat or small-gauge mammalian

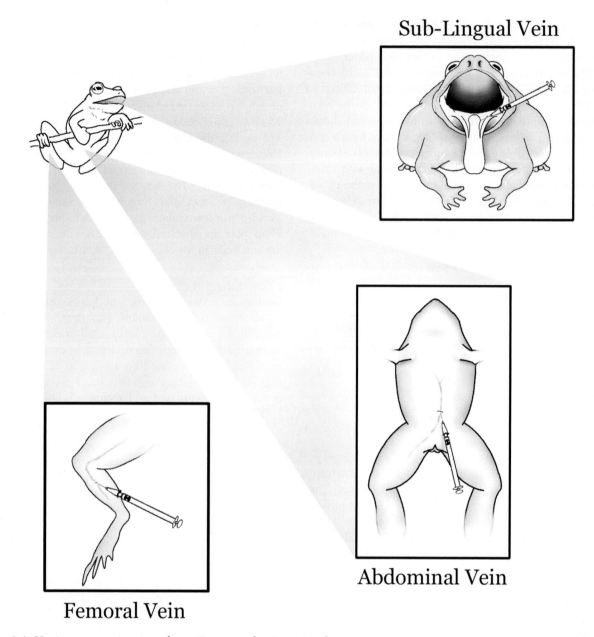

Sub-Lingual Vein

Abdominal Vein

Femoral Vein

Fig. 6.4. Venipuncture sites in a frog. (Drawing by Scott Stark)

intravenous catheter may be inserted into the glottis in the floor of the mouth. Depending on patient size, 0.25 to 0.5 cc sterile isotonic (0.6%) saline is infused and gently retrieved. The sample may then be smeared and stained for microscopic analysis.

Skin Scrape and Impression Smear
These processes are designed to identify fungal, bacterial, and protozoal elements to the skin or wounds on the skin. An impression smear is performed when tissue is damaged or ulcerated and a scraping will only create further trauma. Shed skins are particularly helpful for microscopic analysis and may be fixed in formalin for histopathologic staining to identify certain bacterial and fungal pathogens. A skin scraping is performed with the edge of a coverslip and wetmount examination.

Force-Feeding
Force-feeding is required for amphibians that are diseased and unable or unwilling to voluntarily feed. It is important that the owner understand that this procedure may be stressful on the patient and debilitated

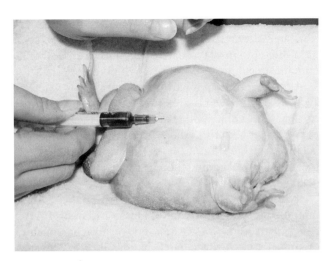

Fig. 6.5. Venipuncture of the midabdominal vein (ventral abdominal vein) in a frog. (Photo courtesy of Dr. Stephen J. Hernandez-Divers, University of Georgia)

patients may not survive repeated handling; nevertheless, this may also be a life-saving procedure designed to return the patient to a normal feeding response. Wright and Whitaker (2001d) list the standard metabolic rates (SMR) for caecilians, salamanders, and frogs at temperatures ranging from 5°C to 25°C and they recommend that caloric intake for diseased animals should exceed the SMR by 50% on a daily basis (Wright 2001d).

An ideal feeding formula for amphibians is Clinical Care Feline Liquid (Pet-Ag, Elgin, IL), which provides 0.92 kcal/ml and has a well-balanced protein to fat to carbohydrate ratio for amphibians (Wright 2001d). This liquid product is easy to administer through a small-bore tube and provides nutrients and calories evenly in suspension. The patient's normal food items are provided daily under observation to assess for a return to normal feeding. Force feedings are not made daily to reduce handling. Instead, the calculated daily dose may be multiplied by the number of days between feedings (3, 5, etc.) and the total dose for those days is administered at one time. Wright and Whitaker recommend that the volume of feeding should not exceed 10% of the patient's body weight in a 24-hour period.

The feeding procedure is accomplished in a manner similar to that of reptiles. A red rubber catheter, intravenous catheter, tomcat catheter, or ball-tipped feeding needle is passed into the stomach and the food preparation is infused. The technician should be aware that the stomach of most amphibians (especially frogs) is relatively proximal in the coelom; thus, passage of the tube no more than one-third to one-half of the patient's body length (excluding the tail) is recommended.

An alternative to Clinical Care Feline Liquid is a mashed or ground mixture of invertebrates such as fruit flies or crickets administered in the same manner. The author has had great success with anorectic dart frogs using this technique on an every 72 hours basis. Several patients have required 2 weeks or more of assist feeding before feeding voluntarily.

Therapeutic Administration

Amphibians present fewer problems than one may expect with medications. The semipermeable skin enables the clinician to apply some medications topically (TO) for systemic absorption, a technique not applicable to reptiles. Additionally, medicated baths may be used to treat both cutaneous and systemic diseases. Oral (PO) administration is possible and standard for some medications such as deworming agents and antibiotics. Injections may also be given intramuscularly (IM) or intracoelomically (ICe) in large amphibians or subcutaneously (SC) in frogs and some salamanders. Intravenous (IV) administration is rare and difficult at best in all but the largest amphibians. Physical restraint of the patient is required for all but the topical route of therapeutic administration.

The application of injectable medications in a topical manner is very practical for amphibians with permeable skin. This method likely results in lower percutaneous absorption rates in toads or in species that produce a waxy skin coating. Antibiotics such as enrofloxacin and ivermectin have been applied topically with great success for various bacterial and parasitic diseases. Baths with medications such as gentamicin, nitrofurazone, itraconazole, sulfamethazine, metronidazole, and other medications have shown success and safety in combating various diseases.

Oral administration is possible in nearly all sizes of amphibians and is the preferred route of treatment when possible to achieve maximum systemic absorption. This route is contraindicated in those species that are refractory to handling or physical manipulation. Metal feeding tubes or rubber catheters are used in large animals and microliter pipettes are used for small patients. Dilution of the commercially available preparations or compounding of medications is required for smaller amphibians. Dosing for most oral medications is daily or less often depending on the drug.

Injections are possible in amphibians, but carry moderate risk of trauma to muscles or internal organs and may result in chemical trauma or excessive pain and disability at the injection site. Many injectable medications applied orally in amphibians show good systemic absorption. This is particularly true of enrofloxacin that may be otherwise irritating to amphibian skin and may cause skin irritation, discoloration, or sloughing from topical administration or injection. The intracoelomic route is preferred for fluid administration in critically ill or dehydrated amphibians. The method of injection is similar to that of celiocentesis.

A considerable benefit to choosing the topical route for medicating the patient is allowing the client to treat at home for noncritical cases. All other routes of administration require hospitalization or repeated visits to the clinic for treatment by the technician or clinician. Medications should be dispensed in individual syringes with the appropriate amount for each dose drawn up and ready to apply. This negates the possibility of inappropriate dosing by the client. The client should return the used syringes for disposal at the end of the treatment period to allow both a recheck of the patient and to assess compliance of therapeutic administration.

An important fact regarding amphibian disease is that pharmaceuticals are not required to treat or cure every disease. It cannot be overemphasized that diseases resulting from improper husbandry comprise a substantial percentage of presenting complaints with amphibians and reptiles. The number-one consideration when choosing pharmaceuticals for diseases management is side effects. Though it may be difficult for the client to appreciate that environmental manipulation alone can correct improper health, it is even more difficult to accept further debilitation caused by unnecessary treatment.

EUTHANASIA

Invariably treatments fail to gain response or patients are too debilitated to withstand treatment and the client elects euthanasia. Amphibians and reptiles can pose some problems with euthanasia in that the heart may continue to beat for some time after neurologic incapacitation or death has occurred.

Reducing patient suffering and pain and client discomfort with the euthanasia process may be difficult. If possible, the patient may be sedated with one of several anesthetic agents prior to administering euthanasia injections. Ketamine at a dose of 100 mg/kg IM or Telazol (tiletamine-zolazepam) at a dose of 10 mg/kg IM (Wright 2001f) is sufficient to achieve sedation for euthanasia. The clinician and technician should understand that both of these injections are likely to

cause pain and discomfort to the patient at the injection site. Alternatively, tricaine (MS-222) may be used as a pre-euthanasia sedative or, if overdosed, as a euthanasia solution (Wright & Whitaker 2001b).

Administration of a barbiturate euthanasia solution such as pentobarbital at a dose of 100 mg/kg intracardiac (if possible) will result in instant death (Wright & Whitaker 2001d). Alternatively the injection may be given intracoelomically or intracranially through the foramen magnum, though cardiac death may be delayed.

If histopathology is required of the patient, then minimizing trauma to vital organs is essential. In this case, an overdose of tricaine given intracoelomically or immersion of the sedated patient in 20% ethanol will result in death (Wright & Whitaker 2001d). Most important, the client should be informed of the euthanasia alternatives and fully understand the procedure to be performed if he or she wishes to be present during the euthanasia process.

REFERENCES

Barnett, S. L. 1996. The Husbandry of Poison-Dart Frogs (Family Dendrobatidae). *Proceed. Assoc. Amphibian and Rept. Veterinarians*, 1–6.

Barnett, S. L., et al. 2001. Amphibian Husbandry and Housing. In: Wright, K. M., and Whitaker, B. R. (ed.), *Amphibian Medicine and Captive Husbandry*. Malabar, FL: Krieger Publishing Co.

Berger, L., et al. 1998. Chytridiomycosis Causes Amphibian Mortality Associated with Population Declines in the Rain Forests of Australia and Central America. *Proc. Nat Acad. Sci.* 95: 9031–9036.

Daly, J. W., et al. 1994. Dietary Source for Skin Alkaloids of Poison Frogs (Dendrobatidae)? *Journal of Chemical Ecology* 20 (4): 943–98.

Daszak, P., et al. 2000. Emerging Infectious Diseases of Wildlife—Threats to Biodiversity and Human Health. *Am Assoc. for the Advancement of Science* 287: 443–449.

de Vosjoli, P. 1996. *Care and Breeding of Popular Tree Frogs*. Santee, CA: Advanced Vivarium Systems, Inc.

Diana, S. G., et al. 2001. Clinical Toxicology. In: Wright, K. M., and Whitaker, B. R. (ed.), *Amphibian Medicine and Captive Husbandry*. Malabar, FL: Krieger Publishing Co.

Donoghue, S., Langenberg, J. 1996. Special Topics: Nutrition. In: Mader, D. R. (ed.), *Reptile Medicine and Surgery*. Philadelphia: W.B. Saunders Co.

Duellman, W. E., and Trueb, L. 1994. *Biology of Amphibians*. Baltimore: Johns Hopkins University Press.

Gagliardo, R. Atlanta Botanical Garden. Personal communication.

Goin, C. J., Goin, O. B., and Zug, G. R. 1978. *Introduction to Herpetology*, 3d ed. New York: W.H. Freeman and Co.

Helfman, G. S. 1990. Mode Selection and Mode Switching in Foraging Animals. *Advances in the Study of Behavior* 19: 249.

Klingenberg, R. J. 1993. *Understanding Reptile Parasites*. Lakeside, CA: Advanced Vivarium Systems.

Lotters, S. 1996. *The Neotropical Toad Genus* Atelopus. Koln, Germany: M. Vences & F. Glaw Verlags GbR.

Mattison, C. 1987. *Frogs & Toads of the World*. New York: Facts on File Publications.

Morell, V. 1999. Are Pathogens Felling Frogs? *Science* 284: 728–731.

Myers, C. W., and Daly, J. W. 1976. Preliminary Evaluation of Skin Toxins and Vocalizations in Taxonomic and Evolutionary Studies of Poison-Dart Frogs (Dendrobatidae). New York, *Bull of Am Museum Natural History* 157(3): 175–262.

Obst, F. J., et al. 1988. *The Completely Illustrated Atlas of Reptiles and Amphibians for the Terrarium*. Neptune City, NJ: TFH.

Petranka, J. W. 1998. *Salamanders of the United States and Canada*. Washington, DC: Smithsonian Institution Press.

Poynton, S. L., and Whitaker, B. R. 2001. Protozoa and Metazoa Infecting Amphibians. In: Wright, K. M., and Whitaker, B. R. (ed.), *Amphibian Medicine and Captive Husbandry*. Malabar, FL: Krieger Publishing Co.

Staniszewski, M. 1997. *Guide to Owning a Mantella*. Neptune City, NJ: TFH Publications.

Stebbins, R. C. 1985. *Peterson Field Guide to Western Reptiles and Amphibians*. Boston: Houghton Mifflin Co.

Stetter, M. D. 2001a. Diagnostic Imaging of Amphibians. In: Wright, Kevin M. and Whitaker, Brent R. (ed.), *Amphibian Medicine and Captive Husbandry*. Malabar, FL: Krieger Publishing Co.

Stetter, M. D. 2001b. Fish and Amphibian Anesthesia. *Veterinary Clinics of North America: Exotic Animal Practice*. 4(1): 69–82.

Taylor, S. K. 2001. Mycoses. In: Wright, K. M., and Whitaker, B. R. (ed.), *Amphibian Medicine and Captive Husbandry*. Malabar, FL: Krieger Publishing Co.

Taylor, S. K., et al. 2001. Bacterial Diseases. In: Wright, K. M., and Whitaker, B. R. (ed.), *Amphibian Medicine and Captive Husbandry*. Malabar, FL: Krieger Publishing Co.

Walls, J. G. 1994. *Jewels of the Rain Forest—Poison Dart Frogs of the World*. Neptune City, NJ: TFH Publications.

Whitaker, B. R. 2001. The Amphibian Eye. In: Wright, K. M., and Whitaker, B. R. (ed.), *Amphibian Medicine and Captive Husbandry*. Malabar, FL: Krieger Publishing Co.

Wright, K. M. 2001a. Amphibian Hematology. In: Wright, K. M., and Whitaker, B. R. (ed.), *Amphibian Medicine and Captive Husbandry*. Malabar, FL: Krieger Publishing Co.

Wright, K. M. 2001b. Anatomy for the Clinician. In: Wright, K. M., and Whitaker, B. R. (ed.), *Amphibian Medicine and Captive Husbandry*. Malabar, FL: Krieger Publishing Co.

Wright, K. M. 2001c. Applied Physiology. In: Wright, K. M., and Whitaker, B. R. (ed.), *Amphibian Medicine and Captive Husbandry*. Malabar, FL: Krieger Publishing Co.

Wright, K. M. 2001d. Diets for Captive Amphibians. In: Wright Wright, K. M., and Whitaker, B. R. (ed.), *Amphibian Medicine and Captive Husbandry*. Malabar, FL: Krieger Publishing Co.

Wright, K. M. 2001e. Evolution of the Amphibia. In Wright, K. M., and Whitaker, B. R. (ed.), *Amphibian Medicine and Captive Husbandry*. Malabar, FL: Krieger Publishing Co.

Wright, K. M. 2001f. Surgical Techniques. In: Wright, K. M., and Whitaker, B. R. (ed.), *Amphibian Medicine and Captive Husbandry*. Malabar, FL: Krieger Publishing Co.

Wright, K. M. 2001g. Taxonomy of Amphibians Kept in Captivity. In: Wright, K. M., and Whitaker, B. R. (ed.), *Amphibian Medicine and Captive Husbandry*. Malabar, FL: Krieger Publishing Co. pp. 3–14.

Wright, K. M., and Whitaker, B. R. 2001a. Nutritional Disorders. In: Wright, K. M., and Whitaker, B. R.(ed.), *Amphibian Medicine and Captive Husbandry*. Malabar, FL: Krieger Publishing Co.

Wright, K. M., and Whitaker, B. R. 2001b. Pharmacotherapeutics. In: Wright, K. M., and Whitaker, B. R.(ed.), *Amphibian Medicine and Captive Husbandry*. Malabar, FL: Krieger Publishing Co.

Wright, K. M., and Whitaker, B. R. 2001c. Quarantine. In: Wright, K. M., and Whitaker, B. R. (ed.), *Amphibian Medicine and Captive Husbandry*. Malabar, FL: Krieger Publishing Co.

Wright, K. M., and Whitaker, B. R. 2001d. Restraint Techniques and Euthanasia. In: Wright, K. M., and Whitaker, B. R. (ed.), *Amphibian Medicine and Captive Husbandry*. Malabar, FL: Krieger Publishing Co.

CHAPTER SEVEN

The Ferret

James R. McClearen and Julie Mays (Techniques)

The art of veterinary medicine extends itself into many families of creatures. The ferret has become one of the more popular pets in today's society. There are a number of similar modalities that transcend from small animal practice to small mammal practice. It is important for both veterinarian and support staff to recognize the similarities and differences. Remember that there are always new ways to approach solutions to problems.

The domesticated ferret found in the United States is commercially raised for the pet industry and medical research. It is conjectured that they arrived in North America as pets from early English settlers over three hundred years ago. They are most likely a domesticated variety of the European ferret (*Mustela putorius furo*). The black-footed ferret (*Mustela nigripes*) is an indigenous species of the southwestern United States. There are strict fish and wildlife regulations that vary from state to state as to the possession of these animals. Veterinary facilities need to be acutely aware of these requirements.

ANATOMY

Conformation

The ferret has an elongated body that allows the animal to enter small areas and holes for the pursuit of prey. This feature provides challenges for both owner and veterinary staff in caging and handling. Remember: wherever the head goes so follows the rest of the body. The males are larger than the females and their weight fluctuations vary according to season, as does that of dogs, cats, and people (Hillyer & Quesenberry 1997, 4).

Skin and Hair Coat

There are three naturally occurring coat color patterns. Sable is the most commonly observed but albino and cinnamon are also seen. The sable ferret, know also as "fitch," has been reported as a cross between the European polecat and ferret. They typically have black-tipped guard hair, cream undercoat, black feet and tail, with a black mask. In the United States, enthusiasts have developed over 30 color combinations. Some of these include silver, chocolate, panda, and Siamese.

One of the first observations handlers of ferrets notice about this animal is that there is a distinct odor. This odor is primarily from the oil glands and not from the anal glands, as many people tend to think. This odor may become more obvious when they are excited or during breeding season. There are numerous commercial bathing products that help to make these creatures more "house friendly." Descenting at a young age is a popular procedure at breeding farms but unfortunately has limited effects in preventing the odor.

Ferrets have no sweat glands in their skin. Due to this the veterinary staff must be aware of the possibility of hyperthermia.

Skeletal

The vertebral formula for the ferret is C7, T15, L5 (6), S3, Cd18 (Hillyer & Quesenberry 1997, 7). The anatomical considerations of interest include a small sternum and thoracic inlet, nonretractable claws and a J-shaped os-penis. Skeletal anatomy is depicted in figure 7.1.

Digestive Tract

The ferret has 30 deciduous teeth and 34 permanent teeth. The permanent teeth erupt between 50 and 74 days. The upper teeth are as follows: incisors: 6, canine: 2, premolars: 6, molars 2. The bottom arcade has incisors: 6, canine: 2, premolars: 6, molars: 4. (Fox 1998, 36). Ferrets have five pairs of salivary glands. Care must be taken not to confuse the mandibular salivary gland with the lymph nodes in that area. The stomach of the ferret is simple and can expand to accommodate large amounts of food (fig. 7.2). The small intestine is short in length and has an average transit time of 3–4 hours (Fox 1998, 36).

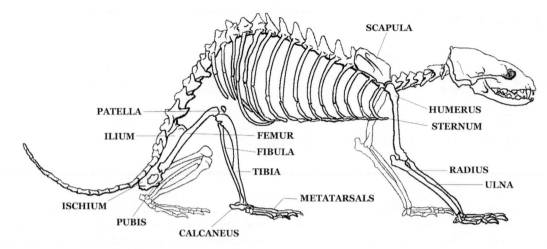

Fig. 7.1. Ferret skeletal anatomy. (Drawing by Scott Stark)

Heart and Lungs

The heart lies approximately between the sixth and eighth ribs. The lungs consist of six lobes. The left lung has two lobes and the right has four (Fox 1998, 51).

Spleen

The ferret spleen varies greatly in size, depending on the animal's age and state of health. When enlarged, the spleen extends in a diagonal fashion from the upper left to the lower right quadrant of the abdominal cavity. The size of the spleen is a very distinct finding during physical examination (Hillyer & Quesensbury 1997, 9).

Urogenital Tract

The right kidney is cranial to the left kidney and is covered by the caudate lobe of the liver. The bladder holds approximately 10 cc of urine. In the male the prostate is found at the base of the bladder.

The gender is easily determined in males by a ventral abdominal preputial opening as in dogs. In females the urogenital opening has the appearance of a small slit (see figure 7.3). During estrus, the vulva becomes enlarged. The natural breeding season is from March to August. Fertility in both genders is dependent on the photoperiod. Females are seasonally polyestrous and induced ovulators. Ovulation occurs 30–40 hours after copulation. Gestation is 41–42 days. If fertilization does not occur, pseudopregnancy often occurs and will last 41–43 days. If these females are not bred, a large percentage of these individuals will remain in estrus with the potential for bone marrow suppression due to elevated estrogen levels (Hillyer & Quesenberry 1997, 10).

Both adrenal glands lie in the fatty tissue anterior to the cranial pole of the kidneys. The left gland is medial to the kidney and is approximately 6–8 mm in length. The right adrenal gland is more dorsal than the left and is covered by the caudate lobe of the liver and is attached to the caudal vena cava. It is larger than the left with an overall length of 8–11 mm. This is important in evaluation of adrenal gland disease.

BIOLOGICAL AND REPRODUCTIVE DATA

Table 7.1 gives helpful information necessary when examining a ferret and answering common client questions.

BEHAVIOR

Ferrets are active little animals limited to the trouble that they can get into only by the size of their head. The adult males are called hobs, intact females are called jills, spayed females are sprites, and juveniles are called kits. The ferret has been and is still used for hunting, biomedical research, and most recently as a pet. The domesticated ferret does not develop fear of humans or of unfamiliar environments, unlike its counterpart the European polecat (Fox 1998, 5). In pairs they constantly play fight expelling sounds from a low growl to high-pitch scream when challenged or in pain. They will continuously roll and bite their opponent on the face and feet with their favorite spot being the nape of the neck. Many times in the heat of play with humans or companions, they will back up across the room chat-

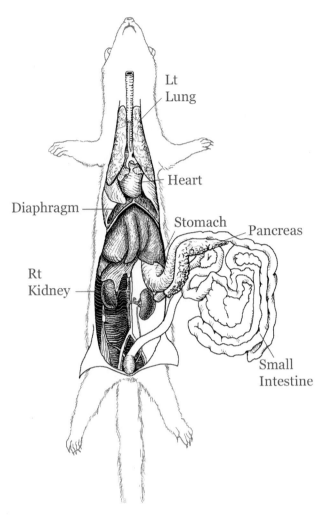

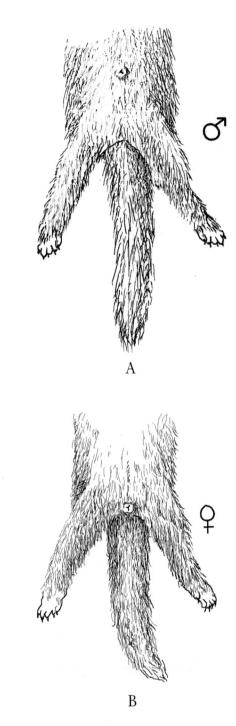

Fig. 7.2. *Ferret visceral anatomy. (Drawing by Scott Stark)*

tering and hissing at the same time. They are attracted to quick movements as they would to prey. Their eyesight is good only at short distances and they depend on their excellent sense of smell and acute hearing to help them maneuver in their environment. Because of their sense of smell, they have their nose close to the ground. This predisposes them to loud sneezing, alerting their owners as to their location. Ferrets are active about 25–30% of the day and asleep the remaining 70–75%(Hillyer & Quesenbury 1997, 12).

HUSBANDRY

One of the meanings of the word "ferret" is to search out something—to ferret it out or find something. This is the meaning of a pet ferret's whole existence and is an extremely important factor in providing a safe and

Fig. 7.3. A. *Male reproductive anatomy.* **B.** *Female reproductive anatomy. (Drawings by Scott Stark)*

an environmentally rich habitat for these animals: Assume that ferrets can go anywhere. The limiting hole diameter for escape is usually less than 1 inch; anything over that they can easily explore. Caging in the home setting and the veterinary hospital must

Table 7.1. Physiologic Values for Domestic Ferrets

Adult weight	
Male	1–2 kg
Female	600–950 g
Life span	5–8 years average in the United States
	Some may reach 12 years of age
Sexual maturity	4–8 months of age (usually reached in first spring after birth)
Gestation period	41–42 days
Normal weight at birth	8–10g
Eyes and ears open	21–37 days of age (usually, 30–35 days)
Weaning age	6–8 weeks
Rectal temperature	37.8–40°C (100–104°F)
Average blood volume	Mature male, 60 mL; Mature female, 40 mL
Heart rate	180–250 beats per minute
Urine volume	26–28 mL / 24 hr

Source: Hillyer & Quesenberry (1997), 10.

reflect this attitude. All potential openings to the outside such as heating and air conditioning vents and tubing, dryer vents, doors, and windows are all routes of escape. A domesticated ferret will not fare well outdoors because of its domestication. Inside the house, furniture, bedding, and appliances offer potential injury and even death as a possibility. Owners must be acutely aware of the dangers of ingestion of household items such as insulation for wiring, pipes, packing material, rubber bands, soft rubber material for shoes or other pet toys. Intestinal obstruction is a common problem in young ferrets.

Caging should be of adequate size with minimum dimensions of 24 × 24 × 18 inches (Hillyer & Quesenberry 1997, 11). Ideal caging should provide a hiding or den area, sufficient area for a litter box, and space for food and water. Food bowls should be made of a nontoxic product and safe water bottles are available commercially. Litter pans in a household setting may consist of a small plastic litter box similar to cat pans but may require lowering one side of the pan for entry. In a veterinary hospital, small, low cardboard boxes are useful with debilitated or postsurgery animals. They are also disposable.

Toys need to be "ferret" approved; hard rubber balls, metal toys that make noise, and "ferret" jungle gyms made of PVC pipe are good entertainment.

NUTRITION

The domestic ferret, European polecat, and blackfooted ferret are predatory animals feeding primarily on small mammals and birds. Early ferreters fed their animals bread or cornmeal soaked with milk. They survived on this diet as long as it was supplemented with fresh meat.

Most ranch ferrets are fed commercial pelleted foods. Initially, mink diets were fed but they lack important nutritional components due to their protein base of fish (Bell 1999, 169).

The ferret is an obligate carnivore with a very short intestinal tract. Compared to a cat, the ferret has about one-half the intestinal length. They are spontaneous secretors of hydrochloric acid, like humans and unlike dogs, cats, and many other predators. These animals will often hide food in various locations in their environment for future consumption. Because of the inefficiency of the ferret's digestive tract, ferret diets need to be high in protein and fat and low in fiber. Ranges for protein go from 30–40% and fat from 15–30% and are dependent on health status, if they are growing kits or lactating jills (Bell 1999, 172).

It is important to feed a high-quality domestic ferret food in dry form. Dry food is preferred over moist due to the health benefit for the mouth, teeth, and gums. Young kits will require some moistening of the kibble foods until they get their adult teeth. At the age of approximately 10 weeks they should begin to handle dry kibble. There are numerous commercial foods available either from pet stores, veterinary clinics, or the Internet. If food availability is difficult, a good dry kitten food can be substituted. Some ferret food manufacturers have senior foods available.

In some situations such as medical problems, surgery recovery, or colder environmental conditions, supplements may be warranted. Products such as Linatone (Lambert Kay) and Nutrical (Evsco Pharmaceuticals; Division of IGI Inc.) are available through veterinary offices. A common over-the-counter product Ferretone (8in1 Pet Products) is also a good choice. Snacks and treats should be held to a minimum since this animal will over indulge on its favorite foods and run the long-term risk of malnutrition. Commercial meat or liver snacks for cats or ferrets are acceptable, and an occasional raisin may add a little variety to a ferret's diet.

Water should be fresh and available at all times.

COMMON AND ZOONOTIC DISEASES

Influenza (orthomyxovirus) is the only documented zoonotic disease of ferrets. In most cases the transmissibility from humans to ferrets is much higher than ferrets to humans. Owners should be aware of that risk to their pets when they have upper respiratory problems. Other potential zoonotic disease includes leptospirosis, listeriosis, salmonellosis, campylobacteriosis, tuberculosis, and rabies. There are no known cases of transmission of rabies to humans from ferrets. Cryptosporidiosis has the potential of transmissibility to immunosuppressed individuals (Hillyer & Quesenberry 1997, 25).

There are many disease syndromes found in ferrets. Upper-respiratory infections are common with ferrets as well as with their owners. Canine distemper is occasionally found manifesting itself in various forms. Early signs include mucopurulent ocular nasal discharge, crusty facial and eyelid lesions, and hyperkeratosis of the footpads. In some individuals there is an orange color change to the skin. These animals are often anorexic, and in advanced cases may show central nervous signs such as ataxia, torticollis, and nystagmus.

Intestinal obstructions are very common in young inquisitive ferrets. These individuals present with or without vomiting, they are lethargic, and in most situations there is a palpable abdominal mass.

ECE (epizootic catarrhal enteritis) or green slime disease is a debilitating disease of young and old ferrets. ECE is usually brought into the house via introduction of a new young ferret. ECE is a highly contagious disease of ferrets characterized by profuse green diarrhea, dehydration, anorexia, and progressive wasting.

Tumors present themselves in many ways with ferrets. The most common tumors involve the adrenal gland (fig. 7.4). These tumors may be benign or malignant. Adrenal gland disease is most often presented as a dermatological concern. Hair loss on the tail, bilateral hair loss along the abdomen, and vulval enlargement in spayed females are consistent findings with adrenal gland involvement. Adrenal tumors can also cause behavior change and generalized muscle wasting. Secondary complications of the disease found in male ferrets involve the prostate in the form of prostatic hyperplasia or cysts and are presented with dysuria. Bacterial or fungal bladder infections can be sequella to prostatic disease in males with adrenal disease. This problem is extremely difficult to treat.

Lymphoma is found in the ferret in numerous forms. It may involve lymph nodes, spleen, liver, intestines, kidneys, lung, and bone marrow.

Squamous cell, mast cell, basal cell, and sebaceous gland tumors are the common tumors of the skin.

Insulinomas are among the more challenging disease syndromes to manage. Ferrets present very weak and sometimes seizuring. Because of the excessive insulin produced by this pancreatic tumor, their blood glucose levels are very low. These animals are often presented extremely depressed or even comatose.

Renal cysts are found in many ferrets and often are only coincidental findings.

Ectoparasites such as fleas, ear mites, sarcoptic mites, and ticks are common in ferrets and are easily treated.

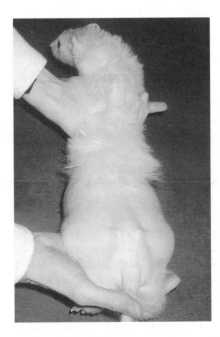

Fig. 7.4. Adrenal gland disease in a ferret. (Photo courtesy of Dr. Sam Rivera)

Endoparasites are uncommon but coccidia and giardiasis are occasionally found. There is some geographic prevalence to ringworm (mycotic) in some individuals.

Posterior weakness is a frequent observation in sick or debilitated ferrets. This is a common sign seen in hypoglycemic animals.

HISTORY AND PHYSICAL EXAMINATION

History taking and physical examination for ferrets should follow routine small animal veterinary protocol. Questions would include: Has your ferret had any coughing, sneezing, vomiting or diarrhea? Has there been any discharge from its eyes, nose, or any other body orifice? What is your pet's diet and how is its appetite? Is your ferret drinking excessive water or is it having increased urination or straining to urinate? Is your ferret active and alert?

Physical examination should always be consistent. Begin at the facial region and work caudally. Look for discharge from eyes, nose, or ears. Does the animal appear normal and of good conformation? Muscle and skeletal systems are symmetric and show no sign of dysfunction. Do they move in a normal manner? Teeth: are all adult teeth present or are there remaining deciduous teeth? Does the rest of the oral cavity appear normal? Are the eyes uniform in appearance and are there any signs of cataracts? Examine the ears for masses or signs of mites. Remember, dirty ears do not necessarily need to be cleaned. A certain amount of discharge is normal and is present for protection. Do you see any signs of lymph node enlargement? Make sure that all areas are searched. Abdominal palpation is best accomplished by elevating the ferret above the examination table by the nape of the neck or gently holding it around the neck. Most of these individuals will accommodate the examination without too much struggle. Keep in mind that the spleen in many ferrets is enlarged with no indication of disease or illness. Examination of the prepuce and penile region in the male and vulval area of the female is important to look for infection and any indication of endocrine problems. Heart and lung fields are evaluated with the same respect as with other small animals. Are the lung sounds normal and is there any indication of heart murmurs? How is the appearance of the skin and hair coat? Canine distemper may cause crusty lesions on the skin or orange color change. Hydration is also measured by skin turgor. Always be aware of masses of the skin and subcutaneous tissue.

PREVENTATIVE MEDICINE

The primary focus for preventative care in ferrets should be centered on yearly or biyearly physical examination. An early vaccination program is imperative in young ferrets. These individuals should be vaccinated at 6–8 weeks, 10–12 weeks, 13–14 weeks, and for distemper (Purevax Ferret Distemper; Merial, Inc. Athens, GA). Rabies vaccination is strongly recommended in environments with risk to infection and may also be required by law in individual states. Rabies vaccine is given at the age of 3 months (ImrabIII, Rhone Merieux Inc., Athens, GA). Both canine distemper and rabies boosters are given yearly along with a physical examination.

Heartworm disease is found in ferrets. Prevention of heartworm disease may be accomplished by off-label use of Heartgard 68 µg (Heartgard-30, Merck Agvet Division, Rathway, NJ). Give one-fourth tablet once monthly. The remainder of the tablet should be discarded since the remaining preparation will deteriorate. A liquid ivermectin preparation may also be used by mixing 0.3 ml of injectable ivermectin (Ivomec 1% Injection for Cattle, Merck Agvet Division, Rathway, NJ) in 28 mL (1 oz) of propylene glycol. Administer 0.2 mL/kg PO (0.02 mg/kg) once per month. This preparation is light sensitive and it is recommended to store it in an amber bottle. Expiration date is 2 years as long as the time period falls within the expiration date of the stock bottle (Hillyer & Quesenberry 1997, 70).

Internal parasites are not common in the ferret but fecal examination is recommended yearly and medicated accordingly.

RESTRAINT

As with many animals, proper restraint involves the humane handling of the patient with consideration for the safety of the assistant. Ferrets are usually active creatures but are easily managed in the clinic setting. Young ferrets and occasional nonhandled adults may have a tendency to nip. Some of these individuals may latch onto a finger and require a gentle extraction.

The preferred method for injections, examination, and fecal examination is scruffing the neck or forming a ring around the neck using your index finger and your thumb (fig. 7.5). The rear legs and rear quarters are firmly pulled caudally but not at full extension.

The second method involves wrapping the ferret in a towel "burrito" style (fig. 7.6). This is very effective for jugular venipuncture.

Many ferrets may be restrained, vaccinated, and

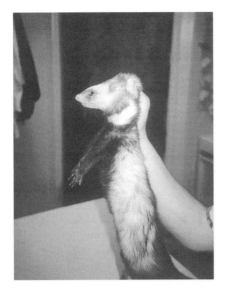

Fig. 7.5. Ferret restraint using the scruffing method. (Photo courtesy of Dr. Sam Rivera)

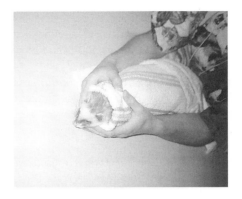

Fig. 7.6. Ferret restraint using a towel. (Photo courtesy of Dr. Sam Rivera)

treated without any physical restraint using a treat to distract these individuals.

RADIOLOGY AND ULTRASOUND

As with many small animals, it is difficult to radiograph a part without radiographing the whole individual. Obviously, one should measure for the body part of interest and set the machine according to the thickness and to the individual machine's technique chart. Small animal technique charts need to be tailored to each clinic's equipment. Contrast radiography is employed as a diagnostic tool in ferrets. The most common use is in GI studies. The protocol is similar to the cat but keeping in mind the fast transit time of the ferret.

Ultrasound studies are easily done and are readily tolerated by ferrets. Whole body scans are performed often with special attention to the kidneys, bladder, prostate in males, and the adrenal glands.

SURGERY AND ANESTHESIA

Inhalation anesthesia is the recommended product for induction of ferrets. Isoflurane is the most common product in use. Sevoflurane has more recently been used due to the fact that it does not have the irritating taste of isoflurane. The main disadvantage is the cost of sevoflurane. Intubation is a little more of a challenge with ferrets but is similar to cats. The technique may require the use of a stylet. Gas anesthesia is then continued for the duration of the procedure. The sup-portive care of warm water heat helps to prevent hypothermia. Pulse oximeters, respiratory monitors, and cardiac monitors work well with ferrets.

Analgesia is an important element in the recovery of postsurgical ferret patients. Butorphanol (0.1 to 0.5 mg/kg IM or SC q12 h) is effective in ferrets.

Common procedures in ferrets include most often gastrotomies, enterotomies, adrenalectomies, cystotomies, and mass excisions of the dermis and visceral organs. Most orchiectomies and ovariohysterectomies are performed at the breeding farms. There are specific regulations as to breeding, spaying, and neutering on a state-by-state basis. Liver and spleen biopsy are employed as diagnostic tools and may be preformed surgically or through the use of ultrasound-guided biopsy. Ferrets are often found to have enlarged spleens that may or may not be the origin of disease. This may require the necessity for a biopsy or spleenectomy. Many orthopedic problems common in dogs and cats are not found in the ferret. However, fractures and dislocations do occur in pet ferrets.

PARASITOLOGY

Fecal examinations are routinely performed in young ferrets and in ferrets presented with clinical illness. Intestinal parasites are uncommon compared to dogs and cats. Coccidiosis (*Isospora* spp.) when found occurs in young animals. They shed oocysts between 6 and 16 weeks of age and can be demonstrated in fecal examination. The *Isospora* spp. that affects cats and dogs may cross-infect ferrets.

Giardiasis can be seen in ferrets in pet store type settings. Cryptosporidiosis is a common finding in young ferrets and may persist in immunosuppressed individuals for months. There is no treatment in ferrets but one must keep in mind the zoonotic potential in the immunocompromised human population.

Ear mites often produce a persistent brown-red aural discharge without clinical significance. These parasites also cross-infect dogs and cats. Ear swabs are the key to diagnosis.

Heartworm disease (*Dirofilaria immitis*) is disease producing in ferrets especially in endemic areas. Heartworm prevention is unapproved but recommended.

Flea infestation (*Ctenocephalides* spp.) is a common finding of household ferrets housed with dogs and cats. Flea control methods for cats are used but not approved. They may be applied but in smaller doses (Hillyer & Quesenberry 1997, 17–18).

URINALYSIS

Collection is achieved by one of three methods. Gentle expression, catheterization, and cystocentesis have all been successfully used. Catheterization is difficult in females and in males due to the size of the urethra and os-penis. There are manufacturers that produce specialized equipment for these purposes (Cooks Veterinary Products, Queensland Australia).

Cystocentesis is best performed under anesthesia, due to the activity of the animal, using a 25 gauge needle and a 1 cc or 3 cc syringe. Care should be taken to not use too large a needle as it may lacerate the bladder.

Urine dipstick, specific gravity, and sedimentation are utilized for standard analysis. Urinalysis normals are presented in table 7.2.

EMERGENCY AND CRITICAL CARE

The normal life span of a ferret is 5–7 years. As with an emergency with any animal, a history and physical examination are crucial in determining the magnitude of the situation. Insulinoma, adrenal gland disease, and cardiomyopathy occur most often in older ferrets. Mediastinal lymphosarcoma or foreign body ingestion are found commonly in emergencies of young animals. Infectious diseases affect ferrets of any age and are a consideration in an environmental setting where people have respiratory illness.

Ill ferrets require minimal handling. Young and old ferrets are susceptible to green slime disease (epizootic catarrhal enteritis). Vaccine reactions were more common with previous vaccine protocols but have improved with the introduction of the new ferret distemper vaccine (Purevax Ferret Distemper, Merial, Inc. Athens, GA).

Table 7.2. Urinalysis Normals for Ferrets

Color	Clear to yellow
Specific gravity	1.015–1.055
Ph	6.0–7.5
Protein	0–1
Glucose	0–Trace
Ketones	Negative
Bilirubin	Negative
Occult blood	Negative
WBC	0–5
RBC	0–3
Casts	Occasional
Crystals	Occasional
Epithelial cells	0–Few
Bacteria	Negative
Urine volume (ml / 24 hr)	8–140 ml (Mean 26–28 ml)

Source: Antech Diagnostics.

Wrapping in a towel or grasping the nape of the neck are standard methods for restraint. TPR, physical examination, and history are important to establish a good baseline.

Hospitalization of critical ferrets requires a quiet, temperature-controlled cage with oxygen capabilities.

Anorexic ferrets are at risk due to hypoglycemia or hepatic lipidosis. Force-feeding A/D Diet (Hill's Pet Nutrition, Inc., Topeka, KS) via syringe or tongue depressor will provide good nutritional support. Other preparations are available or can be formulated in the hospital.

Basic diagnostic tests include blood chemistry, hematology, and fecal examination. Blood glucose can be done best on a glucometer, blood chemistry analyzer, or with less accuracy using a blood glucose stick. The primary venipuncture site is the jugular vein with secondary sites being the saphenous and cephalic veins.

Catheter placement is either IV in the lateral saphenous or cephalic veins. Jugular catheterization can be utilized but is not tolerated well by the ferret. They may become depressed due to the required bandaging around the neck. Cut downs of the jugular and cephalic veins in severely dehydrated ferrets may be a consideration.

Intraosseous catheter placement can be performed in the humerus, femur, or tibia with the femoral placement being the best. This procedure is best done under anesthesia. In animals that are severely debilitated anesthesia may not be a safe option. This procedure is painful and may require local block of the periosteum and soft tissue.

Fluid administration requirement for ferrets is 70

mL/kg/day. Dehydration and losses are the same as other small animals. With critical animals it is important to use the IV or IO route. It is recommended that an IV pump designed for small mammals be used.

Medications are administered via IV or IO catheters, IM injection in the quadriceps, and oral routes. Oral preparations are accepted best in liquid form since pill medication is difficult to administer in ferrets.

Cystocentesis requires sedation due to the thin wall of the bladder and the potential for laceration of the bladder. Ultrasound-guided centesis is also a consideration.

Urethral catheterization requires anesthesia in all patients regardless of condition. Locating the urethral opening is a challenge in both males and females. Male ferrets present more often in an emergency situation due to urethral obstruction from prostatic disease secondary to adrenal gland problems or cystic calculi (Orcutt 1999, 99–107).

SEX DETERMINATION

The sex determination is not as difficult as in many small mammals. Adults are similar to the dog. Neonate males have a urogenital opening on the ventral abdomen. Female ferrets have a narrow anogenital distance (Fox 1998, 106). See figure 7.3.

TECHNIQUES

Urine Collection (Sterile)
1. Cystocentesis: palpation of the bladder or ultrasound-guided use of a 25-gauge needle
2. Urinary catheterization. Materials needed: 3.5 French red rubber catheter or specialty catheter, nasal lachrymal cannula or sterile needle, KY Jelly, sterile gloves, hemostats, gas anesthesia (isoflurane or sevoflurane)

    Males: The male anatomy is complicated by the J-shaped ospenis and the small diameter penile urethra.
    a. Prepare supplies and anesthetize patient.
    b. Estimate length of catheter.
    c. Position ferret into ventral recumbency and retract the prepuce.
    d. Using a nasolacrimal canula or a blunt-tip needle as a stylet, insert the lubricated tip of the canula or catheter into the urethra orifice. Keep in mind the orifice is not directly at the tip of

the penis, but ventral to the end of the penis. There is often a small flap of penile tissue that must be elevated in order to access the urethral opening.
    e. Advance the catheter until urine begins to flow.

Females
    a. Prepare supplies and anesthetize patient.
    b. Place animal in ventral recumbency with elevated hind quarters.
    c. Aseptically prepare vulva and perivulvar area.
    d. Locate urethral opening using vaginal speculum or otoscopic cone.
    e. View the urethral opening on the ventral floor of the vaginal vestibule, approximately 1 to 1.5 cm cranial to the clitoral fosse (Bell 1998, 106–107).
    f. Insert catheter and advance until urine flow is achieved.
3. Collect voided sample from examination table or empty litter box. Many ferrets will urinate and defecate after their temperature is taken.

TPR
The same procedure employed with the dog and cat is used in obtaining these values in the ferret.

Medication Administration
Injectable medications and fluid administration requires proper restraint.
1. IV sites: normally given via IV catheter
    a. Jugular vein
    b. Cephalic vein
    c. Lateral saphenous vein
2. IM sites
    a. Quadriceps
    b. Lumbodorsals
    c. Triceps
    d. Semitendenosus and semimembranosus; Caution is necessary due to the location of the sciatic nerve.
3. Subcutaneous sites
    Can be given in a fold of skin anywhere along the dorsum.
4. Per os
    Administered by tilting head back and placing syringe through the side of the mouth.

Venipuncture
1. Jugular vein
    a. Sternal recumbency with one hand pulling front legs off the table and the other pulling the head back.

b. Using a towel, wrap the ferret tightly with only the animal's head exposed. With the animal in dorsal recumbency the ferret's head is flexed dorsally toward the person responsible for drawing the blood sample. The assistant should apply pressure to the vein on either side and the sample is drawn from the jugular vein.

2. Cephalic vein
   a. Normal restraint using the scruff of the neck
   b. Extend the foreleg.
   c. Hold off the vein.
   d. Draw sample using a 25 or 22 gauge needle.

3. Saphenous vein
   a. Used as last resort
   b. Technique is the same as for the cephalic vein.

4. Cranial vena cava; must only be used in anesthetized or severely debilitated animals.

5. The caudal artery may also be used.

IV Catheter Placement

1. Sites include jugular, saphenous, and cephalic veins (see fig. 7.8)
2. Technique
   a. Materials required: 24-gauge IV catheter, clippers and surgical preparation supplies, tape, flush, tourniquet, if needed
   b. Prepare site using aseptic technique.
   c. Apply tourniquet as needed.
   d. Perform a small cut down using a 22–25 gauge needle. The ferret's skin is a little difficult to penetrate.
   e. After visualizing the vein, begin inserting the needle and advance the catheter until blood enters the hub of the needle.
   f. When the catheter has entered the vein and blood is flowing freely from the catheter, flush the catheter thoroughly and replace the cap.

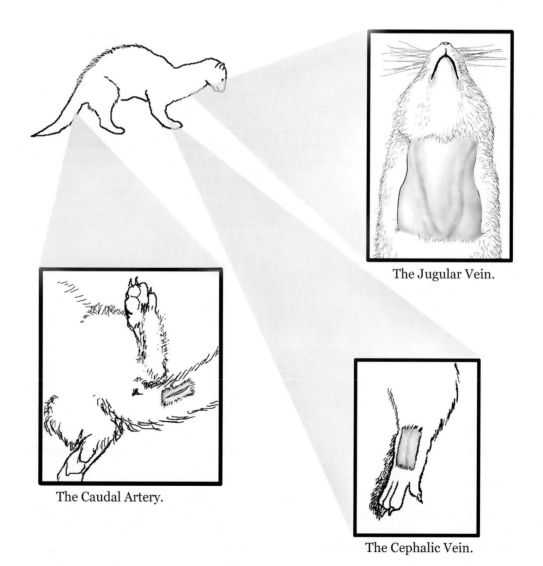

The Jugular Vein.

The Caudal Artery.

The Cephalic Vein.

Fig. 7.7. *Venipuncture sites. (Drawing by Scott Stark)*

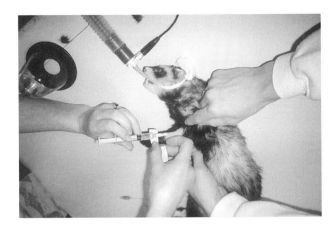

Fig. 7.8. *Cephalic catheter placement. (Photo courtesy of Dr. Sam Rivera)*

g. Begin taping the catheter in securely, with care not to apply tight enough to cause constriction.
h. Connect IV line to patient using a minidrip, IV pump, or other measured IV supply device.

Intraosseous Catheter
1. Sites include humerus, tibia, femur (fig. 7.9).
2. Technique
   a. The femur is the best site causing the least restriction in movement.
   b. Use 20–22 gauge catheters. A stylet or larger needle for a pilot hole may be used to place the catheter.
   c. General anesthesia is recommended except in debilitated individuals. Local anesthetic blocks may be used for the surrounding soft tissue and periosteum.

Enema
1. Materials needed: Small rubber urinary catheter, KY Jelly, enema solution (warm soapy water), syringe
2. Insert lubricated tip of the rubber urinary catheter into the rectum of the restrained animal.
3. Attach syringe full of enema solution to the end of the catheter and flush the colon using constant steady pressure.
4. Remove the catheter and cleanse the surrounding skin.

Bandage and Wound Care
The same procedures used on other small animals and in dogs and cats are used with ferrets.

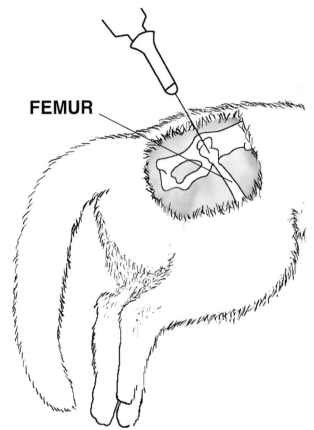

FEMUR

Fig. 7.9. *IO catheter location. (Drawing by Scott Stark)*

Blood Transfusion
Blood transfusions may be used if a local donor system is in place.

EUTHANASIA

Euthanasia is best performed by presedating the patient using IM Telazol (0.2 cc per 10 lb). After the ferret has been sedated, the euthanasia solution can be administrated IV or intracardial.

REFERENCES

Bell, J. A. 1999. Ferret nutrition. *Veterinary Clinics of North America. Exotic Animal Practice, Critical Care,* January, 169–192.

Brown, S. VIN. 2001. Small Animal Series, Midwest Bird & Exotic Animal Hospital, Westchester, IL.

Fox, J. G. 1998. *Biology and Diseases of the Ferret.* 2d ed. Philadelphia: Lea & Febiger.

Hillyer, E. V., Quesenberry, K. E. 1997. *Ferrets, Rabbits, and Rodents, Clinical Medicine and Surgery.* Philadelphia: W.B. Saunders Company.

Orcutt, C. J. 1998. *The Veterinary Clinics of North America. Exotic Animal Practice, Critical Care,* September, 99–126.

CHAPTER EIGHT

The Rabbit

Michael J. Huerkamp

This chapter is dedicated to all of those veterinary technicians with whom I have shared work and through whose dedication, passion, and tireless efforts, we have made a difference together in affecting the health and well-being of people and animals.

INTRODUCTION

The domestic rabbit (*Oryctolagus cuniculus*) is a lagomorph of the family Leporidae that descended from wild rabbits found originally in the area of modern-day Spain. Cottontail rabbits (*Sylvilagus)* are related, but in a different genus. The early domestication of the rabbit began in western Europe and northwestern Africa in the first century B.C. By the mid-1600s, rabbits were raised all over Europe for meat and fur and were in the course of dissemination all over the world via sailing vessels that stocked them as a source of meat supply. Female rabbits are called "does," males are "bucks," and neonates are termed "kits." Those rabbits being raised for food are termed "fryers."

Rabbits are attractive as pets because they are quiet, gentle, rarely bite, are relatively odor free, and can be housebroken and trained to use a litter box. They generally enjoy good health if kept under sanitary conditions, receive adequate water and nutrition, and are protected from predators, environmental extremes, drafts, and trauma. Today, in the United States, in addition to being kept as pets, rabbits are exhibited for showing, used in scientific research, and utilized for food and fur production. Depending upon the locale and nature of the veterinary practice, one could be presented with rabbits from any of these general areas of use.

COMMON TYPES SEEN IN PRACTICE

There are currently 45 breeds in the United States recognized by the American Rabbit Breeders Association (ARBA) ranging in size from 1 kg dwarf/small breeds to 5–8 kg greater giant breeds. Rabbit breeds are made distinctive by a combination of body size and shape,

ear carriage, and pelt coloration. If the ears "flop" down alongside the head, rather than stand erect, the breed is of the lop-eared variety. Some non-show-grade lops may have one or both ears "helicopter" by projecting horizontally. The ARBA currently recognizes 5 breeds of lop-eared rabbits. One lop breed is distinguished from another by a combination of mature size, length of ear, and fur length. The remaining 40 breeds have upright ears and are further distinguished by adult size (at 6–9 months of age), pelt color and patterns, unique attributes of the pelt, and body conformation. Among the more commonly encountered breeds are the Holland lop, Dutch, New Zealand white, Californian, checkered giant, Himalayan, mini-lop, and rex (see table 8.1).

Many rabbits presenting to a veterinary practice, particularly if acquired from a pet store, are not purebreds or are culls and likely do not conform to the "Standard of Perfection" for that breed for show purposes. However, despite cosmetic conformational faults, these "pet quality" animals may still be wonderful pets. The best method to become familiarized with a rabbit breed is to simply visit a rabbit show in order to see first-hand the differences between the many breeds or visit the ARBA web site at http://www.arba.net.

BEHAVIOR

Rabbits are a generally timid and often submissive prey species with a propensity for chewing and gnawing. They are quiet, relatively odor free, and tend to urinate and defecate in a chosen area, which facilitates litter box training. Those of a timid nature retreat to the back of the cage when approached and may thump a hind foot as a general warning or alarm call.

Table 8.1. Common Purebred Rabbit Breeds

Breed	Size range (lb)	Color and markings	Other characteristics
Californian	8–10.5	White with colored nose, ears, tail, and feet	Compact body type and pink eyes
Checkered giant	>11	White with colored nose, ears, eye-rings, cheek spots, a stripe down length of spine, and a pair of spots on each side of body	Harelike posture
Dutch	3.5–5.5	White forequarters and thorax with ears, cheeks, and back half of body colored	Short, blocky, compact body type
Himalayan	4–5	White with colored nose, ears, feet and tail	Small and slender body type with a long pointed head, erect ears, and pink eyes
Holland lop	< 4	Variable	Short, blocky, compact body type
Rex	7.5–10.5	Variable	Short and upright fur
Mini-lop	4.5–6.5	Variable	Short, blocky, compact body type
New Zealand white	9–12	Albino	Compact body type

Aggressive rabbits may growl or grunt, charge, flail with the front feet, and attempt to bite. Biting is fairly rare, but rabbits may scratch especially with their powerful rear limbs. Rabbits are not particularly playful, but may pick up objects and throw or bat at them periodically. While cavorting occasionally, they usually prefer to huddle or rest with intermittent periods of mobility and exploration. They scent mark by rubbing their chins on objects and enjoy chewing on wire, wood, cardboard, paper, hay, or other materials they encounter. Sexually intact rabbits of either gender may fight and this should be taken into account in counseling owners toward neutering or the recommendation of individual housing. Sexually intact, mature rabbits of either gender may also spray urine and mark territory (Stein & Walshaw 1996).

If rabbits are to be mated, this should be done under supervised circumstances as does may be aggressive toward bucks. A buck will circle a receptive doe and then quickly mount and copulate. Mating is an amusing ritual to observe as the postcoital male swoons off of the back of the doe. Kits are born in a nest that the doe makes from hair plucked from the dewlap and other materials that she may scavenge from the cage or environment. The kits are born hairless and blind—an attribute differentiating rabbits from hares, which are born furred and with open eyes. A doe typically nurses the kits only once per day. Lactation peaks at 3 weeks postpartum. The kits start eating solid food at 2 weeks of age and coprophagy commences about a week later. Weaning should be done at 5–6 weeks.

ANATOMY AND PHYSIOLOGY

Rabbits have a number of distinguishing morphophysiologic attributes that make them interesting and differentiate them from more traditional pets. For example, rabbits importantly use cecal bacterial fermentation in digestion, cannot vomit, have a narrow pylorus, and engage in coprophagy. In some part due to the latter three characteristics, they rarely have an empty stomach. They have large, accessible veins and arteries in the ears facilitating fluid administration, intravenous injection of therapeutic agents, blood-gas analysis, and direct blood-pressure measurement. The ears, in addition to high vascularization, serve in sound gathering and heat dissipation and are highly sensitive and fragile. Consequently, rabbits should never be restrained or carried by the ears. Rabbits have a high muscle-to-bone ratio. While 13% of the body weight is made up of bone in the cat, only 8% is bone in the rabbit (Harkness & Wagner 1989). Because they are engulfed in large muscle masses, the long bones and lumbar spine are particularly at risk of fracture or luxation, respectively. For rabbits used as pets and in research, this is an unfortunate characteristic that can be attributed to a heritage of development for maximal meat production. Three in five rabbits will have atropinesterase in the serum, which rapidly hydrolyzes atropine essentially rendering the agent unpredictable to worthless in effect. Like cats, rabbits are prone to laryngospasm and may be a challenge to intubate owing to the combination of a small glottis, narrow oropharynx, relatively large and fleshy tongue, and other anatomic factors. The skeletal anatomy of the rabbit is shown in figure 8.1.

The predominant white blood cells are lymphocytes and heterophils, the rabbit equivalent of a neutrophil, which may be mistaken for an eosinophil because of the presence of numerous small intracytoplasmic eosinophilic granules. Unlike cats and dogs, lymphocytes are generally more common than granulocytic cells (heterophils). Basophils (2–7%) are more common in rabbits than other species (Harkness & Wagner 1989). Reticulocytes also are encountered more frequently in rabbits than dogs or cats.

Clinical chemistry values observed in rabbits are not remarkable as compared to dogs and cats with the exception of serum amylase and calcium levels. Calcium is absorbed from the gut efficiently at a high rate. Consequently, blood levels relate directly to dietary levels often resulting in a dietary nonpathogenic hypercalcemia. Rabbits on high-calcium diets may have blood levels meeting or exceeding 15 mg/dL. Calcium is cleared from the blood by the kidney and excreted in the urine. Most other species excrete calcium primarily in the bile (Cheeke 1987). Rabbits are susceptible to arteriosclerosis as a consequence of dietary calcium imbalance or vitamin D excess. Serum amylase values are considerably lower than those found in dogs and cats (McLaughlin & Fish 1994). Blood gas values of normal rabbits and their interpretation are essentially identical to other species.

Reproductively, does have a duplex uterus with each uterine horn having its own cervix and eight to ten mammary glands. Does can rebreed within 24 hours of parturition, termed "kindling" in the parlance of rabbit users, and produce up to 11 litters per year. Kits may show growth rates of up to 35–40

grams per day. Like cats, ovulation in rabbits is coitus induced. Unlike cats, the receptive does are not likely to drive owners to distraction, but intact bucks, especially those that are house pets, will regularly mount seemingly everything in sight and not uncommonly the owner's slippered foot after sitting down in the evening to relax. The inguinal canals remain open for the life of the buck and the testicles may interchangeably be found to be in the scrotum or retracted into the abdomen. Herniation of other intra-abdominal organs is prevented by large fat depots immediately covering the canals (Swindle & Shealy 1996). Figure 8.2 shows rabbit visceral anatomy.

The rabbit is most interesting and unique from the perspective of digestion. It is a nonruminant herbivore dietarily, preferring the tender, succulent parts of plants. The teeth are open rooted and grow continuously. The normal dental formula is I2/1, C0/0, PM 3/0, M3/3 and is unique because the upper dental arcade includes two sets of incisors with a small, secondary pair, the peg teeth, situated immediately to the lingual side of the larger labial pair. The single pair of lower incisors occlude with the upper secondary incisors. The void between the incisors and premolars that is devoid of canine teeth is called the diastema (fig. 8.3). The incisors may grow at a rate of up to one centimeter per month.

Rabbits have a glandular stomach, which functions essentially as a storage organ. The stomach is never empty and even after a 24-hour fast will typically be more than half full (Griffiths & Davies 1963). The stomach of the adult rabbit is noteworthy for having a gastric pH that is significantly lower than other species (Cheeke 1987). This renders the upper gastrointestinal tract sterile serving partly to protect

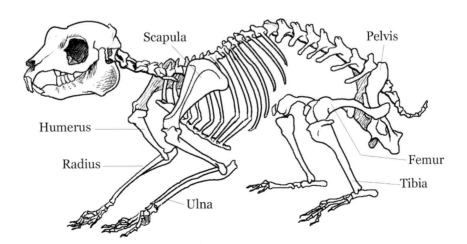

Fig. 8.1. Skeletal anatomy. (Drawing by Scott Stark)

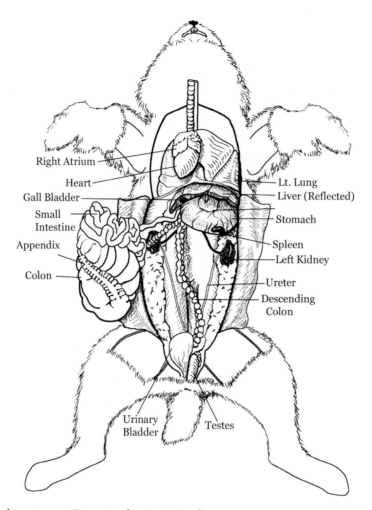

Fig. 8.2. Rabbit visceral anatomy. (Drawing by Scott Stark)

against the oral route of inoculation by pathogens. The gastric pH is higher in sucklings permitting bacterial colonization of the hindgut by feco-oral inoculation from adults in the population. Unfortunately, it also provides a window of opportunity for entry of bacterial gastrointestinal pathogens.

The small intestine, similar to most species, is the major site of acid neutralization, protein and carbohydrate digestion, fat emulsification, and absorption of many nutrients. Rabbits are hindgut fermenters, similar to the horse, with digestion characterized by selective excretion of fiber, cecal fermentation, and reingestion of cecal contents. The spacious cecum, comprising about 40% of the total gastrointestinal capacity, is a site of constant peristalsis with mixing and remixing of its contents, where an intricate and delicate relationship exists between nutrients, the microflora, and motility. It is the primary site of bacterial fermentative digestion and water absorption. The anaerobic flora

important in cecal fermentation are composed of *Bacteroides* and *Acuformis* species (Cheeke 1987).

Fermentation of carbohydrates results in the production of volatile fatty acids, in a process similar to that of rumination, that are absorbed through the cecal wall and used as a source of energy (Cheeke 1987). The colon, characterized anatomically by serial sacculations (termed haustrae), contracts and moves fluid and small digestible particles back into the cecum and propels large pieces of fiber distally where they are formed into the excreted hard pellets that are typically observed in litter boxes and fecal pans. At intervals, the cecum contracts and the fluid-, protein-, and vitamin-rich cecal contents are expelled into the colon, formed into small, soft balls, and consumed directly from the anus by the rabbit. This process is known as coprophagy or cecotrophy and it serves to recycle B vitamins, protein, and vitamin K to the upper GI tract for absorption or further digestion as needed. This

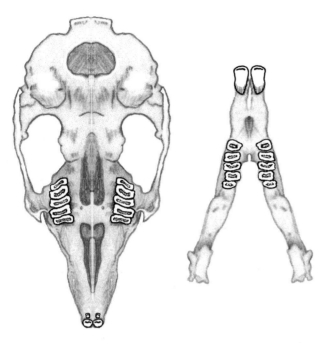

Fig. 8.3. *Rabbit dentition. (Drawing by Scott Stark)*

process allows for more efficient use of forage proteins than rumination. Morphologically, the cecotrophs appear as clumps of smaller, soft, moist fecal pellets that glisten with a gelatinous coat. This mucuslike membrane serves to protect the cecotrophs, and fermentative commensals contained therein, from the gastric pH. Cecotrophs are also called "night feces." Wire caging has no effect upon cecotrophy, but the act can be prevented through the application of an Elizabethan collar.

Anatomically, the rabbit gastrointestinal tract is also unique with respect to the presence of a lymphoid mass, the sacculus rotundus, at the termination of the ileum into the cecum. Lymphoid tissue is also found in the appendix at the cecal tip (fig. 8.4).

BIOLOGIC AND REPRODUCTIVE DATA

In the interpretation of laboratory tests, one should ideally rely upon a normal reference range for the species provided by the diagnostic laboratory that has conducted the test(s). When such values are not provided by the laboratory, the ranges in the tables that follow can be used as an approximation of what can be expected in the normal, healthy rabbit (tables 8.2, 8.3, 8.4). However, one should appreciate that the determination of "normal values" may be subject to laboratory variation, sample collection technique (e.g., extent of restraint, anesthesia, hemolysis), postcollection han-

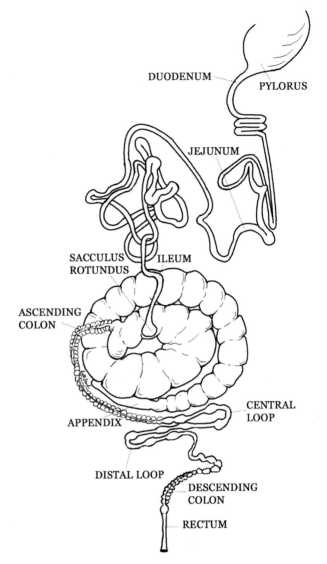

Fig. 8.4. *Rabbit GI tract. (Drawing by Scott Stark)*

dling (e.g., refrigeration, time to centrifugation, centrifugation characteristics), breed and age of the subject, and other factors. The numeric data provided in the tables below are normal values obtained from research populations of rabbits that were of fairly uniform genotype and age and maintained under standard conditions. They are presented as the normal distribution about the mean of a healthy population of rabbits. Presentation of values in this format merits several comments. First, some parameters may not have a Gaussian distribution and a normal distribution may not apply. Second, 5% of normal, healthy animals will have values that lie outside and at the extremes of the normal range. The interpretation of laboratory data, as in any other circumstance with any other species, should take into

Table 8.2. Hematology and Blood Coagulation Values

Parameter	Normal distribution	Reference
Total WBC (10^3/microliter)	4.6–13.2	Wolford et al. 1986
Heterophils (%)	<50%	Wolford et al. 1986
Lymphocytes (%)	>50%	Wolford et al. 1986
Monocytes (%)	0–3%	Wolford et al. 1986
Eosinophils (%)	0–2%	Wolford et al. 1986
Basophils (%)	0–7%	Wolford et al. 1986
Platelets (10^3/microliter)	300–700	Wolford et al. 1986
PCV (%)	33–45	Wolford et al. 1986
RBC (10^6/microliter)	5.5–7.5	Wolford et al. 1986
Hemoglobin (g/dL)	11–15	Wolford et al. 1986
MCV (fl)	56–66	Wolford et al. 1986
MCHC (%)	32–36	Wolford et al. 1986
MCH (pg)	19–22	Wolford et al. 1986
Reticulocytes (%)	<4	Wolford et al. 1986
Bleeding time (min)	0.8–2.0	Livio et al. 1988
Clotting time (min)	1.1–5.5	Livio et al. 1988
OSPT (sec)	7.9–17.9	Gentry 1982
APTT (sec)	19.5–22.5	Gentry 1982
Prothrombin time (sec)	6.9–8.1	Lee & Clement 1990
Thrombin time (sec)	5.7–14.1	Lee & Clement 1990

account the history, findings from a physical examination, and results of any other diagnostic tests.

HUSBANDRY

Rabbits can be housed either indoors or outdoors, the latter with appropriate shelter from the elements. Rabbits can be litter box trained and, for this reason, make suitable indoor pets but their proclivity for gnawing is a drawback. Furniture, carpets, window dressings, toys, electrical cords, and shoes provide numerous indoor targets for gnawing. Wherever they are housed it is critical to protect rabbits from drafts, temperature extremes, predators, flying insects, and environmental intoxicants. Rabbits are cold-weather tolerant and are best kept at temperatures of 55–72°F or slightly below and 30–70% relative humidity (Patton 1994). Rabbits can be housed outdoors if protected from cold below 40°F in the winter and excessive heat in the summer. Protection from cold, drafts, and moisture in winter can be accomplished by providing a covered nesting box containing straw, shavings, or other insulative bedding. In hot weather (generally temperatures above 85°F), rabbits require shade and plenty of cool water. Heat stress is a significant risk at this temperature and above. In extreme heat, consideration should be given to moving the hutch to a breezy garage or patio with a fan. Moving the rabbit indoors to an air conditioned area may be too much of an acute environmental stressor and such drastic actions on the part of an owner should be discouraged.

Plans for rabbit hutches and nesting boxes can be obtained from libraries, extension agents, or feed companies. Assembled cages suitable for rabbits often can be obtained from pet stores. At a minimum, rabbits confined to cages should be given sufficient floor space to stretch out to full length with sufficient head room to permit sitting on the haunches. Hardware cloth of 1.25×2.5 cm grid is suitable for flooring. Wire flooring should be cleaned regularly to remove suspended hair and feces. Sexually mature rabbits, whether male or female, should be individually housed as they may attack one another. Attempts at environmental enrichment should focus on providing hiding places, material for chewing (cardboard, paper), or nutritional supplements such as hay.

NUTRITION

Rabbits should be fed and will readily eat pelleted diets specially formulated for their species. These can be found in feed mills and major pet stores. Pelleted

Table 8.3. Clinical Chemistry Values

Parameter	Normal distribution	Reference
Total protein (g/dL)	5.3–7.6	Yu et al. 1979
Total bilirubin (mg/dL)	0.4–9.2	Yu et al. 1979
Sodium (mEq/L)	138–150	Gillett 1994
SAP (U/L)	0–139	Hewitt et al. 1989
Potassium (mEq/L)	3.5–7.0	Gillett 1994
Phosphorus (mg/dL)	3–5	Yu et al. 1979
Glucose (mg/dL)	86–137	Hewitt et al. 1989
GGT (U/L)	0–8	Hewitt et al. 1989
Creatinine (mg/dL)	0.6–1.5	Hewitt et al. 1989
CPK (U/L)	<700	Hewitt et al. 1989
Chloride (mEq/L)	92–120	Gillett 1994
Calcium (mg/dL)	6–15	Yu et al. 1979
BUN (mg/dL)	9–22	Hewitt et al. 1989
AST (U/L)	0–30	Yu et al. 1979
Amylase (U/L)	270–700	Yu et al. 1979
ALT (U/L)	0–60	Yu et al. 1979
Albumin (g/dL)	3.1–4.7	Yu et al. 1979
		Hewitt et al. 1989
		Gillett 1994

diets should be stored at 72°F or less and used within 3 to 6 months of the milling date (PMI Nutrition International 1998). Pelleted diets are nutritionally complete and typically contain 14–18% crude protein, 40–50% carbohydrate, 2–4% fat, 10–22% crude fiber, and appropriate vitamins and minerals in the proper balance. Indigestible fiber, although discriminately excreted and not an important source of nutrients, is important in digestion, normal health, and the prevention of fur pulling, gastric trichobezoars, enteritis, mucoid enteropathy, and other gastrointestinal maladies (Cheeke 1987). Fiber stimulates ceco-colonic motility promoting the peristaltic activity critical to the hindgut fermentative process. Without sufficient fiber, hypomotility is induced, floral alterations occur, the digestive process grinds to a halt, and disease may be induced. For growth, 10–15% dietary fiber is optimal, while less than 10% predisposes to GI disease. Adult rabbits should be kept on rations containing 15–22% fiber.

Pelleted diets optionally can be supplemented with alfalfa hay cut in the early bloom stage, alfalfa cubes, or succulent, leafy foodstuffs. With respect to the latter, plants of the cabbage family, fresh and washed well, can be offered as a supplement or treat. Suitable greens include cabbage, cauliflower leaves, broccoli leaves, kale, turnip greens, and mustard greens. Other greens, such as sunflower leaves, carrot tops, or green bean vines, can also be offered. There is little to no information on the effect of herbs on rabbit nutrition or health and they should be used with caution. Overfeeding of fresh greens predisposes to starch overload, cecal pH extremes, and enteric diseases. In addition, to prevent gastroenteritis, it is important not to feed spoiled foods or those discarded in the trash at restaurants or groceries. Another option is to permit grazing on clover or dandelions under supervised conditions in a fenced, covered enclosure in the yard. This should only be done in areas where fertilizers, herbicides, and pesticides have not been used and carries some risk of exposure to parasite oocysts shed by wild rabbits, other forms of wildlife, dogs, cats, and other species. Additionally, grazing on forages other than clover or dandelions is not recommended. For example, crown vetch contains glycosides that may be toxic and Bermuda grasses, kudzu, and birdsfoot trefoil have low feeding value (Cheeke 1987). Some rabbits may relish human breakfast cereal products, such as shredded wheat biscuits or grain cereals, as a treat. It is not necessary, and may actually be harmful in some cases, to supplement a sufficient pelleted diet with minerals.

As a rule of thumb, a rabbit generally will consume 5% of its body weight in dry feed and 10% in water. Rabbits kept as pets or used in research typi-

Table 8.4. Normative and Reproductive Values

Parameter	Normal distribution	Reference
Lifespan (years)	5–7 (15 maximum)	Gillett 1994
Gestation (days)	31–32	Gillett 1994
Litter size (kits born)	4–10	Gillett 1994
Weaning age (weeks)	5–6	
Rectal temperature (°F)	101–104	Gillett 1994
Heart rate (bpm)	200–300	Gillett 1994
Respiratory rate (bpm)	30–60	Gillett 1994
Blood pressure, systolic (torr) [1]	90–130	Gillett 1994
Blood pressure, diastolic (torr)[1]	80–90	Gillett 1994
Food consumption (g/kg/day)	50	Harkness & Wagner 1989
Water consumption (ml/kg/day)	100	Harkness & Wagner 1989

[1]Blood pressure values are given for instrumented conscious rabbits with central arterial catheters. Values average 10 torr less if the central auricular artery is used (Edwards et al. 1959).

cally are limit fed, while those grown for food production or lactating are fed ad libitum. Limit or controlled feeding is done by feeding 75% of the ad libitum consumption once per day and is important in preventing obesity, urolithiasis, and otherwise optimizing health. For a medium-sized rabbit (4–6 kg adult), limit feeding is done by providing 120–180 grams of pelleted diet per day. This translates to 3–4 ounces or about two-thirds cup. Administration of the ration by limit feeding encourages daily observation of the pet and prompt detection of anorexia as a tip-off to an underlying health problem. Pregnant does should be fed 175–225 grams per day, and at parturition they should be gradually increased over a few days to ad libitum feeding. Limit feeding is especially important at weaning during the dietary transition from milk-based diet to plant-based food when there may not be sufficient brush border enzymes in the gut to digest plant carbohydrates. Limit feeding of weanlings protects them from osmotic overload, pH extremes, and enteric disease. Weanlings of medium-sized breeds should be given 60 grams per kilogram per day up to a maximum of 120–180 grams per day.

Water should be given free choice and is generally consumed at twice the feed intake quantity or about 100–120 ml/kg/day. Water consumption varies with factors such as environmental temperature, diet composition, and health (e.g., lactation). Does will consume up to 90% equivalent of their body weight daily in water while lactating (Harkness & Wagner 1989).

COMMON AND ZOONOTIC DISEASES

By considering and meeting a few modest details, from a health perspective, the medical management of rabbits can be uneventful. The tenets of preventive care are good nutrition and sanitation combined with protection from predators, drafts, environmental extremes, environmental intoxicants, and trauma.

Rabbits that are commercially reared are often raised in pole barns and, for the most part, are free of infectious agents. *Pasteurella*-free flocks are not uncommon, but most sources have some problems with coccidiosis, encephalitozoonosis and, on occasion, internal and/or external parasites. New Zealand white and Dutch belted rabbits are often available as specific pathogen-free animals from rabbitries. Other outbred stocks or domestic breeds are generally not pathogen-free and typically have *Pasteurella multocida*. Rabbits obtained from pet stores, unless the vendor can make a specific claim otherwise, should be assumed to be *Pasteurella*-infected. Clients considering the purchase of a rabbit should be counseled to obtain it from a source with a *Pasteurella*-free colony or to obtain a kit at weaning or as close to weaning as possible. This is arguably the best advice, from a preventive medicine standpoint, that can be given to a client desiring a pet rabbit.

In private practice, one is most likely to encounter a domestic or wild rabbit in the clinic for interventional purposes rather than preventive medicine. There are no effective vaccines for specific rabbit diseases, for example, and, other than neutering over-sexed males, there is little in the way of preventive medicine procedures that a rabbit owner may seek proactively. However, clients that also own dogs or cats may seek the advice of a clinic in providing proper care for their rabbits. Knowing a little bit about rabbits may not only be good for the occasional rabbit patient, but it may also be valuable in maintaining business.

The most common presentations of a rabbit to a veterinary clinic will be for abscesses, tumors, malocclusion, elective surgical procedures such as ovariohysterectomy and orchiectomy, and possibly nail trimming. The diseases of rabbits of greatest clinical importance are grouped by system into those affecting the respiratory, digestive, and integumentary systems and by cause into those of infectious, inherited, or traumatic/environmental etiology.

Respiratory Infectious Diseases

Pasteurellosis is a chronic, progressive, incurable, fatal multisystemic disease caused by the bacterium *Pasteurella multocida*, which is unarguably the most important pathogen of adult rabbits. In rabbitries where the organism is enzootic, up to 90–100% of adult rabbits will be infected. The organism is part of the normal nasal flora of cats, as well, but the serotypes that cause disease in rabbits differ from those in cats. In terms of causing respiratory disease, all other rabbit pathogens pale in significance as compared to *Pasteurella*. *Bordetella bronchiseptica*, a pathogen of other species such as dogs and cats, is generally benign and clinically silent in rabbits and believed to be part of the normal flora. *Pasteurella* may be transmitted from rabbit to rabbit by direct contact, close contact aerosol, or, less frequently, venereal routes. The disease causes chronic morbidity and shortens life span. *Pasteurella multocida* is harbored in the nasal cavity where it may remain localized causing, at a minimum, frequent sneezing or "snuffles" syndrome characterized by sneezing and mucopurulent nasal discharge. Harborage in the nasal passages protects the bacterium from antibodies and any administered antibiotics. The organism may disseminate from the nasal passages to other parts of the body leading to a constellation of clinical manifestations including conjunctivitis, skin abscesses, inner ear infection, pyometra, orchitis, pneumonia, or septicemia. The diagnosis of pasteurellosis is by the observation of clinical signs confirmed by bacterial culture of lesions. Carriers can be identified by obtaining deep nasal swabs, under sedation/anesthesia, for bacterial culture using an alginate swab (Calgiswab Type 1, Spectrum Laboratories, Inc., 2930 Ladybird

Ln., Dallas, TX 75220). Alternatively, the serum can be assessed for antibodies against *Pasteurella multocida*, which may be suggestive of exposure and infection. Serology for *Pasteurella multocida* is typically not offered by traditional veterinary diagnostic laboratories, but, rather, by those that support veterinary programs in biomedical research such as Taconic AnMed (Rockville, MD). There are no effective vaccines, commercially available or otherwise, to prevent pasteurellosis or control its clinical signs even though a number of vaccine strategies and formulations have been developed and tried. Veterinary care is relatively expensive, primarily supportive and symptomatic, and invariably dissatisfying for all parties. Antibiotics, such as penicillins, tetracyclines, or enrofloxacin (Baytril, Miles Animal Health, Shawnee Mission, KS), may be given for a month or more to improve clinical signs, but upon completion of a course of therapy, symptoms invariably recrudesce and worsen over time. Consequently, antibiotics are part of the end game in buying time for an owner to come to terms with the prospect of euthanasia. Supportive care delivered by a veterinary technician is symptom directed and may include regular cleaning of obstructed nares, flushing of the nasolacrimal duct in cases of severe conjunctivitis, nebulization or vaporizer treatments, and excision or incision/drainage of abscesses.

The proportion of rabbits with pasteurellosis increases as rabbits age. By adulthood, 90% or so of animals from a rabbitry with enzootic infection become colonized. Preweanling rabbits have a low rate of infection and early weaning can be used as a tool to obtain *Pasteurella*-free animals. Additionally, treatment of pregnant does prior to kindling and through lactation with antibiotics, such as furazolidone, oxytetracycline, or sulfaquinoxaline, in the diet or drinking water will suppress the bacterium and promote the weaning of pathogen-free kits.

Diseases of the Digestive System

Enteric diseases have been cited to account for 10–20% of rabbit deaths worldwide (Cheeke 1987) and there are a number of gastrointestinal pathogens of rabbits, the most important of which are enteropathogenic strains of *E. coli*, *Lawsonia intracellularis*, *Clostridium spiroforme*, *Clostridium piliforme*, rotavirus, and coccidia.

Coccidiosis, caused by enteric or hepatotrophic species of the genus *Eimeria*, are arguably the most abundant and important enteric pathogens of young rabbits. Infection is often subclinical or mild, but clinical disease caused by any one of 11 enteric species, characterized by fulminant diarrhea, occurs in juveniles, especially recent weanlings, kept under poor conditions or stressed by transportation. Unlike other species, *Eimeria stiedae* parasitizes the liver and bile duct. Infection is often subclinical, but in young rabbits the agent may cause fatal hepatic failure characterized by icterus, hepatomegaly, elevated hepatic enzymes, wasting, and anorexia. The transmission of coccidia in rabbits is by the feco-oral route and the diagnosis is made by fecal examination for oocysts or made at necropsy. Aggressive sanitation and treatment with sulfa drugs are the focus of treatment. Vitamin E deficiency may potentiate coccidiosis.

Tyzzer's disease is caused by *Clostridium piliforme* (formerly *Bacillus piliformis*), an unclassified gram-negative obligate intracellular bacterium having vegetative and spore forms. Like coccidiosis, it causes disease most commonly in recent weanlings especially in the face of crowding, poor sanitation, or deprivation of food or water. Natural infection is thought to be by ingestion of spore-contaminated food or bedding. The spores are hardy and can persist in the environment for years. Mortality can be acute and high and the diagnosis can be difficult to establish and is often made using special stains (silver) of specimens obtained at necropsy.

Enteropathogenic strains of *E. coli* are also important pathogens of young rabbits. The bacterium is not normally found as part of the commensal flora, but proliferates in the cecum in disease-causing yellow diarrhea and high mortality within 48 hours. Sucklings within 2–8 days of birth and weaned kits less than 3 months of age are most at risk. Good sanitation, fluid therapy, body temperature maintenance, and antibiotics are important in treatment.

Clostridial enterotoxemia is caused primarily by *Clostridium spiroforme*. This gram-positive, anaerobic spore-forming bacterium is not normally a part of the gastrointestinal commensal flora or is suppressed to a very low and nonpathogenic level in healthy adults. Gut colonization may occur by ingestion at weaning, following severe environmental stress, or by disruption of the normal flora through the use of antibiotics with anaerobic and gram-positive spectra. Antibiotics that have been incriminated in the disease include clindamycin, lincomycin, ampicillin, penicillin, metronidazole, and erythromycin. These antibiotics should be used clinically with caution, the informed consent of the client, and not on a herdwide basis. The diagnosis must be made through a combination of clinical signs, culture of the organism, and demonstration of the enterotoxin. Clinical signs may not occur for a period of time after the insult to the flora. For example, enterotoxemia may not become

evident until 12–14 days after the discontinuance of antibiotics (Lipman et al. 1992). Treatment consists of a combination of nursing care, fluid therapy, antibiotics, and cholestyramine (Questran, Bristol-Myers Squibb Company, Princeton, NJ), but mortality is typically extraordinarily high. Cholestyramine also can be used preemptively where it may be required to treat a rabbit with risky antibiotics (Lipman et al. 1992). The importance of sanitation, for removal of spores from the environment, should be stressed to the client.

Rotavirus is enzootic in many rabbitries where it is of mild pathogenicity. It destroys enterocytes that synthesize disaccharidases consequently causing diarrhea due to maldigestion. Infection may be fatal in young kits that are not protected by maternal antibodies under epizootic conditions. Treatment is directed at supportive care as with enteric viral diseases of other species.

Mucoid Enteropathy Syndrome is a mucoid diarrheal disease of grave prognosis that may be common and particularly severe in weanling rabbits. The pathogenesis remains largely conjectural, but the lack of development of appropriate digestive enzymes coupled with dietary transition from milk to plant carbohydrates at weaning are believed to lead to excessive carbohydrate digestion or suboptimal cecal VFA production. This causes extremes of cecal pH resulting in alterations to the fermentative microflora. The imbalance, likely mediated by unknown microorganisms, progresses to profuse, mucoid diarrhea commonly in the face of cecal constipation/impaction and hypomotility. Affected rabbits are often thin, anorectic, dehydrated, hypothermic and mildly bloated. Dietary change and other stressors, such as painful injections, overheating, or inadvertent water deprivation (including excessively warm, yet plentiful, water in the summer months) may also predispose to disease. Treatment is generally unsuccessful with the case fatality rate approaching 100%. This is clearly a disease where an ounce of prevention is worth a pound of cure. Mucoid enteropathy can be prevented by feeding high fiber rations and by restricting the pelleted diet to 60 grams per kilogram body weight.

Lawsonia intracellularis is the cause of proliferative enteropathy and, like mucoid enteropathy, typically afflicts young rabbits. Although infection is characterized by a 1–2 week course of diarrhea, depression and dehydration, it is rarely fatal. The organism is difficult to culture; histopathology or molecular diagnostic assays are usually necessary. Severely diarrheic rabbits require fluid therapy and body temperature management.

Anecdotally, in the author's experience, rabbits that may not be colonized or exposed to pathogenic bacteria develop a constipation/obstipation syndrome, rather than diarrhea, as a consequence of cecal dysbiosis. This probably occurs when there are no pathogens that can effectively exploit niches created by the loss of commensal bacteria when cecal pH derangements occur. Constipation/obstipation syndrome may be particularly common in postoperative rabbits. The treatment regimen consists of fluid therapy, B vitamins, transfaunation with donor night feces, hay, and Fletcher's Castoria. Treatment must be intensive and consistent until normal digestive function resumes.

There are few helminth parasites of importance in domestic rabbits. The rabbit pinworm, *Passalurus ambiguus*, is not contagious for humans and is largely nonpathogenic. It is found in the cecum and large intestine of wild rabbits and occasionally domestic or laboratory rabbits. The life cycle is direct and infection is acquired by ingestion. The diagnosis may be made by demonstration of oocysts by fecal floatation examination techniques or observation of expelled adult nematodes on the feces. The eggs (43 μm x 103 μm, flattened on one side) are laid in embryonated, infective form. Common anthelmintic agents used in dogs and cats, such as ivermectin and fenbendazole, have high efficacy in rabbits (Curtis & Brooks 1990; Düwel & Brech 1981). Thiabendazole (Watkins et al. 1984) and pyrantel pamoate (Carpenter et al. 2001) have also been used safely and effectively in rabbits.

Obeliscoides cuniculi, the rabbit stomach worm, is common in wild rabbits and may be found in laboratory rabbits that are fed contaminated feed or grazed on contaminated forages. It is a trichostrongyle imbedding in the gastric mucosa with a direct life cycle and a 26-day prepatent period (Sollod et al. 1968). Rabbits are infected by ingesting the infective third stage larval form. Infection is usually asymptomatic and self limiting, but can be treated with fenbendazole (Düwel & Brech 1981).

Cerebral larval migrans and fatal central nervous system disease may be seen in rabbits that acquire aberrant infections with *Baylisascaris* species. Disease may occur where raccoons or skunks contaminate stored feed, gain access to pole barns or cages housing rabbits, and defecate from the cage top into the interior of the cage, or where pet rabbits have grazed contaminated forage (Deeb & Digiacomo 1994; Jensen et al. 1983; Kazacos & Kazacos 1983). Signs of infection include progressive torticollis, ataxia, tremors, and falling (Deeb & Digiacomo 1994). The diagnosis is based on clinical signs and histopathology, but fresh-minced brain can be placed in a Baermann apparatus to separate the larvae for specific identification. The condition is untreatable. Rabbits may be an accidental host for the canine heartworm (Narama et al. 1982) and other dirofilarial species if housed outdoors.

The pathogenic consequences of gastric trichobezoars are the subject of considerable debate among rabbit clinicians. In theory dietary fiber deficiency or abnormal grooming habits (boredom, stress) may lead to abnormal fur accumulation in the stomach. Obstruction of the narrow pyloric lumen by the trichobezoar, coupled with the inability of the rabbit to vomit, may lead to gastric obstruction, chronic wasting, and death. In these cases, mortality, without aggressive intervention, may approach 100%. However, in over 15 years of practice in laboratory medicine including the care of thousands of research rabbits, the author knows personally of only two situations where trichobezoars caused disease. One case was of a pet rabbit that ate carpet and window dressings in a home. The second was where rabbits, distressed by the continual barking of dogs in the area, ate hair in large amounts in response to the distressful situation. These experiences affirm the value of feeding high-fiber diets, preventing access to potential foreign bodies, and minimizing the distress invoked by fear of predation in the management of rabbits.

It is important to appreciate, however, that healthy rabbits commonly harbor gastric trichobezoars without pathogenic effect. Slaughter checks of 208 healthy rabbits in one study, for example, showed that 23% had trichobezoars (Leary et al. 1984). In the same study, infusion of rabbit stomachs with latex causing a large space-occupying mass had no effect on the immediate or long-term health of the rabbits. Consequently, trichobezoars are generally incidental findings in rabbits and should not be considered to be pathologic until proven otherwise. Care should be taken in differentiating the effects of a trichobezoar, especially where gastric dilatation is not present, from similar anorexia as a consequence of cecal dysbiosis.

High-fiber diets and prevention of unauthorized chewing on indigestible, fibrous materials such as home furnishings are preventive. Trichobezoars can be digested by oral administration of proteolytic enzymes such as papain or bromelain. These can be obtained in tablet form from health food stores. Oral dosing several times daily with 10 ml raw, fresh pineapple juice, a source of bromelain, for 5 consecutive days or more is reported to be effective (Cheeke 1987). The administration of paraffin oil (10–20ml) by gavage daily with gastric massage may also be curative. Surgery may only be transiently curative—many rabbits will reacquire trichobezoars after an interventional gastrotomy (Leary et al. 1984).

Malocclusion of the incisors (mandibular prognathism, walrus teeth, buck teeth) is the most common inherited disease of rabbits (fig. 8.5). The abnormality is due to shortening of the maxillary skull relative to the mandible of normal length with the lower incisors extending cranial to the upper incisors and growing into the mouth. Malocclusion may also be caused from tooth loss due to trauma. Uncontrolled growth of the incisors will lead to function anorexia and wasting with variable drooling and oral lesions. The treatment for malocclusion is periodic tooth trimming or extraction. In cases where the cause is suspected to be genetic, the owner should be counseled against breeding the animal.

Integumentary Infectious Diseases

The most important integumentary disease of rabbits is ear mite infestation by the ectoparasite *Psoroptes cuniculi* (fig. 8.6). The condition, most properly called otoacariasis, may be referred to as ear mange or ear canker by rabbit keepers. Exudate and inflammation in the ear canal can be extensive and the mites may also parasitize periauricular areas including the face and neck. Transmission of the parasite is direct from rabbit-to-rabbit and the life cycle requires 21 days for completion. Tens of thousands of mites may be found on a single animal (Bowman et al. 1992). Mites can survive off of the host for weeks at a time (Arlian et al. 1981). Infestation causes pruritus, head shaking, stress, and competition for nutrients. The ears may be painful to touch and, in advanced cases, are often heavily encrusted with exudate. The mites are large enough to be seen with the unaided eye, but the diagnosis usually is made by otoscope examination of the large adults (m. 431–547 μm × 322–462 μm; f.

403–749 μm × 351 × 499 μm) in the aural canal or microscopic observation of mites from exudate swabbed from the ear. Treatment is with ivermectin by SC injection given every 2 weeks for a total of three treatments and aggressive environmental sanitation (Curtis & Brooks 1990; Wright & Riner 1984).

Venereal spirochetosis is caused by a spirochete bacterium, *Treponema cuniculi*. The disease is known by a number of synonyms including treponemiasis, cuniculosis, vent disease, and rabbit syphilis. Transmission may be horizontal by the venereal (coitus) or extragenital (facial-genital contact) routes. Fomite inoculation is also a possibility. Few young rabbits or those that are sexually naïve exhibit clinical disease or serologic evidence of infection, but incidence increases with time in a breeding program. Following infectious contact, organisms localize and proliferate at mucocutaneous junctions causing erythema and edema of prepuce, vulva, scrotum, perineum, or anus. The nose, eyelids, lips, and extremities can also be affected. The lesions become vesicular, exude serum, and then become dry, scaly, and crusty. In the natural course of the disease, lesions persist for *at least* 1 to 3 months and often for 5 months or so (Delong & Manning 1994). During the course of infection, the bacterium then colonizes regional lymph nodes where it remains even after lesions fade. Overt clinical disease is then precipitated by stress. Venereal spirochetosis may be confused and should be differentiated from traumatic or chemical dermatitis, localized nontreponemal bacterial pyoderma (e.g., "hutch burn"), dermatophytes, and ectoparasites. The diagnosis of treponemiasis is by history, physical examination, and *in vitro* tests such as darkfield microscopy and various serologic assays. Penicillins, given for

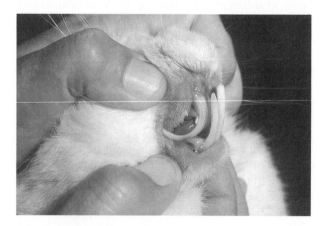

Fig. 8.5. Malocclusion. (Photo courtesy of Dr. Chris King)

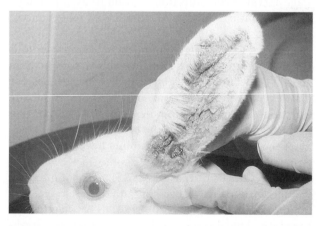

Fig. 8.6. Ear mite infestation. (Photo courtesy of Dr. Mike Huerkamp)

periods ranging from 5 to 28 days, are the treatment of choice. A less-intensive penicillin regimen involving weekly injections for a total of three treatments has also been advocated (Delong & Manning 1994). Lesions generally resolve and the organism will be eliminated within 3 weeks of the start of treatment.

Ulcerative pododermatitis presents as decubital ulcers typically on the plantar surfaces of the hind feet (fig. 8.7). Superficial ulcers and scabs may progress, without intervention, to abscesses or granulomas. The lesions are pressure induced and predisposed commonly by a genetically related decrease in hair density on the feet. Poor sanitation, excessive environmental moisture, foot stomping, large adult size, and shape of the wire all may be contributory factors. Treatment consists of topical application of antibiotic creams with bandaging and rebandaging for weeks at a time. Other interventions should include improving sanitation and changing the flooring from wire to flat metal slatted flooring or solid flooring with use of a litter box. The latter, however, may become soiled and aggravate problems. Where rabbits must be kept on wire, the strategic placement of a flat, solid resting board in an area of the cage the rabbit can use for rest is advisable. Preferably, this should be away from areas used for urination and defecation. Successful treatment is lengthy and the condition often recrudesces.

Moist dermatitis (blue fur disease) may be seen in the perineal area subsequent to urine or diarrhea scald, known colloquially as "hutch burn," or of the face, neck or dewlap as a consequence of malocclusion or continual moisting of the fur in a water crock. The latter presentation may be called "slobbers" by fanciers and breeders. The initial physical insult may lead to secondary bacterial dermatitis often due to pseudomoniasis from the feces or fecal-contaminated drinking water. *Pseudomonas* species elaborate a blue-green pigment that discolors the affected area. Rabbits so affected are often described as having blue fur disease. The treatment is by correcting the initiating cause, drying the environment, clipping fur in the area of any lesions, and treating the lesions with astringents and topical or systemic gentamicin. Prevention is by good sanitation, controlling obesity, and not offering water from bowls or crocks.

Necrobacillosis (Schmorl's disease) is a disease that may be confused, in some cases, with advanced pododermatitis or moist dermatitis. The gram-negative anaerobic bacterium, *Fusobacterium necrophorum*, is a normal inhabitant of the gastrointestinal tract that may cause ulceration and necrosis of the skin and subcutis of the face and neck, plantar areas of the feet, and septicemia. Infection typically is associated with filthy conditions and skin trauma or dental disease. Fecal contamination from coprophagy may be a source of oral inoculation. The diagnosis is made by a combination of clinical signs and anaerobic bacterial culture. Treatment consists of debriding wounds and applying topical antibiotics. Systemic drugs with an anaerobic spectrum such as penicillins, cephalosporins, or chloramphenicol may be used in severe cases. Prevention is by maintaining a high level of sanitation, providing dental care where indicated, and eliminating sources of trauma such as coarse feed or sharp edges in cages.

Fly strike is not uncommon in rabbits housed outdoors. Maggots may be found anywhere on the body, but have a predilection for the perineal skin folds of aged or obese rabbits. The treatment is by removing the maggots and cleaning the wound site under sedation, antibiotics, fluid therapy, and the administration of ivermectin for two doses given at 2-week intervals. Preventive strategies consist of fly control measures including screening outdoor pens.

Mastitis is generally rare except where breeding is done. The offending bacteria are typically staphylococci or coliforms. Treatment consists of antibiotics, warm compresses, fluid therapy, and, where indicated, incision and drainage.

Other Infectious Diseases of Significance

There are a number of other infectious diseases of rabbits that are not likely to be encountered in pet rabbits but are worth mentioning. *Yersinia pseudotuberculosis* is acquired by ingestion and causes emaciation and swollen lymph nodes with variable incidence of septicemia or diarrhea. *Listeria monocytogenes* causes

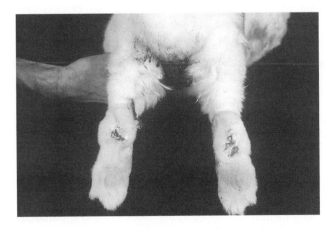

Fig. 8.7. Pododermatitis. (Photo courtesy of Dr. Chris King)

acute, sporadic disease in many species. In rabbits, it most commonly causes septicemia, abortion, and fatality of pregnant does. Staphylococci may cause septicemia, suppurative disease (including cutaneous abscesses or mastitis), and conjunctivitis. It is most severe and common in young or distressed animals. Rabbit Hemorrhagic Disease is caused by a calicivirus and targets rabbits after weaning. The disease is acute and highly fatal showing few clinical signs. Rabbits die from a severe and widespread intravascular coagulopathy (Xu & Chen 1989). Rabbits are also susceptible to toxoplasmosis (Leland et al. 1992).

Inherited Diseases

Buphthalmia (glaucoma, ox eye) is not uncommon in New Zealand white rabbits and is due to inadequate drainage of aqueous from the anterior chamber (Tesluk et al. 1982). It occurs bilaterally and is usually detected by the time the rabbit is 3–5 months old. Buphthalmia in rabbits is characterized by increased intraocular pressure and increased corneal diameter with edema and neovascularization. The condition is generally not painful, at least in the early stages, but may cause blindness. Medical treatment with antiglaucomatous agents generally is not successful. Consequently, regular monitoring of affected rabbits for pain or distress should be done (Cohen 1969).

Rabbits, depending upon the breed and genotype, may be afflicted by any number of other genetic and metabolic diseases including epilepsy, hydrocephalus, arteriosclerosis, cataracts, Pelger-Huet anomaly, cleft palate, lymphosarcoma, and hypertension (Lindsey & Fox 1994). Arteriosclerosis is a polygenic or familial trait that can be seen in all breeds (Feigenbaum & Gaman 1967), although it is more common in Dutch and New Zealand white rabbits with incidences of 10% and 40%, respectively (Gaman et al. 1967; Greene 1965). The condition is generally clinically silent and similar lesions can be induced by vitamin D toxicity. Hydrocephalus is often associated with dwarfism and brachygnathia although vitamin A deficiency in pregnant does will produce identical clinical signs in offspring (Cohen 1969; Lindsey & Fox 1994). Splay leg is not uncommonly seen in Dutch rabbits where the rear limbs of maturing kits splay and will not bear weight (Cohen 1969).

Traumatic and Environmental Diseases

Traumatic vertebral subluxation or compression fractures may occur secondary to struggling against restraint, improper handling, or even overzealous jumping or general rambunctiousness. Injury is predisposed by the high muscle-to-bone ratio in rabbits.

The lumbosacral joint acts as a fulcrum for the hind limbs with subluxation or fracture generally occurring at L7 or the caudal vertebrae. Diagnosis is made by clinical signs (i.e., posterior paresis or paralysis, loss of pain sensation, urinary retention, fecal incontinence), palpation, and/or radiography. Sequellae include decubital sores and perineal dermatitis from urine scald. The condition is incurable, demands extensive nursing care, and requires euthanasia. Rabbits can be provided supportive care for a short period (the condition is nonpainful) before problems due to urinary incontinence, decubital ulcers, and coprophagy prevention set in. Occasionally, affected rabbits recover if the injury is limited to spinal edema without vertebral involvement.

Pregnancy toxemia is uncommon, but may be seen especially in Dutch or Polish breeds. It is most common in pregnant does late in gestation, and may also be seen in pseudopregnant, postparturient, or obese does or bucks, but is most common in does in the last week of pregnancy. Clinically affected animals are depressed, have acetone breath, dyspnea, and decreased urine production. Also abortion, incoordination, convulsions and coma may precede death. Death without premonitory signs can be a presentation. As for other species, the cause of the disease in rabbits is complex and multifactorial. Fasting is a predisposing factor. There is often hepatic fatty infiltration and necrosis. Treatment is recommended to be lactated Ringer's or 5% dextrose, steroids, and empiric use of calcium gluconate, but is rarely successful. Prevention is accomplished by providing an adequate nutritional plane, while preventing obesity.

Neoplasia

Retrospective assessments of tumor incidence in rabbits are confounded by the fact that case reports and retrospective surveys have been largely derived from colonies of research animals where rabbits, for the most part, rarely live longer than 1–2 years of age (Weisbroth 1994). While tumor incidence increases with age, there exists no comprehensive tumor incidence information for aging rabbits.

Uterine adenocarcinoma is the most common neoplasm of female rabbits with a high incidence in the Dutch, Californian, and New Zealand white breeds. The incidence is less than 5% in does under 2 years of age, but in certain populations it may affect 80% of does over 5 years of age (Ingalls et al. 1964). Clinical signs include vulvar bleeding, anemia, and a palpable abdominal mass. The prevention and attempted treatment of the disease is by ovariohysterectomy (OHE). Unless does are to be bred, OHE is recommended universally. Interstitial cell tumors and seminomas have been reported in male rabbits (Weisbroth 1994). Other neoplasms that have been reported with some frequency in rabbits include embryonal nephroma, leiomyoma/leiosarcoma, lymphosarcoma, cutaneous papilloma, and mammary adenocarcinoma (Weisbroth 1994).

Zoonotic Diseases

Domestic rabbits harbor few zoonoses of any significance. Dermatophytosis is arguably the most important zoonotic disease of lapines. *Trichophyton mentagrophytes* is most common, but *Microsporum canis* and other species may cause infection (Bergdall & Dysko 1994; Vogtsberger et al. 1986). There is a demonstrated association with marginal husbandry practices, poor nutrition, environmental or internal stress factors, overcrowding, excessive heat and/or humidity, genetics, ectoparasites, extremes of youth or old age, and pregnancy. Direct contact or fomite transmission is not uncommon and rabbits may be asymptomatic carriers (Lopez-Martinez et al. 1984). The classical signs seen in other species are typical in rabbits and the diagnostic procedures are the same. Individual animals can be isolated and treated with griseofulvin (orally or topically in DMSO) or topical povidone iodine (Bergdall & Dysko, 1994).

Salmonellosis, often presenting as a peracute fatal disease subsequent to a stressor (e.g., anesthesia, environmental extremes), has been reported in rabbits. The diagnosis is based on culture and identification of the organism from blood, bile, feces, lymph nodes, or affected organs. Treatment is ineffective in eliminating the carrier state and infected animals should be euthanized.

Encephalitozoonosis, caused by the protozoan *Encephalitozoon cuniculi*, has a tropism for the brain, kidney, and other tissues and typically does not cause clinical signs in rabbits with the rare exception being encephalitis. It may cause infection in immunocompromised humans, however. Encephalitozoonosis may be found in up to 30% of rabbits in certain colonies. Infection is acquired by ingestion or nasal inoculation. Certain ectoparasites, such as the fur mite *Cheyletiella parasitovorax*, and burrowing sarcoptid mites may be transmissible from rabbits to humans. Of lesser importance are diseases such as leptospirosis, tularemia, and endoparasitism. *Francisella tularensis*, the etiologic agent of tularemia, rarely infects domestic lagomorphs, but may cause acute, febrile disease. It is noteworthy that exposure to wild rabbits is associated with the vast majority of human cases. Zoonoses generally can be prevented by wearing gloves and long-sleeved clinical garments when handling rabbits and hand washing upon the removal of gloves.

TAKING THE HISTORY AND PERFORMING A PHYSICAL EXAMINATION

When it comes to the basic fundamentals of the history, physical examination and treatment, the procedures for rabbits are essentially the same as for cats with a few species-specific differences. As for cats, clients should be advised to bring the rabbit to the clinic concealed in a secure carrier. While in the waiting room, the rabbit should be kept secured in a carrier isolated from predator species such as cats and dogs.

The realities of rabbit medicine are such that virtually all will be presented to a clinic for intervention for a clinical problem and there will be few presentations for wellness exams. Consequently, the most important focus of the history, beyond the signalment (age, breed, gender, etc.), will be the presenting complaint. General areas of questioning important to the history include the source from which the rabbit was acquired, whether it is housed indoors or outdoors, the diet, appetite, frequency of care and observation, and whether the animal has been observed to have frequent sneezing or persistent or intermittent nasal discharge suggestive of pasteurellosis.

A normal rabbit typically will rest compactly on all four limbs with regular twitching of the nostrils. There should be no ocular or nasal discharges and the face should be fully furred up to the periocular margins of the lids. Periocular depilation may be suggestive of chronic epiphora suggestive of pasteurellosis. The pelt, except in certain breeds such as the rex, should be sleek, full, luxurious, and smooth. Hydration is assessed using skin turgor as the index as with other species. The scrotum of mature males and the internal pinnae of the ears are the only hairless areas on a normal rabbit.

The incisors can be easily viewed for length and symmetry by retracting the lips, but not without some resentment. The molars are difficult to see. Except in the hands of experienced and skillful individuals, examination without sedation is out of the question. Rabbits resent and will resist a comprehensive oral examination. Gentle palpation of the trunk should show the vertebrae and ribs to be detectable, but not pronounced. The abdominal organs, such as the stomach, kidneys, and spleen, can be easily palpated. The head and trunk should be free of nodules. The ear canals should be free of crusts, exudate, scabs, and other evidence of inflammation suggestive of otoacariasis. Ocular examinations can be done as for other species, but keeping in mind the caveat that atropine may be unreliable or ineffective as a mydriatic owing to the presence of serum atropinesterase in many rabbits.

The urinary and genital openings are located immediately below the anus. The testes descend at about 12 weeks of age in the buck, but, owing to the open inguinal canals, may be present in the scrotum or retracted partly into the abdomen. During the physical examination, the testicles can be gently forced from the inguinal canals into the scrotum for palpation by applying mild pressure in the cranial inguinal area. In mature animals and those that are obese, it is important to examine the perineal area for evidence of urine scald or the presence of a fecal impaction in the fur and perineal skin folds. The chain of mammary glands of intact does should be palpated for evidence of mastitis. Not only lactating or pseudopregnant does are susceptible to this condition, but also nongravid females with uterine hyperplasia or adenocarcinoma (Mullen 2000).

When it comes to the physical examination, and even as compared to cats, the typical rabbit is not at all agreeable to being rolled onto its back. Consequently, examination of the ventrum should be done by lifting the rabbit, as described in the restraint section, and viewing of the underside at the eye level of the examiner.

With respect to vital signs, the body temperature of the domestic rabbit is significantly higher than that found in cats with the normal range being from 101 to 104°F (Harkness & Wagner 1989). The heart (130–325 beats per minute) and respiratory rates (30–60 breaths per minute) are also more rapid than other more commonly encountered species. Airway sounds are prominent typically upon pulmonary auscultation and are present normally in all lung fields. Auscultated airway sounds should be short, regular, and rapid in progression with obviously dry bronchovesicular sounds. Throughout the examination be mindful of sneezing or evidence of obstructed breathing that may be suggestive of pasteurellosis.

A rabbit presenting with severe pain will show a hunched posture and immobility and may grind its teeth. Those in acute pain or distress may, especially upon handling, emit a haunting high-pitched cry. Many an amiable rabbit will become aggressive, if in chronic pain or distress. Consequently, the existence of underlying health condition should always be explored in cases of behavioral change.

RESTRAINT

Owing to their general timidity and musculoskeletal factors, rabbits are at significant risk of injury from improper handling. Something seemingly as innocuous as permitting a rabbit to leap from one's arms into a cage may result in the exertion of sufficient fulcrum forces upon the lumbar spine to cause a vertebral luxation. Additionally, if rabbits are improperly restrained, they may inflict painful scratches to a handler from the claws on their powerful rear limbs.

The proper manner to carry a rabbit a short distance, such as from a treatment area to an adjacent examination room, is to grasp the scruff of the neck with the dominant hand and support the hindquarters with the other. To traverse a longer distance, the handler should tuck the head of the rabbit into the crook of the elbow of the nondominant limb using that arm to support the body weight. Although the rabbit's eyes and head should be concealed at the convergence of the elbow and body wall of the handler using this technique, continue to grasp the scruff of the neck with the dominant hand in order to maintain control should the rabbit become startled. An alternative for long traverses is to use a carrier box suitable for cats or small dogs. When returning a rabbit to its cage, carrier, or setting it on a surface, such as an examination table, do not allow it to leap or hop from the arms. Rather, continue to grasp the scruff of the neck with one hand and support the hindquarters with the other and place it on the surface with the rabbit facing the handler throughout the process. It will be disinclined to jump and, instead, often will simply turn away from the handler. This technique is far less likely to create conditions for a vertebral luxation.

For examination, rabbits should be placed on an examination table and approached from the side or behind by an examiner or handler. The one restraining a rabbit should stand facing the flank of the patient placing one hand gently over the thorax and the other upon the hindquarters. Most rabbits, provided they are not agitated, will sit quietly in a compact posture occasionally raising the head to look about or sniff. Rabbits are not amenable to being rolled on their sides or backs and will provide vigorous resistance that may lead to catastrophic injury. If one needs to examine the ventrum, the rabbit should be picked up (as described above for short distance carries) and lifted to eye level. Often a second person is necessary to permit effective division of the duties of restraint and examination. Procedures that require lateral or dorsal recumbency, such as radiography, must be done under anesthesia or deep sedation.

The restraint for injection is similar to that for transport, but with the animal resting on a surface such as an examination table. While facing the rabbit from the side, the restrainer should grasp the scruff of the neck with one hand and the other should be cupped over the hindquarters. A second individual gives the injection by immobilization of a hindlimb or location of the epaxial muscles and administers the injection. When working alone, the rabbit should be approached from the side and rotated one-quarter turn toward the handler. The maneuver should be finished by tucking the head of the rabbit between the nondominant arm and side of the handler. The nondominant arm is used to compress the side of the rabbit toward the handler. Likewise, using the nondominant hand, gently abduct and immobilize the pelvic limb adjacent to the nondominant hand and deliver the injection with the syringe held in the dominant hand. Fractious or aggressive rabbits may be restrained in a cat bag or have a towel rolled about them, but with the forewarning that struggling against such restraint, even if the rabbit is seemingly immobilized, may also be a source of injury (figs. 8.8 and 8.9).

For oral medication administration, the rabbit should be placed on a smooth examination table and approached from the rear. While using the nondominant forearm and elbow to press the flank of the rabbit against the body of the restrainer, grasp the head with the nondominant hand positioning the fingers under the mandible and the thumb in the occipital region. With a catheter-tipped syringe in the contralateral hand, insert the syringe tip into the commissure of the mouth at the proximity of the diastema and administer the agent. Often it is preferable to kneel on the floor and use knees and thighs to laterally restrain the rabbit as it faces away. A syringe tip can then be

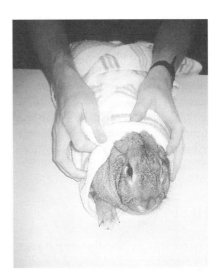

Fig. 8.9. Restraint using a towel. (Photo courtesy of Dr. Sam Rivera)

maneuvered to the oral commissure and the agent administered. The procedure for passage of a stomach tube, including restraint, is described below under "Clinical Techniques."

RADIOLOGY

The most likely indications for radiography include confirmation or evaluation of dental disease, vertebral luxation, limb fracture, obstructive trichobezoar, pregnancy, pneumonia, and intra-abdominal disease such as uterine adenocarcinoma. Positioning for radiography must be facilitated by the use of anesthesia, typically with xylazine:ketamine, or deep sedation. Otherwise it will not be possible to stretch the rabbit and properly position for lateral or ventrodorsal views without risking serious injury to the animal or movement during the exposure, which may degrade the quality of the image. The DV view, rather than the VD, is preferred in rabbits because it minimizes the risk of torso rotation along its sagittal axis and enhances spinosternal alignment. In general, and because of the relatively rapid respiratory rate, short exposure times (0.017 sec) are most desirable (Morgan & Silverman 1984). If the practice encounters a significant number of lapine patients, it is most advantageous to develop a technique chart for the various anatomic structures given the capacity of the X-ray generator, the film speed commonly available, and the qualities of the intensifying screen. An alternative is to use a feline technique chart, but to shorten the exposure time, compensate with increase mA, and,

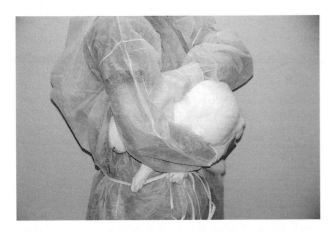

Fig. 8.8. Restraint for transport. (Photo courtesy of Ryan Cheek)

given the less-dense bones, reduce the KVp to preserve resolution. Without a custom technique chart, a good starting point for rabbits is to use a focal film distance of 40 inches and an intensifying screen. For a thoracic exposure, use 60 kilovolts, 300 milliamperes, and an exposure time of 0.008 seconds for an 8 cm thick chest (Morgan and Silverman 1984). For a similarly thick abdomen, increase the exposure time to 0.034 seconds, reduce the mA to 100, and reduce kVp to 58 (Morgan & Silverman, 1984).

ANESTHESIA

Rabbits may present an anesthetic challenge to veterinarians or veterinary technicians unfamiliar or inexperienced with them. However, because virtually all drugs, equipment, and resources necessary for safe and humane anesthesia of rabbits are available in most veterinary clinics, this does not need to be the case. The rumors regarding rabbit anesthesia, for example, that rabbits are difficult to intubate, can be overcome by a veterinary technician who is knowledgeable and balances caution with confidence. It is important to keep the rabbit calm and isolated from perceived threats especially noisy dogs, cats and humans. A frightened rabbit can be so permeated with catecholamines that anesthesia can be adversely affected (Jenkins 2000). A formulary is found at the end of the chapter, which gives dosages of drugs that are recommended in this chapter.

Preanesthesia

As with other companion animals, obtaining a thorough history and a preanesthetic physical examination are important in detecting underlying medical conditions, such as rabbit pasteurellosis, that may complicate anesthesia. For rabbits, examination of the nares for rhinorrhea suggestive of bacterial respiratory disease, careful auscultation of the thorax for evidence of cardiac or pulmonary disease, and determination of the rectal temperature should be done. Once admitted to the clinic, rabbits should be kept in escape-proof cages in a quiet area. Rabbits have high metabolic energy requirements and are unable to vomit. Mature, nonobese rabbits may be fasted for 12 hours to decrease the amount of ingesta in the cecum and stomach that may result in anesthetic overdosages due to overestimating the real body weight. Since rabbits breathe primarily by diaphragmatic movement, fasting to decrease stomach volume will enhance respiration during anesthesia. However, this may have variable effect due to coprophagy and given that rabbits will drink water to excess when fasted (Chew 1965). Fasting may also cause mild metabolic acidosis. Some advocate a period of preoperative fasting as short as 1–2 hours (Jenkins 2000). Fasting in excess of 12 hours is contraindicated as it may promote hypoglycemia and more severe metabolic acidosis and, in young rabbits or adults of small breeds, fasting for more than a few hours may induce the same conditions. Fasting of obese, pregnant, or pasturient rabbits may predispose to ketosis and liver necrosis.

Preanesthetic medications are not recommended, with the exception of anticholinergic drugs, because single injection anesthesia techniques have been developed that minimize the handling stress and eliminate the discomfort associated with multiple injections. Serum and tissue atropinesterases found in many rabbits render the use of atropine sulfate unpredictable or labor intensive at best in rabbits. In the presence of atropinesterase, atropine must be given in high doses (1–2 mg/kg) with redosing every 10–15 minutes (Lipman et al. 1997). Therefore, 0.01–0.02 mg/kg subcutaneous (SC) administration of glycopyrrolate (Robinul, A.H. Robins Company, Richmond, VA), a quaternary ammonium parasympatholytic, should be given to reduce salivary and bronchial secretions and prevent vagal bradycardia.

Anesthesia

For practical purposes, anesthetics used in rabbits can be divided into injectable and inhalation agents. Historically, injectable drugs have been popularly used for anesthesia of rabbits because they are inexpensive, avoid the technical demands of gas anesthesia, and have been generally safe, effective, and easy to administer. However, disadvantages attendant to anesthesia by injection include the lack of precision in controlling anesthetic depth, prolonged recovery time, and physiologic changes such as hypotension, hypoxemia, and acid-base disorders. For uncomplicated procedures involving healthy animals, these drawbacks may not be of consequence, but their safety and predictability when used in ill animals is not known, because injectable anesthetic techniques have been largely developed for use in healthy experimental animals.

Ketamine HCl (Ketaset, Aveco Co. Inc., Fort Dodge, IA) is the most common anesthetic used in rabbits, but as a sole agent, it does not provide sufficient analgesia or muscle relaxation for surgical purposes at any dose. For minimally invasive diagnostic procedures requiring immobilization (i.e., radiography), surgical procedures of moderate intensity (i.e., wound suturing, tissue biopsies) lasting less than 30–45 minutes, or anesthesia permitting preparation of a surgical field, placement of intravascular catheters and intubation for subsequent administration of gas, anesthetics is necessary. Ketamine is most commonly combined with xylazine HCl (Rompun, Miles Animal Health, Shawnee Mission, KS) or medetomidine (Domitor, Pfizer Animal Health, Lee's Summit, MO) and given intramuscularly as a single injection into the caudal muscles of the thigh or the lumbar epaxial musculature. The ketamine dose is 35–45 mg/kg with xylazine (5 mg/kg) and 25 mg/kg with medetomidine (0.5 mg/kg) (Flecknell 1996). Anesthesia is fully induced within 10–15 minutes and typically lasts 25–45 minutes, but total time unconscious may be up to 2 hours (Flecknell 1996). Because of inherent variability in rabbits, the combination of xylazine and ketamine alone may be unreliable in inducing and/or maintaining an adequate anesthesic plane for an appreciable period of time and will not provide adequate analgesia for procedures with intense sympathetic stimulation such as laparotomy and thoracotomy. In these cases, 0.1 mg/kg butorphanol tartrate (Torbutrol, Aveco Co., Inc., Fort Dodge, IA) or, less ideally, 0.75 mg/kg acepromazine maleate (Promace, Aveco Co. Inc., Fort Dodge, IA) should be given at the time of anesthesia induction with xylazine (5 mg/kg) and ketamine (35 mg/kg). These triple combination regimens will provide anesthesia lasting 60–90 minutes. Acepromazine should be used with caution in ill animals, however, because it may further contribute to hypotension, bradycardia, and respiratory depression. If it is necessary to further extend anesthesia, incremental doses of one half the original ketamine dose can be given. The tiletamine given in combination with zolazepam in the product Telazol (Aveco Co. Inc., Fort Dodge, IA) has been shown to be nephrotoxic for rabbits at doses of 7.5 mg/kg and its use should be avoided unless further studies show its safety (Brammer et al. 1991; Doerning et al. 1992). Consequently, while popularly used in many species, Telazol is contraindicated in rabbits.

For procedures anticipated to last 1–4 hours where inhalation anesthesia is unavailable and the patient is healthy, administration of a constant infusion of xylazine and ketamine can be done. Over comparable periods of time, anesthesia by controlled infusion provides stable anesthesia with a decreased total anesthetic drug requirement and reduced recovery time as compared to anesthetics given periodically by multiple bolus (Wyatt et al. 1989). Rabbits to be anesthetized by intravenous infusion are first given xylazine (5 mg/kg) and ketamine (35 mg/kg) by intramuscular injection to induce anesthesia. Following placement of an indwelling catheter in a lateral ear vein, as described elsewhere, a constant infusion of xylazine (0.04 mg/kg/minute) and ketamine (0.4 mg/kg/minute) can be given in 0.9% saline. A working infusion solution is made by adding 4 ml of ketamine HCl (100 mg/ml) and 2 ml of xylazine (20 mg/ml) to 94 ml 0.9% saline. The infusion solution is given at a rate of 6 ml/kg/hr to maintain anesthesia. This method of anesthesia should be done with an infusion pump or precisely controlled use of a minidrip (60 drops/ml) and vital signs should be monitored closely.

Inhalation anesthesia is technically feasible in rabbits and preferred because it is precise, rapidly adjustable, and safe and effective for procedures lasting 2 or more hours (fig. 8.10). An Ayre's T-piece or other nonrebreathing circuit is most appropriate for rabbit inhalational anesthesia (Flecknell 1996). Postoperative recovery is more rapid and less complicated than with injectable anesthetics.

For anesthetic induction, an intravenous injection of propofol (1.5 mg/kg slowly to effect) or a SC or IM injection of xylazine and ketamine are preferred. Inhalation induction, using a mask or induction chamber, is not a preferred method because of the high incidence of struggling, distress vocalization, and breath-holding (Flecknell 1996). Xylazine-ketamine or propofol induction is also preferred over intravenous injection of ultra-short acting thiobarbiturates, which have a narrow margin of safety, are slowly eliminated in obese animals, and may cause marked respiratory

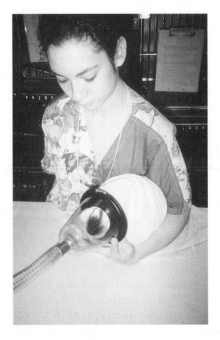

Fig. 8.10. *Inhalation anesthesia using a face mask. (Photo courtesy of Dr. Sam Rivera)*

depression or fatal apnea if intubation is not done immediately.

If, for some reason such as debilitation or disposition, injection is not feasible, the intranasal route is an option for administration of induction agents (Robertson & Eberhart 1994). The onset of effect is generally rapid (less than 3 minutes) and the duration of effect may be 30 minutes or more. Midazolam alone for sedation and xylazine-ketamine for low-grade anesthesia can be given effectively by this route (Robertson & Eberhart 1994).

The anatomy of the rabbit oropharynx makes endotracheal intubation somewhat of a challenge. The oral cavity is long and narrow, the mandible has a limited range of abduction, and entry into the oral cavity is partially occluded by the large incisors and cheek teeth. The tongue protrudes dorsally, the epiglottis is relatively large, U-shaped, soft, and flexible, and the larynx slopes ventrally. Just beyond the epiglottis is a deep sagittal niche, bordered on both sagittal recesses by the friable hamuli epiglotti, which are easily damaged. Additionally, laryngeal tone and the propensity to laryngospasm is high. All of these factors combine to obscure visualization and access to the glottis and make endotracheal intubation of the rabbit challenging.

These drawbacks aside, rabbits can be reliably and easily intubated by an experienced technician. The key to intubation by direct visualization is to bring the mouth, larynx, and trachea into linear alignment by positioning the rabbit in dorsal recumbency and hyperextending the head by placing a rolled towel under the cervical spine or permitting the head to overhang a table edge. The tongue should be retracted laterally through one of the diastema, the bilateral spaces between the incisors and premolars, to prevent laceration on the incisors and an inverted laryngoscope with a #1 Miller blade (Baxter Health Care Corporation, McGaw Park, IL) should be inserted into the contralateral diastema and maintained either between the incisors in alignment with the midline or lateral to the incisors at a slight angle to the sagittal plane of the body. Gentle pressure should be directed ventrally with the blade tip while slight rostrodorsal traction is placed on the head until the epiglottis and arytenoid cartilages are seen.

There is no consensus on the use of topical anesthetics to enhance intubation. While spraying of the pharynx, larynx, and trachea will reduce the risk of laryngospasm and enhance passage of the tube, it also suppresses the convenient forward motion of the glottis during swallowing that may enhance intubation. If a topical anesthetic is desired, lidocaine 10% oral spray (Xylocaine, Astra Pharmaceutical Products, Inc., Westborough, MA) should be judiciously misted on the glottis to prevent laryngospasm and facilitate intubation. Topical benzocaine should not be used, because it may cause methemoglobinemia.

In cases where relaxation of the musculature is not sufficient to permit intubation, additional propofol or 1 mg/kg slow boluses of either diazepam (Valium, Roche Products, Inc., Manati, PR) or midazolam (Versed, Roche Laboratories, Nutley, NJ) can be given IV to effect. Intubation should be done with a transparent, cuffed, 14 cm long, 3.0–4.0 mm internal diameter endotracheal tube (CT Cuffed Tracheal Tube Murphy Eye, Sheridan Catheter Corp., Argyle, NY) for rabbits weighing 3–6 kg or an uncuffed 1.0–2.5 mm endotracheal tube for rabbits weighing less than 3 kg. Using a metal dowel or cotton-tipped applicator as a stylet to prevent bending of the tube, intubation should be done by advancing the endotracheal tube through the diastema until it is immediately rostral to the epiglottis. As the tip of the endotracheal tube approaches the epiglottis, visualization will be impaired and the final passage must be done blindly during inspiration when the vocal cords are abducted. If a 3.0 mm or larger internal diameter endotracheal tube is used, intubation can be done using the polypropylene guide technique (Gilroy 1981). A 56 cm, 8 French polypropylene catheter (Sovereign Urinary Catheter, Sherwood Medical, St. Louis, MO) should be passed through the endotracheal tube lumen from the connector to the distal end until the blunt catheter tip extends 15–20 cm past the bevel. Under direct visualization, the tip of the catheter should be cautiously advanced through diastema, past the vocal folds and into the trachea. Once the guide is in the trachea, the laryngoscope can be removed and the endotracheal tube advanced as a sheath over the stationary catheter into the trachea.

If a sufficiently small laryngoscope blade is not available, intubation can be attempted blindly. After anesthesia is deepened by delivery of gas from a mask until the rabbit is completely relaxed and areflexic, it should be placed in sternal recumbency with the head extended dorsally such that the alignment of mouth, larynx, and trachea is perpendicular to the table surface. An endotracheal tube should then be advanced to the proximal aspect of the larynx. This can be confirmed by visualizing the fogging of the tube interior with every exhalation and listening for respiratory sounds through the endotracheal tube. The position of the tube should be adjusted pos until the sounds are at maximal intensity. At this point, the endotracheal tube should be gently advanced into the trachea. If breaths are shallow, it is sometimes helpful to have an assistant administer gentle chest compressions and to advance the tube timed with the release of a compression (inhalation). A cough reflex often confirms correct insertion. A capnograph, with the alarm temporarily disabled, also can be used to confirm proximity of the tube tip to the oropharynx. This blind technique carries a risk of trauma and should be abandoned in favor of direct observation if intubation is not successful after several gentle attempts. Regardless of the intubation technique, intubation should never be forced, because the trachea, tracheal bifurcation, and tissues of the oropharynx are easily damaged and the vagus nerve may be stimulated. Following intubation, the stylet or guide should be immediately removed and the endotracheal tube secured. Correct placement in the trachea should be further confirmed by visualizing the respiration-associated condensation of water vapor on the internal surface of the endotracheal tube, by auscultation in conjunction with manual respiration using an Ambu bag, or capnography. Mechanical ventilation should not be done until intubation is confirmed, because overzealous ventilation into the stomach can lead to acute dilatation and rupture.

The intubated rabbit should be connected to a gas anesthesia machine with a closed breathing circuit for ventilation with a mechanical respirator at a rate of 30–40 breaths per minute and a tidal volume of 11–15 ml/kg. The inspiration-to-expiration ratio should be 1:2 or 1:3 and airway pressures should not be permitted to exceed 20 cm H_2O. If mechanical ventilation is not available, spontaneous ventilation should be accommodated with a semiclosed pediatric breathing circuit. Spontaneous respirations should be regular and deep and occur at a rate of 15 or more breaths per minute. The anesthetist should be cognizant of the risk of apnea in this circumstance and be prepared to evaluate the depth of anesthesia and assist ventilations. Anesthesia should be maintained with 2–3% isoflurane or 1.5–2.5% halothane in 100% oxygen. The higher requirement for isoflurane in rabbits may come as a surprise to persons used to using equivalent concentrations of the gases in other species. Although not routinely done because combination anesthetic regimens contribute to the reduction of gas concentration needed to maintain anesthesia, yohimbine (Yobine, Lloyd Laboratories, Shenandoah, IA) or atipamezole (Antisedan, Pfizer Animal Health, Lee's Summit, MO) can be given shortly after gas anesthesia is commenced to reverse the hypotensive effects of xylazine or medetomidine.

Perioperative Considerations

While anesthetized, rabbits should have bland ophthalmic ointment placed in the eyes to prevent exposure keratitis and should be maintained on a water-circulated heating pad to prevent hypothermia. Other means of promoting euthermia include using Bair Huggers, warmed solutions for irrigation and, where inhalation anesthesia is done, humidifying inspired gases. The marginal lateral ear vein of rabbits should be catheterized for administration of parenteral fluids. Because fasting generally induces mild metabolic acidosis, warmed lactated Ringer's solution, provided the kidneys are functioning normally, or half-strength saline-dextrose solutions with sodium bicarbonate supplementation are most ideal for fluid administration in surgery. These should be given at a rate of 10–20 ml/kg/hr via a 60 drop/ml intravenous fluid administration set. If it is desirable to gain arterial access for blood gas analysis or blood pressure monitoring, a 22 gauge catheter can be placed in the central auricular artery and secured with a heparin-lock (for blood gases) or connected to a transducer (for continuous arterial pressure monitoring).

Anesthesia Monitoring

Because controlled ventilation may increase mean intrathoracic pressure, decrease venous return, compromise cardiac output, and cause hypotension, blood and airway pressure monitoring should be done. The systolic/diastolic arterial pressure of an anesthetized rabbit is approximately 95/75 (Huerkamp 1995). As a rule, arterial pressures should not be permitted to decrease below 80/60. Intubated animals undergoing lengthy procedures should have cuffed tubes deflated, rotated, and reinflated hourly while those that are not intubated should be positioned to maintain an open airway. Alterations in heart rate and blood pressure are the most reliable indicators of anesthetic depth with changes of 20% or more from baseline usually dictating modifications in anesthetic management. The monitoring of heart rate and rhythm can be done with an esophageal stethoscope or electrocardiography. In addition to direct blood pressure monitoring via the central auricular artery, indirect monitoring can be attempted with cuffs placed on a limb. Capnography (end tidal CO_2 determination), blood-gas analysis, and pulse oximetry are useful in evaluating the adequacy of ventilation. Ventilation-perfusion efficiency can also be assessed through observation of mucous membrane color and capillary refill time.

Where sophisticated cardiovascular monitoring is not practical, reflex assessment is the most accurate determinant of adequate anesthesia. Traditional reflexes used in the monitoring of rabbit anesthesia include righting, palpebral, corneal, pedal withdrawal, and pinna reflex. The pinna reflex is the most accurate measure of depth of anesthesia followed by pedal withdrawal, corneal, and palpebral reflexes, in that order. Corneal reflex may be preserved until very deep levels of anesthesia are reached. Muscle tone, jaw tone, and purposeful movements in response to surgical stimuli may also be used as indicators of anesthesia depth. When reflex assessment is used as the sole determinant of anesthetic depth, more than one reflex should be monitored to insure adequate anesthesia. At a minimum, anesthetic depth should be monitored temporally by constantly assessing reflexes, cardiac rate and rhythm, and respiratory rate.

Analgesia

Well-established studies have shown repeatedly that effective analgesia enhances locomotion, increases appetite, and reduces the time of postoperative recovery. Rabbits, in particular, benefit from pain-killing medication because they are sensitive to pain due to inflammation at the site of a surgical wound, which can lead to self-mutilation and distress, which may also result in cecal hyperacidity precipitating a syndrome of anorexia, ileus, dysbiosis, and impaction. To preclude these effects, the use of a 12-inch Elizabethan collar (Ejay International, Inc., Glendora, CA) to prevent self-mutilation in conjunction with administration of analgesics for discomfort is helpful. Long-term maintenance of an Elizabethan collar will prevent coprophagy and could lead to B vitamin and other nutritional deficiencies.

As a general rule, analgesics should be first administered before the animal is fully recovered from anesthesia, but stable, and should be continued for the next 48–72 hours. Nonsteroidal anti-inflammatory drugs (NSAID) inhibit the production of chemical mediators that activate peripheral nociceptors and are sufficiently potent to treat musculoskeletal, incisional, and acute, mild visceral pain. Flunixin meglumine (Banamine, Schering Corporation, Kenilworth, N.J.) should be given by IM or SC injection every 12 hours at a dose of 1.1 mg/kg.

For the control of acute or chronic visceral pain, opioids are the most powerful and effective analgesics. However, the use of traditional, parenterally administered opioid analgesics such as morphine, meperidine, and pentazocine are impractical in rabbits because of their high metabolic rates which necessitates intensive dosing schedules to maintain therapeutic blood concentrations. Morphine also carries the risk of inducing ileus and nausea/anorexia. Moderate pain relief can be obtained by giving a banana-flavored preparation of meperidine HCl (Demerol Hydrochloride Syrup, Winthrop Pharmaceuticals, New York, NY) in the drinking water at a concentration of 0.2 mg/ml. Opioid agonist-antagonists, such as butorphanol, or buprenorphine (Buprenex, Reckitt and Colman Pharmaceuticals, Inc., Richmond, VA), have relatively long half-lives and offer the advantage of attenuating or ablating visceral pain while minimizing the undesirable respiratory and cardiovascular side effects associated with opioids. Buprenorphine, a Class V controlled substance, should be given by injection every 6–12 hours to rabbits (0.01–0.05 mg/kg IM, SC). Administration of buprenorphine per rectum (0.5 mg/kg) will diminish the degree of analgesia, but extend the duration of effect to a minimum of 12 hours (Wootton et al. 1988). This route may be useful where rabbits resent injections. Anecdotally, the author has observed frequent cases of postoperative anorexia and ileus in rabbits given intensive treatment with buprenorphine injections. In these cases, appetite return was associated with discontinuance of analgesic treatment. Buprenorphine given at the high range of recommended levels in rats has been shown to cause anorexia and weight loss (Jablonski et al. 2001). Others have also questioned the efficacy of buprenorphine in rabbits (Wixson 1994). Until these issues can be resolved, buprenorphine should be used under close observation in rabbits and with some suspicion of efficacy.

An interesting attribute of rabbits is the propensity with which they can be hypnotized. Unfortunately, however, the induction of hypnosis, much as in humans, is subject to individual variability. The condition is characterized by a lack of spontaneous movement, failure to respond to overt external stimuli, and mild analgesia lasting for several minutes. The condition can be induced by grasping the awake rabbit around the back of the neck with the thumb and forefinger hooked under the mandible. The rabbit is then lifted from a resting position into a vertical position and steadied with the contralateral hand around the hindquarters. Using this technique, a considerable portion of the body weight is exerted on the spine and this induces immobility and the hypnotic response (Danneman et al. 1988).

Acute Postanesthetic Care

Following completion of surgery under inhalation anesthesia, recovery is rapid and rabbits typically are conscious and regain the righting reflex within 20–30 minutes. The most likely causes of delayed or complicated recovery from general anesthesia are hypothermia and anesthetic overdosage followed by complications related to lengthy procedures or poor presenting medical conditions such as hypoglycemia and dehydration. Anesthetic agents directly affect central and peripheral thermoregulatory mechanisms and rabbits, similar to cats, are highly prone to radiative and conductive heat losses because of their high body surface area to body weight ratio. Because the pharmacokinetics of anesthetic metabolism are partially temperature dependent, maintaining body temperature is critical to recovery from anesthesia. Ideally, recovering animals should be kept in an escape-proof incubator on a clean, dry towel or blanket. The use of an incubator permits careful control of the ambient temperature and enables supplemental oxygen administration. Recovery should not be done on metal flooring or in suspended wire cages because heat loss will be accelerated. Where an incubator is not available, supplemental heating can be provided with a water-circulated heating pad or a heat lamp judiciously placed outside of the cage. It is important to remember that rabbits are gnawing species that, left unattended following recovery, may mutilate heating pads or wiring. The ambient temperature in the recovery area should be 84–89°F. Temperature monitoring of the animal and the recovery area should be done as regularly as for dogs and cats.

Animals slow to recover from anesthesia should be turned every 30–60 minutes to prevent hypostatic lung congestion and should be given warmed, parenteral fluids to compensate for metabolic needs and for losses during surgery. Extubation should be done only when chewing begins or coughing is elicited. If not done beforehand, yohimbine or atipamezole can be given to reverse the effects of xylazine and medetomidine. Where reversal is not possible, respiratory depression can be treated with 2–5 mg/kg doxapram (Dopram-V, Aveco Co. Inc., Fort Dodge, IA) given SC or IV every 15 minutes.

COMMON SURGICAL PROCEDURES

The duties of a veterinary technician supporting a surgical procedure for a rabbit are identical to those for other species with the focus on preoperative preparation of the surgical patient and intraoperative support of the procedure including anesthesia management. The surgeon and operating room attendants should prepare and dress as for procedures done on other pet species. Sterile instruments and draping should be used. Where post-op care is expected to be extensive, a nasogastric tube can be placed to permit feeding of liquid diets and evacuation of any gastric gas (Mullen 2000). Rabbits with a history of pasteurellosis should be started on a preoperative course of antibiotics for a duration sufficient to suppress any clinical manifestations (days) or prevent septicemia (1–2 hours preoperatively IV).

The fur at the surgical site should be clipped and the skin should be decontaminated with alcohol and disinfectants as for like procedures done on other species. Some persons prefer to wear a mask while shaving a rabbit to preclude floating hair from entering their mouth or nose. Rabbits have thick hair coats and thin skin, which renders clipping of the hair from a surgical site more time-consuming and puts a premium on clipper blade sharpness. It is critical that sharp spare blades be available and that all clipper blades be properly cleaned and restored after use. The rabbit skin easily lacerates or tears in cases where clipping is done hurriedly or carelessly or where dull clipper blades are used. The technician should concentrate on keeping the skin taut in front of the clipper blade and the head of the blade flat against the skin. The best skin preparation comes from using a combination of no. 10 and no. 40 blades to prepare the skin. This is an area where patience and careful attention to detail are most important. In fact, gentle handling of the skin preoperatively and all tissues intraoperatively are critical in reducing the incidence of postoperative automutilation of incisions for which rabbits are notorious.

The most common surgical procedures in rabbits include spay, castration, drainage of abscesses, cutaneous mass excision, and exploratory laparotomy. Enucleation, perineal dermatoplasty in cases of relentless urine scald, and cystotomy have also been described in rabbits (Mullen 2000). These surgical procedures are typically done using the positioning, approaches and techniques similar to cats. This is the case with castration, which is most commonly done by the scrotal approach (Jenkins 2000), but also may be done by the prescrotal approach, as for dogs, or by abdominal midline incisions for cryptorchidism (Swindle & Shealy 1996). Castration should be recommended to clients as a preventive measure for bucks housed indoors to prevent urine spraying and mounting, fighting among those housed in groups, and elimination of the risk of testicular cancer.

Ovariohysterectomy is done with the doe in dorsal recumbency and with preparation of the abdominal skin as for other conventionally encountered species. The procedure is the same as for dogs and cats and is recommended as a preventive measure for group-housing and uterine disease and as a treatment for uterine adenocarcinoma. Technicians expressing the urinary bladder in preparation for this procedure should be aware that is easy to unintentionally force urine into the vagina and uterus. This urine may contaminate the abdomen later during resection of the uterus. Because the urinary bladder and cecum are thin-walled and easily punctured upon initial penetration into the abdomen, extra care is taken when making this incision. The bicornuate uterus is also fragile relative to other species (Jenkins 2000).

Cystotomy is indicated for urolithiasis. Although the bladder wall is thin which may be discouraging to some surgeons, it holds suture well (Mullen 2000) and can be closed in a single layer (Swindle & Shealy 1996). Despite the daunting apparent thinness of the bladder wall, veterinarians with cystotomy experience in other species can easily do this procedure. Most rabbits with urolithiasis are overweight and probably overconsuming calcium (Mullen 2000). Consequently, the postoperative instructions given to the owner should include an exhortation to limit feed and not provide mineral supplementation.

Exploratory laparotomy is required in cases of gastrointestinal obstruction from trichobezoars, other foreign bodies, or space-occupying lesions. As with other intra-abdominal procedures, the surgeon should be gentle with the friable cecum and urinary bladder.

Enucleation may be necessary for ocular trauma, severe buphthalmia, or retrobulbar abscess. This procedure is contraindicated with inexperienced surgeons and might best be referred to a veterinary specialty surgical practice. The retrobulbar venous sinus is extensive and the risk of severe and difficult-to-control hemorrhage exists (Mullen 2000). If the procedure is to be done, it is important to have considerable sterile methylcellulose on hand to pack the ocular defect. Likewise, bulla osteotomy for drainage of middle ear infections, such as for pasteurellosis, is fraught with risks of postoperative pain and drainage complications (Swindle & Shealy 1996) and is a procedure probably best referred to a specialty surgical practice.

Absorbable polymer suture materials, such as monofilament polyglyconate, are preferred for internal use, owing to their less-reactive nature, and for closure of the skin. Because they are not exposed and are less likely to be chewed, subcuticular sutures are preferred for skin closure. Generally, sutures in sizes appropriate for cats (3-0, 4-0, 5-0) are most appropriate for rabbits. Cyanoacrylate tissue adhesives also provide satisfactory closure provided they are used in clean, dry incisions. Steel sutures or wound clips, although advocated by some for skin closure, can be easily chewed from the incision. The risk of self-mutilation of suture lines will be minimized using these techniques and with gentle, atraumatic handling of the tissues in general.

Rabbits are gnawing species and fastidious groomers. Exposed sutures and dressings, especially if irritating or pruritic, may be removed in short order with considerable collateral self-mutilation. Fitting the post-op rabbit with a 12-inch Elizabethan collar (Ejay International Inc., Glendora, CA) will prevent or break any cycle of irritation and self-inflicted injury. However, if the collar is to remain in place for more than a few days, consideration should be given to supplementing B vitamins and vitamin K. Alternatively, attempts can be made to hand-feed cecotrophs.

Extraction of incisors for malocclusion is done by using the standard flap and elevation techniques for other species. It is important, however, to ream and thoroughly remove residual tooth from the evacuated cavity. If this is not done, the tooth will regrow (Swindle & Shealy 1996). As the teeth are constantly growing, extraction of a damaged or maloccluded tooth must be accompanied by the extraction of any opposing teeth to prevent their uncontrolled overgrowth.

Following acute recovery from anesthesia, the most reliable indicator of postoperative well-being, including the effectiveness of analgesia, is the daily assessment of body weight and food and water consumption. As rabbits are prone to hypoglycemia because of high metabolic rates and, in juvenile animals, limited fat reserves, a nutritious pelleted diet should be provided as soon after surgery as feasible. Inappetent animals can be offered supplements such as hay, other supplements, or treats as described above under "Nutrition," or herbivore liquid dietary products. In some cases, the stress associated with surgery will cause pH changes in the cecum that result in alterations of commensal and fermentative bacteria. Where this results in chronic anorexia and ileus that is nonresponsive to treatments described above, specific bacteriotherapy, as described below in the "Emergency and Critical Care" section, may be useful in recolonizing the gastrointestinal tract.

PARASITOLOGY

The most important diagnostic tools used in the diagnosis of parasitism in rabbits are essentially the same as for dogs and cats. These comprise the fecal floatation examination, fur exam, skin scraping, and the examination of the ear canals. With respect to skin scrapings, bear in mind that the skin of rabbits is thin relative to dogs and cats and may lacerate easily. The examination of the ear canals should be done using an otoscope. This is sufficient in many cases to diagnose aural acariasis. The mites typically are easily seen with low magnification crawling in the beam of light emitted from the otoscope. The diagnosis can be confirmed, and mites demonstrated for the owner, by swabbing exudate from the canal with a cotton-tipped applicator and mineral oil and examining it under a microscope. For rabbits housed outdoors, one important consideration is that flies are attracted to rabbit droppings and owners may confuse recently hatched fly larvae with parasites.

URINALYSIS

The urine pH ranges from 6 to 8.2 with alkaline urine (pH > 8) generally associated with good health and acidic pH with anorexia or fasting. The normal range of urine specific gravity is 1.003 to 1.036 with 1.015 representing the normal mean in a healthy population of rabbits (McLaughlin & Fish 1994). The urine typically is turbid due to calcium carbonate excretion and is also pigmented ranging from light yellow to orange to various combinations of red with brown. Certain porphyrin pigments in the urine may cause a reddish appearance and elicit concerns of hematuria (Garibaldi et al. 1987). Consequently, any suspected cases of hematuria in the rabbit should be confirmed by complete urinalysis. The most likely causes of hematuria are from uterine adenocarcinoma, uterine polyps, uterine hyperplasia, abortion, urolithiasis, cystitis, septicemia, DIC, and certain renal diseases.

The urine should be free of protein, casts, blood, glucose, ketones, and bilirubin. An occasional white blood cell per high-powered field in an examination of the sediment is within the realm of normal. The urine output ranges from 20–350 ml/kg/day range and is influenced by many factors related to the diet, animal and environment (McLaughlin & Fish 1994). Ammonium magnesium phosphate (struvite) and calcium carbonate are the two most common uroliths of rabbits (Bergdall & Dysko 1994). Struvite uroliths are usually the consequence of urinary tract infection. Calcium carbonate uroliths may precipitate and form uroliths when the urinary pH exceeds 8.5 (Leck 1988). Infection, inadequate water intake, genetic predisposition, metabolic disturbances, and nutritional imbalances enhance the development of urolithiasis.

EMERGENCY AND CRITICAL CARE

As with other species, emergency and critical care are action oriented and immediate with the goal of interventions being to stabilize the rabbit and afford the opportunity to then pursue the diagnosis of the primary problem. There may be any number of presentations requiring critical care including trauma, environmental exposure (hypothermia, hyperthermia), severe diarrhea, internal hemorrhage, intoxications, or nutritional deficiencies. Identical presentation-directed interventions constitute the tenets of care including fluid therapy, body temperature maintenance, oxygen administration, and control of hemorrhage.

Hypothermia is a risk in sucklings, those rabbits housed outdoors in winter, and those recovering from anesthesia. The goal in treating hypothermia, as it is with other species, is to raise the body temperature slowly (<0.5°F per minute). Otherwise, in theory, the cure may be worse than the disease. A rapid rise in body temperature without control may increase brain metabolic demands above that which can be provided and expose the heart, liver, and lungs to cold, acidotic blood from the periphery. Overzealous body warming also could result in hyperthermia. As with other species, therapy centers on slow rewarming using warm water immersion, massage, water-circulated heating pads, an incubator, padding with hot water bottles, or a Bair Hugger. Thermal blankets and camper's heat pouches may also be useful in body heat restoration. Less preferable, because of the risk of overheating without close supervision, is the use of a heat lamp. The administration of warm, isotonic fluids to restore circulation, aid rewarming, and restore intravascular fluid volume, is warranted. Failure to restore fluids in any hypothermic animal can result in acute tubular necrosis.

Hypoxemia should be considered as a possible complication in downer and hypothermic animals. The intervention should be to ensure a patent airway and provide supplemental oxygen delivered via intubation with an Ambu bag or ventilator, face mask, nasal cannula, or a bag placed over the head (a crude oxygen tent).

Hypoglycemia is generally a risk in neonatal or small-breed animals either on an inadequate nutritional plane or recovering from surgery. High metabolic energy demands and low depot fat reservoirs coupled with preoperative fasting and postoperative anorexia make these animals particularly at risk. It could be a companion to hypothermia and ideally should be confirmed by laboratory test. In a pinch, however, response to glucose therapy can be used as a diagnostic tool. Acute hypoglycemia should be treated acutely as for other species by intravenous or oral bolus of 50% dextrose (e.g., 2 ml/kg). Parenteral administration of glucose is preferred because excessive administration of oral carbohydrates may create conditions that upset the enteric microflora and predispose to cecal dysbiosis. For those animals that are both hypoglycemic and hypothermic, intravenous glucose will provide fuel to the brain during rewarming.

Hyperthermia is usually encountered as a consequence of outdoor housing in the summer without adequate protection from heat. It may also be caused iatrogenically by overzealous rewarming during anesthetic recovery. The treatment, as for other species, is to cool the rabbit slowly in alcohol or ice water baths.

Diarrhea, with or without other conditions such as hypothermia or dehydration, is not an uncommon presentation given the susceptibility of young animals to colibacillosis, coccidiosis, and rotavirus-induced diarrheas. Additionally, diarrhea is not uncommon given the intricate, complex, and delicate interrelationship between diet, other environmental factors, the commensal, fermentative microflora and gut motility in rabbits of all ages. Diarrhea should be treated symptomatically with fluids, dietary restriction, and antibiotics, anthelmintics, or other agents specifically related to etiology. Transfaunation with cecotrophs collected from a healthy donor rabbit to reestablish the enteric flora should be considered. It should be noted that yogurt and many ruminant probiotics, containing lactobacilli, have not been shown to be effective in floral reconstitution.

Traumatic presentations may include fractured limbs, traumatic vertebral subluxation or luxation, and fight-related lacerations, including those of the scrotum. The former should be treated by splinting, but with as little handling as possible. Radiography should be done to characterize the fracture and permit the development of a plan for reduction and stabilization. The basic principles of fracture management in other species apply keeping in mind that the cortices of rabbit bones may be somewhat less. Unfortunately, vertebral injuries are rarely curable and usually result in euthanasia. Rabbits presenting acutely for vertebral injury should be radiographed to confirm the diagnosis and should be kept clean, padded to retard the development of decubital ulcers, and provided fluid and dietary therapy as needed. Trauma to the scrotum or testes may require surgical castration.

In some cases, distress may cause pH changes in the cecum that result in alterations of commensal and fermentative bacteria leading to a vexing clinical syndrome characterized by anorexia, ileus with obstipation/constipation, and, given sufficient time, dehydration and weight loss. This is often a diagnosis based upon lack of defecation and appetite in an otherwise seemingly normal rabbit and of exclusion of other causes. Where this results in chronic anorexia and ileus that is nonresponsive to treatments described above, specific bacteriotherapy may be useful in recolonizing the gastrointestinal tract. Parenteral fluids, B

vitamins, and vitamin K should also be provided. Nutritional supplementation should be provided using an appropriate liquid diet given by oral syringe feeding or, in extreme and unresponsive cases of anorexia, by force-feeding using a stomach or nasogastric tube. Critical Care for Herbivores (Oxbow Pet Products, 29012 Mill Road, Murdock, NE) is a palatable, nutritionally complete formula designed for syringe feeding of convalescing herbivores. It is easy to mix, is packaged for resale to clients, and contains microencapsulated anaerobic bacteria.

Hemorrhage should be controlled by providing hemostasis, including surgical interventions, if needed. Fluid therapy should be given for rabbits that are shocky or in shock. Transfusion should be considered for those rabbits that are profoundly anemic although blood typing and blood transfusion of rabbits, if ever attempted or reported, remain obscure. Rest, oxygen therapy, and nutritional support and supplementation are also important in the treatment of anemia. The most likely causes of hemorrhage are trauma from a predator species, cutaneous neoplasms, and internal hemorrhage and hematuria in intact does from uterine adenocarcinoma.

SEX DETERMINATION

Gender determination in rabbits is similar to cats with the exception that does also show sexual dimorphism by virtue of a pendulous fold of skin at the caudal mandibulocervical region. This redundant skin is termed the "dewlap." The vulva in does is located directly below the anus. The ensheathed penis of the buck is also located directly below the anus similar to cats, but bucks do not have a dewlap and they have an obvious scrotum with palpable testes. However, due to open inguinal canals, the testes may migrate back and forth from the scrotum to the abdomen (figs. 8.11 and 8.12).

CLINICAL TECHNIQUES

Placing a Catheter
The marginal lateral ear vein of rabbits is accessible and can be catheterized without difficulty and without the need for sedation or a high degree of restraint. To enhance visualization, the thin coat of fur should be shaved or plucked from the site. Topical vasodilating agents such as 70% ethanol, d-limonene (citrus oil), or methylsalicylate (oil of wintergreen) can be applied to the skin overlying the vessel to enhance venous access

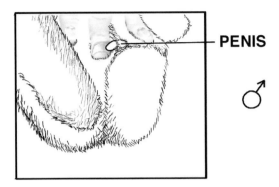

Fig. 8.11. *Sex determination of a male rabbit. (Drawing by Scott Stark)*

by increasing the vessel diameter. Vasospasm occurs at a high incidence and is a confounding factor for vascular access in rabbits. Additionally, a combination of butorphanol and acepromazine (Flecknell 1996) or midazolam alone (Robertson & Eberhart 1994) can be given to induce tranquilization, obviate vasospasm, and enhance blood flow. See color plate 8.1.

As for obtaining venous access in any species, it is important to engorge the vessel with blood by obstructing flow toward the heart. This should be done by compressing the vessel at the base of the ear with the thumb and forefinger of the nondominant hand. This can be done by the person giving the injection or an assistant. A 22 gauge, 25 mm catheter (Jelco catheter, Critikon, Tampa, FL) can be placed without difficulty in a 2–5 kg rabbit. Smaller catheters should be used for rabbits of correspondingly smaller size. After puncture of the vessel wall, the catheter should be advanced over the stylet and into the vessel lumen. The thin walls of the vessel make it easy to visualize the threading of the catheter into the lumen of the vein to the hub. Owing to the relative small volume of blood in the vein and the low venous blood pressure,

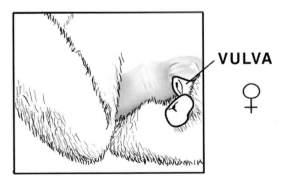

Fig. 8.12. *Sex determination of a female rabbit. (Drawing by Scott Stark)*

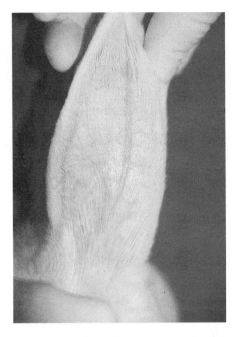

Plate 8.1. *Marginal lateral ear vein on the left and the prominent central auricular artery. (Photo courtesy of Ryan Cheek) (See also color plates)*

it is unlikely to obtain a backflow of blood into the catheter flange or hub. If in doubt, a small quantity of heparinized saline can be injected via the catheter for observation of the telltale blanching of the vessel with infused fluid. Once a patent catheter is established, it should first be secured to the convex surface of the ear by taping to the skin in butterfly fashion. A roll of four to five gauze 4 × 4 sponges should be placed in the concave pinna and the IV line should be secured with a circumferential wrap of tape. If the line is not needed for fluid administration, a heparin lock can be placed. If it is desirable to maintain the catheter for a period of time in the conscious rabbit, the catheter should be protected by use of an Elizabethan collar. The principles of fluid therapy are identical to those for other species. See figure 8.13 for the procedure for placing a catheter in the marginal lateral ear vein.

Catheters can be maintained for longer periods of time for regular arterial or venous access in hospitalized rabbits. The general technique is to tranquilize the rabbit if feasible with butorphanol-acepromazine, fully shave the convex surface of the ear, apply a vasodilating agent topically, and insert a 22 gauge catheter as close to the tip of the ear as possible (Smith et al. 1988). An alternative is to thread sterile PE-10 tubing through a 20 gauge needle 2–3 cm into the vessel (Melich 1990). After appropriately attaching an injection cap, glue the catheter hub or PE-10 tubing to

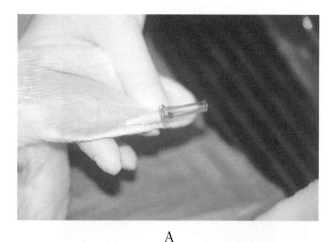

A

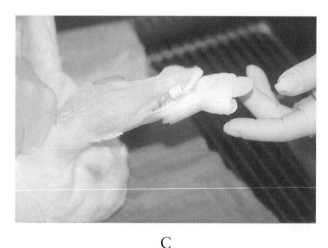

B

C

Fig. 8.13 A. Initial insertion of the catheter in the vein; note the "flash." B. The catheter seated into the vein and cap has been applied. C. A tongue depressor was added for additional support. (Photos courtesy of Ryan Cheek)

the skin using tissue adhesive (VetBond, 3M, St. Paul, MN) and tape circumferentially to secure the device to the ear with medical adhesive tape. The final step is to bind both ears together with full-length circumferential wraps of cast padding and roll gauze followed by adhesive tape while leaving the injection cap exposed (Smith et al. 1988). This prevents the rabbit from scratching the ears and stripping the catheter. The catheter should be infused with heparinized saline (100 U/ml).

Intraosseous infusion is indicated in situations where intravenous access is not possible because of the small size of the patient or where a delay in access may affect survival. The procedure is done using a similar approach and equipment as for cats and can be done in kits as small as 200 grams (Bielski et al. 1993). Under anesthesia, the stifle area should be shaved and prepared aseptically. A 20–22 gauge, 1–1.5 inch spinal needle should be inserted at the medial aspect of the proximal tibia of the flexed stifle at an angle of about 30° through a nick in the skin (Anderson, 1995; Bielski et al. 1993; Otto & Crowe 1992). The needle should be advanced in a distal direction away from the physis until there is a dramatic reduction of resistance indicating penetration of the marrow cavity. At this point, one should aspirate slightly to obtain marrow for cytology to confirm that the needle is in the desired location. If a spinal needle is not available, use an appropriately sized hypodermic needle. If the hypodermic needle plugs, a thinner, sterile Kirschner wire can be used as a plunger to push bone cortex from the needle lumen (Anderson 1995). Once in the marrow cavity at the desired depth, the needle should be sutured to the skin and protected and further immobilized with a sterile wrap and bulky bandage. Any drug, agent, or fluid that can be safely given intravenously can be given by the intraosseous route. The maximal rate of infusion is about 10 ml/min by this route (Anderson 1995).

Venipuncture/Arterial Puncture

For purposes of blood collection or sampling, puncture of the central artery of the ear (central auricular artery) is the easiest, most effective and reliable technique in rabbits. Consequently, there is rarely a need for venipuncture of other vessels. However, if there are compelling reasons to do so, the jugular vein, lateral marginal ear vein, and cephalic vein all can be accessed in rabbits(fig. 8.14). See color plate 8.1.

The technique for access of the central auricular artery is the same as that for venous access with a few qualifiers. The thin coat of fur should be shaved or plucked from the region of the artery to enhance visu-

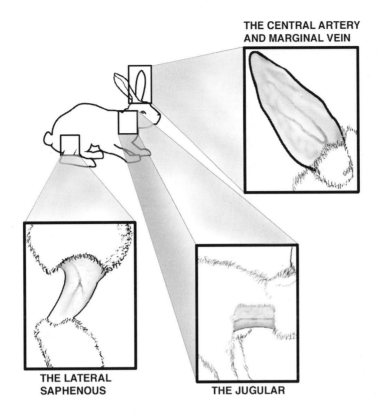

THE CENTRAL ARTERY AND MARGINAL VEIN

THE LATERAL SAPHENOUS

THE JUGULAR

Fig. 8.14. Venipuncture sites. (Drawing by Scott Stark)

alization. Topical vasodilating agents should also be applied to the skin overlying the vessel to promote dilation. A 21–23 gauge needle should be inserted through the artery wall and into the vessel lumen. Provided the animal is not hypothermic or distressed, blood will flow freely from the needle or can be gently aspirated into a syringe. Where the rabbit is fractious or there is a need to collect more than a few milliliters of blood, such as for transfusion, a combination of butorphanol and acepromazine can be given to sedate the animal, promote arterial vasodilation, and preserve blood pressure (Flecknell 1996). Upon removal of the needle, it is necessary to apply pressure for 3–5 minutes to the artery at the site of the puncture and monitor thereafter for 10–15 minutes for recrudescence of bleeding.

If it is desirable to gain arterial access for blood-gas analysis, blood pressure monitoring, or periodic sample collection, the central auricular artery is similarly easily accessible. A 22 gauge catheter can be placed in the vessel and secured as for an auricular intravenous catheter using tape in a butterfly application and a circumferential wrap of tape over a roll of gauze in the ear. The catheter can be prepared with a heparin-lock, to facilitate periodic sampling as for blood-gas analysis in surgery, or connected to a transducer for continuous arterial pressure monitoring.

The technique for venipuncture of the lateral marginal ear vein is the same as that described previously for catheter placement (fig. 8.15). Jugular and cephalic venipuncture or catheterization are also options, but, given the ease of accessibility of the auricular blood vessels, are rarely needed in rabbits.

Bandaging and Wound Care

The principles of bandaging and wound care are essentially the same for rabbits as for other species. The usual indications for such are trauma of limbs or trunk such as from fighting or pododermatitis. Foot bandages, providing they are secured so as not to be kicked off, are generally well tolerated by rabbits being treated for pododermatitis. However, an Elizabethan collar should be used where gnawing is a concern to protect the bandage. Bandages of the feet should be extended above the hock and should be secured at the proximal aspect of the bandage with loosely wrapped adhesive tape extending from the bandage to the fur. This anchoring will protect the bandage from being kicked off, but the staff and clients, upon discharge of the patient, should be mindful of monitoring the bandage to make sure that it does not become too tight.

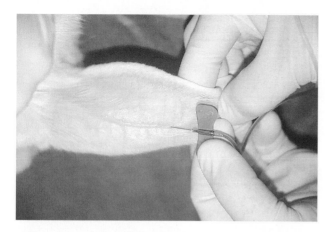

Fig. 8.15. Venipuncture of the marginal lateral ear vein using a butterfly catheter. (Photo courtesy of Ryan Cheek)

Urine Collection

Urine may be collected from rabbits into a clean cage pan, by catheterization as for cats, cystocentesis, or, from anesthetized rabbits by expression. As the bladder wall is thin and susceptible to trauma or puncture, cystocentesis, manual expression, or catheterization should be done with care.

TPR

The temperature, pulse, and respiration are obtained from rabbits as from more conventionally encountered pet species using a rectal thermometer and thoracic auscultation.

Administration of Medication (IV, PO, SC, IP, IM)

Intravenous Injection

The lateral veins of the ears are well suited for injection of materials. The technique is the same as that described above for placement of an intravenous catheter. They can be entered without trouble using 21–23 gauge needles or catheters. Typically volumes of up to 5 ml can be given by bolus by this route (Flecknell 1987).

Per Os

Small volumes of palatable fluid, not to exceed 5 ml, can be gently given by syringe or plastic dropper to awake rabbits. Larger volumes of liquid, unless readily accepted, should be given by stomach tube or small bore endoscope to an appropriately sedated or restrained animal. In some cases it may be tempting to give drugs via the drinking water or feed, however, it

is imprecise. Depending on their level of consumption, animals may be over- or underdosed. Medicated food or water should only be used where animals are consuming normally and should not be used where healthy companions may consume it. To achieve an effective dose, the animal must be consuming food and/or water and drug concentrations should be at maximal safe levels (based on estimated consumption), freshly prepared and renewed on a daily basis, with all residual feed or water being discarded.

Subcutaneous Injection

Subcutaneous injection is the most frequently used and easiest injection route provided that the agent is not excessively irritating. The methodology for a subcutaneous injection is the same as that for other species with the interscapular region preferred. A 21–25 gauge needle should be inserted under the lifted loose skin over the scapulae and parallel with the underlying muscle. Volumes of 30–50 ml can be given by this route (Flecknell 1987).

Intraperitoneal Injection

This route is rarely used in rabbits, but should be considered in neonates or moribund, hypothermic animals where vasoconstriction may be pronounced and there is a need to rapidly attempt fluid therapy or administer medications. For intraperitoneal injection, the rabbit ideally should be held on its back with the head slightly lower than the hindquarters to allow the stomach and intestines to fall cranially. A second individual should insert a 21–23 gauge needle at a 45° angle through the skin and abdominal wall slightly to the right of the midline at a midpoint between the xiphoid process and cranial wings of the ilium. However, if dorsal recumbency is at all resisted, the animal can be positioned on its side or in ventral recumbency. For fluid therapy or injection of a volume of material in excess of a few milliliters and to prevent accidental laceration of the internal organs, a catheter can be inserted and the stylet immediately removed after puncture of the abdominal wall. Volumes of up to 100 ml of warmed fluids can be given to a 4–5 kg rabbit by the IP route (Flecknell 1987).

Intramuscular Injection

In rabbits, the semimembranosus and semitendinosus muscles, found on the caudal aspect of the rear legs, and the epaxial muscles can be used as injection sites. A 20 gauge needle is recommended and volumes of up to 1.0 ml can be given (Flecknell 1987). The same principles for avoidance of injection into or around nerves apply as for other species.

CSF Collection

The collection technique for cerebrospinal fluid from rabbits is identical to that used for dogs and cats. The cisterna magna is the preferred site. The anesthetized rabbit is placed in lateral recumbency, with the dorsal cervical region shaved and aseptically prepared, and the neck flexed ventrally. The head with the ears reflected rostrally are grasped with one hand and the free hand is used to insert a 22 gauge spinal needle at the atlanto-occipital articulation. Contamination of CSF samples with blood from dural injury may be frequent (Bivin 1994).

Teeth Trimming

The technique used traditionally to clip excessively long incisors in cases of malocclusion has been to use a conventional dog nail trimmer such as a Resco. This may be an acceptable acute and short-term solution, but is unacceptable for long-term health maintenance for a number of reasons. Longitudinal fissures, predisposing to periodontal abscesses, may be induced, the trimmed teeth may be left with sharp edges that may lacerate the tongue, cheek, or lips, and the periapical germinal tissues and periodontal ligament may be damaged (Gorrel 1996; Malley 1996). Consequently, either extraction of the maloccluded teeth or gentle burring to shorten the teeth should be done. The latter procedure may require sedation, but, where the veterinary personnel are facile and the rabbit is accustomed to restraint, it may be possible to rapidly trim the incisors in an awake animal. This should be done, however, with great caution and the obvious consent of the owner. Using a low-speed drill and a diamond bur, the incisors should be trimmed and shortened to their normal height (Gorrel 1996; Malley 1996). It might be useful to insert the barrel of a 3 or 5 milliliter syringe through the diastema to serve as a gag to open the mouth slightly. Dental care of the premolars and molars requires general anesthesia and is difficult and confined work probably best referred to a veterinary dental specialist. In cases of malocclusion, teeth trimming must be repeated every 6–8 weeks for the lifetime of the animal (Swindle & Shealy 1996).

Nail Trimming

Nail trimming can be done with any conventional nail trimmer used for dogs or cats. The quick is generally easy to visualize and overly aggressive trimming leading to bleeding should be managed as for dogs and cats. Owners can be taught to trim the nails of their pets as nails may grow long with rapidity in sedentary animals.

Force-feeding

The cases where medication or nutritional support must be given by stomach tube must be facilitated by sedation if done by one individual or reliable restraint provided by an assistant if the animal is to remain awake. Prior to the start of the procedure, the substances to be administered should be preloaded in catheter-tip syringes. An additional empty syringe should be handy for air bolus injection to confirm placement of the tube in the stomach. The distance from the stomach (last rib) to the incisors should be measured and the stomach tube should be marked at this distance from its tip to serve as a guide for insertion of the tube. Soft pliable rubber or plastic tubs 1.5 to 6 mm in diameter can be used for force-feeding.

To restrain a conscious rabbit for passage of a stomach tube, the rabbit should be placed on a smooth examination table and it and the restrainer should face the same direction. The rabbit should be gently slid toward the edge of the table. While using the forearm to press the flank of the rabbit against the body of the restrainer with the elbow pressing the pelvic limbs, grasp the head with the hand of the same limb positioning the fingers under the mandible and the thumb in the occipital region. One then folds the contralateral arm over the spine and uses the hand to gently compress the hindquarters. The second person inserts a gag into the mouth of the rabbit through the bilateral diastemae. When the gag is adequately positioned and provided the rabbit remains adequately restrained, the assistant (restrainer) removes the hand compressing the pelvis and takes control of the gag. The coworker passes the stomach tube via the aperture in the gag from the mouth into the stomach. In cases where gastric intubation is not obvious, proper placement can be confirmed by injecting 5–10 ml of air through the tube while auscultating the stomach for the telltale sounds of bubbling fluid or turbulent airflow. The administration of liquid agents follows immediately. Upon completion of the administration of the prescribed substances, the tube should be kinked and withdrawn. If the rabbit gags, is overly resentful, or if the restrainer is losing control, the procedure should be halted, the tube removed, and the procedure should be attempted again. The tube should be easy to pass and should never be forced or tissue damage or fatal pulmonary administration will result.

If a suitable mouth gag is not present on the premises, a gag can be made by taping two tongue depressors (0.75 in. width) in flat alignment with medical adhesive tape. A hole should be bored through the center of the taped tongue depressors, using a scissors tip or other sufficiently sharp instrument, of such size to permit passage of the stomach tube. An alternative is to remove the plunger from a syringe, bore a hole through the cylinder walls, and use the empty barrel as a gag. Mouth gags for rabbits should be of sufficient height or diameter to prohibit occlusion of the incisors and sectioning or damage to the tube. Tongue depressors that are 0.75 in. wide or the barrel of a 10 ml syringe are generally sufficient as gags for rabbits 4–6 kg in weight.

Force-feeding is indicated for administration of liquid nutritional supplements, medical treatment of trichobezoars, and transfaunation in cases of cecal dysbiosis. The latter procedure is accomplished by outfitting a healthy donor rabbit with an Elizabethan collar overnight to prevent coprophagy. The collected cecotrophs should be mixed and suspended in warmed (98.6°F), nonbacteriostatic saline and strained through gauze prior to administration with a stomach tube. A volume of 40–60 ml of this suspension can be safely given to a 4–5 kg rabbit using a 12 French, 16 inch Sovereign feeding tube (Kendall Co., Mansfield, MA).

EUTHANASIA

Methods should conform to those listed as acceptable by the most recent guidelines of the AVMA Panel on Euthanasia. In a practice setting, the most preferable method is by injection of a barbiturate overdose (50–100 mg/kg) into the lateral marginal ear vein. This can be facilitated by first sedating or anesthetizing the rabbit as described in the preceding section on surgical anesthesia.

REFERENCES

Anderson, NL. 1995. Intraosseous fluid delivery in small exotic animals. In *Kirk's Current Veterinary Therapy XII: Small Animal Practice*,1331–35. Philadelphia: W.B. Saunders Co.

Arlian, LG, et al. 1981. Infestivity of *Psoroptes cuniculi* in rabbits. *Amer J Vet Res* 42: 1782–1784.

Belluco, C., et al. 2001. Prevention of postsurgical adhesions with an autocrosslinked hyaluronan derivative gel. *J Surg Res* 100(2): 217–21.

Bergdall, VK, Dysko, RC 1994. Metabolic, traumatic, mycotic and inherited diseases and variations. In *The Biology of the Laboratory Rabbit*, 2d ed., edited by PJ Manning, DH Ringler, CE Newcomer, 293–319. Orlando: Academic Press.

Bielski, RJ, et al. 1993. Intraosseous infusions: Effects on the immature physis–an experimental model in rabbits. *J Ped Orthopedics* 13(4): 511–15.

Bivin, S. 1994. Basic biomethodology. In *The Biology of the Laboratory Rabbit*, 2d ed., edited by PJ Manning, DH Ringler, CE Newcomer, 71–86. Orlando: Academic Press.

Bowman, DD, Fogelson, ML, and Carbone, LG. 1992. Effect of ivermectin on the control of ear mites (*Psoroptes cuniculi*) in naturally infested rabbits. *Amer J Vet Res* 53: 105–9.

Brammer, DW, et al. 1991. Anesthetic and nephrotoxic effects of Telazol in New Zealand white rabbits. *Lab Anim Sci* 41(5): 432–35.

Carpenter, JW, Mashima, TY, Rupiper, DJ 2001. *Exotic Animal Formulary*. 2d, 301–26. Philadelphia: W.B. Saunders Co.

Cheeke, PR. 1987. *Rabbit Feeding and Nutrition*. Orlando: Academic Press.

Chew, RM. 1965. Water metabolism of mammals. *Physiol Mammal* 2: 43–178.

Cloyd, GC, Moorhead, DP. 1976. Facial alopecia in the rabbit associated with *Cheyletiella parasitovorax*. *Lab Anim Sci* 26: 801–803.

Cohen, C. 1969. Genetics of the rabbit. In *Laboratory Animal Medicine*, NAS Publication 1724, Washington, DC.

Curtis, SK, Brooks, DL. 1990. Eradication of ear mites from naturally infested conventional research rabbits using ivermectin. *Lab Anim Sci* 40: 406–8.

Danneman, PJ, et al. 1988. An evaluation of analgesia associated with the immobility response in laboratory rabbits. *Lab Anim Med* 38(1): 51–57.

Deeb, BJ, Digiacomo, RF. 1994. Cerebral larval migrans caused by *Baylisascaris* species in pet rabbits. *JAVMA* 205: 1744–47.

Delong, D, Manning, PJ. 1994. Bacterial diseases. In *The Biology of the Laboratory Rabbit*, 2d ed., edited by PJ Manning, DH Ringler, CE Newcomer, 131–170. Orlando: Academic Press.

Doerning, BJ, et al. 1992. Nephrotoxicity of tiletamine in New Zealand white rabbits. *Lab Anim Sci* 42(3): 267–69.

Düwel, D, Brech K. 1981. Control of oxyuriasis in rabbits by fenbendazole. *Lab Anim* 15: 101–5.

Edwards, AW, Korner, PI, and Thornburn, GD. 1959. The cardiac output of the unanesthetized rabbit, and the effects of preliminary anesthesia, environmental temperature, and carotid occlusion. *Q J Exp Physiol* 44: 309–21.

Feigenbaum, AS, Gaman, EM. 1967. Influence of mother's milk on incidence of spontaneous aortic lesions in weanling rabbits. *Proc Soc Exper Biol Med* 124:1020–1022.

Flecknell, PA. 1987. *Laboratory Animal Anaesthesia: An Introduction for Research Workers and Technicians*. London: Academic Press.

Flecknell, PA. 1996. *Laboratory Animal Anaesthesia*. 2d ed. London: Academic Press.

Gaman, EM, Feigenbaum, AS, Schenk, EA. 1967. Spontaneous aortic lesions in rabbits: Part 3. Incidence and genetic factors. *J Athero Res* 7:131–141.

Garibaldi, BA, et al. 1987. Hematuria in rabbits. *Lab Anim Sci* 37: 769–74.

Gentry, PA. 1982. The effect of administration of a single dose of T-2 toxin on blood coagulation in the rabbit. *Can J Comp Med* 46: 414–19.

Gillett, CS. 1994. Selected drug dosages and clinical reference data. In *The Biology of the Laboratory Rabbit*, 2d ed., edited by PJ Manning, DH Ringler, CE Newcomer, 467–72. Orlando: Academic Press.

Gilroy, BA. 1981. Endotracheal intubation of rabbits and rodents. *JAVMA* 179: 1295.

Gorrel, C. 1996. Teeth trimming in rabbits and rodents. *Vet Rec* 139(21): 528.

Greene, HSN. 1965. Diseases of the rabbit. In *The Pathology of Laboratory Animals*, edited by WE Ribelin and JR McCoy, 330–350. Springfield: CC Thomas.

Griffiths, M, Davies, D. 1963. The role of soft pellets in the production of lactic acid in the rabbit stomach. *J. Nutr* 80: 171–80.

Harkness, JE, Wagner, JE. 1989. *The Biology and Medicine of Rabbits and Rodents*, 3d ed. Philadelphia: Lea & Febiger.

Hewitt, CD, et al. 1989. Normal biochemical and hematological values in New Zealand White rabbits. *Clin Chem* 35: 1777–79.

Huerkamp, MJ. 1995. Anesthesia and postoperative management of rabbits and pocket pets. In *Kirk's Current Veterinary Therapy XII: Small Animal Practice*. Philadelphia: W.B. Saunders Co.

Ingalls, TH, et al. 1964. Natural history of adenocarcinoma of the uterus in the Phipps rabbit colony. *J Nat Canc Inst* 33: 799–806.

Jablonski, P, Howden, BO, and Baxter, K. 2001. Influence of buprenorphine analgesia on post-operative recovery in two strains of rats. *Lab Anim* 35: 213–22.

Jenkins, JR. 2000. Surgical sterilization in small mammals. Spay and neuter. *Vet Clin N. A. Exot Anim Pract* 3(3): 617–27.

Jensen, LJ, et al. 1983. Natural infection of *Obeliscoides cuniculi* in a domestic rabbit. *Lab Anim Sci* 30: 231–233.

Kazacos, KR, Kazacos, EA. 1983. Fatal cerebrospinal disease caused by *Baylisascaris procynosis* in domestic rabbits. *JAVMA* 183: 967–71.

Leary, SL, Manning PJ, Anderson LC. 1984. Experimental and naturally-occurring gastric foreign bodies in laboratory rabbits. *Lab Anim Sci* 34: 58–61.

Leck, G. 1988. Removing a calculus from the urinary bladder of a rabbit. *Vet Rec* 83: 64–65.

Lee, MJ, Clement, JG. 1990. Effects of soman poisoning on hematology and coagulation parameters and serum biochemistry in rabbits. *Mil Med* 155: 244–49.

Leland, MM, Hubbard, GB, Dubey, JP. 1992. Clinical toxoplasmosis in domestic rabbits. *Lab Anim Sci* 42: 318–19.

Lelkes, L, Chang, C-L. 1987. Microbial dysbiosis in rabbit mucoid enteropathy. *Lab Anim Sci* 37: 757–64

Lindsey, JR, Fox, RR. 1994. Inherited diseases and variations. In *The Biology of the Laboratory Rabbit*, 2d ed., edited by PJ Manning, DH Ringler, CE Newcomer, 293–319. Orlando: Academic Press.

Lipman, NS, Marini, R, Flecknell, PA. 1997. Anesthesia and analgesia in rabbits. In *Anesthesia and Analgesia in Laboratory Animals*, edited by DF Kohn, SK Wixson, WJ White, GJ Benson, 205–232. Boston: Academic Press.

Livio, M, et al. 1988. Role of platelet-activating factor in primary hemostasis. *Am J Physiol* 254: 218–23.

Lopez-Martinez, R, Mier, T, Quirarte, M. 1984. Dermatophytes isolated from laboratory animals. *Mycopathologica* 88: 111–113.

Malley, D. 1996. Teeth trimming in rabbits and rodents. *Vet Rec* 139(24): 603.

McLaughlin, RM, Fish, RE. 1994. Clinical chemistry and hematology. In *The Biology of the Laboratory Rabbit*, 2d ed., edited by PJ Manning, DH Ringler, CE Newcomer, 111–127. Orlando: Academic Press.

Melich, D. 1990. A method for chronic intravenous infusion of the rabbit via the marginal ear vein. *Lab Anim Sci* 40(3): 327–8.

Morgan, JR, Silverman S. 1984. *Techniques of Veterinary Radiography*. 4th ed. Davis: Veterinary Radiology Associates.

Mullen, HS. 2000. Nonreproductive surgery in small mammals. *Vet Clin N. A. Exot Anim Pract* 3(3): 629–45.

Narama, I, et al. 1982. Pulmonary nodule causes by *Dirofilaria immitis* in a laboratory rabbit. *J. Parasitol.* 68: 351–352.

Otto, CM, Crowe, DT. 1992. Intraosseous resuscitation techniques and applications. In *Kirk's Current Veterinary Therapy XI: Small Animal Practice*. Philadelphia: W.B. Saunders Company.

Patton, NM. 1994. Colony husbandry. In *The Biology of the Laboratory Rabbit*, 2d ed., edited by PJ Manning, DH Ringler, CE Newcomer, 27–45. Orlando: Academic Press.

PMI Nutrition International. 1998. LabDiet: Product Reference Manual, SL1-5.

Robertson SA, Eberhart S. 1994. Efficacy of intranasal route for administration of anesthetic agents to adult rabbits. *Lab Anim Sci* 44(2): 159–65.

Smith, PA, et al. 1988. A method for frequent blood sampling in rabbits. *Lab Anim Sci* 38(5): 623–5.

Sollod, AE, Hayes, TJ, Soulsby, EJ. 1968. Parasitic development of *Obeliscoides cuniculi* in rabbits. *J Paras* 54: 129–132.

Stein, S, Walshaw, S. 1996. Rabbits. In *Handbook of Rodent and Rabbit Medicine*, edited by K Laber-Laird, MM Swindle, P Flecknell, 183–217. Tarrytown: Elsevier Science, Inc.

Swindle, MM, Shealy, PM. 1996. Common surgical procedures in rodents and rabbits. In *Handbook of Rodent and Rabbit Medicine*, edited by K Laber-Laird, MM Swindle, P Flecknell, 239–54. Tarrytown: Elsevier Science, Inc.

Tesluk, GC, Peiffer, RL, Brown D. 1982. A clinical and pathological study of inherited glaucoma in New Zealand white rabbits. *Lab Anim* 16: 234–9, 1982.

Vogtsberger, LM, et al. 1986. Spontaneous dermatophytosis due to *Microsporum canis* in rabbits. *Lab Anim Sci* 36: 294–297.

Watkins, AR, Slocumbe, JO, Fernando, MA. 1984. The effects of single and multiple doses of thiabendazole on growing and arrested stages of the rabbit stomach worm *Obeliscoides cuniculi*. *Vet Parasitol* 16: 295–302.

Weisbroth, SH. 1994. Neoplastic diseases. In *The Biology of the Laboratory Rabbit*, 2d ed., edited by PJ Manning, DH Ringler, CE Newcomer, 259–92. Orlando: Academic Press.

Wixson, SK. 1994. Anesthesia and analgesia for rabbits. In *The Biology of the Laboratory Rabbit*, 2d ed., edited by PJ Manning, DH Ringler, CE Newcomer, 87–109. Orlando: Academic Press.

Wolford, ST, et al. 1986. Reference range data base for serum chemistry and hematology values in laboratory animals. *J Toxicol Environ Health* 18: 161–88.

Wootton, R, Cross, G, Wood, S, West, CD. 1988. An analgesiometry system for use in rabbits with some preliminary data on the effects of buprenorphine and lofentanil. *Lab Anim* 22: 217–22.

Wright, F, Riner, J. 1984. Comparative efficacy of injection routes and doses of ivermectin against *Psoroptes* in rabbits. *Amer J Vet Res* 46: 752–754.

Wyatt, JD, Scott, RW, Richardson, ME. 1989. The effects of prolonged ketamine-xylazine intravenous infusion on arterial blood pH, blood gases, mean arterial blood pressure, heart and respiratory rates, rectal temperature, and reflexes in the rabbit. *Lab Anim Sci* 39: 411–16.

Xu, ZJ, Chen, WX. 1989. Viral hemorrhagic disease in rabbits: A review. *Vet Res Commun* 13: 205–12.

Yu, L, et al. 1979. Biochemical parameters of normal rabbit serum. *Clin Biochem* 12: 83–87.

FORMULARY

A formulary for agents recommended in this chapter is provided below (tables 8.5–8.9). However, excellent and affordable formularies for rabbit medicine and many other exotic species exist (Hawk & Leary 1999; Carpenter et al. 2001). Where no recommended dose exists or can be found, as a rule of thumb, given their equivalent body sizes, feline doses and administration schedules for most agents are appropriate for rabbits.

The only agent commonly used in cats and contraindicated in rabbits is Telazol. However, antibiotics with gram-positive and anaerobic spectra should be used with caution and under close supervision owing to the risk of clostridial enterotoxemia. See tables 8.5, 8.6, 8.7, 8.8, 8.9.

ABBREVIATIONS

BID = every 12 hours
CRI = constant rate infusion
IM= intramuscular
IN= intranasal
IP = intraperitoneal
IT = intratracheal
IV = intravenous
PO = per os
PRN = use as needed
QOD = every other day
SC = subcutaneous
SID = every 24 hours

GENERAL REFERENCES

Carpenter, JW, Mashima, TY, Rupiper, DJ. 2001. *Exotic Animal Formulary*. 2d ed. Philadelphia: W.B. Saunders Co.

Hawk, CT, Leary, SL. 1999. *Formulary for Laboratory Animals*. 2d ed. Ames: Iowa State Press.

SPECIFIC FORMULARY REFERENCES

Bergdall, VK, Dysko, RC. 1994. Metabolic, traumatic, mycotic and inherited diseases and variations. In *The Biology of the Laboratory Rabbit*, edited by PJ Manning, DH Ringler, CE Newcomer, 2d ed., 293–319. Orlando: Academic Press.

Blake, DW, Jover, B, McGrath, BP. 1988. Haemodynamic and heart rate reflex responses to propofol in the rabbit. *Br J Anaesth* 61: 194–99.

Bowman, TA, Lang, CM. 1986. Drug therapy in laboratory animals. In *Veterinary Pharmaceuticals and Biologics*, edited by AJ Weber, K Grey, et al, 5th ed. Lenexa: Veterinary Medicine Publishing.

Broome, RL, Brooks, DL. 1991. Efficacy of enrofloxacin in the treatment of respiratory pasteurellosis in rabbits. *Lab Anim Sci* 41: 572–76.

Cabellos, C, et al. 2000. Evaluation of combined ceftriaxone and dexamethasone therapy in experimental cephalosporin-resistant pneumococcal meningitis. *J Antimicrob Chemotherap* 45: 315–20.

Carpenter, JW, et al. 1995. Caring for rabbits: An overview and formulary. *Vet Med* 90(4): 340–64.

Curtis, SK, Brooks, DL. 1990. Eradication of ear mites from naturally infested conventional research rabbits using ivermectin. *Lab Anim Sci* 40: 406–408.

Flecknell, PA. 1987. *Laboratory Animal Anaesthesia: An Introduction for Research Workers and Technicians*. London: Academic Press.

Flecknell, PA. 1991. Post-operative analgesia in rabbits and rodents. *Lab Anim* 20(9): 34–37.

Flecknell, PA. 1996. *Laboratory Animal Anaesthesia*. 2d ed. London: Academic Press.

Gillett, CS. 1994. Selected drug dosages and clinical reference data. In *The Biology of the Laboratory Rabbit*, 2d ed., edited by PJ Manning, DH Ringler, CE Newcomer, 467–72. Orlando: Academic Press.

Harkness, JE, Wagner, JE. 1989. *The Biology and Medicine of Rabbits and Rodents*. 3d ed. Philadelphia: Lea & Febiger.

Huerkamp, MJ. 1995. Anesthesia and postoperative management of rabbits and pocket pets. In *Kirk's Current Veterinary Therapy XII: Small Animal Practice*. Philadelphia: W.B. Saunders Co.

Lacy, MJ, Kent, CR, Voss, EW, Jr. 1987. D-Limonene: An effective vasodilator for use in collecting rabbit blood. *Lab Anim Sci* 37: 485–87.

Liles, JH, Flecknell, PA. 1992. The use of non-steroidal anti-inflammatory drugs for the relief of pain in laboratory rodents and rabbits. *Lab Anim* 26: 241–55.

Lipman, NS, Marini, RP, Erdman, SE. 1990. A comparison of ketamine/xylazine and ketamine/xylazine/acepromazine anesthesia in the rabbit. *Lab Anim Sci* 40: 395–98.

Lipman, NS, et al. 1992. Utilization of cholestyramine resin as a preventative treatment for antibiotic (clindamycin) induced enterotoxemia in the rabbit. *Lab Anim Sci* 26: 1–8.

Lipman, NS, Marini, R, Flecknell, PA. 1997. Anesthesia and analgesia in rabbits. In *Anesthesia and Analgesia in Laboratory Animals*, edited by DF Kohn, SK Wixson, WJ White, GJ Benson, 205–232. Boston: Academic Press.

Marini, R, et al. 1992. Ketamine/xylazine/butorphanol: a new anesthetic combination for rabbits. *Lab Anim Sci* 42: 57–62.

McDuffie, RS, Jr., Heddleston LN, Blanton SJ, Gibbs RS. 1995. A comparison of aztreonam and two regimens of gentamicin in a rabbit model of intra-amniotic infection and sepsis. *J Soc Gynecol Invest* 2: 23–5.

McKellar, QA. 1989. Drug dosages for small mammals. *Practice* (March): 57–61.

Robertson SA, Eberhart S. 1994. Efficacy of intranasal route for administration of anesthetic agents to adult rabbits. *Lab Anim Sci* 44(2): 159–65.

Wootton, R, Cross, G, Wood, S, West, CD. 1988. An analgesiometry system for use in rabbits with some preliminary data on the effects of buprenorphine and lofentanil. *Lab Anim* 22: 217–22.

Table 8.5. Analgesics, Anesthetics, Sedatives, and Tranquilizers

Agent	Dosage	Reference
Acepromazine	0.75 mg/kg–5 mg/kg IM	Flecknell 1987; Lipman et al. 1990
	0.5 mg/kg IM (with butorphanol for phlebotomy)	Flecknell 1996
Buprenorphine	0.01–0.05 mg/kg SC q 12 hours	Flecknell 1991
	0.5 mg/kg per rectum	Wootton et al. 1988
Butorphanol	0.1 mg/kg IM, SC (as an anesthetic supplement to xylazine:ketamine)	Marini et al. 1992
	0.1–0.5 mg/kg IM, SC q 4 hrs (postoperative analgesia)	Carpenter & Mashima 1995
	0.5 mg/kg IM (with acepromazine for phlebotomy)	Flecknell 1996
Diazepam	0.5–2 mg/kg IV	Flecknell 1996
Flunixin meglumine	1.1 mg/kg SC q 12 hours	Liles & Flecknell 1992
Halothane	1.5–2.5% (maintenance)	Huerkamp 1995
Isoflurane	2–3% (maintenance)	Huerkamp 1995
Ketamine	35–45 mg/kg (with xylazine)	Flecknell 1996; Huerkamp 1995
	25 mg/kg (with medetomidate)	Flecknell 1996
Medetomidate	0.5 mg/kg IM (with ketamine 25 mg/kg)	Flecknell 1996
Meperidine	0.2 mg/ml in drinking water (postoperative analgesia)	Huerkamp 1995
Midazolam	0.5–2 mg/kg IM, IV, IN	Flecknell 1996 Robertson & Eberhart 1994
Propofol	1.5 mg/kg IV bolus (induction)	Blake et al. 1988
	0.2–0.6 mg/kg/min (CRI)	Blake et al. 1988
Xylazine	5 mg/kg (with ketamine)	Flecknell 1996

Table 8.6. Anthelmintic Agents

Agent	Dosage	Reference
Fenbendazole	20 mg/kg PO SID x 5 days	McKellar 1989
Pyrantel pamoate	5–10 mg/kg PO	Carpenter et al. 2001
Ivermectin	400 mcg/kg SC SID q 15–17 days	Curtis & Brooks 1990
Thiabendazole	50 mg/kg PO SID q 21 days	Carpenter & Mashima 1995

Table 8.7. *Anti-infective Agents*

Agent	Dosage	Reference
Chloramphenicol	30–50 mg/kg/day (enterotoxemia risk; use with caution)	Harkness & Wagner, 1989
Enrofloxacin	5 mg/kg IM,SC BID	Broome & Brooks 1991
Furazolidone	200–800 mg/L in drinking water	Gillett 1994
Gentamicin	6 mg/kg/day IM, SC	McDuffie et al. 1995
Griseofulvin	25 mg/kg PO SID × 14 days	Bergdall & Dysko 1994
	1.5% in DMSO topically SID	Bergdall & Dysko 1994
Oxytetracycline	400 mg/L in drinking water	Bowman & Lang 1986
Penicillin G, procaine	42,000–84,000 U/kg IM SID (enterotoxemia risk; use with caution)	Gillett 1994
Penicllin G, benzathine and procaine	42,000–84,000 U/kg IM QOD (enterotoxemia risk; use with caution)	Gillett 1994
Sulfaquinoxaline	100 mg/kg SC	Gillett 1994
	0.1–0.15% in drinking water	Gillett 1994

Table 8.8. *Autonomic Drugs*

Agent	Dosage	Reference
Atropine	1–2 mg/kg IM, SC q 15 minutes	Lipman et al. 1997
Glycopyrrolate	0.01–0.1 mg/kg SC PRN	Flecknell 1996

Table 8.9. *Other Agents*

Agent	Dosage	Reference
Atipamezole	1 mg/kg IV (medetomidate reversal)	Flecknell 1996
Cholestyramine	0.5–0.8 g/kg SID PO	Lipman et al. 1992
d-Limonene	20–40% in ethanol topical (for local vasodilation)	Lacy et al. 1987
Dexamethasone	0.25 mg/kg/day IM, SC, IV	Cabellos et al. 2000
Doxapram	2–5 mg/kg IV, IM, IN, IT PRN	Huerkamp 1995
Methlysalicylate	Topical application (to induce local vasodilation)	Huerkamp 1995
Povidone iodine	10% solution topical SID-BID	Bergdall & Dysko 1994
Prednisone	0.5–2.0 mg/kg PO	Carpenter et al. 2001
Yohimbine	0.2 mg/kg IV (xylazine reversal)	Flecknell 1996

CHAPTER NINE

The Mouse, Rat, Gerbil, and Hamster

Anne Hudson

This chapter will focus on the mouse (*Mus musculus*), rat (*Rattus norvegicus*), gerbil (*Meriones unguiculatus*), and hamsters: golden or Syrian hamster *(Mesocricetus auratus),* European hamster *(Cricetus cricetus),* and Russian dwarf hamster *(Phodopus* spp.).

ANATOMY AND PHYSIOLOGY

Basic anatomy and physiology of rodents is like that of other mammals, so only the significant differences will be addressed in this section (fig. 9.1).

Rodents all share a dental formula of 2 (I 1/1, C 0/0, P 0/0, M 3/3), with hamsters having incisors at birth (Harkness & Wagner 1989, 28). The incisors are open rooted and grow continuously; the molars do not. Incisors will develop a yellow-orange color as the animal ages. Gnawing wears down the surface of the teeth, but a malocclusion of the incisors precludes normal wear and clipping or cutting the teeth down will be necessary.

Rats, mice, and gerbils possess long tails; hamsters have very short tails. It is very important to exercise caution when handling the tail since improper restraint can cause trauma. In gerbils the skin can actually "slip" or deglove with improper handling.

Mammary tissue is extensive, reaching cranially between the front legs and up over the shoulders, and caudally toward the inguinal area. For this reason, mammary masses can be located well away from the teats. The mammary glands are paired, with rats having four to six pair, mice having five pair, gerbils four pair, and hamsters six to seven pair (Lawson 2000, 149–151).

Harderian glands are specialized glands located behind each eye. These glands secrete a substance containing porphyrin, giving the secretion a red tinge. An animal experiencing stress or illness may have a buildup of the secretions around the eyes, and due to the red color, the animal may appear to the client to be bleeding from the eyes and the nares. This collection of secreted material is also referred to as "red tears."

Additional glandular structures include bilateral flank glands in the hamster, and a ventral gland in the gerbil (Harkness & Wagner 1989, 28, 34.) These sebaceous glands are brown in color and play a part in mating behavior and territorial marking behavior. The animals will spend time grooming these areas and will often be observed rubbing the glands over surfaces.

Small rodents are seasonally polyestrus and are spontaneous ovulators. Mating behavior results in the production of a whitish-tan collection of secretions called a copulatory plug often found lying in the bedding of the cage (Lawson 2000, 35). Most male rodent species have an os-penis and open inguinal canals allowing them to retract the testicles into the abdominal cavity (Lawson 2000, 150). Gentle pressure to the caudal abdomen will force the testicles into the scrotal sac.

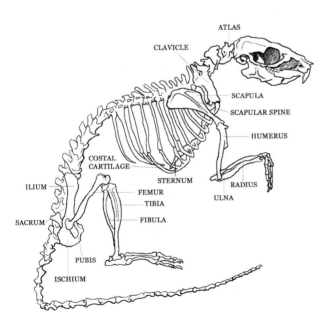

Fig. 9.1. *Rodent skeletal anatomy. (Drawing by Scott Stark)*

Hamsters possess large cheek pouches extending back to the scapula. These pouches can distend to quite a large size, allowing the hamster to transfer food and bedding from one point to another. A startled mother may also move offspring from one area to another via the cheek pouches (fig. 9.2).

The digestive systems of rodents have some differences from other mammals, including an inability to regurgitate. Hamsters have an esophageal pouch that allows for pregastric fermentation of food prior to reaching the stomach (Lawson 2000, 150). Rodents are monogastric, with their stomachs divided into two areas: one glandular portion, and one nonglandular portion. The practice of coprophagy is believed to assimilate certain nutrients, such a B vitamins, that are produced by bacterial action in the colon (Hillyer & Quesenberry 1997, 296). Rats do not have a gallbladder; therefore bile continuously flows into the duodenum. The pancreas of rodents is arranged in diffuse lobes, making palpation difficult. Brown fat in rodents seems to provide a source of energy, and is found deposited around the kidneys and thymus, and between the shoulders (Lawson 2000, 149–151). The rodent's visceral anatomy is shown in figure 9.3.

BIOLOGIC AND REPRODUCTIVE DATA

It is important that a technician know physiologic data for small rodents. This aids in determining an animal's state of health and also helps answer questions owners commonly ask. See table 9.1.

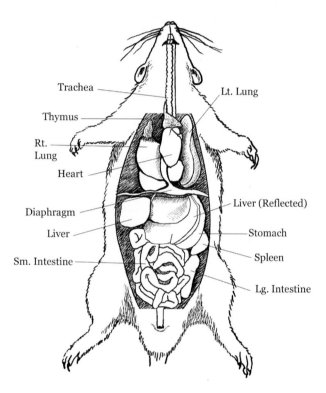

Fig. 9.3. *Rodent visceral anatomy. (Drawing by Scott Stark)*

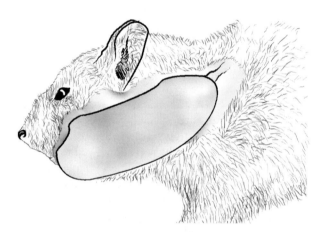

Fig. 9.2. *Cheek pouch. (Drawing by Scott Stark)*

Table 9.1. Physiological Data of Selected Rodents

Physiological data	Mouse	Rat	Gerbil	Hamster
Lifespan	1–3 years	2–4 years	3–4 years	18–24 months
Adult weight M/F	20–40 g / 25–40 g	300–400 g / 250–300 g	80–120 g / 70–95 g	85–130 g / 95–150 g
Body temperature °F	98–101	99.5–100.6	101–103	101–103
Heart rate (bpm)	300–750	250–450	360	300–500
Respiratory rate (bpm)	60–220	70–115	90	
Puberty	35 days	37–67 days	70–84 days	45–75 days
Estrous cycle	4–5 days	4–5 days	4–7 days	3–4 days
Gestation	19–21 days	21–23 days	24–26 days	15 days
Weaning age	19–28 days	21 days	21 days	20–25 days
Average litter size	10–12	6–12	3–7	5–9

HUSBANDRY

Rodent housing should be escape proof, chew proof, and easily cleaned. A variety of metal and plastic caging is available. Solid flooring is easy to clean and may help prevent trauma to the limbs. Breeding animals should be housed on solid flooring. Adequate ventilation is important since the buildup of ammonia from urea breakdown will contribute to upper respiratory disease (Harkness & Wagner 1989, 2). Wire caging promotes better ventilation than plastic-shoe-box-type or tunnel-type caging, but cleaning the cages frequently will solve most of the ventilation problem. Plastic caging with tunnels provides more environmental enrichment for the animal than a simple wire cage.

A variety of bedding material is available including pine shavings and corncob products. The use of cedar shavings is controversial; the aromatic oils they contain may be irritating. If cleaning is performed adequately (one to two times a week at least), scented bedding is not required. The most important consideration is that the bedding be clean, dry, nonabrasive, and supplied in enough quantity that the animal can dig or burrow. Breeding animals should be provided with some form of nesting material. Commercial products are available, or tissue paper and the empty cardboard tubes from paper towels can be shredded by the rodent. Don't use old toweling because the animal can get entangled in the fibers. Lack of appropriate nesting material can result in the death of any offspring (Harkness & Wagner 1989, 32), either through abandonment or cannibalism, as can disturbing the nest in an effort to clean the cage. For this reason, cages should be cleaned just prior to parturition if at all possible. Ensure the animal has enough food to last about a week, and do not disturb the nest in any way. Do not handle the young at all during this time unless absolutely necessary.

Exercise wheels and balls are popular with pet owners and provide the animal with an activity. Routinely check the wheels for any rough or sharp areas, and caution owners using plastic balls to keep them away from stairs and other pets. Most rodent species will be more active at night, so placing the animal in another area than the bedrooms might be a good idea. A small amount of vegetable based oil applied on the axle of a metal wheel will help temporarily eliminate any squeaking.

NUTRITION

Pelleted diets like those utilized for laboratory animals are preferable to seed mixtures, which contribute to nutritionally related diseases. Seeds can be given, but are best saved for an occasional treat. Some fresh foods can be given as snacks (carrot, raw potato, sliced apple) but should be removed at day's end if not eaten to prevent spoilage. Crocks or hoppers may be used to provide feed. If using a hopper for a hamster, which possesses a blunt nose, make sure the hamster can fit its nose in the hopper spaces (Harkness & Wagner 1989, 32). Crocks are preferable to plastic bowls that the animal may chew on, and wire hoppers, which may cause facial abrasions. Mothers with litters should have their food placed in a crock or directly in the cage for easier access. Fresh water should be provided daily, and water bottles need to be checked each day for proper function. Sipper tubes may become clogged with bedding or other foreign material preventing the animal from having access to water. Alternately, a malfunctioning water bottle may leak all over the cage. The bottle should mount on the outside of the cage with only the metal tube extending into the cage in order to prevent the animal from chewing any plastic or rubber parts.

COMMON PARASITES, DISEASES, AND ZOONOSES

Rodents can be affected by several species of skin mites, which are spread through exposure to infected animals and bedding. Signs include alopecia, dermatitis, rough hair coat, and skin lesions from excessive scratching. Some mite species can be visualized with a hand lens, or microscopically with a skin scraping. Ectoparasites can be treated with a variety of antiparasitic agents including ivermectin and Amitraz (Mitaban) (Hillyer & Quesenberry 1997, 313). Caging must be concurrently cleaned. Alopecia in mice housed in groups may be a result of barbering rather than an infestation with an ectoparasite. Barbering behavior, when dominant mice chew the fur around the faces of the subordinate mice, should be suspected if one mouse in an affected group is not suffering from hair loss (Lawson 2000, 105). Mange in a rat is shown in figure 9.4.

Common endoparasites include pinworms and tapeworms. Clinical signs may not be present, but could include weight loss, diarrhea, and rectal prolapse in young animals. Detection of parasites is performed either through examination of a fecal floatation or cellophane tape preparation.

Cellophane Tape Preparation
Use these steps for cellophane tape preparation.

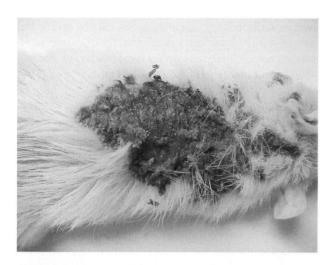

Fig. 9.4. Mange with a bacterial infection in a rat. (Photo courtesy of Dr. Stephen J. Hernandez-Divers, University of Georgia)

1. The following supplies should be assembled: cellophane tape, microscope slide, microscope.
2. A small piece of the cellophane tape should be pressed against the perianal area.
3. The tape should then be placed on a microscope slide sticky side down for examination (Hillyer & Quesenberry 1997, 313–14).
4. The slide should be examined for the slightly banana-shaped pinworm ova.

Neoplasia does occur in rodents, with mammary tumors a common finding (fig. 9.5). Extensive mammary tissue may result in the tumor being located on the abdomen or on the shoulders. The tumors often interfere with the animal's ability to walk normally, and chronic mechanical irritation can cause them to become ulcerated (Harkness & Wagner 1989, 165).

Malocclusion results when the continuously erupting incisors do not meet properly, and signs include weight loss, drooling, and oral trauma. Causes include genetics, malnutrition, disease, or injury (Harkness & Wagner 1989, 165). Periodic trimming with a dental burr or clippers must be done carefully to avoid splitting the tooth. Splitting teeth can result in the formation of abscesses. Clippers should be very sharp and all rough edges need to be filed smooth.

Moist dermatitis commonly occurs in rodents who are chronically exposed to wet conditions, or in those with trauma to the skin from urine scald, diarrhea, abrasions, cuts, or other breaks in skin integrity. Gerbils may have lesions on the face and nose caused by an accumulation of harderian gland secretions (Hillyer & Quesenberry 1997, 323). Other causes should be ruled out, such as malocclusion, damaged crockery or caging, and abrasive bedding. Treatment involves clipping the hair from the lesion, cleaning the area, and removing any known causative agents. The veterinarian may prescribe systemic or topical antibiotics.

Hamsters with diarrhea are often referred to as having "wet-tail" (fig. 9.6). Young animals are particularly sensitive to proliferative ileitis, especially if recently weaned. Multiple bacteria are implicated in the cause, as well as improper diet and stress. Signs are hunched posture, matted hair, watery diarrhea, lethargy, rectal prolapse, and death. Careful husbandry may help prevent the disease, and the veterinarian may prescribe antibiotic therapy (Harkness & Wagner 1989, 178–179).

Gerbils are susceptible to epileptiform seizures that can result from excitement related to handling. The

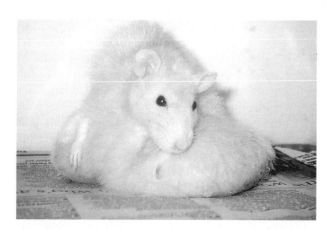

Fig. 9.5. Neoplasia in a rat. (Photo courtesy of Ryan Cheek)

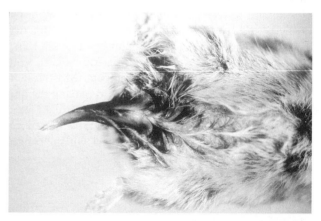

Fig. 9.6. Wet tail. (Photo courtesy of Dr. Chris King)

seizures can be mild, resulting in a dazed or hypnotic appearance, or severe and the activity may last only a few seconds to a minute or more. There is no treatment and anticonvulsant drugs are not indicated. Exposure to frequent handling at a young age may help prevent the seizures from occurring (Harkness & Wagner 1989, 139).

Infectious diseases affecting rodents include mouse hepatitis virus (MHV), mouse parvovirus (MPV), Sendai virus, mycoplasmosis, sialodacryoadenitis virus, and lymphocytic choriomeningitis (LCM) (Lawson 2000, 101–102).

MHV is a highly contagious disease that can cause severe diarrhea and death in very young (1–2 weeks old) mice. Mouse parvovirus also results in enteritis but is usually subclinical.

Sendai virus is a respiratory virus that can spread quickly and is often fatal in neonatal mice. Older animals may have an active immunity to the disease and not show clinical signs. Because morbidity is close to 100%, the disease is of great significance to research colonies. Signs include rough hair coat, hunched posture, dyspnea, weight loss, and chattering. Animals showing signs need to be handled very carefully since the added stress of handling may result in the patient's death.

Chronic respiratory disease in rodents may be caused by *Mycoplasma pulmonis*. This disease may also be referred to as murine respiratory mycoplasmosis. Signs will include general upper respiratory signs described above, as well as rhinitis and a possible head tilt associated with otitis. Antibiotics can be employed to help control the signs, but will never completely eradicate the disease.

Sialodacryoadenitis virus is a coronavirus related to MHV, and is spread through respiratory secretions. Infection causes the cervical lymph nodes to swell and the salivary glands to become inflamed. Affected animals may continue to eat despite swelling in the neck. A very noticeable sign will be chromodacryorrhea, or "red tears." The animal may be sensitive to light and develop ophthalmic lesions.

Lymphocytic choriomeningitis (LCM) is found naturally in wild mouse populations and can be passed via arthropod vectors, through bodily secretions, and through bite wounds. Animals may be asymptomatic, or can present with a hunched posture, unthrifty appearance, photophobia, and convulsions. LCM is zoonotic; humans can become infected through contact with infected tissue, urine, or a bite wound. Symptoms are similar to those associated with influenza and include headache, fever, muscle aches, malaise, and meningitis.

Hamsters and gerbils may also contract a fatal hepatoenteric infectious disease called Tyzzer's disease, which is caused by *Bacillus piliformis*. Signs include sudden death, listlessness, rough hair coat, and weight loss. Stress is a major contributing factor in addition to exposure to infected bedding.

There are diseases with zoonotic potential aside from LCM, many of which are more common in wild rodent populations than in domestic rodents. According to the Centers for Disease Control, the risk of a human contracting Korean hemorrhagic fever or the organism responsible for bubonic plague from a pet rodent is extremely remote in the United States (CDC, personal communication). People with immunosuppression are at higher risk, and practicing good hygiene is essential. Salmonellosis in humans will cause vomiting, diarrhea, fever, and in severe cases, death. Rat bite fever is a bacterial infection causing chills, fever, myalgia, localized swelling at the wound site, and headache. It is also possible to contract hymenolepid tapeworm infection, which causes enteric disease in humans (Lawson 2000, 101–102; Hillyer & Quesenberry 1997, 315–317; Harkness & Wagner 1989, 121).

BEHAVIOR

Most rodents are nocturnal but are easily awakened during the day. Gentle handling will prevent a startled animal from biting out of defense. Male mice, gerbils, and hamsters will fight with each other, and should be housed alone. Hamsters of either sex are better housed singly than in groups, and should only be brought together for mating. Gerbils have been known to establish monogamous pairs, but fighting in older gerbils that previously seemed to peacefully coexist may develop, and they can inflict serious wounds on each other. Since many rodents are kept as pets for small children, separate housing is recommended since witnessing such activity could be traumatic. The exception to the housing recommendation is the rat. Rats of both sexes can be grouped together, and females with litters can be left in communal housing with relative safety, provided conditions are not overcrowded. Females will share in caring for and nursing young animals.

Cannibalism of young may occur if nests are disturbed or the mother is overly nervous. This behavior is most often associated with hamsters; gerbils seem less sensitive to disturbance and rats rarely cannibalize offspring. It is imperative to ensure the cage is supplied with clean bedding, and adequate food and water prior to parturition to prevent having to disturb the nest once the offspring have been born.

HISTORY AND PHYSICAL EXAMINATION

Rodents should be brought to the hospital in the cage in which they are normally housed. The person scheduling the appointment should advise the client not to clean the cage prior to coming into the hospital. This allows the staff to observe the condition of the cage, the presence of fecal material, type of bedding, and so on. Ideally, have the client sit away from cats and dogs once at the hospital to prevent further stress. The exam room should be stocked with urine dipsticks for immediate sampling since most rodents urinate as soon as they are handled (Hillyer & Quesenberry 1997, 310).

As with any patient, clients should be asked where they obtained the pet, how long they have had it, what they feed it, and if this is the first time they have owned this particular species. Discuss with clients when they first noticed any signs of illness, how long the problem has existed, and what, if anything, they have done in response to the signs. Rodents can accurately be weighed using a gram scale. The animal may need to be in a small container when weighed to prevent escape; a plastic margarine tub with holes punched in the lid works well to keep the animal confined. Unless the practice has a thermometer specifically designed for use in rodents, forgo obtaining a rectal temperature. Standard thermometers are too large to use safely.

RESTRAINT AND HANDLING

Firm but gentle handling is important when working with rodents. They will bite out of fear, and also jump or run quickly in an effort to escape. Most rodents are amenable to being gently scooped up into the hands in order to lift them from their cages. Rats, mice, and gerbils can be briefly lifted by the base of the tail onto a table or other surface. Prolonged handling of the tail can cause trauma, such as sloughing of the skin and exposing the vertebrae. A towel or the screened lid of the animal's cage gives them something to hold on to when being restrained on a table. Rodents showing signs of aggression or agitation (chattering, vocalizing, rolling onto their backs, and in gerbils, thumping the hind feet) can be picked up with an empty can or plastic container, or lifted with a small towel folded for thickness. Gloves may be needed to handle some rats, but they are often unwieldy and can make it difficult to feel what the animal is doing. For this reason, care must be taken to observe the animal for any respira-

tory difficulty. There are plastic restraint devices available from laboratory animal supply companies (i.e., Kent Scientific, Torrington, CT).

Gerbils, Mice, and Rats

1. The animal should be grasped firmly at the base of the tail.
2. The animal should then be lifted out of its enclosure, and the animal's body allowed to rest on a table, hand, or arm. A hold should be maintained on the tail while supporting the animal's body to prevent escape (gerbils are excellent jumpers) (fig. 9.7).
3. Rats can alternatively be lifted by placing a hand over the dorsum and gently pressing the forelimbs together under the rat's chin with a thumb and index finger.

Hamsters

1. If the animal is awake, it can usually be scooped up gently using both hands; use caution if the hamster is sleeping as startled hamsters may bite.
2. If there is concern that the hamster may react aggressively, a piece of toweling or a can may be used to lift the animal up.

For injections or other procedures that the rodent may object to, the animal may be scruffed:

1. It is helpful to place the rodent on a towel or the top of a wire cage while maintaining a gentle hold on the tail.
2. Slight traction should be applied to the base of the tail, which will encourage the animal to grip onto the surface with its front feet.

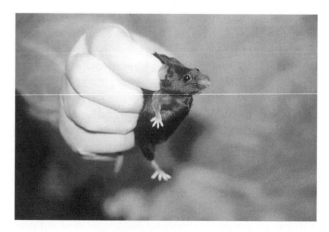

Fig. 9.7. Mouse restraint. (Photo courtesy of Ryan Cheek)

3. One should grasp the loose skin over the neck, using the little finger of the restraining hand to hold the tail.
4. Scruffing a hamster can be more difficult; the abundance of loose skin can still permit the animal to turn and bite if the restrainer has not grasped a sufficient amount. An indication of a sufficient amount of skin grasped is when the hamster "smiles" (figs. 9.8 and 9.9).

RADIOLOGY

Sedation is usually needed for most radiography in order to have proper positioning. Due to the size of the patient, whole-body studies are often employed. Animals may be placed in radiolucent tubing, or briefly positioned with paper or masking tape. Exposure times of ¹⁄₆₀ of a second or shorter will be necessary due to the rapid respiratory rate.

SURGERY AND ANESTHESIA

Common surgical procedures include ovariohysterectomy, castration, excision of tumors, and draining of abscesses. Surgical preparation is similar to that of any small animal, except fasting the animal prior to anesthesia is not necessary. Surgical scrub solutions should be warmed prior to use to prevent unnecessary heat loss to the patient. All rules of aseptic technique apply, and the surgical suite and equipment should be prepared with this in mind.

A warm water circulating pad or similar device to prevent heat loss should be placed on the surgical table with a small towel or similar material between

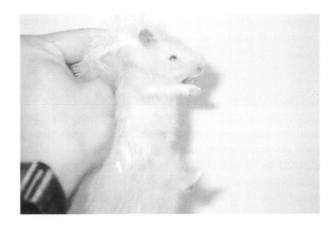

Fig. 9.9. Restraint of hamster. (Photo courtesy of Dr. Chris King)

the patient and the heating pad. Surgical tape can be used to restrain the animal on the table.

Rodents can be chamber or face-mask induced using isoflurane gas. Intubation is difficult in rodents, but they can be maintained using a face mask, or a plastic syringe case modified to use as a nose cone. A rebreathing system should be used (Hillyer & Quesenberry 1997, 283). The veterinarian may choose injectable induction agents such as thiopental, ketamine, or acepromazine (contraindicated in gerbils due to risk of seizures) (Harkness & Wagner 1989, 64).

The technician should monitor the depth and quality of respiration. The deeper the animal's anesthetic plane becomes, the more the abdominal muscles will move with each breath. Lightly anesthetized rodents will still blink when the eyelashes are touched. The palpebral reflex will be diminished as the animal enters a surgical plane. The toes can be pinched to evaluate the animal's ability to retract the limb; if the animal pulls the limb away when the toes are pinched, the plane of anesthesia is still light (Hillyer & Quesenberry 1997, 389). Mucous membranes should be pink, and the color can be evaluated using the pads of the feet, ears, eyes if albino, and gingiva. Pulse oximeters are commonly found in most small animal hospitals and can be placed on the tail or tongue.

Recovery from surgery should be provided in a warm, quiet area. The technician should gently turn the animal from side to side every few minutes to prevent pooling of blood on the dependent side. Rodents will attempt to chew sutures and bandages; surgical glue or subcuticular sutures are a better option. There are commercially available Elizabethan collars, but these are often not well tolerated. The sedative effects of opioid analgesics, such as Buprenex, often are enough to prevent self-trauma to the surgical site.

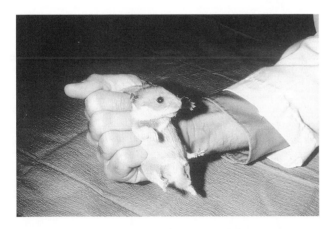

Fig. 9.8. Hamster restraint. (Photo courtesy of Dr. Sam Rivera)

Nonsteroidal anti-inflammatory drugs, like ketoprofen, may also be used in rodents. A recommended formulary is included at the end of the chapter.

BANDAGING AND WOUND CARE

Rodents easily become stressed and daily wound care may do more harm than good. Wounds should be cleaned as thoroughly as possible during the initial treatment phase. Advise the owner to increase the frequency of bedding changes to keep the healing wounds as clean as possible.

EMERGENCY AND CRITICAL CARE

Unfortunately, many of the infectious diseases can be difficult to treat; several antibiotics can cause fatal reactions in rodents. Supportive care in the form of fluid therapy, adequate dietary support, and comfort measures is vitally important. Because some of the diseases have zoonotic potential, the veterinarian may recommend the pet be euthanized.

Proliferative ileitis in hamsters may respond to improved diet, sanitation, and tetracycline (450–540 mg/L) in the drinking water, but the animal's prognosis is guarded (Plunkett 1993, 177).

Animals suffering from bite wounds or lacerations may be extremely stressed and vocalizing. Be cautious when attempting to pick up an animal in this condition, as it may respond aggressively. The patient should be kept warm and quiet until it can be sedated for wound care.

SEX DETERMINATION

Males and females can be distinguished by comparing anogenital distance, and the lack of nipples in the male. The distance from the anus to the genital papilla will be greater in the male than in the female. This can be difficult to assess if there are no other animals present for comparison purposes. In hamsters, the male will have a rounded posterior when viewed from above due to the scrotum, whereas the female's will appear more square (fig. 9.10). Male gerbils will have a larger midventral scent gland.

TECHNIQUES

Administration of Medications
Parenteral administration sites include IV, IM, and IP, SC (Lawson 2000, 18–25).

IV
Intravenous injection of drugs is difficult to accomplish in rodents. The most commonly used site for intravenous injection is the lateral tail vein in mice, rats, and gerbils.

1. Assemble supplies: 23–25 gauge needles, tuberculin syringes, and alcohol swabs.
2. Unless a restraint device is used, a second individual will need to restrain the animal.
3. Clean the venipuncture site with alcohol. Warming the tail with a focal heat light (penlight) may be useful to help visualize the vein.
4. Always gently aspirate to ensure proper placement.
5. Once the injection is completed, apply gentle pressure as the needle is removed to allow for clot formation.

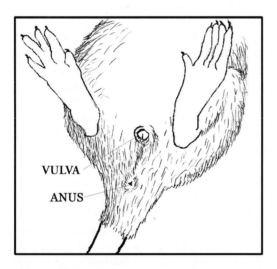

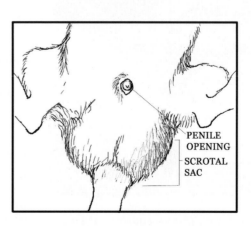

Fig. 9.10. Sex determination. A. Female.   *B. Male. (Drawing by Scott Stark)*

6. Dispose of the needle into a puncture-proof bio-hazard container.

IM

The quadriceps muscle can be used to administer injections in all four rodents discussed. Only very small amounts of drug can safely be injected into this site due to the small size of the patient (0.05 ml in mice, up to 0.3 ml in rats). Care must be taken not to inject into the posterior thigh since irritation of the sciatic nerve may result. It may help to "pinch up" the muscle mass between the fingers of one hand while injecting with the other.

1. Assemble your supplies: 23 gauge needles for mice, up to 21 gauge for larger rats, tuberculin syringes, and alcohol swabs.
2. Have an assistant restrain the animal if a commercial restraint device will not be used.
3. Always aspirate prior to administering any medication to ensure correct placement.
4. Inject drug and withdraw the needle.
5. Dispose of needle into a puncture-proof biohazard container.

IP

IP injections allow for larger volumes of drug to be injected than what can be safely given IM or IV. Care must be taken not to puncture any abdominal organs. IP injections in rats require injecting into the *left* caudal quadrant, rather than the right, as in gerbils, mice, and hamsters (fig. 9.11). The rat's cecum is located in the right caudal quadrant. Slight resistance may be felt as the needle penetrates the abdominal muscles.

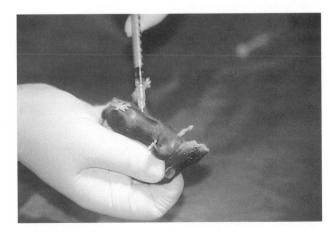

Fig. 9.11. *IP injection in a mouse. (Photo courtesy of Ryan Cheek)*

1. The following supplies should be assembled: 21 gauge needles, syringes, and alcohol swabs.
2. Restraining the animal in one hand by scruffing the loose skin over the back of the neck and shoulders is required. The little finger of the same hand can be used to keep the tail pressed against the palm of the hand.
3. The animal's head should be tilted lower than the rest of the body to cause the abdominal organs to fall forward.
4. The needle should be inserted bevel up at an angle of about 20° into the right caudal quadrant *unless* it is a rat, in which case use of the left caudal quadrant is required.
5. The syringe should be aspirated to ensure no organs have been punctured with the needle. If any yellow or greenish-brown fluid or any blood is aspirated, the needle and syringe should immediately be withdrawn and discarded. The procedure should be attempted again with a new needle and syringe.
6. The needle should be disposed of into a puncture-proof biohazard container.

SC

Larger drug volumes can also be given subcutaneously (2–3 ml in mice, up to 5–10 ml in rats). The injection can be given in the skin along the flank, or in the loose skin of the neck being scruffed for restraint purposes.

1. The following supplies should be assembled: a needle of 20 gauge or smaller, syringes.
2. The animal's loose skin over the neck should be scruffed if performing injection alone, or the loose skin along the flank tented if an assistant is restraining.
3. The needle should be inserted into the tented skin between the fingers. It is often easier to position the syringe over the animal's head and point the needle toward its hindquarters if doing this alone.
4. One should aspirate prior to injecting the medication to ensure proper placement.
5. The needle should be disposed of into a puncture-proof biohazard container.

Oral Administration

Medications mixed into food or water often affect the taste, leading to the animal's refusing to eat or drink. Liquid medications can be more accurately administered to awake animals using a gavage needle affixed to a syringe. Gavage needles have ball-like tips to prevent trauma to the animal, and may be straight, curved, or bent (depending on the operator's preference).

1. The following supplies should be gathered: a gavage needle attached to a syringe large enough to hold the entire dose of medication.
2. The top of the needle should be lined up with the animal's nose, and the ball of the needle lined up with the animal's last rib to gauge depth of insertion.
3. Wetting the ball of the needle with water may help it slide down more easily.
4. The animal should be restrained by scruffing the loose skin over the back of the neck, tucking the tail under the little finger. The animal should be held vertically with the head up.
5. The gavage needle should be inserted into the space behind the incisors, and the needle gently pushed into the animal's mouth, allowing it to follow the curve of the mouth down into the esophagus.
6. If any resistance is felt, or the animal becomes cyanotic (indicating you are probably in the trachea), immediately remove the needle and start again.
7. When inserted to the level measured in step 2, inject the contents of the syringe and withdraw the needle.

Blood Collection

In all rodents except the hamster, blood can be collected from the tail veins located on each side of the tail. It is recommended that no more than 0.14 ml of blood be collected from mice, 0.3 ml collected from a gerbil, 0.65 ml from a hamster, and 1.3 ml from a rat (Hillyer & Quesenberry 1997, 301).

1. The following supplies should be assembled: 23–25 gauge needles, tuberculin syringes or 3 cc syringe if a rat, alcohol swabs, restraint device if available (rodent restrainers that leave the tail free are commercially available).
2. Have an assistant restrain the animal if no restraint device is available.
3. Warming the tail with a warm water compress or low-wattage light may help to visualize the vein.
4. Pressure must be applied proximally to the venipuncture site, and can be accomplished using a rubber band and hemostats.
5. The needle should be inserted bevel up into the vein and gently aspirated in order to prevent collapsing the vessel.
6. After blood collection, apply pressure to the venipuncture site as the needle is withdrawn to prevent hematoma formation.

Blood can also be collected retro-orbitally by puncturing the venous sinus or plexus with a microhematocrit tube inserted in the medial canthus of the eye, a procedure requiring the animal be anesthetized (fig. 9.12). There is a risk of causing damage to the eye, and this procedure should not be performed with the owner present.

1. The following supplies should be assembled: microhematocrit tubes, gauze sponges, ophthalmic ointment.

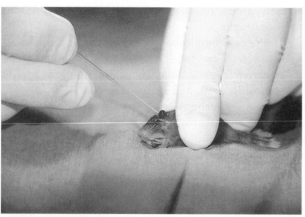

A   B

*Fig. 9.12. Blood collection from the venous sinus. **A.** Restraint of a mouse during the initial insertion of a microhematocrit tube into the medial canthus. **B.** Blood collection after successful puncture of the venous sinus with the microhematocrit tube. (Photos courtesy of Ryan Cheek)*

2. Insert the microhematocrit tube into the eye at the medial canthus, rotating the tube gently in order to puncture the sinus.
3. Blood will fill the tube by capillary action.
4. Following the collection of blood, the tube should be removed, excess blood wiped from the site and the eyelids gently held shut until hemostasis occurs.
5. Apply a sterile ophthalmic ointment into the eye (Hillyer & Quesenberry 1997, 301; Lawson 2000, 23).

While not a common venipuncture route, blood can be drawn from the anterior vena cava in rats. Anesthesia is required, however. See figure 9.13.

EUTHANASIA

As with any pet, the owner may request to be present during the euthanasia procedure. An overdose of inhalant anesthetic is effective. If the chamber is relatively large, prefill it with the anesthetic to decrease the amount of time it will take before having the desired effect. Intraperitoneal injections of barbiturate anesthetics may also be administered, with the understanding that the results will not be immediate as with IV administration. A combination of the two may be less traumatizing to the client since some rodents struggle during injections. Staff members not fond of rodents must keep in mind that pet rodent owners can be just as emotionally attached as the more familiar

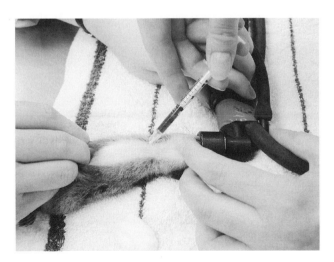

Fig. 9.13. Blood being drawn from a rat using the cranial vena cava, an uncommon route. (Photo courtesy of Dr. Stephen J. Hernandez-Divers, University of Georgia)

dog and cat owner can. Remains should be treated with the same respect afforded all deceased pets.

REFERFENCES

Harkness, JE, Wagner, JE. 1989. *The Biology and Medicine of Rabbits and Rodents*. 3d ed. Philadelphia: Lea & Febiger.

Hillyer, EV, Quesenberry, KE. 1997. *Ferrets, Rabbits, and Rodents Clinical Medicine and Surgery*. Philadelphia: W.B. Saunders Co.

Holmes, DD. 1984. *Clinical Laboratory Animal Medicine, An Introduction*. Ames: Iowa State University Press.

Lawson, PT, ed. 2000. *American Association for Laboratory Animal Science LATG and LAT Training Manuals*. Memphis, TN: AALAS.

Plunkett, SJ. 1993. *Emergency Procedures for the Small Animal Veterinarian*. Philadelphia: W.B. Saunders Co.

FORMULARY

Hawk, CT, and Leary, SL. 1999. *Formulary for Laboratory Animals*. 2d ed. Ames: Iowa State University Press.

Web Sites with helpful links:

American Association for
Laboratory Animal Science
    9190 Crestwyn Hills Dr.
    Memphis, TN 38125
    http://www.aalas.org

Net Vet
    http://netvet.wustl.edu/ssi.htm

University of Florida Animal Care Services
    http://www.health.ufl.edu/acs/index.htm

Laboratory Animals Ltd.
    http://www.lal.org.uk/laban.htm

Laboratory Animal Supply Companies
    Harvard Apparatus, Inc.
    84 October Hill Road
    Holliston, MA 01746
    http://www.harvardapparatus.com

Biomedical Research Instruments, Inc.
    12264 Wilkins Ave.
    Rockville, MD 20852
    Phone: 301-881-7911
    Phone2: 301-881-8762
    Toll Free: 800-327-9498
    E-mail: contact@biomedinstr.com
    Web: http://www.biomedinstr.com

CHAPTER TEN

The Chinchilla

Trevor Lyon

TAXONOMY/COMMON SPECIES SEEN IN PRACTICE

The chinchilla is classified as a rodent and is most closely related to the guinea pig. There are three subspecies of chinchilla with *Chinchilla langier* being the most commonly available in the pet trade. These animals inhabit the Andes Mountains of South America and are adapted well to living on cold and rocky slopes. As they are closely related to the guinea pig, similarities in their physiology, care, and treatment will be apparent.

ANATOMY AND PHYSIOLOGY

External Anatomy
There are two distinctive features in the external anatomy of the chinchilla. The first is the very dense fur that covers the entire body. It is so dense, in fact, that up to 90 individual hairs can come from each root (Hayes 2000). Second is the locomotory apparatus, which can be compared to the rabbit but is closer to that of the nutria. Chinchillas have very short front legs that are used for support and to hold food. These small legs have four digits (numbers 2, 3, 4, and 5. Digit 1 is lost). The rear legs, however, are very large and powerful. Designed for jumping, they have three digits varying in size (numbers 2, 3, 4). The first and fifth digits are rudimentary only.

Digestive Tract
The mouth is largely filled by the tongue. The two lateral areas of the tongue are wider than the dorsal side, giving it an unusual shape.

The adult chinchilla has 4 incisors and 16 molar-type teeth. The upper incisors usually have a right angle indentation, while the lowers are ground down to a point. Only about one-third of the incisors protrude from the jaw. The grinding and cutting teeth have open roots, which means that they are growing continuously. Therefore, the correct positioning of each tooth is crucial as it assures that each tooth is being constantly ground down. There may be slight differences in dentition among the different species. The most distinctive part of the mouth is the palatal ridges. Each chinchilla, no matter how closely related, has palatal ridges that distinguish it from any other chinchilla (Kraft 1987).

The stomach is located in the abdominal cavity behind the diaphragm. It is similar in shape to that of a horse or pig. The duodenum has several afferent ducts from the pancreas as well as the bile duct. The longest portion of the small intestine is the jejunum and in conjunction with sections of the large intestine, it takes up a large portion of the abdominal cavity. The ileum is the shortest section of small bowel that makes up the transition to the cecum. The cecum in chinchillas is similar to that in other rodents as it is located on the left side of the abdomen and under normal conditions, its contents are of liquid consistency. The cecum and the ascending colon help to fill the remainder of the abdomen, as it is the segment with the greatest volume. The ascending portion of the colon is also the longest section of the large bowel. The descending portion of the bowel and the rectum are usually filled with compact fecal matter and can be easily palpated if the animal is relaxed. It is difficult to determine the end of the colon and the beginning of the rectum. The end of the rectum widens slightly before reaching the anus. The posterior end of the rectum is surrounded by glandular packets; these packets in females appear to be thicker ventrally. In males, these packets are twice the circumference of the females' packets. The skeletal anatomy is shown in figure 10.1; the visceral anatomy is shown in figure 10.2.

Liver
The liver is located between the diaphragm and the stomach. There is very little lobulation visible and the

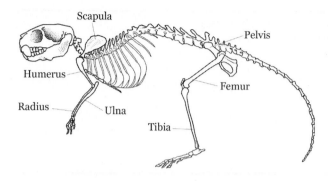

Fig. 10.1. *Skeletal anatomy. (Drawing by Scott Stark)*

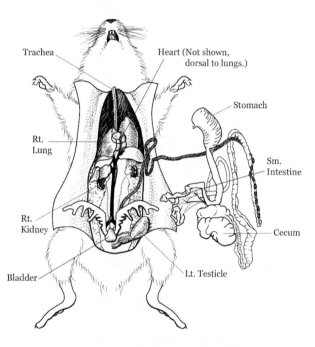

Fig. 10.2. *Visceral anatomy. (Drawing by Scott Stark)*

gallbladder is located between the right and median sides. In the adult chinchilla, the liver weighs about 8–10 grams (Kraft 1987).

Pancreas

In the chinchilla, the pancreas can be difficult to locate as it has many lobes. In addition, the surrounding fatty tissue and lymph nodes can make it difficult to distinguish with the naked eye.

Spleen

The spleen is of similar shape and location of other rodents. It is triangular in cross section and in the shape of an "L." The bottom of the "L" is located near the last rib on the left side.

Respiratory Tract

Starting with the head of the chinchilla, the first portion of the respiratory tract visualized are the nostrils. To the outside of each narrow nostril is a "false" nostril. The nasal cavities arch upward and are interconnected along the upper portion. The chinchilla's nasal cavity is very large for an animal of this size. The trachea is dorsoventrally compressed as it moves down toward the lungs. The trachea splits at the level of the fourth and fifth vertebrae, descending toward the lungs. The right lung has four distinct lobes and the left only three.

Reproductive Organs

Female sex organs (ovaries) are located just below each kidney and are very small, about the size of a grain of rice. As the female reaches maturity, small lumps appear on the ovary giving it an unusual shape. These lumps are caused by eggs migrating to the surface of the ovary. Several eggs mature at the same time, which means that several eggs can be fertilized at the same time. Unlike other mammals, as the eggs migrate down the oviduct they do not go into the ovarian pouch. They remain in the wall of the pouch where they are fertilized. After fertilization, the eggs move via peristaltic action to the uterus. The reproductive tract ends with the vagina, which becomes very visible when the animal is in heat. It is visualized as a horizontal slit between the anus and the urethra. Unlike many other mammals, the urethra of the female chinchilla terminates outside the vagina. There are no labial folds present.

The male sex organs are somewhat different from most other mammals. The testicles do not descend down into the scrotum and are considered incomplete. Only the epididymis is located outside the abdominal cavity and there is no scrotum. The sperm cells mature in the epididymis before they move to the sperm duct, and from there, they move across the mesentery of the urinary bladder. The sperm ducts open right next to each other into the urethra, along with the openings of the other sex glands. The penis is S-shaped when in the normal resting position, with the glans penis terminating below the anus. Since the foreskin extends all the way to the anus the actual opening is very narrow. A small bone about 1 cm long supports the penis during copulation. As blood fills the penis pushing the tip forward, small backward facing spines can be seen. These assure better attachment during copulation.

Urinary Tract

The chinchilla's urinary system is similar to that of other mammals, in that it has two kidneys, two ureters, a bladder, and a urethra.

Anal Sacs

Located just inside the lower corner of the anal slit is a yellow nodular anal sac. Similar to dogs and cats, the chinchilla can expel the contents of this sac. It is a foul smelling substance, which is probably used as a defense against natural enemies.

REPRODUCTION

These are average numbers for the different species of chinchillas:

First "heat": 3 to 4 months of age
Gestation period: 110 to 138 days
Number of young: 1 to 3 per pregnancy
Number of litters: 1 to 2 per year

The female will go back into heat every 25 to 35 days if she does not conceive.

The most reliable method of determining if the female is in heat is the behavior of the male (Johnson-Delaney 1996; Kraft 1987).

HUSBANDRY

Since the chinchilla's normal habitat is the Andes Mountains in South America, it does not tolerate heat or humidity. Therefore, they should not be housed in a location where there is no protection from the heat. The enclosure must have ample hiding places as chinchillas in the wild live mostly in caves. Since it is in their nature to jump, it is recommended that the enclosure have multiple levels. Small platforms on which they can perch are also helpful.

Since the teeth of the chinchilla are constantly growing, they need ample objects to gnaw on. Branches, wood blocks, pumice stones, and salt blocks are all good choices.

The most specific requirement for chinchilla care is making a "dust bath" available to them on a daily basis. This helps to keep the coat and skin healthy. There are several commercial dust baths on the market. However, you can make your own by using cornstarch or unscented talc powder mixed with sand. One can also use diatomaceous earth in place of sand. The bath mixture should be dry before allowing the chinchilla to use it. The mixture of choice should be placed about 1–2 inches deep in the bottom of a litter box, large bowl, or glass jar (one gallon or larger).

NUTRITION

Chinchillas are herbivorous and as their digestive tract is similar to that of the horse, they need large amounts of roughage. As in other rodents, chinchillas are coprophagic. In captivity a diet of hay supplemented with a good quality pelleted diet should be offered. If not enough hay is made available, the low amount of fiber may lead to enteritis. The quality of the hay must be monitored closely. Small amounts of fruits, veggies, seeds, and grains may be offered as treats. Last, as with all animals, fresh water must be made available at all times.

COMMON AND ZOONOTIC DISEASES

Dental Diseases

A common problem in chinchillas is "slobbers," or malocclusion (Hayes 2000). This can occur in the incisors, premolars, or molars. As the teeth overgrow, they cause ulcers of the buccal mucosa and the tongue. Clinical signs may be drooling, pawing at the mouth, weight loss, anorexia, and decrease in stool volume. Malocclusion can be caused by hereditary factors or a lack of objects in the environment to gnaw on. Routine teeth trimmings may be necessary in cases of hereditary problems.

Skin Diseases

Husbandry issues are the leading cause of skin disorders in chinchillas. Bite wounds, traumatic injuries, fur chewing and unthrifty coat can all occur when the environmental conditions are poor. Housed in a cage that is too small or if two incompatible animals are housed together, these disorders can appear rapidly. The animals may chew on themselves or their cage mates, which may lead to other injuries. Inadequate access to a dust bath may also cause a poor coat quality.

Dermatophytosis is a disease usually caused by the introduction of contaminated hay or bedding to the chinchilla's housing. As in other species, scaly, circular areas of hair loss around the face, feet, and ears are the most common presentation. A fungal culture should be done to confirm the diagnosis. This disease does have zoonotic potential.

Gastrointestinal Diseases

Choke
Like rabbits and rats, chinchillas cannot vomit, so esophageal choke can result if the animal ingests an object too large to swallow. The most common objects are bedding and treats. The animal usually presents with excessive salivation, dyspnea, and anorexia. The object may be palpated on physical exam or diagnosed with radiographs.

Bloat
Bloat can occur for many reasons as in other species. The chinchilla will present similarly to other animals with a distended and painful abdomen, dyspnea, and reluctance to move. There are many treatments recommended, from exercise in mild cases to decompression by transabdominal trocar.

Hairballs
Hairballs are as common a problem in chinchillas as they are in rabbits. They are usually caused by excessive fur chewing in combination with low dietary fiber. The animal usually presents with lethargy, reluctance to move, and anorexia. The hairball may be palpated on physical exam or diagnosed with contrast radiographs. Treatment protocol are similar to that for rabbits, fluid therapy, feline laxatives, increased dietary fiber, and proteolytic enzymes (pineapple juice) (Hayes 2000). If the animal is anorectic, then force-feeding may also be necessary.

Enteritis
Proper diet for chinchillas is one of the most important factors when discussing their care. An improper diet can be one of the most likely causes of enteritis, although a sudden diet change may also be a factor (Hayes 2000; Kraft 1987; Ritchey et al. 1994). If the animal is not offered hay, the hay is of poor quality, or it is eating a large amount of pellets or fruit and green vegetables, this may cause a change in the normal flora and fauna of the gastrointestinal tract. The motility of the gut and the fermentation process may also be altered, leading to an overgrowth of pathogenic bacteria. Other less-common causes of enteritis are parasitic infection and prolonged or inappropriate use of antibiotics (Hayes 2000; Lightfoot 1999). Animals may present with anorexia and bloating. Those who have had chronic enteritis may present with constipation, impactions, intussusceptions, and rectal prolapse.

Determining the cause may be difficult because of the multiple factors involved. Radiographs, fecal floatation for parasites, and fecal cultures may be needed to determine an etiology. Symptomatic treatment is usually best with fluid therapy, antibiotics, and antiparasitics given as indicated.

Constipation
As mentioned before, improper diet is one of the most common problems associated with caring for a chinchilla. In most cases owners feed a diet of pellets almost exclusively, which can lead to many of the problems mentioned before. The pelleted diets are high in protein as well as calories, but are low in fiber. This low-fiber diet can also lead to constipation, which may be seen more often than diarrhea (Hayes 2000; Kraft 1987; Johnson-Delaney 1996). Clinical signs are straining to defecate and fecal pellets that may be small, hard, and in some cases, bloodstained. Treatment involves slowly increasing the amount of fiber in the chinchilla's diet by feeding a small amount of fresh vegetables or good quality hay.

Respiratory Diseases
Chinchillas are susceptible to pneumonia, however these cases usually occur when there are large numbers of animals housed together and the husbandry is poor (Kraft 1987). Most pet owners should not have any problems in this area. Clinical signs would be depression, dyspnea, and a nasal discharge. The treatment protocol includes antibiotics administered by nebulization if conditions allow.

Neurologic Diseases
Chinchillas are highly susceptible to *Listeria monocytogenes* infection, however it is unlikely that pet chinchillas would be exposed (Hayes 2000). Ataxia and circling are usually followed by convulsions and death. Treatment protocols have been ineffective once clinical signs are noticed.

Pet chinchillas may be exposed to *Baylisascaris procyonis* in contaminated hay (Ness 1999). This nematode infects the cerebrospinal fluid causing ataxia, torticollis, and paralysis. There is no treatment for this condition and there is zoonotic potential for anyone handling the contaminated bedding and feed.

BEHAVIOR

Chinchillas are usually nocturnal, but may be active during daylight hours. They have become popular as pets because of their curious personality, gentle nature, and the fact that they rarely bite.

TAKING THE HISTORY AND PERFORMING THE PHYSICAL EXAM

An accurate history is vital when working with chinchillas, as husbandry is often the most significant factor. These animals can be difficult to handle, as they are very quick and agile, and in most cases do not want to be touched. A good preliminary exam should be done prior to actually handling the animal. If the owner has brought the pet in a wire cage, a visual exam may be performed. If not, then placing the chinchilla on the floor of the exam room and allowing it to move around normally is the best option. One should be sure that all doors are closed, as they are very curious about their surroundings. A healthy chinchilla should be alert with bright eyes and a twitching nose. It may be breathing rapidly, but should not be open-mouth breathing. The tail should be erect and its hair-coat should be thick, soft, and smooth.

HANDLING AND RESTRAINT

Chinchillas can be very difficult to restrain and should be handled with care. Because they are very excitable and nervous, handling a sick or debilitated patient can pose a challenge. The base of the tail and hind legs should be held gently with one hand while the other hand supports the chest and shoulders (fig. 10.3). Some patients may be easier to handle if allowed to hide their face in the bend of the handler's elbow. Making the patient feel secure is of the utmost importance, if not they may attempt to jump from the handler's grasp. If this is the case, sitting on the floor while completing the exam may be necessary. This allows for better support and if they do get away, they will not fall and sustain a traumatic injury. If they are frightened while being restrained, they may release a large portion of fur in areas where they are being held. This is called a "fur-slip" (Lightfoot 1999). As you do not want to have a hairless patient leave your facility, great care should be taken while handling them.

Once the patient is comfortably restrained, the examination can begin. The average weight of a chin-

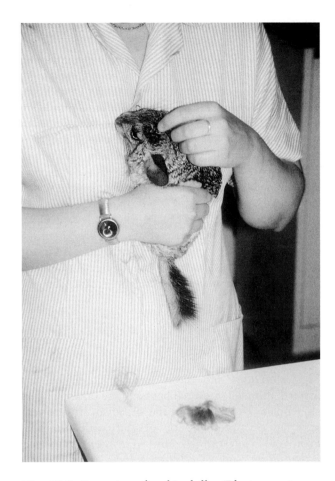

Fig. 10.3. *Restraint of a chinchilla. (Photo courtesy of Dr. Stephen J. Hernandez-Divers, University of Georgia)*

chilla is 400–600 grams with the male usually being smaller than the female (Johnson-Delaney 1996; Lightfoot 1999). The temperature can be taken rectally, although they may object to this procedure. The normal temperature is 97–102°F (Johnson-Delaney 1996; Lightfoot 1999). Heart rate and respiratory rate can be obtained by normal means. The normal HR is 200–350 beats/min and normal RR is 40–80 breaths/min (Johnson–Delaney 1996; Lightfoot 1999).

RADIOLOGY

If the circumstances allow, radiographs will be most easily obtained if the animal is anesthetized, as the chinchilla may be difficult to restrain. The most noticeable difference on a radiograph is the very small thorax in comparison to the abdomen.

ANESTHESIA AND SURGERY

There are very few surgical procedures performed commonly on chinchillas. However, on occasion there may be need to neuter a male chinchilla in order to allow it to be housed with others. With this procedure and some of the others listed above, isoflurane or sevoflurane gas is the preferred anesthetic agent. A face mask or induction chamber should be used to administer the anesthetic gas. Intubation is not recommended as blind intubations can cause trauma, which can lead to epiglottal edema and dyspnea.

Injectable anesthetics can be used such as acepromazine, butorphanol tartrate and ketamine hydrochloride in combination with diazepam or xylazine. However, gas is highly preferred for surgical procedures, venipuncture, radiographs, and catheter placement.

PARASITOLOGY

Fecal flotations and direct smears should be performed although intestinal parasites are uncommon in chinchillas. Depending on the organism, the patient may be asymptomatic or present with diarrhea. Protozoal infestations by *Trichamonas* spp., *Balantidium* spp., *Cryptosporidium*, and *Eimeria chinchillae* may occur. The latter being the chinchilla coccidian that has been shown to be transmissible to other rodents. Nematode infestations by *Physoloptera* and *Haemonchus contortous* have been reported. Since it is also possible for chinchillas to have flea infestations, they may also have tapeworms, usually *Hymeolepsis nana* (Ness 1999). One unusual aspect of the life cycle is that the same animal can be the intermediate and permanent host.

URINALYSIS

Normal urine values are listed here:

Color: Yellow to slightly red
Turbidity: Most often cloudy
pH: 8.5
Protein: Negative to trace
Glucose: Negative
Ketones: Negative
Bilirubin: Negative
Urobilinogen: 0.1–1.0 ng/dl
Nitrates: Negative
Blood: Negative
Specific gravity: Usually >1.045

During a urine sediment examination of a normal chinchilla, some calcium carbonate crystals may be found along with amorphous debris. Casts, bacteria, erythrocytes, and leukocytes are rare in a normal patient, but occasional squamous epithelial cells are common (Ness 1999).

EMERGENCY AND CRITICAL CARE

In the diseases and ailments discussed previously, most are not considered emergencies. However, in the case of an emergency with a chinchilla, protocols similar to those of other small mammals should be followed. For example, an IV catheter can be very helpful in an emergency as well as in a critically ill patient. Once the patient has been stabilized, a calm and quiet environment is also very important for the recovery process.

SEX DETERMINATION

Determining the sex of a chinchilla can be very difficult, especially in young animals. One can visualize the testicles in adult males but the lack of a scrotum can make this more of a challenge. The fact that the clitoris, because of its size and shape, can often be mistaken for a penis provides another obstacle when sexing chinchillas. The location of the penis versus the clitoris can often be the determining factor as the distance from the rectum to the penis is greater than that of the clitoris.

TECHNIQUES

Venipuncture

For a procedure of this nature, the preferred method is to have a chinchilla anesthetized. There are several sites for venipuncture, with the jugular vein being the most common site. Accessing the jugular vein allows larger blood volumes to be obtained. There are six other sites for venipuncture: the cephalic, saphenous, femoral, dorsalis penis, lateral abdominal, and tail vein (fig. 10.4).

The process for collecting blood from the jugular is as follows (Ness 1999):

1. Place the patient in sternal recumbency.
2. The head and neck are extended to make the lateral aspect of the lower cervical region accessible.
3. Apply gentle pressure to one side of the thoracic inlet to occlude the vessel.

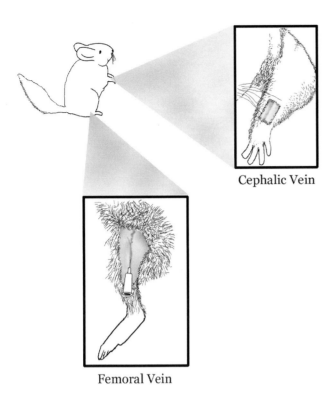

Cephalic Vein

Femoral Vein

Fig. 10.4. Venipuncture sites. (Drawing by Scott Stark)

4. Wet the area with an alcohol swab and visualize the distended vein.
5. Using a 23–25 gauge needle attached to a 1–3 ml syringe, insert the needle into the vein at approximately a 45° angle.
6. Draw back slowly if using a 3 ml syringe so as not to collapse the vein.

A 25–27 gauge needle on a 0.5–1.0 ml syringe should be used to collect samples from the other sites mentioned above. The femoral and cephalic veins are the most commonly used of those mentioned.

Intravenous Catheter Placement

The cephalic vein is the most common site used for catheter placement. The procedures are the same as in any other small animal. See chapter 7 in the technique section for ferrets. Note that a small cutdown may not be necessary.

Intraosseous Catheter Placement

While in most cases the chinchilla's peripheral veins are readily accessible, in an emergency it may be necessary to place an intraosseous catheter. In critical patients, sedation or anesthesia is not usually required

for this procedure. The steps for placement are as follows:

1. Locate the site for placement of the catheter. The two sites used in chinchillas are the femur or tibia. The femur is preferred due to its size and location, so this one will be discussed.
2. Locate a syringe needle or catheter stylet of the largest bore possible for the patient (usually a 22 gauge is of sufficient size). A spinal needle may also be used. A syringe of heparinized flush will also be needed.
3. Clip and surgically prep the site.
4. Once the site has been prepped, the greater trochanter should be palpated and stabilized for insertion of the needle. The needle is then inserted and with a gentle twisting motion, advanced slowly. The needle should continue to be advanced through the bone and into the marrow cavity. Aspiration with the flush syringe until blood is visualized in the hub should be performed. It should be flushed quickly as the marrow can clot the needle.
5. The needle should be secured with tape and in some cases, it may need to be sutured in place to provide more stability.
6. This catheter may be used for up to 72 hours, after which a replacement in another location will be required.

Once the catheter is in place, great care must be taken to maintain it. Its location may inhibit normal movement and cause some discomfort. This in turn may cause the patient to attempt to remove the catheter by chewing or rubbing.

Administration of Medication

In the event that medications need to be given, there are several routes of administration. As with many other exotics, one must make sure to downsize the equipment and the volume of medications used.

Per Os: Usually medication will be liquid and can be given by needle-less syringe in the side of the mouth just behind the incisors.
Subcutaneous: 23–25 gauge needle under the skin in the flank or neck area.
Intravenous: 25–28 gauge needle, preferably an insulin syringe in the lateral saphenous or cephalic.
Intramuscular: 23–25 gauge needle with no more than 0.3 ml per site. Recommended sites include the semimembranosus, quadriceps, and semitendinosus muscles (Ness 1999).

EUTHANASIA

As with most other small animals, the preferred method of euthanasia is lethal injection. If an IV catheter has been placed in the cephalic vein, it can be used for administration of the euthanasia solution. If a catheter is not available, either an IV or intracardiac injection with a syringe can be used.

REFERENCES

Hayes, PM. 2000. *Diseases of Chinchillas*. Philadelphia: W.B. Saunders Company.,

Johnson-Delaney, CA. 1996 *Exotic Companion Medicine Handbook for Veterinarians*. Lake Worth: Wingers Publications.

Kraft, H. 1987 *Diseases of Chinchillas*. Neptune City: T.F.H. Publications.

Lightfoot, TL. 1999. Clinical Examination of Chinchillas, Hedgehogs, Prairie Dogs, and Sugar Gliders. *Veterinary Clinics of North America: Exotic Animal Practice* 2(2): 447–54.

Ness, RD. 1999. Clinical Pathology and Sample Collection of Exotic Small Animals. *Veterinary Clinics of North America: Exotic Animal Practice* 2(3): 591–619.

Ritchey, L, Cogswell, EL, Cogswell, M. 1994. *Joy of Chinchillas*.

CHAPTER ELEVEN

The Guinea Pig

Anne Hudson

COMMON TYPES

The domestic guinea pig *Cavia porcellus*, also referred to as a cavy, has been raised as a meat animal in South America. Guinea pigs are considered rodents despite several differences between guinea pigs and other common pet rodent species. They are grouped as hystricomorphic rodents along with porcupines and chinchillas. Male guinea pigs are called boars, and females are called sows. Most commonly seen in companion animal practice are the American or English variety, the Abyssinian, and the Peruvian. English cavies have short, smooth hair coats. Abyssinians have a rougher coat that looks swirled. The hair is described as growing in rosettes. Peruvian guinea pigs have long hair coats that require grooming to maintain good condition. Guinea pigs are available in a wide variety of colors and combinations of colors.

BEHAVIOR

Guinea pigs are docile animals that rarely bite. They are sociable and will share housing with another if introduced at an early age, however crowded animals or breeding animals may fight. Cages with tops are not needed if the sides are 8–10 inches high since jumping seldom occurs.

A wide variety of vocalization patterns have been demonstrated, and cavies will vocalize in response to hearing their food being prepared, lights being turned on, and so forth.

They are neophobic animals, mistrusting any new foods or changes in their normal routine. For this reason it is important to gently handle young animals on a regular basis, and to expose them to a variety of certain foods. Trying to change feed types for a mature animal will be nearly impossible. When frightened, guinea pigs may "stampede" in an effort to escape, bolting around the cage. Another typical response is to suddenly freeze and remain immobile for a brief period of time.

ANATOMY AND PHYSIOLOGY

Guinea pigs have short, stocky, tailless bodies with one pair of inguinal teats. The legs are short with the front feet having four toes and the rear feet having three toes. Like all rodents, they have open rooted incisors. Guinea pigs also possess open-rooted premolars and molars, and malocclusions seem to occur more frequently with these teeth than the incisors. The dental formula is 2(I—1/1, C—0/0, P—1/1, M—3/3) (Harkness & Wagner 1989, 21).

The soft palate is continuous with the tongue forming a membranous covering of the posterior pharynx. Food, water, and air pass through an opening called the palatal ostium. The cecum in the guinea pig is very large, occupying a large portion of the abdominal cavity.

Male guinea pigs have open inguinal canals allowing them to retract their testicles into the abdominal cavity, and an os-penis. Females possess two uterine horns and a single cervix. A thin membrane covers the vagina except for during estrus and parturition. The symphysis pubis of the guinea pig is fibrocartilaginous and is capable of separating during parturition. Failing to breed a female prior to 6 months of age may lead to dystocia as the symphysis will be less able to separate. Physiological data are contained in table 11.1.

BIOLOGIC AND REPRODUCTIVE DATA

Guinea pigs reach breeding age at approximately 3 months of age. Females housed with other females will mount each other if in heat. It is possible to keep breeding pairs together long term; breeding may take place during the postpartum estrus. Evidence of breeding is

Table 11.1. Physiological Data for the Guinea Pig

Physiological data	Range
Lifespan	5–7 years
Average adult weight (M/F)	900–1,200g/ 700–900g
Puberty	45–70 days
Breeding age	3–4 months
Estrous cycle length	15–17 days
Gestation period	63–68 days
Litter size	2–5 pups
Weaning age	21 days
Respiratory rate per minute	70–130
Heart rate	230–300
Rectal temperature °F	99.0–103.1

Source: Harkness & Wagner (1989), 21; Hillyer & Quesenberry (1997), 248.

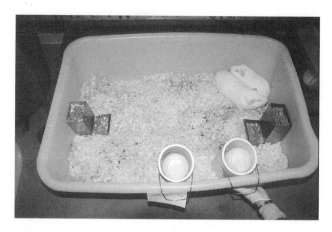

Fig. 11.1. An appropriate housing setup for guinea pigs. (Photo courtesy of Ryan Cheek)

finding a copulatory plug in the bedding of the cage. This plug is an accumulation of secretions that will fall from the vagina shortly after breeding takes place.

Sows do not build nests like other rodents, and young are born precocious. Litters of two to five pups are typical, although larger litters are possible (Hillyer & Quesenberry 1997, 248). Pups are born fully furred, with eyes open, all teeth erupted, and able to walk. Within a few hours, pups will be able to begin eating from a bowl.

HUSBANDRY

Guinea pigs can be messy, often tipping over food crocks and scattering food throughout the cage. They defecate throughout the cage as well. Water should be provided in a bottle with a sipper tube. Fresh water may need to be provided more frequently than for other rodents due to the guinea spitting food particles into the bottle, and their tendency to play with the sipper tube. Bedding changes and cleaning of the cage surfaces will need to be done more frequently as well.

Cages do not need lids if the sides are tall, unless the owner has a dog or cat; a secure lid would then be a requirement. Solid flooring is preferable to wire mesh in order to prevent trauma to the feet. Wire cages with deep solid bottoms are nice since the tray will contain scattered bedding material, and the open sides allow the guinea pig to see out and observe what is going on around it. Nonaromatic wood shavings or shredded paper can be used as bedding material.

Guinea pigs are comfortable at a normal room temperature of about 70°F. Good ventilation is essential to

help prevent respiratory diseases. Owners should be cautioned to keep cages away from drafty areas, windows, and home heating sources (fig. 11.1).

Abyssinian and Peruvian guinea pigs will benefit from gentle grooming. Fecal pellets may become stuck in the longer fur of these animals. If needed, they can be bathed with a mild shampoo as long as they are dried carefully and not subjected to chilling.

NUTRITION

A variety of food items including some fresh vegetable material needs to be offered from an early age to prevent rigid food preferences from forming. Fresh hay, apple, oranges, spinach, kale, broccoli, or other dark, leafy green vegetables should be provided daily, removing uneaten matter to prevent spoilage. Vegetables should be washed thoroughly prior to feeding to remove any pesticide residue.

Like primates, guinea pigs cannot synthesize vitamin C and must be supplemented with this nutrient. A reputable brand of pelleted food specifically formulated for guinea pigs should be used. Pellets should be utilized within 90 days of manufacture or the vitamin C content will begin to break down. Pellets will also help wear down the teeth through chewing activity.

Supplementation of vitamin C in the water ration will ensure the animal receives adequate amounts. One gram of vitamin C per liter of water mixed fresh daily is recommended. Pregnant animals will have a higher (30 mg/kg/day) vitamin C requirement than nonbreeding adults (5 mg/kg/day) (Harkness & Wagner 1989, 24).

COMMON AND ZOONOTIC DISEASES

Stress is a major factor in developing illness. Poor diet or sudden dietary changes, overcrowding, and failure to maintain clean caging will all result in stress.

Failure to receive adequate vitamin C supplementation may result in the development of scurvy. Guinea pigs with scurvy are lethargic, anorexic, and may actually bite due to painful joints. Diarrhea and weight loss may also be evident. Supplementation with appropriate amounts of ascorbic acid (10 mg/kg body weight) (Plunkett 1993, 175) coupled with good supportive care usually result in a rapid recovery.

Common respiratory diseases seen in guinea pigs include those caused by *Bordetella bronchiseptica*, and *Streptococcus pneumoniae*. Transmission is via aerosolization, fomites, direct contact with another sick guinea pig, or in the case of *Bordetella*, any animal capable of carrying the bacteria: dogs, cats, rabbits, and nonhuman primates. Signs of respiratory disease include anorexia, ocular-nasal discharge, dyspnea, and death. Treatment with antibiotics and increased vitamin C, as well as supportive care, is needed. The animal may also require force-feeding.

Guinea pigs may contract salmonellosis and clostridial infections through fecal contamination of food. Signs include rough hair coat, weight loss, and diarrhea. Again, treatment involves antibiotics and supportive care.

Swellings on the neck are usually due to inflamed or abscessed lymph nodes caused by *Streptobacillus* spp. or *Streptococcus* spp. infection. Cervical lymphadenitis, or "lumps" as it is commonly called, may result from a bite wound, abrasion from bedding or caging equipment, or trauma from malocclusion. Abscesses are usually drained and flushed, followed by systemic antibiotic therapy. Contact with the drainage will infect any other guinea pigs housed with the affected animal so isolation is necessary until wound healing has occurred.

Pododermatitis is often associated with animals housed on wire flooring. The surfaces of the feet become irritated, thickened, and ulcerated. A secondary staphylococcal infection may ensue. The animal will vocalize and be unwilling to move due to pain.

Antibiotic therapy in guinea pigs must be undertaken with great care, as many of the antibiotics effective against gram-positive organisms, such as penicillin, can lead to enterotoxemia.

The significant reproductive problems in guinea pigs are dystocia, common if females are not bred prior to reaching 6 months of age, and pregnancy ketosis. Obesity also puts the female at risk for problems during parturition. Straining, abnormal vaginal discharge, depression, and/or failure to produce a pup within 30 minutes after onset of contractions are all indications of dystocia (Hillyer & Quesenberry 1997, 265). Cesarean sections are often necessary. Ketosis is most commonly associated with obesity and stress. Rapid onset of signs including anorexia, dyspnea, convulsions, and death may occur. The problem is easier to prevent through proper diet and husbandry than to treat.

Zoonotic diseases include salmonellosis, sarcoptic mange, ringworm, and lymphocytic choriomeningitis.

HISTORY AND PHYSICAL EXAM

Questions to ask when interviewing a client are the basic signalment questions asked with all species:

- the chief complaint
- where they obtained the pet and how long they have owned it
- their past experience, if any, in keeping guinea pigs

Ideally, the pet is brought into the clinic in the cage it is normally housed in, allowing staff to see what type of bedding and equipment the patient is exposed to. When scheduling appointments, advise the owner not to clean the cage prior to the appointment.

Information as to appetite, type of diet, fecal pellet production and quality, and overall attitude should be obtained. Observe the animal in its cage; healthy guinea pigs are active and vocal. The patient should be weighed on a gram scale, and while gently restraining the guinea pig, a rectal temperature can be obtained with a standard rectal thermometer. The technician will need to restrain the guinea pig in order for the veterinarian to examine the mouth and teeth, and should be prepared for the patient to squirm and vocalize its objection to the exam.

RESTRAINT

Guinea pigs respond well to gentle restraint; inappropriate handling can cause damage to the internal organs. Always use two hands to restrain a guinea pig (fig. 11.2).

1. Gently place one hand under the thorax of the guinea pig, just caudal to the front limbs.
2. Support the hindquarters of the patient with the other hand.

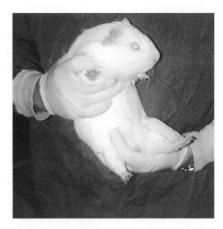

Fig. 11.2. Proper guinea pig restraint. (Photo courtesy of Ryan Cheek)

3. The guinea pig may also have the dorsal thorax supported in one hand in a cradling fashion while supporting the hind limbs with the other hand. This placement may be more comfortable for pregnant animals by avoiding any pressure on the abdomen.

Restraint for jugular venipuncture is similar to that used on cats in that the animal's forelegs are extended over the edge of a table while the head is gently extended up. Stop the procedure immediately if the animal becomes stressed (Hillyer & Quesenberry 1997, 256).

RADIOLOGY

Whole body studies are common in guinea pigs, and may require anesthesia to prevent movement during exposure. Exposure times of $\frac{1}{60}$ of a second or less will be necessary. Masking tape can be used to secure the sedated animal in position. For ease in tabletop technique, taping the animal to a small sheet of Plexiglas rather than directly to the cassette prevents having to retape the patient each time cassettes are changed (Imaging Resources 1995, 42). The general references listed at the end of this chapter have excellent recommendations for radiology techniques.

SURGERY AND ANESTHESIA

Guinea pigs should be fasted for 2–4 hours prior to surgical procedures. Induction with isoflurane gas via face mask is recommended, and the animal can be maintained on gas administered by face mask and a nonrebreathing circuit (Hillyer & Quesenberry 1997, 283).

Depth of anesthesia in most rodents can be evaluated partially by pinching of toes or gently pinching the ear for reaction to pain, however, there has been concern that pedal reflexes may not be reliable depth indicators in guinea pigs and may actually indicate the animal is too deeply anesthetized (Plunkett 1993, 173).

Doppler monitors and pulse oximeters are helpful in monitoring the patient in addition to watching the chest wall for movement related to respiration.

Take care to keep the animal warm perioperatively, and turn the animal from side to side every 15–30 minutes to prevent fluids from pooling on the dependent side. Once fully recovered, ensure the client keeps the cage and bedding fresh and clean to prevent any surgical wound contamination.

PARASITOLOGY

Guinea pigs may be parasitized without showing any clinical signs, however infection from *Cryptosporidium wrairi* may result in diarrhea, weight loss, and death (Hillyer & Quesenberry 1997, 262). Animals tend to recover on their own after a period of weeks. There is a zoonotic risk from this parasite so owners should be cautioned.

Fleas, mites, and lice are ectoparasites that can infest guinea pigs, causing intense itching, alopecia, and excoriation of the skin. Humans may be affected by the sarcoptic mange mite. The veterinarian may prescribe ivermectin or topical pyrethrin products safe for use in cats (fig. 11.3).

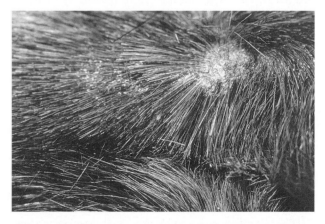

Fig. 11.3. A guinea pig with mange. (Photo courtesy of Dr. Chris King)

URINALYSIS

Because of the potential of urinary calculi and cystitis in the guinea pig, the veterinarian may request a urine sample be obtained by cystocentesis in order to perform a urinalysis. The technique is like that used in other small animals, except a 25 gauge needle should be used and anesthesia may be required (Hillyer & Quesenberry 1997, 256).

EMERGENCY AND CRITICAL CARE

Pregnancy toxemia may occur in later days of gestation and does not respond well to treatment. The condition is usually fatal (Plunkett 1993, 173).

Dystocia is an emergency that usually requires an immediate cesarean section. If the animal had several successful litters previously, demonstrating the pelvic canal is capable of separating, the veterinarian may try oxytocin prior to surgery (Plunkett 1993, 173).

SEX DETERMINATION

Anogenital distance is not a reliable method for sexing animals. To sex a guinea pig, gently restrain the animal and examine the external genitalia. In the female, the genital area will have a "Y" shape. The male will appear to have more of a straight slit. Applying gentle pressure caudally and cranially to the genitals will cause the penis of the male animal to extrude.

TECHNIQUES

Techniques for administration of medication, venipuncture, catheter placement, bandaging, and wound care are discussed in this section (Lawson 2000, 16–22).

Administration of Medication

Subcutaneous, intramuscular, or intraperitoneal administration of drugs is often used due to the difficulty of administering drugs intravenously. Many drugs given intramuscularly may lead to irritation of the tissue surrounding the injection site (Hillyer & Quesenberry 1997, 386). Exercise caution when administering IP injections to avoid damaging internal organs.

SQ

Subcutaneous injection of medications allows for slightly larger volumes (5–10 mls) to be administered than with IM administration. Fluid therapy may also be administered via the subcutaneous route. Most guinea pigs will rest on the exam table and can be restrained by cupping your hands around them. A towel placed on the table gives the animal some traction.

1. Use a 20 gauge or smaller needle.
2. Tent the skin away from the underlying muscles over the scruff of the neck.
3. Insert the needle into the tented area at a slight angle, being careful not to pass all the way through the skin.
4. Administer the medication.
5. A butterfly catheter may be easier to use if the animal is very active.
6. Dispose of the needle into a puncture-proof biohazard container.

IM

Intramuscular injections are usually given in the large muscles of the hind limbs, such as the gluteal muscles. To avoid tissue damage, use needles of less than 21 gauge, and do not inject volumes of greater than 0.3 ml into any one site.

1. Place a towel on the table and gently restrain the animal or restrain it with your hands, being sure to support the hind end.
2. It may be helpful to "pinch" the muscle tissue with one hand while administering the injection with the other hand.
3. Aspirate the syringe prior to injection to avoid injecting into a blood vessel.
4. Administer the medication.
5. Dispose of the needle in a puncture-proof biohazard container.

IP

1. Place the guinea pig gently onto its back, supporting the animal in one hand.
2. Tilt the animal's head down and insert the needle at an approximate 45° angle into the lower right quadrant of the abdomen.
3. Aspirate prior to injection to ensure you are not in the bladder or digestive tract. If any blood or fluid enters the syringe, withdraw and discard the syringe before starting over.

4. Administer the medication.
5. Dispose of the needle in a puncture-proof biohazard container.

IV

Intravenous injection is difficult; the saphenous vein is the easiest to use.

1. Use a needle size of 23 gauge or smaller.
2. Shave the area and clean with alcohol or other antiseptic solution.
3. Applying a low-watt lightbulb (such as a pen light) or a warm-water compress to the area prior to the procedure may help to distend the vein slightly.
4. Apply pressure proximal to the injection site to distend the vein.
5. Aspirate prior to injection to ensure proper placement.
6. Inject medications slowly after releasing proximally applied pressure.
7. Apply direct pressure to venipuncture site as the needle is withdrawn to prevent formation of a hematoma.
8. Dispose of the needle in a puncture-proof biohazard container.

Venipuncture

Small quantities of blood can be taken from the ear veins or saphenous veins (fig. 11.4). Larger amounts of blood can be obtained using jugular venipuncture, extending the guinea pig's forelegs over the edge of an exam table as you would a cat. Jugular venipuncture can be stressful and should not be performed on very ill animals. The amount of blood that can safely be collected from guinea pigs is approximately 0.5–0.7 mL/100 grams body weight (Hillyer & Quesenberry 1997, 255–256).

1. Use a 23 gauge or smaller needle attached to a tuberculin syringe, or a 3 mL syringe if performing jugular venipuncture.
2. Shave the proposed venipuncture site and prep with alcohol to make it easier to visualize the vein.
3. Applying a low-watt lightbulb (such as a pen light) or a warm-water compress to the area prior to the procedure may help to distend the vein slightly.
4. Apply pressure as described above for IV administration of medications, however maintain pressure to keep the vessel distended.

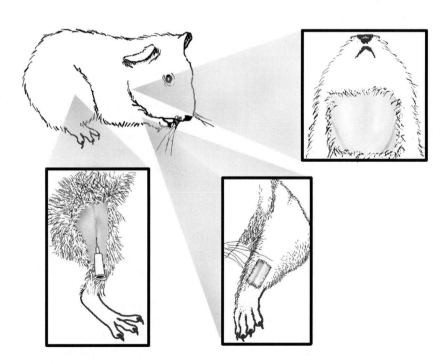

Fig. 11.4. Venipuncture sites on a guinea pig. (Drawing by Scott Stark)

5. After collecting the sample, withdraw the needle as you apply pressure to the venipuncture site.
6. Dispose of the needle in a puncture-proof biohazard container.

Catheter Placement

Intravenous catheterization in guinea pigs is difficult, and is more commonly performed in a research setting. Indwelling catheters meant for long-term use may need to be surgically placed under anesthesia. Catheter supplies are available from Harvard Apparatus. Intraosseous administration of medications can be performed and the technique would be the same as for a chinchilla (see chapter 10).

Bandaging and Wound Care

Minor wounds are best cleaned as thoroughly as possible during initial treatment to avoid repetitively stressing the animal. The risk of wound infection will be decreased if the patient's caging receives regular bedding changes. External sutures and bandages are not usually well tolerated; subcuticular sutures and surgical glue are better alternatives (Hillyer 1997).

1. Keep the animal as comfortable as possible.
2. Gently clip hair from around the wound and clean with an antiseptic solution.
3. The wound can be temporarily covered with a sterile dressing until surgically closed.

More serious wounds and fractures can be quite difficult to manage.

EUTHANASIA

Guinea pigs can be euthanized using an overdose of barbiturate anesthesia administered intraperitoneally as described above.

REFERENCES

Harkness, JE, Wagner, JE. 1989. *The Biology and Medicine of Rabbits and Rodents*. 3d ed. Philadelphia: Lea & Febiger.

Hillyer, EV, Quesenberry, KE. 1997. *Ferrets, Rabbits, and Rodents: Clinical Medicine and Surgery*. Philadelphia: W.B. Saunders Co.

Holmes, DD. 1984. *Clinical Laboratory Animal Medicine*. Ames: Iowa State University Press.

Imaging Resources, Inc. 1995. *An Overview of Small Animal Radiology*. 3d ed. Corvallis State: Imaging Resources.

Lawson, PT, ed. 2000. *American Association for Laboratory Animal Science; LAT and LATG Training Manuals*. Memphis: AALAS.

Plunkett, SJ. 1993. *Emergency Procedures for the Small Animal Veterinarian*. Philadelphia: W.B. Saunders Co.

CHAPTER TWELVE

The Hedgehog

Michael Duffy Jones

TAXOMONY, ANATOMY, AND PHYSIOLOGY

Hedgehogs belong to the order of Insectivora, which includes the most primitive of all living placental mammals today (Storer 1994, 14). There are many different species of hedgehogs, including the European, African, Pruner's, Algerian, long-eared or Egyptian, and Ethiopian or desert hedgehog. There are slight differences between these species, including ear size and times of hibernation. For the most part, the various species can be treated medically in a similar way. The Egyptian hedgehog is noted for its surly disposition (Lightfoot 1997, 100). African hedgehogs are slightly different from their European cousins in the fact that they do not hibernate (Storer 1994, 21).

Their brains are small and primitive and are smooth, not fissured. The sensory parts of the brain, including the olfactory and tactile areas, are very well developed. They have vibrissae, which are long stiff hairs around the mouth and nostrils used for their sense of touch (Storer 1994, 14).

Most species of hedgehogs have five toes on each foot, except for the four-toed hedgehog, which only has four toes on the back feet (Storer 1994, 43). They have very strong legs used for digging, and have a nonexistent tail.

The urogenital opening of females is not connected to the anus but is directly anterior (toward the animal's head). The male's penis is more anterior than the female's genitalia (Storer 1994, 43) (fig. 12.1).

Dentition in these animals is unique because they

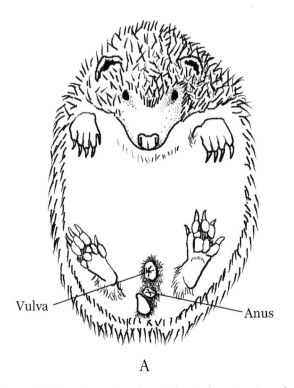
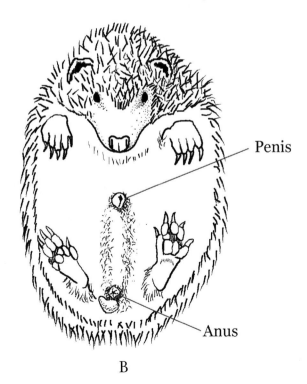

Fig. 12.1. Sex determination in hedgehog. A. Female. B. Male (Drawing by Scott Stark)

are insectivores (fig. 12.2). The top row of teeth includes 3 incisors, 1 canine, 3 premolars, and 3 molars on each side, and the bottom consists of 2 incisors, 1 canine, 2 premolars, and 3 molars for a total of 36 (Storer 1994, 43). The incisors are sharp, while the canines are small and the molars and premolars are broad and flat for grinding. The first set of incisors has a large gap for appending and killing insects. Their teeth are very small and sharp. The baby teeth erupt at about 23 days and permanent teeth erupt at 7 to 9 weeks (Storer 1994, 44). Skeletal anatomy is shown in figure 12.3.

Their senses, including smelling and hearing, are very developed. Their eyesight is of moderate ability with limited color vision. They are highly resistant to many toxins (Storer 1994, 45).

Their face, underbody, and legs are covered with cream to brown colored soft hairs. The rest of the body is covered with quills (also called spines). Each

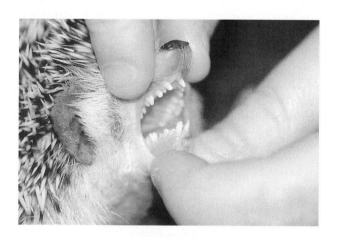

Fig. 12.2. Dentition. (Photo courtesy of Ryan Cheek)

quill is connected to a small muscle, which can help pull the quill erect. When the animal is frightened, the quills are erect and crossed, making a very formidable barrier (Storer 1994, 45).

Hedgehogs are mostly terrestrial. They tend to walk slowly looking for food, but can scurry at about 6 feet per second (four miles per hour). They can also use their spines as a cushion for rolling or dropping from high places (Storer 1994, 47).

BIOLOGIC AND REPRODUCTIVE DATA

Table 12.1 includes biological and reproductive information. Clinical pathology data are also included.

BEHAVIOR

Hedgehogs are usually solitary animals and they can be aggressive when housed together. However, captive animals can become quite tame over time (Storer 1994, 48).

Typical defense postures include rolling into a ball with erect spines. Hedgehogs will hiss and spit to try and scare off potential predators. The spines will stay erect and will vibrate, to try and drive the spine into anything that touches it. This posture makes it very difficult for them to be picked up either by a human or another animal (Storer 1994, 49).

Hedgehogs are also good at wedging themselves into very small places. This can make it difficult to examine these pets. It is a good idea not to have owners bring them in balls or other transport apparatuses that will make it difficult to remove them if they become frightened.

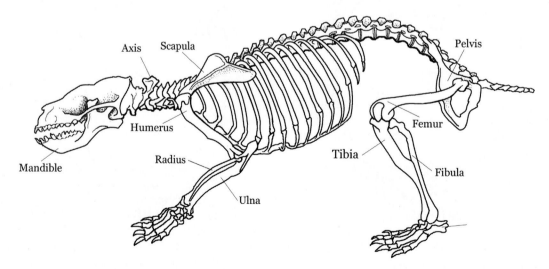

Fig. 12.3. Skeletal anatomy. (Drawing by Scott Stark)

Table 12.1. *Biologic and Reproductive Data*

Sexual maturity	3–9 months (Storer 1994, 53)
Litter size	2 to 6 (Storer 1994, 53)
Gestation	32–48 days (Storer 1994, 53)
Weaning	5– 6 weeks (Storer 1994, 53)
Breeding	1– 2 times a year spontaneous ovulates, but depends on environmental conditions (Storer 1994, 54)
Life span	3–4 years in the wild (Gregory 1992, 63)
WBC	5.8–21 × 103/ml (Ness 1999, 596)
Neutrophils %	49–70
Lymphocytes	22–38
Monocytes	0
Eosinophil	2–11
Basophils	0–5
Hematocrit	28–38
Hemoglobin	9.9–13.1
RBC (×106/ml)	4.4–6.0
MCV (fL)	60.0–67.4
MCHC (g/dl)	25.1–48.3
Platelets (×103/ml)	200–412
MCH (pg)	21.2–23.4
ALT(IU/L)	39.7–68.9 (Ness 1999 2:3, 600)
T. Bill (mg/dl)	0.0–0.1
T. Protein (g/dl)	5.3–6.3
Albumin (g/dl)	2.6–3.4
Glucose (mg/dl)	81.5–116.1
BUN (mg/dl)	21.3–32.9
Creatinine (mg/dl)	0.2–0.4
Phosphorus (mg/dl)	4.7–6.5
Calicium (mg/dl)	9.5–10.9

Hedgehogs can become excited when encountering smells or substances. They will engage in a behavior that is called self-anointing. When they encounter a small animal or substance they can become stiff, and they make licking motions with their tongues (which are very long). They can start to bite or tug and start producing large amounts of saliva. They can then get into extremely contorted positions by stiffening their front legs and pinning their head back between their shoulder blades. This behavior can look much like a seizure, and can continue for a long period of time. There is much controversy about this behavior, and most people believe that it may be a sexual reaction or a self-defense behavior (Storer 1994, 50).

HUSBANDRY

Optimal temperature is between 65 and 90°F, with the best temperature at 80°F. If the temperature is too low, these pets may start to hibernate, and if too high, they can have significant health problems related to heat stress. Hedgehogs can tolerate temperatures of 100°F for short periods of time (Storer 1994, 70).

It is best to keep adults in individual cages, because if housed together they can become aggressive. Plastic or fiberglass crates are good due to ease of cleaning. Aquariums make great housing, but one must be careful to monitor for overheating. Twenty-gallon aquariums are of adequate size and can be purchased with wire covers. Pine and aspen shavings are a very good substrate, and should be changed twice a week (Storer 1994, 78). Litter box training is possible and hedgehogs tend to use the bathroom in one area of the cage. Once that area is found, a small litter pan can be placed in the cage. Dust-free litter seems to work best since these pets will roll and scratch the litter (Storer 1994, 80). The self-clumping litter can pose a problem for hedgehogs, because if they become wet for any reason, the litter can stick in the spines and be very difficult to remove.

Hedgehogs like security and they feel quite secure if they have a place to hide. One can use a piece of PVC piping for sleeping quarters. One side of the tube can be capped off, providing a small and secure place for them to sleep. However, should more than one hedgehog be housed together, the tube should not be capped, as they may pile on top of one another and become trapped inside (Storer 1994, 82).

Regular rabbit or guinea pig water bottles work well. Bowls or saucers are potentially hazardous, since hedgehogs may climb inside and could drown.

NUTRITION

Hedgehogs are insectivores, which means that they have a high-protein diet (Storer 1994, 94). For non-breeding hedgehogs, feeding live food is acceptable. Crickets, mealworms, grasshoppers, pinkie mice, or small nontoxic frogs are good sources. Feeding live food can also add interest to their lives.

Nonbreeding hedgehogs can become fat on regular diets, so care must be taken on how much to feed these pets. Kitten food (wet or dry) may be used, as well as high-quality dog food mixed with cottage cheese in a 5 to 1 ratio (Storer 1994, 96). Chopped meat or hard-boiled eggs can be given as an occasional treat.

COMMON DISEASES

Lameness

Often hedgehogs are presented for reluctance to move or weak gait. There are many causes of lameness, including overgrown toenails, constriction of toes with foreign material, fracture of long bones from trauma, and even neoplasia. Systemic disease causing weakness can be perceived as lameness (Lightfoot 1999, 458).

Anorexia

Since hedgehogs do not have continuously erupting teeth, malocclusion is a problem seldom seen. However, gingival and periodontal disease does occur in older hedgehogs. Many times, husbandry problems are the cause of anorexia, such as changing food. If this does not seem to be the case, then blood work may be needed to see if there are any significant liver problems, such as hepatic lipidosis or neoplasia (Lightfoot 1999, 458).

Diarrhea

Diarrhea can be caused by many types of problems from husbandry, parasites, bacterial infection, and even salmonellosis. After reviewing correct feeding techniques and food with the owner, other appropriate diagnostics, such as fecal floats, should be taken. There can be other systemic illnesses that can present with diarrhea as well.

Dermatologic Problems

There are many forms of diseases that can cause problems with skin or quill loss (fig. 12.4). The problems can range from ectoparasites, hypersensitivity, dermatophytosis, and neoplasia. Fungal infection can be found with normal fungal culture techniques and is most likely to be *Trichophyton* (Lightfoot 2000, 163).

Neurological Problems

Progressive paralysis has been noted in hedgehogs. A viral encephalopathy has been noted in European hedgehogs (Ness 1999). Nutritional deficiencies can also cause many of the same signs. Included in the causes of neurologic disease is rabies as well as *Baylisascaris* migration and polioencephalomyelitis.

Ophthalmologic Trauma

Due to the fact that these pets ball up, eye problems are usually associated with trauma and are not noticed until later in the course of the disease. These pets are also very difficult to treat. Enucleation is common and they do quite well with only one eye (Lightfoot 2000, 158–59).

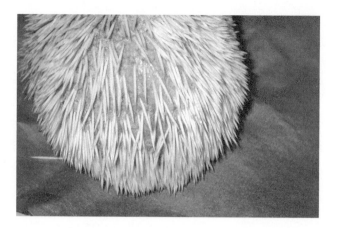

Fig. 12.4. Mange. (Photo courtesy of Dr. Sam Rivera)

OBTAINING A HISTORY AND PHYSICAL EXAMINATION

It is important to obtain as much information as possible about the pet before any actual handling takes place. Because hedgehogs get frightened very easily, it is better to observe the pet while taking a thorough history including what the pet eats and drinks, its cage environment, or any other significant finding. Much of the physical examination will need to be performed under anesthesia to prevent the pet from balling up.

Hedgehogs can be difficult pets to pick up, but one can use an object like a spoon or litter box scooper to pick them up. One must be very gentle and make sure that a finger does not get caught if the pet is trying to ball up.

There are many techniques to get hedgehogs to unroll. One method is to hold the hedgehog over a flat surface with the head pointing downward. With time, the hedgehog will unroll and reach for the table. Once the pet has unrolled, one can gently grab the back legs and hold the animal suspended by the back legs over the table (Gregory 1992, 63). If this fails, anesthesia will be necessary. Isoflurane is very well tolerated by these pets (Lightfoot 1999, 454). A mask or tank is the most effective way to administer anesthesia. Salivation is often encountered with isoflurane.

RADIOLOGY

For accurate radiographs, anesthesia is needed. Positioning would be similar to other small animals.

ANESTHESIA AND SURGERY

Anesthesia is an important part of the physical exam (fig. 12.5). Isoflurane is well tolerated and is best accomplished by using a large dog mask and removing the diaphragm. Place the entire mask over the hedgehog and then wait for sedation to occur. Once it uncurls, switching to a smaller mask is preferable (Lightfoot 1999, 454).

The most common surgical procedure is toe amputation, secondary to a foreign body that cuts off circulation.

URINALYSIS

Extensive analysis of the urine of the African hedgehog has not been done but one can extrapolate from the research done on the European hedgehog. Research showed that the urine was negative for glucose, acetone, and acetoacetic acid. Albumin was present in about half of the animals (Ness 1999, 610).

PARASITOLOGY

Mites are a common problem with hedgehogs. The two major parasites commonly seen are the *Caparinia* and *Chorioptic* species. *Caparinia* is usually distributed over a significant portion of the body, and one may suddenly notice that it looks as if the entire hedgehog's skin is moving. Ivermectin is commonly used, but must be used with proper shampoos as well. For the *Chorioptic* species, it usually presents as moderate to severe skin infection around the face and ears.

Ivermectin is very effective (Lightfoot 2000, 162–63).

Dermatophytes are also common causes of quill loss. *Trichophyton* is the most common dermatophyte found.

A variety of nematode, cestode, and protozoan parasites have been found in hedgehogs. Coccidia is present in as much as 10% of wild hedgehogs (Ness 1999, 612). *Crenosoama striatum* is a common lungworm of the wild hedgehog.

EMERGENCY AND CRITICAL CARE

Many of the same techniques used in small mammals can be used in hedgehogs, yet with hedgehogs, anesthesia is still needed to perform a good physical examination. Intraosseous catheters are very useful in these small patients. Many of these patients must be monitored carefully because they will start to curl up and make further diagnostics quite difficult.

SEX DETERMINATION

Figure 12.6 shows reproductive anatomy of the hedgehog (see also fig. 12.1). Note that the distance from the penis to the anus is much greater than the distance from the vulva to the anus.

TECHNIQUES

Venipuncture
Venipuncture is next to impossible in the awake hedgehog. Supplies needed include a large face mask

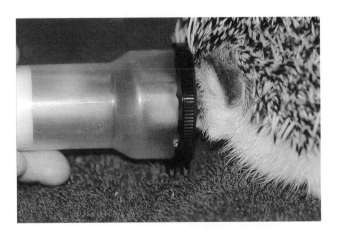

Fig. 12.5. *Maintenance of anesthesia after initial induction by placing patient in a face mask. (Photo courtesy of Ryan Cheek)*

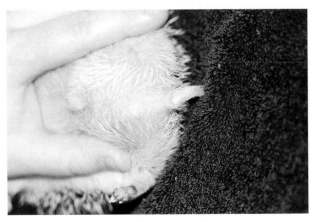

Fig. 12.6. *Male hedgehog. (Photo courtesy of Ryan Cheek)*

(diaphragm removed), small face mask, anesthesia machine, 1 ml 25 gauge needle syringe, 3 ml 22 gauge needle syringe, and blood collection tubes (preferable small tubes). The technique for a jugular venipuncture is as follows:

1. A large anesthetic face mask with diaphragm removed is obtained.
2. The patient is placed under facemask with opening of face mask tight against table.
3. Oxygen and anesthetic gas is turned on.
4. Wait for patient to become anesthetized.
5. Once patient is asleep the face mask is changed to a smaller one.
6. The patient is placed in dorsal recumbency.
7. Gentle pressure is applied to thoracic inlet.
8. A 3 cc 22 gauge, or 1 cc 25 gauge needle is inserted into jugular vein inserting caudally and directing cranially to point of jaw. Alternately, the needle could be inserted into the proximal vein with the needle directed caudally. See figures 12.7 and 12.8. Gentle negative pressure is applied until blood is seen. Note: Many of these patients are obese so this technique is performed blindly.

TPR

Much of this information can be obtained while looking at the patient before it is handled. Many times anesthesia is required. A large face mask with the diaphragm removed is placed over the patient and held tight to the table. Once the patient is anesthetized, a small face mask can be applied. The TPR can then be obtained along with a physical examination.

Urine Collection

The patient is anesthetized as described for the previous techniques. The patient is placed in dorsal recumbency once it is anesthetized. The bladder is palpated and stabilized while a 3 cc 22 gauge needle is placed through the skin and body wall and then into the bladder. Once sample collection is complete the needle and syringe are withdrawn.

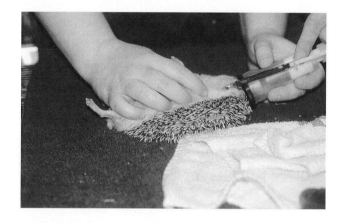

Fig. 12.7. Jugular venipuncture. (Photo courtesy of Ryan Cheek)

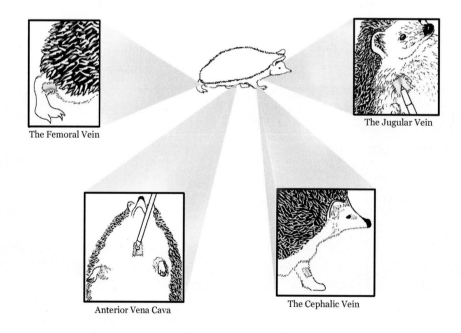

The Femoral Vein

The Jugular Vein

Anterior Vena Cava

The Cephalic Vein

Fig. 12.8. Venipuncture sites. (Drawing by Scott Stark)

Administration of Medications

Administration of fluids can be difficult. When hedgehogs are older they do not take to oral fluids easily, and they must be eating well if moistening the food is considered. Some oral medications can be injected into food but one must be sure that the patient is eating.

Injectable medications are tolerated well by these pets. Medications can be injected into the quill area subcutaneously (Lightfoot 2000). This is a high fat area of the hedgehog but absorption is sufficient.

Subcutaneous injections can be made in the rear legs or back. This is performed by carefully picking the patient up. A 25 gauge needle with a syringe is inserted between the quills and then under the skin. The medication is injection and then the needle and syringe removed.

Intravenous catheter placement can be done with the cephalic vein, but can be very difficult due to size of the patient. When the pet awakens from anesthesia, it may curl up and cause the catheter not to function properly.

Bandaging and Wound Care

This is very difficult in these pets and one must be aware of what will happen to the bandage as the pet curls up. Anesthesia is required and normal bandaging techniques are used.

In all, many of the techniques used in small animal medicine can be used in hedgehogs, however one must always consider the possible complications if the animal should curl up.

BIBLIOGRAPHY

Antinoff, N. 1998. Small Mammal Critical Care. In *Veterinary Clinics of North America Exotic Animal Practice* 1(1): 153–75.

Gregory, M. 1992. Hedgehogs. In *Manual of Exotic Pets*, edited by P. Beynon and J. Cooper. Gloucestershire: British Small Animal Veterinary Association.

Lightfoot, T. 1997. Clinical Techniques of Selected Exotic Species: Chinchilla, Prairie Dogs, Hedgehogs, and Chelonians. In *Seminars in Avian and Exotic Pet Medicine* 6(2): 96–105.

Lightfoot, T. 1999. Clinical Examination of the Chinchillas, Hedgehogs, Prairie Dogs, and Sugar Gliders. In *Veterinary Clinics of North America Exotic Animal Practice* 2(2): 447–69.

Lightfoot, T. 2000. Therapeutics of African Pygmy Hedgehogs and Prairie Dogs. In *Veterinary Clinics of North America Exotic Animal Practice* 3(1): 155–72.

Ness, R. 1999. Clinical Pathology and Sample Collection of Exotic Small Mammals. In *Veterinary Clinics of North America Exotic Animal Practice* 2(3):591–620.

Storer, P. 1994. *Everything You Wanted to Know About Hedgehogs But You Didn't Know Who to Ask*. Columbus, TX: Country Store Enterprises.

CHAPTER THIRTEEN

Other Species Seen in Practice

Samuel Rivera

SKUNKS

Introduction

Skunks are commonly kept as pets. They belong to the family Mustelidae. Other members of this family are ferrets, weasels, badgers, mink, and otters. The striped skunk (*Mephitis mephitis*) is the most common species found in the pet market. It is native to North America, ranging from southern Canada into the United States and northern Mexico. The most popular color pattern is brown fur with white stripes along the dorsum. The skunks in the pet market are usually descented at 2–4 weeks of age. Contrary to popular belief, skunks are usually not neutered at an early age. They have extremely sharp teeth and their bite can cause severe injuries.

Skunks adapt well to life in captivity and can be litter trained and harness or leash trained. They are nocturnal animals but can adjust to a diurnal cycle. Even though they have poor sight their hearing and sense of smell are very good. In the wild, skunks do not undergo true hibernation.

Skunks have unique health and dietary needs. Furthermore, there are limited resources describing their health and nutritional needs. In many states it is illegal to keep skunks as pets and it is essential for all the veterinary personnel to be familiar with the state and local regulations on keeping them as pets.

Anatomy and Physiology

The anatomy and physiology of skunks are similar to that of other carnivores. One difference is the highly developed anal sacs, which can eject their contents for a distance of 3 meters (Fowler 1986).

Biologic Data

Average lifespan: 10–12 years
Body temperature: 102°F (38.9°C)
Heart rate: 140–190 beats per minute
Respiratory rate: 25–50 breaths per min
Average body weight: 4.5 kg
Gestation: 63 days
Litter size: 4–10
Urine pH: 6.0

Husbandry and Nutrition

In the wild, adult males are solitary except during the winter months when they may share a den with several females (Wallach & Boever 1983). Young skunks can be housed together, but as they get older they should be kept in separate enclosures. The cage should have a nest box and a litter box. Skunks have a natural instinct to dig and should be closely monitored when outside the cage.

Wild skunks are omnivores. Their natural diet consists of insects, rodents, small vertebrates, fruits, green vegetables, and grain. In captivity, skunks have been fed a variety of diets. To date there is not a formulated diet specifically designed for skunks. Light dog food or a zoo omnivore diet supplemented with fruits and vegetables has been recommended. A varied diet consisting of fruits, vegetables, eggs, a small amount of dog and cat food, yogurt, cottage cheese, mice, cereal, and insects should be provided. It is important to remember that skunks will eat anything in sight and as a result become obese. Dairy products are a good source of calcium but should be fed in limited amounts as they can cause gastrointestinal upset. Skunks tend to gain weight in the fall and are less active during the fall and winter months. Feeding an adequate diet will decrease the development of obesity and the associated health problems.

Common Health Problems

Obesity

This is the most common clinical presentation and the leading cause of morbidity in skunks. Most pet skunks are kept inside and fed an inadequate diet that leads to obesity. In some cases, correction of the diet and adequate husbandry practices can help to maintain a skunk in an ideal body weight.

Hepatic Lipidosis

This disease is caused by an increased accumulation of triglycerides in the liver, which is due to an increased mobilization of fat from the body stores and the inability of the liver to process it expeditiously. The end result is the buildup of fat within the hepatocytes leading to compromised normal function. There is a close relationship between obesity and the development of hepatic lipidosis. Clinical signs include prolonged anorexia, lethargy, vomiting, weight loss, and jaundice. The presumptive diagnosis of hepatic lipidosis is based on the history, physical exam findings, and serum chemistry abnormalities. A definitive diagnosis is based on the cytological evaluation of a liver fine-needle aspirate or biopsy. The treatment involves primarily supportive care.

Amyloidosis

This disease is characterized by the buildup of insoluble fibrillar proteins (amyloid) in multiple organ systems leading to compromised function. The clinical signs are nonspecific and will vary depending on which organ system is affected. The diagnosis is based on a histopathological evaluation of the affected tissue. There is no treatment reported in skunks.

Cardiomyopathy

Cardiac disease is commonly seen in obese skunks. The clinical signs are exercise intolerance, weight loss, dyspnea, lethargy, anorexia, coughing, ascites and/or edema, pale mucous membranes, and cold extremities. The diagnosis is based on radiographs, electrocardiogram, and echocardiogram. Cardiomyopathy is treated the same as in ferrets.

Dental Disease

The dental formula of skunks is 2(I3/3, C1/1, PM3/3, M1/1). Common dental conditions seen in skunks are advanced periodontal disease and fractured teeth. Common clinical signs are change in eating habits, halitosis, pawing at the mouth, hypersalivation, or facial swelling. Periodontal disease is usually a result of a poor diet. Treatment involves dental cleaning, antibiotics, and diet correction where appropriate.

Dermatitis

Skin problems are common in skunks, particularly in obese ones. Some of the most commonly seen lesions are dry, scaly skin, alopecia, papules, pustules, and excoriations. Dermatitis can be caused by nutritional deficiencies, ectoparasites, and fungal or bacterial infections.

Canine Distemper

Canine distemper has been reported in the ferret, skunk, mink, badger, weasel, sable, and grison (Wallach et al. 1983). The clinical signs are fever, hyperemia of the face and ear, scleral inflammation, ocular discharge, depression, anorexia, diarrhea, dyspnea, hyperkeratosis of the foot pads, and neurologic signs. The incubation period is 5 to 7 days for the acute phase. The diagnosis is based on clinical signs and serologic testing. Treatment involves mostly supportive care. Fluids support and broad-spectrum antibiotics should be initiated. Unvaccinated skunks that contract canine distemper have a poor prognosis.

Feline Panleukopenia

Feline panleukopenia has been reported in several mustelid species (Wallach et al. 1983). This is an acute viral disease that can lead to high mortality in skunks. The clinical signs are hemorrhagic enteritis, anorexia, and depression. Death usually occurs within 3 to 5 days after the onset of the clinical signs. A presumptive diagnosis is based on the characteristic clinical signs accompanied by a low white blood cell count. The best treatment is supportive care.

Zoonotic Diseases

Baylisascaris columnaris is a roundworm found in skunks. This parasite can cause serious visceral larva migrans in humans. The usual contamination is through the fecal-oral route. Strict hygiene to decrease exposure to contaminated material is the best prevention.

Rabies is a serious human health problem. The rabies virus can be transmitted to humans through bites from infected skunks. In North America, the wild striped skunk is the most important wildlife reservoir of rabies (Drenzek & Rupprecht 2000). The clinical signs of rabies in skunks are varied. Generally, any behavior considered abnormal for the particular animal should be considered suspicious. The incubation period for rabies is from 2 weeks to 6 months. In the furious form of the disease, the virus can be shed in the saliva 1–6 days prior to death.

The diagnosis of rabies is based on the identification of viral antigen and/or characteristic lesions in the brain. Public health officials do not accept vaccination against rabies in pet skunks and the animal may need to be euthanized and tested for rabies if it is involved in a biting incident. Even though rabies is a concern in the wild skunk population, the disease is relatively rare in pet skunks. Pet skunks, as any other pet, can become infected with rabies if exposed to a reservoir in the wild.

Physical Examination

A healthy skunk should have a glossy, thick coat and bright clear eyes. Yellow coloring of the white fur is considered abnormal. The stools should be formed. Obesity or an underweight patient should raise a red flag as to the health status of the pet.

Signs of illness in a skunk include change in stool consistency, dry dull hair coat, yellowing of the white fur, obesity, dry cracked feet, ocular or nasal discharge, coughing, sneezing, and bad breath.

Vaccinations

Pet skunks should be vaccinated against canine distemper, feline panleukopenia, and rabies (Miller 1995). There are no vaccines licensed for use in skunks. However, vaccines licensed for use in ferrets can be used in skunks. It is important to remember that if a skunk bites a person, public health officials will not accept rabies vaccination and the animal may need to be euthanized and tested for rabies.

Restraint

Skunks can be restrained in a manner similar to cats. One difference is that many skunks lack a significant scruff, making scruffing behind the neck difficult and painful to the skunk. Most tame skunks can be picked up by placing one hand on each side of the body caudal to the axillary region. The animal can be restrained in this manner for taking the temperature or clipping the nails. The skunk's primary defense is the expression of its anal sacs. Because of this they tend to be less likely to bite as their primary means of defense. Leather gloves can be used for handling fractious animals, but one must keep in mind that skunks have sharp teeth that can bite through leather gloves causing severe injuries. Many fractious skunks will need chemical immobilization prior to handling.

Radiology

The radiographic techniques and positioning are similar to those used in domestic animals. Many skunks require sedation in order to obtain good quality radiographs.

Anesthesia

Gas anesthesia is most commonly used in skunks. Sevoflurane and isoflurane are among the safest anesthetic agents used. The skunk can be anesthetized by placing it in an induction chamber. The animal can be maintained on gas anesthesia via a face mask or endotracheal intubation. Fractious animals that are difficult to handle can be anesthetized with parenteral drugs. If the animal cannot be safely contained, it can be transferred to a squeeze cage for intramuscular injection. Ketamine and medetomidine are commonly used together for induction of anesthesia.

Parasitology

Skunks are susceptible to a variety of parasites including roundworms, tapeworms, and coccidia. Roundworms and tapeworms are managed similar to an infestation in domestic animals. Coccidiosis can cause severe disease in skunks. The clinical signs commonly seen are diarrhea, weight loss, anorexia, dehydration, and depression. The diagnosis is based on the identification of oocysts in the feces. Treatment involves the administration of antiprotozoal agents similar to those used in domestic species.

Toxoplasmosis has been reported in skunks, ferrets, and weasels. The clinical signs are fever, lymphadenopathy, splenomegaly, myocarditis, pneumonitis, hepatitis, hydrocephalus, encephalitis, dermatitis, and enlarged lymph nodes. The antemortem diagnosis is based on serologic testing. Antiprotozoal drugs are used to treat toxoplasmosis.

The lungworm *Crenosoma mephitidis* is a parasite that can affect the lungs of skunks. The clinical signs are coughing, dyspnea, depression, anorexia, and depression. The diagnosis is based on the identification of the infective larvae in the feces.

Clinical Techniques

Blood Collection

Blood sampling is an important diagnostic tool particularly when assessing a sick skunk. The sites most commonly used are the jugular, cephalic, lateral saphenous, and femoral veins. Manual restraint for blood collection is appropriate for tame skunks used to handling or with extremely debilitated animals. Fractious animals will need sedation for safe venipuncture. It must be kept in mind that skunks have sharp teeth and can cause severe damage when they bite. The supplies needed include 25 to 22 gauge needles, 1 to 3 ml syringes, 70% isopropyl alcohol, and blood collection tubes. The size of the needle used will depend on the size of the animal and the vein used.

Jugular Vein. Skunks usually resist restrain for jugular venipuncture more than they do for cephalic or lateral saphenous collection. The restraint is similar to that used for cats. The animal should be restrained in sternal recumbency, with the front legs held over the edge of the table (fig. 13.1). The assistant can hold the head with one hand extended by holding the head

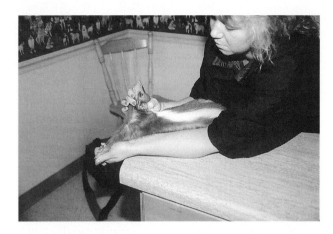

Fig. 13.1. Restraint for jugular venipuncture of the skunk. (Photo courtesy of Ryan Cheek)

from the dorsum, use the thumb and fingers and wrap the head in the palm, placing the thumb and fingers in opposite sides of the head under the temporomandibular joint. Gentle pressure is applied at the thoracic inlet lateral to the trachea. The needle is inserted bevel up at a 25° angle into the vein. After the sample is collected, pressure is released, the needle is withdrawn, and digital pressure is applied at the venipuncture site for 30 seconds.

Cephalic Vein. The animal is restrained in sternal recumbency (fig. 13.2). An assistant should restrain the head by the scruff of the neck with one hand and the forelimb extended by the elbow. Alternatively the head can be restrained as described for jugular venipuncture. Pressure is applied with the thumb around the elbow, rotating gently laterally. The limb is

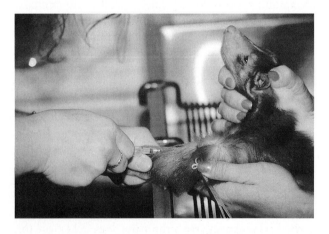

Fig. 13.2. Cephalic venipuncture in a skunk. (Photo courtesy of Ryan Cheek)

held with a free hand and the thumb is used to stabilize the vein. The needle is inserted at a 20–25° angle. Once the vessel is entered, gentle suction is applied until the desired amount is obtained. Too much suction can cause collapse of the vein. Once the needle is withdrawn gentle pressure should be applied to the venipuncture site.

Lateral Saphenous Vein. This vein is located in the lateral aspect of the hind limb. This is the third option if the other two vessels are not accessible. This vein is small and often yields a small volume of blood. The assistant can hold the skunk in lateral recumbency by holding the scruff of the neck with one hand and the venipuncture leg with the other hand. The leg is held around the stifle with the leg extended. The leg is grasped around the tarsus and the skin gently pulled to stabilize the vein. The needle is inserted at a 20° angle and the blood sample is collected. Digital pressure is applied for 30 seconds afterward to prevent hematoma formation.

Femoral Vein. The femoral vein is located in the medial aspect of the thigh. Collection from this vein is performed similar to the cat. In obese skunks the femoral vein can be very difficult to find.

Urine Collection
Urinalysis is an important part of the health assessment in skunks. The techniques to collect urine are similar to those used in dogs and cats.

Voided urine: Urine can be collected from the bottom of the cage using a syringe. The disadvantage of this technique is that fecal and litter contamination affects the results.

Manual expression: With the animal sedated, transabdominal pressure is applied to the urinary bladder to overcome the sphincter pressure. The urine can be collected into a sterile container or from the tabletop.

Cystocentesis: With the animal sedated, the bladder is gently isolated. A 25 to 22 gauge needle on a 3 to 5 ml syringe is inserted into the bladder and the urine collected. This is the preferred method when performing a culture and sensitivity on the urine.

Fecal Analysis
The flotation and direct fecal smear techniques are done the same as for domestic species.

Administration of Medications
There are several routes for administration of medications.

Oral route: Liquids or powders mixed with food are the most common forms of oral medications. In many cases the skunk's sharp teeth precludes the use of tablets. Liquid medications can be placed in the side of the mouth with a syringe. Powder medications can be mixed with a favorite treat or a small amount of soft food such as yogurt or cottage cheese.

Intramuscular route: Parenteral medications can be given in the thigh musculature or the biceps.

Subcutaneous route: This site is most commonly used for the administration of fluids to sick animals. The intrascapular and lateral flank regions are the best sites for the administration of subcutaneous fluids.

Intravenous route: The cephalic, jugular, and saphenous veins can be used for the administration of medications. In most cases the skunk has to be sedated to facilitate intravenous medications, unless the animal is severely debilitated.

PRAIRIE DOGS

Introduction

The black-tailed prairie dog (*Cyonomys ludovicianus*) is a rodent native to North America, more specifically to the western plains of the United States. Over recent years prairie dogs have become common in the pet trade. Prairie dogs are diurnal social animals that live in large groups in the wild. The ownership of wild-caught prairie dogs should be discouraged due to serious zoonotic potential. It is important to be aware of the fact that owning prairie dogs is illegal in certain states.

Husbandry and Nutrition

Prairie dogs are very social animals that are best kept in pairs or more. Prairie dogs require adequate room for digging. The enclosure should be made of heavy-gauge wire or stainless steel. It is important to provide a thick layer of substrate to allow the animals to burrow. Adequate bedding includes recycled paper, nonaromatic wood shavings, and hay. The larger the enclosure the better. The enclosure should be provided with a suitable hiding box. The cage should also be well ventilated.

Prairie dogs are not true hibernators. When exposed to low ambient temperature they may undergo torpor, a state in which the body's physiological activities are greatly reduced to conserve energy. The environmental temperature should be kept between 69 and 72°F (20.5–22°C) and the humidity at 30–70% (Johnson-Delaney 1996).

Prairie dogs are mostly herbivores. They should be fed high-quality grass hay ad lib, supplemented with a commercially formulated diet. Fresh water must be provided on a daily basis

Common and Zoonotic Diseases

Barbering

This condition often presents as areas of abnormal fur appearance with underlying healthy skin. It can be caused by the animal or a cage mate chewing the fur. It is often related to stress, and husbandry practices must be evaluated to help minimize fur barbering.

Obesity

Obesity is commonly seen in prairie dogs. As with other unusual pets, this condition is often due to inadequate diet and lack of proper exercise. Diets high in fat such as seeds and nuts lead to obesity and should be avoided. Obesity predisposes prairie dogs to other conditions such as heart, respiratory, and liver disease.

Nasal Dermatitis

This is a common condition in captive prairie dogs. It is most often due to rubbing the face on the cage wire. This results in abrasions and inflammation leading to secondary bacterial infections.

Dermatomycosis (ringworm)

Prairie dogs are susceptible to *Microsporum canis* and *Trichophyton mentagrophytes*. The most common clinical sign is alopecia. The diagnosis is based on a positive fungal culture. The treatment is similar to that of domestic animals and involves the administration of systemic antifungal drugs in addition to topical antifungal treatment.

Respiratory Disease

Respiratory disease is relatively common in prairie dogs. Obesity and poor ventilation are two common predisposing factors. Cedar bedding contains aromatic oils that can lead to irritation of the respiratory tract. Nasal foreign bodies (cage litter, hay, carpet fibers) are common presentations. Overgrowth of the maxillary incisors teeth roots can lead to increased pressure and irritation in the nasal sinus passages. Pneumonia is often associated with bacterial and viral agents. The clinical signs of respiratory disease are similar to those seen in dogs and cats. They include dyspnea, nasal or ocular discharge, cyanosis, anorexia, and lethargy. The treatment includes appropriate antibiotic therapy and supportive care. Appropriate husbandry is important in the prevention of respiratory disease.

Odontomas

This is a common cause of upper respiratory symptoms in captive prairie dogs (Phalen 2000). Odontomas are caused by an inflammation of the periodontal bone as a result of dental disease or trauma. This inflammation leads to narrowing of the nasal passages. The diagnosis is based on radiographic abnormalities of the incisor's root and surrounding soft tissue. Treatment involves removal of the affected teeth and debridement of the abnormal tissue.

Heart Disease

Obesity is a predisposing factor for the development of heart disease. Clinical signs are lethargy, syncope, cyanosis, dyspnea, and cold extremities. The diagnosis is based on auscultation, radiography, echocardiography, and ultrasonography.

Pododermatitis (bumblefoot)

This condition is usually the result of poor husbandry. Animals kept on wire-bottom cages can develop small ulcers on the footpads that become infected. The infection results in severe swelling and abscess formation in the affected foot. In severe cases tendonitis and osteomyelitis can develop. Bumblefoot is treated by debriding the affected lesions in conjunction with topical and systemic antibiotics. Correction of the underlying husbandry problem is essential for resolution and/or prevention of bumblefoot.

Zoonotic Diseases

Prairie dogs, particularly wild-caught animals, can be reservoirs of *Yersinia pseudotuberculosis*, *Yersinia pestis*, and *Baylisascaris procyonidae*. *Yersinia pseudotuberculosis* can cause severe illness in humans. Affected humans can develop acute mesenteric lymphadenitis, fever, anorexia, vomiting, enteritis with diarrhea, and dehydration. This bacteria is transmitted to humans through the ingestion of contaminated material. *Yersinia pestis* is the causative agent of Sylvatic Plague in humans. This bacteria is transmitted to humans through the bite of fleas from carrier prairie dogs. Humans can also contract the infection from handling tissues from affected animals during necropsy. Flea control is essential to eliminate the human risk of exposure.

Baylisascaris procyonidae can cause serious visceral larva migrans in humans. This parasite is transmitted to humans through the ingestion of contaminated material or contact with open wounds on the skin.

Anatomy and Physiology

The anatomy and physiology of prairie dogs are similar to that of other rodents of comparable size. They are hindgut fermenters. The male has a prominent scrotum and the penis is relatively easy to exteriorize. The female has a short distance between the anus and the vaginal groove. Prairie dogs have a characteristic set of scent gland papillae that can be visualized on the anal margin when the animal is stressed.

Biologic Data

Average weight: 0.5–2.2 kg
Average lifespan: 6–10 years
Temperature: 95.7–102.3°F (35.4–39.1°C)
Heart rate: 83–318/min
Respiration: 40–60/min
Gestation: 30 days

Restraint

Prairie dogs are difficult to restrain. Animals that are used to frequent handling can be quite tame and examined awake. In many cases sedation is needed to perform a thorough physical exam. They do not have much loose skin around the neck making it difficult to scruff. Prairie dogs have sharp claws and teeth that can cause severe wounds to the handler. Tame animals used to being handled can be restrained by placing one hand around the chest and supporting the hind end with the other hand. Alternatively, the animal can be grabbed at the base of the tail and lifted gently with the forelimbs resting on a flat surface. The free hand is used to grab the animal on the back of the neck. This technique can be used to move the animal or to perform minor procedures such as nail clipping. Additionally, a thick towel can be used to wrap the animal. This allows for closer examination of the head and the administration of intramuscular injections in the hind limbs. The towel also protects the handler from been scratched.

Radiology

The radiographic techniques and positioning are similar to those used in domestic animals. Prairie dogs, unless severely debilitated, require sedation in order to obtain good quality radiographs. The radiographic techniques are similar to those used in other small rodents.

Anesthesia

Sevoflurane and isoflurane gas are the most commonly used anesthetic agents. Induction can be accomplished by chamber induction. Tracheal intubation is difficult in prairie dogs. As a result, the animal can be maintained via a face mask. When the animal is anesthetized, its anterior end should be kept slightly elevated so the extensive viscera do not put excessive pressure on the diaphragm.

Clinical Techniques

Venipuncture

Many animals require sedation for blood collection. The jugular vein is the preferred site for blood collection. In obese prairie dogs this vein can be difficult to visualize and is often approached blindly. The sedated animal is restrained in dorsal recumbency. The animal is kept with the anterior end elevated to facilitate breathing. In prairie dogs the pressure from the abdominal organs on the diaphragm can compromise respiration. With the animal in dorsal recumbency, the forelimbs should be extended caudally. Gentle pressure should be applied at the thoracic inlet. The fur along the jugular groove should be moistened. A 23 to 25 gauge needle in a 1 to 3 ml syringe should be used. The needle should be inserted at a 45° angle and suction applied as the needle is advanced forward. In some cases the needle may need to be redirected to either side in order to find the vein. Blood will immediately fill the syringe as the needle enters the vein.

Venipuncture from the cephalic and lateral saphenous veins is done similar to the way blood is drawn in other animals of comparable size. The cephalic vein is located on the dorsal aspect of the front leg and the lateral saphenous vein is located in the lateral aspect of the hind limb, just above the tarsus.

Urine Collection

Urinalysis is an important part of health assessment in sick prairie dogs. The techniques to collect urine are similar to those used in dogs and cats.

Voided urine: Urine can be collected from the bottom of the cage using a small syringe. The disadvantage of this technique is that fecal and litter contamination affects the results.

Manual expression: With the animal sedated, gentle transabdominal pressure is applied to the urinary bladder to overcome the sphincter pressure. The urine can be collected into a sterile container or from the tabletop. Excessive pressure should not be applied as this can lead to rupture of the urinary bladder.

Cystocentesis: With the animal sedated, one should gently isolate the bladder. A 27 to 25 gauge needle on a 0.5 to 1 ml syringe is inserted into the bladder and the urine collected. This is the preferred method when performing a culture and sensitivity on the urine.

Fecal Analysis

The flotation and direct fecal smear techniques are performed the same as for domestic species.

Administration of Medications

There are several routes for administration of medications.

Oral route: Liquids are the most common forms of oral medications. The prairie dog's small mouth and sharp teeth precludes the use of tablets. Liquid medications can be placed in the side of the mouth with a syringe.

Intramuscular route: Parenteral medications can be given in the thigh musculature or the biceps.

Subcutaneous route: This site is most commonly used for the administration of fluids to sick animals. The intrascapular and lateral flank regions are the best sites for the administration of subcutaneous fluids.

Intravenous route: The cephalic, jugular, and saphenous veins can be used for the administration of medications. In most cases, the prairie dog has to be sedated to facilitate intravenous medications, unless the animal is severely debilitated.

SUGAR GLIDERS

Introduction

Sugar gliders (*Petaurus breviceps*) are small marsupials native to Australia and New Zealand (fig. 13.3). They are nocturnal arboreal animals. In the wild, sugar gliders live in groups of up to 12 individuals (Booth 2000). They are very social animals that are best kept in pairs or small related groups and require a large enclosure with branches, nest boxes, and hiding areas. Proper husbandry and diet are essential for a healthy pet. During extreme weather conditions or food shortages, sugar gliders conserve energy by going into torpor for up to 16 hours per day (Booth 2000).

Husbandry and Nutrition

Sugar gliders need a lot of room. The larger the enclosure the better. An enclosure measuring 2 × 2 × 2 meters is adequate for housing up to six animals (Dunn 1982). A nest box for sleeping and hiding must be provided. The nest box can be lined with a piece of cloth, shredded bark, or dried leaves and should be changed weekly. Newspaper and pine or cedar wood shavings are not recommended. Sugar gliders are arboreal animals, therefore branches for climbing are essential. A pair is the minimum number to keep together.

The environmental temperature should be between 64 and 75°F (18–24°C). They can withstand temperature in the mid to high 80s but higher temperatures can predispose them to hyperthermia.

In the wild, sugar gliders eat sap and gum from

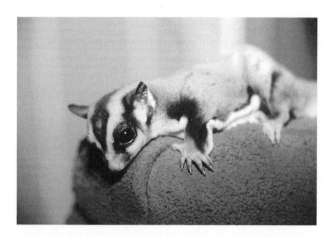

Fig. 13.3. Sugar glider. (Photo courtesy of Ryan Cheek)

eucalyptus and acacia trees, nectar from eucalyptus blossom, and a variety of insects (Henry 1984). The diet in captivity consists of a variety of fruits, commercial sugar glider pellets, commercial insectivore diets, insects supplemented with vitamin and minerals, nectar, and small invertebrates. They are mainly insectivores but also eat sugar-containing sap from several sources. Food and water should be provided in an elevated location. Nectar should be provided in covered feeders to keep the nectar from getting on the fur. The ideal amount of food to offer is 15–20% of their body weight (Booth 2000).

Anatomy

Sugar gliders have blue-gray fur with a dark line extending from the nose to the lower back. Each foot has five digits. The second and third digits of the hind feet are partially fused. They do not have the eupubic bones that support the pouch characteristic of marsupials. Sugar gliders have a membrane (the petagium) that extends from the lateral aspect of the forelimb to the tarsus. This membrane allows the sugar glider to glide a fair distance. Males have frontal, sternal, and urogenital scent glands. The females have a pouch and urogenital glands. Scent glands are also found on the paws, corners of the mouth, and external ears. The scent glands are used for marking territory and members of the same group (Smith 1984). The males have a pendulous scrotum located cranial to the penis. The female have a ventral abdominal pouch that opens cranially. Sugar gliders have a cloaca where the gastrointestinal, urinary, and reproductive tracts empty. They have a large cecum that may assist in digestion of the sap eaten in the wild (Henry & Suckling 1984).

Sugar gliders have a short gestation period with a longer development within the pouch.

Biologic Data

Weight range: 95–160 grams
Body length: 16–21 cm
Heart rate: 200–300 beats per minute
Respiratory rate: 16–40 breaths per minute
Rectal temperature: 96.5–97.9°F (35.8–36.6°C)
Gestation 15–17 days, young leave the pouch at 70 days
Weaning age: 110–120 days
Lifespan: 9–12 years

Common Diseases

Nutritional Osteodystrophy

This is one of the most common diseases seen in captive sugar gliders (Pye & Carpenter 1999). The clinical signs include acute onset of hind limb paresis or paralysis. This disease is believed to be caused by feeding an inadequate diet low in calcium and vitamin D_3 and high in phosphorus. Too much fruit and muscle meat can predispose animals to this disease. The diagnosis is based on a thorough history and radiographs. The treatment includes cage rest, parenteral calcium, diet correction, and calcium and vitamin D_3 supplementation.

Trauma

Trauma is most common in wild sugar gliders. In captivity the most common cases of trauma involve cat and dogs attacks. Some of the common injuries are lacerations, pneumothorax, hemothorax, spinal trauma, and ocular trauma.

Dental Disease

Tartar buildup associated with periodontal disease is often seen. This has been associated with feeding carbohydrate-rich diets (Booth 2000). The teeth can be cleaned as needed. Feeding insects with a hard exoskeleton can help minimize tartar buildup.

Obesity

Obesity is seen in sugar gliders fed an inadequate diet. Diets high in fat and proteins predispose animals to obesity. Lack of exercise can also contribute to obesity. Obese animals are predisposed to cardiac and hepatic disease.

Stress-related Disease

Animals under constant stress are prone to developing behavioral problems. Some of the clinical signs of stress-related disorders include alopecia, self-mutilation, coprophagia, hyperphagia, polyuria, pacing, and cannibalism. The source of the stress must be identified and eliminated to help correct the problem.

Neoplasia

Neoplastic disease is relatively common. Lymphoid neoplasia is the most common type of tumor reported (Booth 2000). Other tumors reported include mammary gland tumors, bronchogenic carcinoma, and chondrosarcoma.

Malnutrition

Malnutrition is frequently seen in sugar gliders fed an inadequate diet. As a result, malnutrition leads to hypocalcemia, hypoproteinemia, and anemia. The clinical signs of malnutrition are nonspecific and include lethargy, weakness, dehydration, pale mucous membranes, cachexia, and in some cases seizures and pathologic fractures. The owner should be educated as to what the appropriate diet is. Treatment involves correction of the dietary inadequacies and supportive care.

Physical Examination

Sugar gliders can be challenging to examine without sedation. A thorough history should be taken first. One should ask about the number of animals kept and the enclosure size. The diet should be recorded. The owner should be asked whether there are other pets in the household, and where the animal was obtained. While taking the history, the animal's motor function and disposition can be observed. If a weight is needed, many times the owners can place the animal on the scale and then the weight can be recorded. If the animal is fractious, the weight can be obtained by placing it in a cloth bag.

Restraint

The best way to restrain sugar gliders is by holding the head between a thumb and middle finger and using the index finger to restrain the top of the head. The body is then placed in the palm of the restrainer's hand. Fractious animals can be restrained using a cloth bag. To accomplish this the owner should place the animal in a small enclosure (scale basket or nest box). Then a cloth bag is placed over the hand that will grasp the animal. The animal is then grasped and the bag slipped over the whole body. Once in the bag one can gently expose the head and restrain it. It is important to keep the seam of the bag toward the outside to keep the animal from injuring itself with the small threads.

Radiology

The radiographic techniques are similar to those used in other domestic animals. Because of their small size, high-definition radiograph film offers the best detail.

Anesthesia

Gas anesthetics are most commonly used. Sevoflurane and isoflurane are most commonly used. Induction can be accomplished by either face mask or chamber induction. A large face mask can be used as an induction chamber. The animal can be maintained via a face mask.

Parasitology

Coccidia and *Giardia* spp. have been identified in captive sugar gliders (Ness 1999). The diagnosis is based on the identification of the oocysts or trophozoites in the fecal sample. There is limited information on the incidence of gastrointestinal parasites in sugar gliders.

Clinical Techniques

Blood Collection

The blood volume that can be safely collected is up to 1% of the body weight. Because of their active nature, sugar gliders often require sedation for blood collection, unless the animal is severely debilitated. They can be sedated using isoflurane or sevoflurane via a mask or chamber induction.

Supplies needed include 27–30 gauge needles, 0.5–1 ml syringes, and 0.5 ml collection tubes.

Jugular vein: The animal is placed in dorsal recumbency. The forelimbs are aimed caudally. Gentle pressure is applied in the thoracic inlet. The fur is moistened along the jugular groove to allow better visualization. The needle is then inserted at a 30 to 45° angle in the jugular groove. Negative pressure is applied as the needle is advanced. The syringe will fill with blood as the jugular vein is entered.

Cranial vena cava: The animal is placed in dorsal recumbency. Both forelimbs are extended caudally. The needle is inserted at the angle formed by the manubrium and the first rib. The needle is aimed toward the contra-lateral hip joint at a very shallow angle. Suction is applied as the needle is advanced. It will fill with blood as soon as the vessel is entered. It is important not to reposition the needle in an attempt to find this vessel. If the vessel is missed, the needle should be withdrawn and another attempt made. There are other vessels and nerves that can be damaged inadvertently by excessive manipulation of the needle.

Medial tibial artery: The hind limb is held in the extended position with the medial aspect exposed. The fur is slightly moistened with alcohol. The artery runs superficially from the stifle to the tarsus. The vessel should be visualized and the needle then inserted at a 30° angle. After the blood is collected, gentle pressure should be applied to the site to avoid hematoma formation.

Other sites for blood collection include the cephalic, lateral saphenous, femoral, ventral coccygeal, and lateral tail veins. The main disadvantage is that only very small amounts of blood can be collected from these sites due to their small size. In some cases, a small-gauge heparinized needle can be inserted into the vein and the blood collected directly from the hub using small collection containers or capillary tubes.

Urine Collection

Urinalysis is an important part of the health assessment in sugar gliders. The techniques to collect urine are similar to those used in dogs and cats.

Voided urine: Urine can be collected from the bottom of the cage using a small syringe. The disadvantage of this technique is that fecal and litter contamination affects the results.

Manual expression: With the animal sedated, gentle transabdominal pressure is applied to the urinary bladder to overcome the sphincter pressure. The urine can be collected into a sterile container or from the tabletop.

Cystocentesis: With the animal sedated, one should gently isolate the bladder. A 27 to 25 gauge needle on a 0.5 to 1 ml syringe is inserted into the bladder and the urine collected. This is the preferred method when performing a culture and sensitivity on the urine.

Fecal Analysis

The flotation and direct fecal smear techniques are done the same as for domestic species.

REFERENCES

Booth, RJ. 2000. General husbandry and medical care of sugar gliders. In *Kirk's current veterinary therapy XIII*, edited by JD Bonagura. Philadelphia: W.B. Saunders Co.

Drenzek, CL, and Rupprecht, CE. 2000. The rabies pandemic. In *Kirk's current veterinary therapy XIII*, edited by JD Bonagura. Philadelphia: W.B. Saunders Co.

Dunn, RW. 1982. Gliders of the genus Petaurus: their management in zoos. In *The management of Australian mammals in captivity*, edited by DD Evans. North Melbourne, Australia: Ramsay Ware Stockland.

Ellis, C, Mori, M. 2001. Skin diseases of rodents and small exotic mammals. In *The Veterinary Clinics of North America Exotic Animal Practice*, edited by RE Schmidt 4(2): 493–542.

Fowler, ME. 1986. Descenting carnivores. In *Zoo and Wild Animal Medicine*, 2d ed., edited by ME Fowler. Philadelphia: W.B. Saunders Co.

Henry, SR, Suckling, GC. 1984. A review of the ecology of the sugar glider. *Possums and gliders*, edited by PA Smith, ID Hume. Australian Mammal Society. Sydney, Australia.

Johnson-Delaney, CA. 1996. *Exotic companion medicine handbook for veterinarians*. Lake Worth: Wingers Publishing.

Lightfoot, TL. 1999. Clinical examination of chinchillas, hedgehogs, prairie dogs, and sugar gliders. In *The Veterinary Clinics of North America Exotic Animal Practice*, edited by CJ Orcutt 2(2): 447–69.

Miller, E. 1995. Immunization of wild animal species against common diseases. In *Kirk's current veterinary therapy XII*, edited by JD Bonagura. Philadelphia: W.B. Saunders Co.

Ness, RD. 1999. Clinical pathology and sample collection of exotic small mammals. In *The Veterinary Clinics of North America Exotic Animal Practice*, edited by DR Reavill 2(3): 591–620.

Nowak, RM. 1991. *Walker's mammals of the world*, 5th ed., vol 1. Baltimore: The Johns Hopkins University Press.

Phalen, DN, Atinoff, N, Fricke, ME. 2000. Obstructive respiratory disease in prairie dogs with odontomas. In *The Veterinary Clinics of North America Exotic Animal Practice*, edited by DN Phalen 3(2): 513–17.

Pye, GW. 2001. Marsupial, insectivore, and chiropteran anesthesia. In *The Veterinary Clinics of North America Exotic Animal Practice*, edited by DL Heard 4(1):211–37.

Pye, GW, Carpenter, JW. 1999. A guide to medicine and surgery in sugar gliders. *Veterinary Medicine*, Oct., 891–905.

Smith, MJ. 1984. *The reproductive system and paracloacal glands of Petaurus breviceps and Gymnobelideus leadbeateri (Marsupalia: Petauridae)*, edited by PA Smith, ID Hume. Australian Mammal Society. Sydney, Australia.

Wallach, JD, Boever, WJ. 1983. *Diseases of exotic animals medical and surgical management*. Philadelphia, PA: W.B. Saunders Co.

Williams, CSF. 1976. *Practical guide to laboratory animals*. Saint Louis, MO: C.V. Mosby, Co.

CHAPTER FOURTEEN

The Role of the Veterinary Technician in Wildlife Rehabilitation

Melanie Haire

INTRODUCTION

Wildlife rehabilitation is the process of rescuing, raising, and treating orphaned, diseased, displaced, or injured wild animals with a goal of releasing them back to their natural habitats. For rehabilitation to be deemed successful, these released animals must be able to truly function as wild animals. This includes being able to recognize and obtain the appropriate foods, select mates of their own species and reproduce, and show the appropriate fear of potential dangers (people, cars, dogs, etc.) (Pokras 1995).

The veterinary technician is on the front line for receiving injured and/or orphaned wildlife. A background in veterinary medicine and animal husbandry makes veterinary technicians perfect candidates for this rewarding endeavor. If fact, the general public often assumes that the veterinary technician is knowledgeable about all species. This assumption could be detrimental to the wild animal's welfare if the technician does not have access to the proper instruction, facilities, and materials needed to care for these unique individuals.

This chapter is a compilation of pertinent information that will provide the veterinary technician with the resources and guidelines needed to provide temporary care for many of the wildlife species that are encountered in veterinary hospitals today. The chapter includes charts, instructional articles, networking contacts, product sources, suggested readings, and references taken from numerous literary sources on the topic of rehabilitation of North American wildlife. Interested technicians should note there are many books, seminars, web groups, and related organizational memberships available for anyone interested in quality wildlife care and a list of a suggested few is provided in appendix 11.

The information in this chapter is primarily to be used as a starting reference point for the wild animal care technician working in a small animal clinic. It provides immediate information that can be used until more detailed information is obtained or the animal is transferred from the veterinary clinic to a licensed rehabilitator for long-term care and release.

GETTING STARTED

For a veterinary technician, the level of involvement in wildlife rehabilitation can range from the care of an occasional orphan discovered by a hospital client to a career on staff at a wildlife center. The technician can rehabilitate wild animals as a full-time occupation, as a volunteer at a wildlife center, on the job at a veterinary clinic, or at home in addition to a separate career. Many zoological parks and aquariums also provide care to injured and orphaned wildlife and have separate facilities and staff designated for such activity.

Although the numbers and types of animals received by different wildlife technicians will vary, legal obligations are relatively consistent. To keep or possess in captivity any sick, orphaned, or injured wildlife, one must first obtain a wildlife rehabilitation permit from the state and/or federal government. Everyone, including the veterinarian, must have his or her own permit or be listed on someone else's permit to rehabilitate wildlife. Each state has its own laws and requirements but most require a permit to work with any indigenous species. A federal permit is required in addition to a state permit to work with migratory birds. A list of governmental departments that issue applications and permits is provided in appendix 1 at the back of this book. The permitee is responsible for knowing what species are covered on the permit and their individual regulations. The rehabilitator is responsible for keeping records on each animal and knowing its current listed status (non-threatened versus endangered).

It is very important for anyone doing rehabilitation to build a reference library. The collection should contain literature on three basic topics: natural history, wildlife rehabilitation, and veterinary medicine as rehabilitation, which is a combination of all three. The veterinary technician should always keep in mind, when reading articles and talking to other rehabilitators, that there is more than one way to do things. New information is always coming out and it is the veterinary technician's responsibility to keep current as well as to learn to recognize what techniques might work better in different situations. Common sense and experience are the best ways to sort out contradictory suggestions and inaccurate information.

Networking with other rehabilitators is one of the most important sources for information. A list can be obtained from your state's special permits department with the names and contact numbers of all the rehabilitators in your state. These contacts can prove helpful for answering questions as they arise, helping to place animals that aren't covered by your permit, placing animals when the clinic has reached a full capacity, and building a network team to help with long-term animal care and releases.

REHABILITATING WILDLIFE IN A SMALL ANIMAL VETERINARY HOSPITAL

If the staff at a veterinary practice is interested in wildlife rehabilitation, it needs to establish a set of protocols. To accomplish this, the staff needs to first understand all that is involved. Rehabilitation can be both expensive and time-consuming. Profit making is not a valid or realistic reason to do rehabilitation. Currently there is no monetary assistance provided by any governmental departments to cover or reimburse rehabilitators for the costs of wildlife care.

Another crucial and difficult point that needs to be understood and accepted is that half of the animals that come in for rehabilitation will die or need to be euthanized. This is often extremely taxing emotionally on veterinary personnel, people who chose their profession in order to save lives. Deciding to euthanize an animal that could otherwise be saved but not returned to the wild with a good quality of life (such as releasing a one-legged hawk) may just be too hard for some individuals. Euthanasia is never an easy choice but keeping a wild animal alive because one "can not handle" putting it to sleep is selfish and inhumane. Occasionally, nonreleasable wildlife can be placed in appropriate educational facilities but quality of life should always be the highest priority.

Another issue concerns zoonotic diseases and learning to recognize them. Injured wildlife may expose hospital staff and animals to new risks. Proper personal hygiene as well as facility disinfecting techniques and protocols are critically important. Separate housing areas and separate clothing available for these areas provide safeguards against infectious or zoonotic cases. One method is to always treat the sick animals last so as not to transmit diseases to any other patient.

Hospital staff that has any contact with the wildlife should consider having the appropriate prophylactic vaccinations, such as tetanus and rabies, to protect them. Consultation with a personal physician is recommended.

Despite these cautions, there are many reasons to consider this volunteer work. It generates good clinic PR, provides a valuable service to the community and the clinic's clientele, is a kind act of giving something back to nature, and offers a personal reward for giving a living creature a second chance that it otherwise may not have had. Veterinarians benefit by gaining skill at performing new procedures (i.e., IM pin in an owl) by first learning on wildlife patients. Veterinary technicians can gain valuable experience in exotic animal handling from wildlife work such as restraint, anesthesia, blood collecting, bandaging, radiology, and necropsy.

CLINIC PROTOCOLS

Selecting Types of Wildlife to Care For
If the decision to do rehabilitation is made, clinic procedures and protocols must be clear and written down. Among the decisions to make are what types and how many animals the practice can reasonably take in. Taking in more animals or more species than personnel are prepared to properly and safely handle can easily overwhelm a clinic. One way to set limits is to specialize in a particular species or area (i.e., take in only birds of prey or injured wildlife, no orphans, etc.) and refer the other calls to another qualified recipient.

Above all, the motto "Do No Harm" should always be remembered when working with animal patients and wildlife is no exception. Wildlife rehabilitation should not be attempted at a clinic without sufficient staff to do the feedings, treatments, cage cleanings, and so forth, as the animals will be the ones that suffer. The ability to realize one's limits shows professionalism. Hospital managers and owners need to make a clear decision about animal limits based on costs and expenses. Staffing and other business costs are very real factors that should be discussed ahead of time to help avoid staff "burn out" or resentment.

Stabilization or Long-Term Rehabilitation—An Important Decision

Temporary stabilization verses long-term care should be determined by examining the layout of the buildings and grounds, available facilities, and the number and experience of participating staff. Barking dogs, staring cats, ringing phones, and exposure to people are unacceptable conditions for long-term rehabilitation. A treatment room might be a marginally acceptable area to keep an orphaned 2-week-old squirrel (both eyes and ears are closed at 2 weeks) but not a high-stress, imprintable, or easily habituated animal such as a deer fawn or raptor. Very few veterinary hospitals have flight cages of appropriate sizes and materials to adequately recondition a red-tailed hawk for release. Wildlife must be respected as wild and provided with suitable housing to reduce additional stress and fear and to promote natural behaviors that are necessary for successful release.

If there is no dedicated space for them, the clinic should provide temporary care only until the animal is stable and can be safely transferred to another rehabilitator. Veterinary hospitals without adequate facilities for rehabilitation can still perform a vital function for wildlife by becoming a drop-off and/or referral site for the public. This arrangement can benefit both the animal, by providing it proper temporary care away from the well-intentioned, but often detrimental, handling of the rescuer, and the rehabilitator by providing a valuable time-saver of a one stop "pick-up" location.

Oftentimes the single most crucial role for the technician in a veterinary practice is simply to give the public accurate names and phone numbers of the appropriate rehabilitator. Putting the public in direct communication with the rehabilitation facility that will provide the long-term care can eliminate the sometimes-fatal animal stress and delay of using the hospital as a drop-off site. This system allows the rehabilitator to be the clearing point and to have the opportunity to advise the finder how to return the animal if care is not truly needed or to have the caller transport the needy animal directly to the appropriate care provider. If the caller is willing to bring the animal to the clinic, chances are the caller will be willing to transport the animal directly to the rehabilitator. This method promotes the best use of time for both the veterinary staff and rehabilitators, thus allowing the medical personnel to best utilize their valuable expertise by caring mainly for the injured wild patients that must receive immediate medical attention.

Whether a hospital chooses to be a drop-off site, a referral center, or both, a current list of participating rehabilitators' names, locations, phone numbers, and species covered under each permit is a prerequisite. A prearranged plan for informing rehabilitators when a pick up or transport needs to be scheduled is a must to prevent unnecessary and often detrimental time delays before an animal can receive adequate care.

On the other hand, if the practice can provide adequate staff time and housing for the wildlife patients, then the hospital can consider becoming more involved in longer-term care such as surgery, wound care, emaciation, and hand rearing.

Choose your hospital's role wisely putting the animal's best interest foremost in the decision-making process.

Euthanasia

Before receiving animals, the hospital must have a clear euthanasia policy. Who will make the decision and do the actual procedure, what techniques will be used, and what criteria are used should be included in these protocols. There is a section on nonreleasable criteria and euthanasia later in this chapter to help with this difficult topic.

Phone Protocols

So often overlooked, one of the most important areas in which the wildlife veterinary clinic personnel must be trained is the telephone procedure. Posting a clear protocol for handling wildlife calls near every phone will help ensure that the information received is accurate and consistent. The development of a wildlife phone call protocol should be a combined effort between the veterinary staff and the participating wildlife rehabilitators. Many animals come into rehabilitation that never should have been removed from the spot in which they were found. Educating the public is part of the responsibility of anyone participating in wildlife rehabilitation. Taking proper animal history information before the animal is even touched will drastically reduce the number of "orphans" that are kidnapped and end up needing to be hand raised, thus reducing wasted time, money, and energy.

The caller should be asked if the animal appears to be orphaned or injured. What brought the finder to this conclusion? Many times it turns out that a little education in animal natural behavior can turn a "needy" or "nuisance" animal call into a lesson in living with wildlife. If the animal does appear to need assistance and the caller cannot handle it, advise the person to bring it in. One should never instruct or allow the caller to take care of the foundling himself or herself. If the caller cannot bring the animal in to the clinic, the caller should be provided with phone numbers from the contact list for a rehabilitator, rescue volunteer, or a wildlife center in the caller's area.

Handling Phone Calls

In most instances, if an adult wild animal can be caught and picked up by a person, it has sustained some type of injury, shock, or is sick and is in need of some type of rehabilitation.

   Conditions that require immediate medical attention include:

- Unconsciousness
- Bleeding
- Cold body temperature
- Open fracture
- Weakness, inability to stand (emaciated)
- Head swelling
- Head/eye twitching
- Eyes closed or matted shut
- Shock
- Puncture wounds from cat/dog bite
- Broken bones
- Flies, fly larva, or eggs present

   If the animal found is an infant, have the caller describe the baby and its condition. It should be determined if the animal is truly an orphan. If warm, strong, and apparently healthy, the baby is probably not an orphan and every attempt should be made to return it to its mother or nest. If the baby is cold, weak, emaciated, or if there are dead siblings nearby, the animal is probably orphaned. *Mother animals do not abandon their young because humans have touched them.*

Baby Songbirds

If the bird is naked or has a few body feathers but no tail feathers, the baby should be put back in the nest if at all possible. If the nest cannot be reached, instruct the caller to hang a homemade nest made from a basket or container near the old nest. The "surrogate" nest should be placed up off of the ground and protected from direct sunlight and rain. If the mother does not return by dark, advise the caller to bring the baby in to the clinic. If the bird has body feathers with one inch or longer tail feathers, is hopping around and chirping, it is probably a fledgling. These youngsters have left the nest but the parents are still providing them with food. Instruct the caller to look around for a parent bird. If the baby is picked up and it vocalizes and attracts an adult bird's attention, leave it alone. If there are no parent birds in sight, the bird should be

left and checked on several hours later. It may take 3–4 days for a "grounded" fledgling to learn to fly but a healthy one should be active, very mobile, and left where it was found.

Baby Raptors

If the nestling has eyes closed or has no feathers, return it to the nest if at all possible or make a surrogate nest. If the juvenile is hopping around or perching, has wing feathers and a short tail, it should be left alone. "Branchers" are young raptors that have left the nest but cannot yet fly. Both parents are still providing care to these birds on the ground or in low trees and shrubs. The only time to bring in a nestling raptor is if the caller cannot return it to its nest or secure a surrogate nest to the nesting tree. Refer the caller to a raptor rehabilitator for further instructions on how to replace a baby in its nest or make a surrogate one.

Baby Squirrels

Young squirrels are independent when they are about half the size of the adult and have bushy tails. If the baby does not yet have a fluffy tail, is crying or is cold, it might be orphaned. Mother squirrels often move their babies from nest to nest so a baby found at the base of a tree is not automatically an orphan. Even if there is no adult squirrel visible but the caller can stay nearby and watch for the mother, leave the baby unmoved. If the caller cannot watch, advise the caller to tie a small basket or box up off of the ground, with the baby inside, onto the possible nest tree out of reach of ground predators. The caller or someone must check the nest before dark and make sure that the infant has been reclaimed. If it is still in the box by dark, have the caller bring it in. Infant squirrels make a very high-pitched squeal or "chirp" when they are frightened, hungry, or cold and the mother can hear it from quite a distance.

Baby Rabbits

Baby cottontail rabbits should be left alone if uninjured and found in the nest. Even if the nest has been disturbed, the mother will usually come back. The deciding factor seems to be the extent of the nest disturbance. If the nest has sustained minimal disturbance of the nesting material, the babies should be covered back up and left alone. If the nest site has been destroyed or dug up by a predator, the mother may not come back. An attempt can be made to put the nest back together and a string placed on top of the nest. If, by morning, the string has been disturbed and the babies are warm and plump, the mother has come back to feed them. However, if the string is undisturbed over night or the babies are cold or look thin, the babies should be brought in. If the location of the nest is unknown and the baby's eyes are closed, it should be brought in. But if the young rabbit's eyes are open and its ears are upright and capable of rotating, they should be left undisturbed. Mother rabbits will not pick up and carry a baby back to the nest. Infants only feed at dusk and dawn and the mother will leave the nest in between feedings but stay nearby. Due to rabbits' secretive nature and infrequent visits to their nests, one should not automatically assume the babies are orphaned.

Baby Opossums

If an infant opossum is found that is less than 6 inches long and alone advise the caller to bring it in. Baby opossums that are old enough to leave the mother's pouch should cling to the mother's coat or follow along behind her. If they fall off or cannot keep up, they are sometimes left behind.

Baby Deer

Fawns should be left alone unless injured. The doe often leaves the fawn alone for hours at a time while she feeds.

Baby Raccoons

Baby raccoons are usually on their own by the time they are 4–5 months old and weigh 8–12 pounds. If a younger raccoon is discovered alone, the caller should leave the youngster where it was found and check on it periodically. Although nocturnal, the mother raccoon will look for her missing infant during the daytime as well as during the nighttime. If 24 hours passes with no sign of the mother, the licensed rabies vector rehabilitator should be called for instructions. One should be careful in advising the public to handle any rabies vector species.

Reuniting diurnal species' (active during the day) babies during the day light hours and nocturnal species' (active at night) babies during the night should be practiced. If the infant gets cold while waiting for the parent, a warm water bottle should be provided and placed with the baby. It may take several hours for a mother to reclaim its baby. If a diurnal species is found at night, it may be worth a try in the morning to reunite it with its parent.

Orphans that are brought in to the hospital will probably need to be taken home at night by a caretaker and brought back in the morning in order to provide the young animals with enough nourishment.

If the caller wants to try to take care of the animal themselves, explain to them why that is not in the animal's best interest. Some points to be made to argue this point include:

1. The problems of *imprinting*—the rehabilitators probably have more infants of the same species that they can put with the caller's animal and raise together as siblings.
2. The possibility of *zoonotic* or *infectious diseases*.
3. It is *illegal* for them to care for the animal without a permit.
4. Using the *wrong formula* or feeding technique can cause harm to or even the death of the animal.
5. Hand raising is very *time-consuming*—they should be given an idea of how often the animal needs to eat and how long the care time may be.
6. Acquiring and preparing the proper foods may be *difficult, expensive,* and *not always pleasant* (mealworms, grubs, killing mice, etc.).

If the caller has a raccoon, fox, bear, bobcat, owl, hawk, or any rabies vector species, or potentially dangerous animal, the name and phone number should be taken immediately in case he or she decides to keep it and not bring it in. This information should then be turned over to the appropriate authorities (county game protector, federal wildlife agent, etc.).

INTAKE PROCEDURES

Under no circumstances should animals be handled or looked at in between the necessary feedings and treatments intervals. This rule needs to begin in the reception room with the arrival of the animal. Without lifting the lid or opening the transport cage, the receptionist should immediately transport the animal to the examination area while the rescuer fills out an intake form. This form should include the rescuer's name, address, phone number, animal type and numbers, and finally the animal's circumstances for needing care. A detailed account of how, when, and where the animal was found can help determine the nature of the animal's problem. Also, information should be recorded as to how long the rescuer had the animal and if he or she attempted to medicate or feed the patient. This information helps the caretaker to investigate what happened to the animal and what the correct form of treatment should be. This form should be used as one would a pet's chart and record the physical exam findings, treatments, observations, and final disposition. The state and/or federal permit issuing departments also require this information. A copy should be made and turned in to the rehabilitator who receives the animal to provide the new caretaker with all the available information. The original copy should be filed at the facility and used to help make the end-of-year report required by most states (see appendix 2).

Meanwhile, back in the treatment room, the animal should have a quick visual exam to check for emergency conditions such as shock, hypothermia, or bleeding. If the animal appears stable and is not in a critical position, the animal should be allowed a little time to calm down from the previous handling and car ride before pulling it out of the box.

ETHICAL CONSIDERATIONS AND REDUCING STRESS IN CAPTIVE WILDLIFE

"It is incumbent upon a person who takes the responsibility of manipulating an animal's life to be concerned for its feelings, the infliction of pain, and the psychological upsets that may occur from such manipulation" (Fowler 1986).

The wild nature of these animals should always be respected and one should be sensitive to the unique needs of these unusual patients. The number-one reason wild animals under human care die is from stress. All sick or injured animals need their strength to recover and cannot afford to use it up in attempts to escape from captive stress. Learning to recognize signs of early stress, with each species as well as between individuals, may possibly prevent or at least reduce such fatalities. Many birds have a natural escape pattern of moving up and away from danger and they feel threatened if they are housed down low and looked at from above. Typically, they are calmer if their cage is placed level with or above human eye level.

All prey animals fear direct eye contact or being stared or even looked at. One should consider the animal's viewpoint as typically the first thing a predator does while hunting is to keep its eye on the prey and then move directly toward it. When humans do this, it mimics the predator's behavior and frightens the animal. When walking past wildlife cages, it is a good idea to look in another direction.

Housing for different species is discussed further in each of their sections but a note on stress-reducing environmental factors should be mentioned here. Within each animal's enclosure, using something natural and familiar to the patient will help decrease stress. Housing away from sight or sound of predators (humans, domestic animals, wild predators—i.e., avoid housing hawks and cottontails in the same

room) is of foremost importance. Second, providing something of a natural setting is calming to many species of captive wildlife. Many bird species need to feel hidden or protected from view by vegetated plant cover. By cutting a few small leafed branches off of a nearby tree or shrub and placing them inside the animal's enclosure (preferably before placing the animal inside), one can provide naturalistic hiding places for the recovering patient. Animals such as rabbits, squirrels, opossums, and chipmunks seek refuge by hiding under or inside something that cannot be seen through. Providing these types of patients with a nest box, hollow log, plastic tube, or even layers of cloth that they can burrow in will increase their sense of security and well-being as well as the chance of keeping them alive. Animals also equate having choices with comfort. Offering a bird several perches provides them with the opportunity to feel as if they have some control in their strange new captive world.

INITIAL EXAM

The visual exam is the first part and perhaps one of the most important parts of the examination. Before even touching the patient, observe its posture, color, behavior, and stool quality. Look for discharges, level of alertness, body conditioning, head tilts, nystagmus, limping, or wing droops. Record all observations either on the intake sheet or on the examination form, whichever one the hospital's wildlife protocol calls for. There is an example of each form provided in appendix 2. Many of these signs are not as obvious once the animal has been picked up and is held in an unnatural position. Also, an animal will try its best to conceal these "signs of weakness" to a predator if it knows it is being watched, so try to be sly about the visual exam. Sometimes using binoculars and watching from across the room gets the best results.

When performing the hands-on part of the examination, the examiner should be swift and thorough, reducing the handling time and the animal's psychological stress. Restraint should be performed on the animal quickly and with confidence, without a lot of repositioning. Prey animals view a predator's grip as fatal and frequent shifting of the animal's position only draws out the suffering.

Use of a systematic approach when doing exams insures that no area gets overlooked. Even though it may be obvious that the patient has a wing injury the exam should be performed in a systematic manner and all the animal's systems evaluated in order. The animal's eyes, ears, mouth, nose, skin turgor, limbs, body condition, and reflexes should be checked. Respiratory sounds should be observed and noted as well as any signs of bleeding. All anticipated supplies and medications must be ready before handling the animal so the patient does not have to wait unnecessarily. It is not uncommon to find secondary problems days later because they were initially overlooked due to the examiner's mistake of starting right at the big problem and then forgetting to follow through with the rest of the exam.

Restraining and examination techniques should be practiced as often as possible as this is the only way to become fast and efficient. Examine healthy live animals whenever possible to become familiar with "normals" in order to recognize the "abnormals." Information obtained from examining dead animals should not be underestimated. One can practice restraint positions, palpation, injection training, IO or IV catheter placement, bandaging, tube feeding, necropsy, and even surgical techniques on deceased patients.

CHOOSING TREATMENT ROUTES

When choosing appropriate treatment regimens, one should take into consideration the differences between the wild animal patient versus the domestic animals that are more routinely worked with. Domesticated animals can withstand more extensive procedures done with manual restraint alone. On the other hand, the use of anesthesia (i.e., isoflurane) should be considered when obtaining quality radiographs or performing even minor but painful procedures on wildlife.

Routes and frequencies of medication need to be carefully compared as well. Oral medications should be chosen, when appropriate, that can be injected into food items and fed to the patient. For example, enrofloxacin can be injected into a cricket and fed to a blue jay, or into a minnow and be fed to a heron. Every effort should be made to weigh the stress of handling and administering treatments against the benefits they provide. Although the first treatment of choice may recommend BID-TID treatments, realize that with wildlife this may not always be practical or possible. Wildlife medicine is a balance between what is effective and what the patient can tolerate. This sometimes calls for some creative medicine delivery ideas. Raptors can receive treatments of dexamethasone, LRS, vitamins, or antibiotics injected into a small or pinkie mouse that the bird can swallow whole

at its normal eating time. Some pediatric suspensions have a more palatable taste and may be more readily eaten either right out of the medicine dropper or when mixed in with a favorite food item (i.e., Clavamox drops mixed in with fruit yogurt offered to an opossum). Another option is to have, frequently used, oral medications specially flavored or concentrated at a compounding pharmacy. Banana flavored dewormers, meat flavored antibiotics, alfalfa flavored anti-inflammatories just to name a few, have been very useful in both zoological and wildlife medicine.

Animals that do not swallow their food whole or eat food items in which medications are not easily hidden (i.e., adult squirrels, rabbits) may need to be hand injected. In these cases, effective medications with the longest action time to reduce multiple daily "catch ups" should be chosen. Ideally, medications that need to be given only once daily should be sought.

In conclusion, it is not the role of veterinarians to know the best way to rehabilitate every wild animal. Their expertise is in anatomy, surgery, diagnostics, and treatment, not necessarily the natural history and behavior patterns of a southern flying squirrel. To assist the veterinarian in making more informed decisions, the technician should collect as much information as possible pertaining to the types of wildlife that the clinic decides to work with. Teamwork is crucial and the combined efforts of many individuals make up the best rehabilitation team. Each wildlife technician needs to form good working relationships with several veterinarians. One veterinarian cannot be expected to look at every baby squirrel, but can advise on general treatment regimes and drug dosages.

A technician should always realize his or her limits and should never feel as if networking makes one look incapable. Utilizing the experience of others is the best way to learn and can also prevent animals from suffering unnecessarily. No one should ever reinvent the wheel at the animal's expense. Always remember that the ultimate goal is to release the animal back into the wild with the best possible chance of survival. A technician can offer this to each and every animal that he/she works with if he/she learns to recognize when someone else may be more qualified. This may even mean transferring the animal to another person who may have a better rehabilitation setup, more experience or time, animal conspecifics, or better release sites.

While wildlife rehabilitation can be difficult, time-consuming, expensive, and many times downright frustrating, the benefits and personal rewards gained from this unselfish kind deed can be life changing.

RELEASE CRITERIA VERSUS EUTHANASIA

Some animals arrive at the clinic with injuries that warrant euthanasia. Other injuries and illnesses may not present themselves as life threatening but in fact are just as profound in terms of release and survivability in the wild. The veterinary technician should learn to recognize these less-obvious conditions that will ultimately lead to death of the animal if released back into the wild.

Merely saving a life for survival in captivity is not the goal. The animal must be capable of recognizing, obtaining, and processing food; recognizing and evading or defending against predators; acquiring shelter; acquiring and defending territories; performing normal seasonal movements and dispersal; and be capable of normal socialization with conspecifics (Diehl & Stokhaug 1991). Each type of animal, depending on its natural history and what it needs to do to survive, has different criteria, so a handicap considered relatively minor for one species may be life threatening to another. For instance, a bird of prey must be capable of hunting and catching prey animals that may be as quick and fast as they themselves are. If a Cooper's hawk was released with any degree of flight defect, it would not be able to obtain prey that is often caught in midair. On the other hand, a mallard duck with a slight wing defect but flight capability, may be considered for release because it acquires its food while swimming and dabbling in the water, breeds in the water, and can also escape predators by diving as well as flying. Also, in some areas mallards do not have to migrate so the need to fly great distances would also be reduced. Another example would be of an animal with impaired vision. An animal that does not depend on excellent sight to obtain food and avoid predation could also be considered releasable. For instance, a one-eyed, adult opossum might be considered releasable because in the wild it has few predators and relies on its sense of smell to find food items (carrion, insects, vegetation) that do not require a great deal of visual acuity to acquire. However, a fox needs perfect vision to obtain its mainstay diet of live and very quick prey animals such as mice, chipmunks, birds, and rabbits.

The species of the animal involved should also be considered. An opossum with a fractured limb has a good chance for recovery. Opossums tend to tolerate bandages and splints well plus they are relatively inactive, which provides for optimal recovery. A deer with a fractured limb, on the other hand is a challenge. Many hospitals or centers do not have the facilities to deal with an injured deer. At best, these animals, even with adequate facilities, are difficult to maintain in captivity and they tend to further injure themselves trying to escape.

The potential for current handicaps to create new problems for an animal must be considered. For example, is a one-footed bird likely to develop bumblefoot or frostbite on the remaining foot? The bottom line is that the animal must have enough of the equipment and capabilities necessary to survive by means natural to its species if it is to be released (Diehl & Stokhaug 1991).

Being a careful observer, understanding the animal's natural history, performing a thorough physical exam and being knowledgeable of the release requirements could spare an animal hours or days of suffering. Each animal deserves a careful and unbiased evaluation. If the releasability is in question, contact a rehabilitator immediately so a speedy decision can be made and the animal can begin to receive the treatment it deserves whether it turns out to be freedom by release or euthanasia.

Situations that may require euthanasia include:

- Compound or open fracture more than 48 hours old. These old injuries rarely can be properly repaired and the animal would lose full function of the limb making the animal nonreleasable.
- Complete loss of sight or hearing in any animal.
- Impaired vision in both eyes. Depending on the species, some animals can be considered for release if only one eye is affected.
- Nocturnal owls with hearing impairment.
- Amputated wings or legs: "Any birds that have sustained injuries requiring amputation of a wing at the elbow (humero-ulnar) or above, a leg or a foot ... should be euthanized" (U.S. Fish & Wildlife—Rehabilitation regulation 50 CFR 21.27 #8). No animal should be put through the stress and pain of surgery only to be euthanized later because it can never be released.
- Raptors need unimpaired function of their feet to grasp, kill, and carry prey; therefore any injury involving the unilateral loss of both the hallux (digit 1) and digit 2 on the same foot or the bilateral loss of both hallux.
- Fractures involving the wing or leg joints (or very near the joint) will never heal sufficiently enough for the animal to have normal use of the limb. The joint will heal by fusing in place and not allow for normal movement thus preventing the animal from flying or walking.
- Fractures with a significant piece of bone missing.

- Some wing fractures can heal out of alignment and result in a wing droop. Although flight may be possible, the wing cannot be allowed to drag on the perch/ground. The feather tips will become damaged and soiled and over time the bird may become nonflighted or develop an infection in the damaged follicles.
- Head trauma that results in abnormal posture in any animal.
- Back injuries that have resulted in loss of limb function in any animal.
- Animals imprinted on humans should never be released. These animals are not able to behaviorally fit into their own natural population and they could be dangerous to the public.
- Animals that have a highly incurable infectious disease.
- A rabies vector species from a rabies endemic area (follow current state guidelines) should never be released.
- Mammals with two or more nonfunctional legs.
- Rodents or rabbits with a fractured jaw or any facial injury leaving permanently unaligned incisors. (Opposing incisor teeth must be able to be normally worn down or they will overgrow and eventually kill the animal.)

Nonreleasable animals can sometimes be placed in an approved educational, research program or breeding facility. There are now several nonreleasable animal placement programs designed to help place these animals. Do not euthanize an endangered species without first contacting your local and federal authorities for authorization.

"We look to wildlife for the rules that we follow. Wildlife leads a life of quality, or it isn't alive—it's one or the other for wildlife" (Moore & Joosten 1995a).

IMPRINTING AND TAMING

Imprinting

The veterinary technician's code of ethics to "do no harm" could not be more pertinent to this subject. Understanding the definitions and what these two things mean to a wild animal under a technician's care can make the difference between life and death.

Imprinting is a socialization process by which an individual animal learns to identify itself with a species. This is a natural psychological process, which occurs early in life, during a restricted period of time called a critical period. Once this has occurred, the animal now identifies with the adult of its own species and learns by imitation and observation the methods for acquiring shelter, food, mates, and proper behaviors.

The route in which a mammal, bird, or reptile imprints is different and still not completely understood. In the area of wildlife rehabilitation, imprinting is probably only relevant to birds. The critical periods for most species of birds have not yet been determined. With ducks and geese it occurs within the day of hatching and with smaller raptor species between day 8 and 21 after hatching. Larger raptor species usually imprint between day 12 and 28. The variations of days between species are largely due to their different rates of development. The most important period seems to be when the bird's visual focus develops. Before their eyes open, neonates also imprint on their parents' calls and vocalizations.

What this all means for the wildlife caregiver is that the animal could be improperly imprinted on humans if a great deal of care is not taken. Imprinting is not believed to be reversible so if the process is transferred to a person the animal will have a poor chance to survive. Birds that do not imprint on their own species will lack the survival skills they need, will not reproduce in the wild, and are often killed outright by their own species. A bird that has imprinted on a human is not releasable and will probably need to be euthanized.

To reduce the chances of improper imprinting, the baby should be returned to its nest and/or parents if at all possible. Sometimes orphans can be placed in foster nests and raised with like species of similar age. Many rehabilitation centers have nonreleasable surrogate parents (most commonly birds of prey) that raise same species' orphans that are not their own. If that is not possible, care should be taken to be sure all animals are raised with at least one other member of the same-aged species. Rehabilitators and nature centers that have permanent nonreleasable raptors can also house the young beside the adults to allow the juveniles a chance to observe, listen, interact, and possibly imitate the same species adult. With some birds, a mirror may be helpful if the baby has no nest mates.

Birds (especially raptors) should be fed during their critical period, from behind a curtain-type blind or while wearing a hooded poncho with a mask to hide the human shape. By also using a hand puppet shaped like the head of the adult to feed raptor chicks, the young do not associate food with humans. Wildlife should be handled as little as possible, with limited talking, and housed out of sight or sound of humans, dogs, cats, and pet birds.

Taming

Taming is the process of an animal becoming socialized to humans by association with foods or other comforts over a prolonged period of time (Beaver 1984). Baby animals in a wide range of species are especially easy to tame. These tame animals have properly imprinted and identify with their own species but socialize with humans. Taming differs from imprinting in that the bond to humans is not as strong, takes longer to establish, and is more readily lost once human contact no longer occurs (Klinghammer 1991). The lack of fear tame animals show toward humans often leads to their deaths. These animals often get shot or trapped as few people trust a "friendly raccoon" and often misinterpret it to be diseased or rabid. Tame game species are often easy targets for hunters and trappers. Tame animals are also unsuitable for release due to possible dangerous encounters with humans. This process is usually reversible but should be done by a person other than the one who caused it, before the animal is released. Taming can be avoided by minimizing human contact, especially human-associated positive stimuli such as food (Diehl & Stokhaug 1991). Wild animals no longer requiring hand-feeding should never be fed by hand. Food should be scattered around the enclosure when animals are sleeping and not likely to see the provider (i.e., feed opossums and flying squirrels 1–2 hours before dark when they are still asleep and out of view).

It is critical that the distinction be made between a true human imprint and a tamed animal with regard to the release potential. The animal's history must be traceable from the day it came in. Again, good record keeping is essential as it will help determine if improper imprinting is even a possibility. If the animal can be proven to be tame but not imprinted on humans, it may still have a chance to be released.

TRANSPORTING WILDLIFE

A variety of containers can be used to transport wildlife. The two main considerations for choosing the appropriate transport container are the animal's safety and comfort. If someone is on the phone asking for advise on how to bring an animal in to the clinic, someone should always ask for information about the animal such as, what type of animal is it, is it conscious, and is it a baby or adult? Each call should be taken on a case-by-case basis to determine what is the safest way to capture and transport each animal. After determining that the animal needs assistance, it should also be determined if the caller has the tools on hand to safely get the animal into the transport container, such as gloves, a blanket, or a broom. The caller's confidence and experience level should be ascertained before even suggesting that he or she attempt to handle a potentially dangerous animal. Human safety comes first. If in doubt, referring the caller directly to the rehabilitator may be the safest thing to do.

After capture an animal should be placed in a suitable lidded container with holes and kept in a quiet area before and during the transport. Unnecessary talking or playing the radio in the vehicle during transport should be avoided. Extreme temperatures should also be avoided by providing ventilation, shade from the sun, or extra heat if needed. Cardboard boxes make good temporary cages and can be quickly altered to suit many different types of animals. Ideally, the size of the container should be just large enough for the animal to comfortably fit into but not large enough for a great deal of activity. Cardboard boxes and pet carriers make the best types of transport containers because they offer solid sides and tops, which reduce visual stress for the patient and are also disposable after use. Placing wildlife in a clear aquarium or plastic tote should only be done if there is a towel or blanket available to cover the enclosure to block out light and remove visual stimuli.

Proper nonslip material should be placed on the enclosure bottom to ensure proper footing and reduce stress as a result of slipping and sliding during the transport. Also the cage should be secured down so it does not slide or flip over. No food or water should be provided during the time of the transport because the animals are usually too stressed to eat and the bowls often end up tipping over and spilling their contents getting the animal wet or dirty.

Adult Birds

Open-wire bird/rodent cages are not advisable for transporting because they need to be covered with a towel and the wire can be very damaging to the flight feathers. Songbirds can be placed in a wide open paper bag with the top rolled tightly shut and clipped with a paper clip or clothespin. Several pencil-sized air holes should be provided in the bag for fresh air and ventilation. Plastic pet carriers work well for waterfowl, raptors, and the larger songbird species (i.e., blue jays, robins), but care should be taken with the smaller species (i.e., wrens, warblers) that can fit through the holes on the cage door. Appropriate sized cardboard boxes work equally well for small sparrows on up to large herons.

Carpet pieces, paper towels, or cloth towels serve as good cage flooring. Newspaper is too slippery as is the plain plastic bottom of a pet carrier. Alert and standing adult birds might use a perch to stand on if it is securely fastened and of proportional size to the bird's foot size. Tightly wedging a tree branch down low inside of a box before placing the bird inside can give the animal an option to perch. Raptors need a branch about 2–3 inches in diameter to properly perch on.

Provide soft material (i.e., rolled towel) to prop the animal up on if it is not capable of standing on its own.

If the rescuer describes a heron-type bird, warn the person of the dangers of the spearlike beaks and advise them not to go near the bird without eye protection such as safety glasses.

If the caller describes a bird of prey, first warn them about the dangerous talons. It may be best to refer the caller directly to a raptor rehabilitator for an on-site rescue.

Baby Birds

Young featherless birds need supplemental heat and can be transported using a warm water bottle or a ziplock bag (double bagged to prevent leaks) filled with warm water placed under or next to the baby's enclosure. The nestling bird can be placed in a small box, berry basket, or any plastic margarine-sized container lined with nonscented toilet or facial tissues as nesting material. The artificial nest, not the infant itself, should be placed on the heat source to prevent the chance of skin burns. It should be kept in mind that these types of portable warming devices stay warm for only 30–60 minutes. Covering the nest/carrier with a light cloth reduces drafts and helps hold the warmth inside. These young animals need to be transferred as quickly as possible to prevent chilling or further dehydration.

If the baby's nest fell also, advise the rescuer against bringing it with the baby due to the strong possibility of unwanted parasites living in the nest.

Adult Mammals

A wire cage or live trap is suitable to transport an adult squirrel, raccoon, opossum, fox, or groundhog, to name a few. Most of these animals can chew out of cardboard or plastic kennels in a surprisingly short period of time. The transporter's safety is of foremost importance so do not advise them to put themselves at risk over the animal. Also be informed as to the status of rabies in the caller's area and of the vector species that carry the disease so the caller can be warned of any potential danger.

Injured medium to large mammals such as deer, coyotes, and bobcats may need chemical immobilization and special capture equipment, such as punch poles, dart guns, and snare poles, to prevent injury to the animal or the handler.

Flying squirrels and chipmunks are escape artists and need to be contained in a box or solid sided container with the lid taped or snapped shut. Instruct the caller to make the air holes on the lid only and no larger around than a pencil or they could chew and enlarge the air holes to escape through them.

The cage bottom should be lined with ravel-free cloth and the entire cage draped for privacy. The cloth inside the cage provides better footing and a layer to hide under, which greatly reduces their stress. The transporter can be advised to protect the vehicle's floor or seats by placing an old blanket, if available, down first before setting the cage inside. The rescuer should be warned to use caution when handling these potentially dangerous animals and their cages.

Baby Mammals

Cardboard boxes and pet carriers work well to transport these animals. Soft ravel-free cloth should be placed inside the cage and a heat source (warm water bottle) provided for hairless babies or those whose eyes are closed. The heat source should never go directly against the baby's skin but rather under the cage to warm up the cage bottom.

Turtles

Cardboard boxes or plastic buckets work for transporting these animals. Do not transport water turtles in a container filled with water because the turtle will bump against the sides of the container as it is moved about.

Snakes

Snakes are best transported in a pillowcase with the opening tied in a knot. The bag can then be placed into a box, cooler, or bucket. The handler should carry the bag by the tip of the knot because the snake could bite through the cloth bag. Snakes can also be gently swept with a broom into a lidded box or small trash can. Unless the caller has experience in identifying venomous snake species from nonvenomous ones, care should be taken in advising anyone to handle any snake. This may be a job for animal control or a reptile rehabilitator.

See appendix 3 for additional information on handling and restraint of wildlife species.

RAPTOR CARE

Birds of prey include eagles, falcons, condors, vultures, harrier, hawks, kites, osprey, owls, and the caracara. Raptors are legally protected by a number of federal acts such as the migratory bird treaty act of 1918, bald eagle protection act of 1940 and endangered species act of 1973. Many federal bird rehab permits do not automatically include birds of prey due to the special training and housing needed to work with these animals.

Raptor Handling
When handling any of these species of birds always keep in mind that their first line of defense is their talons. Be careful to safely secure the raptor's feet and legs before attempting to pick up or move the bird. Heavy gauntlet-type welding gloves, such as the type used for restraining aggressive cats, should be worn to catch a medium- to large-sized raptor. Small raptors such as screech owls and kestrels can be caught up using leather work gloves.

If a raptor feels trapped, it may either roll onto its back with feet up and talons ready or make a bold dash at its restrainer. A gloved hand should be kept ready at all times to deflect or grab such a bird in midair. If the bird flips onto its back, a rolled towel or a spare glove can be handed to it to grab with its feet and distract it long enough to allow a gloved hand to slip under the barrier and grab the animal by its legs.

To remove a raptor from a cage, one gloved hand should be used to block the bird from darting out around the other gloved hand as one reaches in. It is often helpful to drape a towel over the door to prevent the bird's from seeing a "get away" space around the restrainer's body. With medium and large birds of prey, it is best to grab both legs, up high against the bird's body, with one hand keeping a finger between the birds legs. Once the legs are both contained, the wings can be folded up against the body with the other hand as the bird is pulled out. Every attempt should be made to avoid allowing the bird to beat its wings against the cage as it is extracted through the door.

When only one leg is grabbed, the natural reaction of the raptor is to grab back at the handler with its free foot. If the raptor manages to talon and hold onto a glove either the restrainer or someone else must first fully extend the leg in order for the toes to be opened back up. Then one by one each nail is removed with care taken to locate each of the other needle sharp talons. It is very difficult to open up a foot on a raptor with a flexed leg.

Some birds will also attempt to bite, so securing the head or covering it with a towel may be necessary. The head must be secured when the eyes, mouth, nares, and ears are being examined. The handler needs to distract the bird with one hand and quickly grasp the head from behind with the other. Head restraint is accomplished by firmly holding the head between the thumb and index finger at the articulation of the mandible. Covering their eyes also tends to relax many raptor species and allows minor procedures to be more easily accomplished (giving injections, weighing, taking radiographs, or collecting blood). The use of an orthopedic stockinet to cover the head and body is another useful technique for raptor restraint when weighing. A Velcro strip can be used as leg restraints by first attaching around one leg, just above the feet, then wrapping around both legs.

If the bird is on the ground or in a large open-top box, a towel, blanket, or net can be draped over the bird and then the bird picked up after first feeling for and securing the legs through the draped material with a gloved hand. See figure 14.1.

Raptor Initial Exam
Birds of prey are most commonly brought into veterinary hospitals with wing and/or leg fractures due to

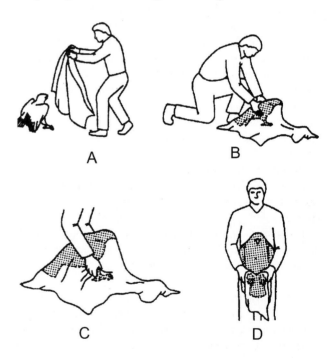

Fig. 14.1. Picking a raptor up from the ground. A. Blanket technique used to cover and catch a raptor. B. Covered raptor is initially grasped with both hands over back shoulders. C. Both hands secure legs just above the feet. D. Restrain and carrying method with raptor held between arms against handler's body. (Permission for drawing use granted by the National Wildlife Rehabilitators Association)

their frequency of colliding with motor vehicles. These birds tend to survive many of these collisions and due to their large size are more easily noticed along side the road and thus rescued by other passing motorists. Two other common presentations are head or eye injuries.

Some of these animals, when presented to the hospital, may be in shock and will need to be treated accordingly. Usually dexamethasone and lactated Ringer's solution is the treatment of choice but only after first checking with the veterinarian. During the initial examination on any wild animal, one should be quick but thorough. A systematic method of examination that covers the patient from head to toe in the shortest time possible should be developed. Decreasing the handling time will dramatically reduce the bird's stress and increase its survival chances. Any cold bird should be placed on or under heat to allow the body temperature to reach normal range (98°F–102°F) before continuing with the exam.

Since raptors receive most of their water intake from the prey they eat, they easily become dehydrated when they are undernourished. Signs of dehydration include sunken eyes and thick, cloudy strands of mucous in the mouth. These birds should to be immediately treated with warmed lactated Ringer's solution by the oral, subcutaneous, intravenous, or intraosseous routes. One method is to tube feed small amounts of lactated Ringer's solution with 5% dextrose into the bird's crop every 15 minutes for the first hour or two (see fig. 14.2).

Next, the bird should be examined for fractures by palpation and radiology. Many raptors will tolerate a quick radiograph without sedation if properly held to the table with a combination of manual and paper tape restraint. Any potentially repairable broken limbs should immediately be stabilized with the proper splints or bandages. A bandage should be chosen that immobilizes the joint above and below the fracture site. The figure-eight bandage is good for immobilizing the wing and then can be wrapped to the body to eliminate joint movement (see fig. 14.12).

If there is a fracture found in or very near any limb joint or if any two or more limbs contain a break, euthanasia should be strongly considered. These types of injuries often result in a nonreleasable animal and immediate euthanasia would be the most humane treatment. If the veterinarian is unsure of the releasability of any injured raptor, a raptor rehabilitator should be called first to help make the decision.

The bird's feather and muscle condition are two clues that are useful in determining the reason why the

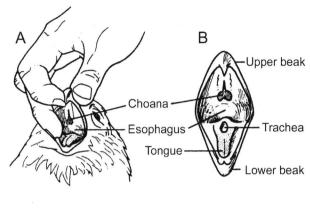

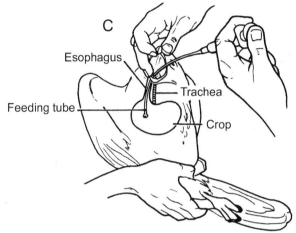

Fig. 14.2. *Anatomy of the avian oral cavity and technique for assisted feeding in birds. A. Beak is held open by placing a finger in the corner of the mouth. B. Close-up view of oral anatomy showing the esophagus at the back of the throat and trachea at the base of the tongue. C. Proper placement of feeding tube in crop. (Permission for drawing use granted by the Georgia Department of Natural Resources and Branson Ritchie, DVM, MS)*

bird may have come in. If the feathers are ragged and soiled, that is evidence that the bird has probably been "grounded" for a long period of time so any injury is not likely to be fresh and wounds should be examined for fly eggs or larva. Any raptor that has been on the ground for several days or more will be dehydrated and potentially emaciated since these birds are unable to acquire live prey without flight. Dark green mutes (feces) are another sign of starvation. The bird's keel (sternum) can be palpated with fingertips to help assess the bird's level of health. A thin or emaciated bird's keel will feel "sharp" to the touch meaning that the keel bone is prominent and the breast muscles are atrophied. See figure 14.3.

*Fig. 14.3. Subjective evaluation of a bird's condition based on pectoral muscle mass. **A.** Severe muscle atrophy indicating a substantial amount of weight loss. **B.** Moderate weight loss. **C.** Severe weight loss, mild muscle atrophy. **D.** Excellent condition with no detectable muscle atrophy. (Permission for drawing use granted by the Georgia Department of Natural Resources and Branson Ritchie, DVM, MS)*

Use a combination of physical condition, body weight, and degree of muscling on the keel to evaluate the bird.

Another all too common reason birds of prey end up in rehabilitation is gun shot injuries. Poisoning, whether intentional or unintentional, is also worth mentioning here because the veterinarian can sometimes determine toxicities with specific blood tests. Due to the nature of a raptor's eating habits, these birds may end up consuming a rodent or bird that ate poisoned bait and thus become secondarily poisoned. Emaciated juvenile birds often end up in hospitals and wildlife care centers during their first winter due to their inexperienced hunting skills and the difficulties of surviving without an established hunting territory in the months when prey is most scarce.

Once the bird has been examined, it should be weighed (ideally in grams) so the medication, fluids, and food dosing will be accurate. The animal's weight is often the best indicator of how it is doing overall after being admitted for medical care. Good medical records that include all procedures, treatments, food intake, and weights should be maintained daily. A copy of these records can be made to give to the rehabilitator when the bird is transferred.

All treatments should be done as quickly as possible and with minimal talking. If any food, fluids, or medications are needed to be given orally, this should be done last after everything else has been done (injections, radiographs, venipuncture, etc.) to lessen the chances of regurgitation.

IM injections can be given in the leg or breast muscle. SQ fluids can be administered in either the axilla (wing web), lateral flank, or inguinal areas, doses divided into several sites, to provide maintenance or mild dehydration fluids. Intraosseous (IO) fluids are most often delivered via sterile catheter placed into the hollow cavity of the distal ulna or tibia for severe dehydration. This technique is described in chapter 2 in this text. IV injections are given in the medial metatarsal or the right jugular vein. Once the patient is self-feeding, many medications can be injected or pilled into a food item that the bird can swallow whole, such as a pinkie or small mouse, and offered as part of the daily meal.

Raptor Caging

Most veterinary clinics can do short-term convalescent care with birds of prey but do not have the proper facilities for any long-term care or housing. All housing for raptors, as well as all wildlife, should be separate from the domestic patients and in a quiet area away from people and animal traffic.

Feathered healthy birds can be comfortably maintained at 60°F–85°F. Cages should have solid sides such as the stainless sterile hospital rack cages or a large plastic pet kennel. A towel should be draped over the inside of the door opening to provide a complete visual barrier for the patients and to prevent them from catching their wings on the vertical door bars. The cage size should be large enough to allow the bird of prey to stand, turn around, and step up on a perch without touching its head or tail feathers yet not big enough for the bird to fly within and potentially further injure itself. Newspapers are adequate for lining the bottom of the cage.

Proper perching should always be provided for rehabilitating birds. Perches need to be of appropriate size and well secured to the floor or cage sides. Large wooden tree branches or small logs can be used if the bird is only staying for several days. Cage perches can be made by combining PVC pipes into a "T" shape and then mounting it to a block of wood. These plastic perches should be wrapped with outdoor carpet or Astroturf and can be cleaned and reused. Raptors that require longer-term hospital stays should have padded perches to stand on to reduce foot injuries caused by the pressure of standing for long periods of time. The technician can wrap the perches with Vetrap to add cushioning and to provide an easy gripping surface. The perches should be secured at a height to prevent the bird's tail from dragging on the cage bottom but low enough to be easily stepped up on to.

The nature of the bird's injury should determine perch placement. No high perches should be available to a bird with a limb injury. To avoid any additional trauma, the perch should be 6–12 inches off the ground to begin with and gradually raised as the bird learns to step up and hop down from the perch. Ramped perches can cause problems if the injured bird climbs up to the top but "forgets" its handicap and jumps off. Most raptors never learn to descend from these learning perches the same gentle way they climbed up them.

A towel should be provided for padding to protect the bird's sternum if it is unable to stand. A rolled-up towel can be used to prop a weak bird up on its stomach at a 45° angle. The head should be level to prevent any fluids from the bird's nose or mouth from draining down into the lungs. Another caging method used for birds too weak to stand or with fractured legs is to place them in a box half full of shredded newspapers. This material not only supports the bird's body but also allows the feces to fall away from the bird.

The importance of keeping the feathers in good condition cannot be stressed enough. Wing and tail feathers, especially, are easily damaged if the birds are improperly housed. Even if the clinic is only holding the bird for a day or two, housing the bird in any cage where the feathers or feather tips can stick out will do some degree of damage. It only takes two or three broken flight feathers to deem an otherwise fit bird temporarily nonreleasable. If the damage in any way interferes with normal mobility, the bird must remain in captivity until it undergoes a molt and replaces the broken feathers with new ones. This is a normal process but may take up to a year to naturally occur.

In addition to proper housing, a tail guard can be easily applied. Some rehabilitation centers and veterinary clinics wrap tails as a common intake procedure. A tail-wrapping method is reprinted with permission from the North Carolina Raptor Center in Charlotte, North Carolina. (See appendix 4.)

Raptor Feeding

As with any animal, the bird should be warm and hydrated before you offer solid food. If the bird appears in good condition and is not emaciated, it can be offered a natural prey item for its diet. Healthy diurnal birds of prey (hawks, falcons) need to be fed once a day during the daylight hours. Nocturnal birds (owls) should be fed once a day but only in the evening.

These birds eat a variety of rodents, birds, rabbits, fish, insects, and snakes in the wild but in short-term hospitalization, fresh-killed or thawed adult mice will do. In some cases it may take the new patient several days to accept the new surroundings and food. As long as the bird came in at a good weight this should not be a problem and the bird will start to eat when it gets really hungry. The food presentation may also confuse the bird and it may not recognize a dead white lab mouse as a food item. Offering brown or black mice sometimes helps, as well as cutting open the mouse cavity to reveal the organ tissue, which often stimulates the bird's appetite.

Occasionally a raptor needs a little help with one or two hand-feedings to get started. A mouse may need to be cut into small bite-size pieces depending on the size of the bird. The pieces can be offered from a hemostat while leaving the bird inside the cage. One should be quiet and not stare at the bird or make sudden movements. The food should be slowly held up to and allowed to touch the bird's beak. Sometimes the bird will bite at the food defensively and accidentally take the offering. One should stay still until the bird swallows it, which could take a minute or two for the first bite. This can be repeated several times, and then the remaining part of the meal can be left inside the cage with the bird. If the bird will not swallow the food or is too aggressive and tries to foot and bite the feeder, then it may need to be force-fed.

With the bird wrapped securely in a towel and properly restrained, the beak should be opened and pieces carefully placed one by one into the back of its mouth (past the glottis) with fingers or blunted hemostats. The bird needs to be allowed to swallow each bite one at a time. Care should be taken to open the beak at the base and not the biting curved tip. Once the beak is open, it can be kept open long enough to place the food by wedging a finger inside at the extreme base of the mouth. It should always be remembered that these birds can be dangerous and will foot or bite at any given chance. Once a stubborn raptor swallows several pieces of delicious rodent, even if it is a white one, it usually gives the bird incentive to start self-feeding.

If the bird is emaciated, dehydrated, or too weak to eat solid whole items, then tube feeding may be needed. Start first with SQ LRS fluids and then switch to the oral route once the bird has stabilized. Continue with liquid formula feeding (such as Emeraid II or Isocal) until the bird has gained strength. Next, bites of skinless and boneless pieces of muscle or organ meat such as raw beef liver or muscle meat from a cut-up mouse or rat can be offered. Only after the bird has recovered its strength, which can take up to 3–4 days, should it be offered solid whole foods. Table 14.1 provides a feeding guideline for birds of prey.

Raptor Orphan Initial Care

The intake of many of raptor "orphans" into the veterinary hospital can often be prevented by good phone protocols and animal history taking. Raptors have a stage of development between the nestling and fledgling stage referred to as "branching." At this age,

Table 14.1. Recommended Feeding Guideline for Birds of Prey

Species	Avg. male/female wt (g)	Food type	Amount
American kestrel	M-111 g / F-120 g	1 mouse	25 g
Bald eagle	M-4,123 g / F-5,244 g	2 rats	200–300 g
Barn owl	M-442 g / F-490 g	2–3 mice	50–75 g
Barred owl	M-632 g / F-801 g	2–3 mice	50–75 g
Broad winged hawk	M-420 g / F-490 g	2 mice	50 g
Cooper's hawk	M-349 g / F-529 g	2–3 mice	50–75 g
Great horned owl	M-1318 g / F-1769 g	3–5 mice or 1/2 rat	75–125 g
Peregrine falcon	M- 611 g / F-952g	4 mice	100 g
Red-tailed hawk	M-1,028 g / F-1,224 g	3–5 mice or 1/2 rat	75–125 g
Rough-legged hawk	M-1,027 g / F-1,278 g	4 mice	100 g
Saw-whet owl	M-74.9 g / F-90.8 g	1 mouse	25 g
Screech owl	M-167 g / F-194 g	1 mouse	25 g
Sharp-shinned hawk	M-103 g / F-174 g	1–2 mice	25–50 g
Red-shouldered hawk	M-475 g / F-643 g	2–3 mice	50–75 g
Turkey vulture	1,467 g	6–8 mice or 1 rat	150–200 g

young birds are feathered, still being fed by the parents, have left the nest, but are not flighted. Well-meaning people often discover these birds and believe them to be orphaned or injured because they will not fly away and there is no nest in sight. Because these birds are so easily captured, they are usually first picked up before the rehabilitator is notified. By asking the right questions, many of these "kidnapped" birds can be returned to the founding sight before any harm is done. If the clinic receives these calls, the best thing to do is to instruct the caller to leave the bird where it is and have the person call one of the raptor rehabilitators (on the referral phone list) to determine if the bird is truly orphaned or not.

Raptors are hatched with down but unable to leave the nest (semi-altricial). While hawks are born with their eyes open, owls are born eyes closed. Hatchling- and nestling-stage babies found on the ground should be replaced into the nest if at all possible. Some rehabilitators, nature centers, or wildlife agencies may have individuals to help with this process. If returning to the original site is not possible, the orphan should be temporarily cared for until a foster nest or captive foster parent can be found. Many of the larger wildlife rehabilitation centers have permanent foster parent birds that willingly feed many orphans each year.

Initial temporary care of orphaned raptors is similar to the care of all animal species (make sure they are warm and hydrated). The chick should first be provided with heat if it is not old enough to regulate its own body temperature.

One accepted rule for raptor brooding temperature is:

- Unfeathered birds should be kept at an ambient temperature of 85°F–90°.
- Downey chicks with quills present can be kept at 80°F–85°F.
- Birds with feather quills and small feathers should be kept at 75°F–80°F.

Estimating actual raptor-chick age is beyond the scope of this chapter due to the sheer number of species and classifications of birds of prey. The raptor rehabilitator can be called with the bird's description and weight for age estimate and feeding instructions. After the chick is warm and active, provide hydration fluids orally by carefully placing two to four drops of solution into the throat beyond the glottis every 15–20 minutes until the bird becomes active.

Raptor Orphan Feeding

If the chick's transportation cannot be arranged before it needs to eat, the technician can offer it small pieces of rodent from a tweezers or hemostats. Caution should be taken to avoid improper imprinting from the chick watching hand-feeding (refer to imprinting section). Imprinting within raptors occurs anywhere between 5 and 15 days of age. Raptor chicks do not gape for food like songbird babies do but they readily take food with the tips of their beaks and sometimes will even nibble on the feeding tool as they would their parent's beak.

If the chicks eyes are closed, it is safe to hand-feed by touching the bird's beak with the feeding instrument containing small bites of food and trying to imitate the parents' feeding calls by whistling or chirping quietly. Because the chicks cannot see the person feeding it, one need only be concerned about the chicks' not hearing the person feeding talking.

If the bird's eyes are open and it demonstrates no fear or aggression, this is within the dangerous critical imprinting period and much care should be taken to prevent the youngster from seeing or hearing a human or any animal in the hospital. Some centers feed these birds with gloves and ski masks to partially hide the human shape or better yet feed with a hand puppet of a raptor-type bird (rubber bird hand puppets can sometimes be found at gift shops of nature stores and zoos; fig. 14.4). Another option is to hang a towel, sheet, or curtain, to serve as a kind of blind, in front of the infant and feed by reaching around and peeking through a hole in the blind. These animals must never be available for "show and tell," and should be disturbed only for care taking until they can be transferred to the rehabilitator.

A juvenile raptor that shows fear or aggression is beyond the critical imprinting stage and, one hopes, has properly imprinted on its own species by now. These birds may also be capable of self-feeding, so try placing small pieces of food in with the bird. If it refuses to pick up the food on its own after several feedings, refer to the above section on feeding adult raptors for hand-feeding ideas.

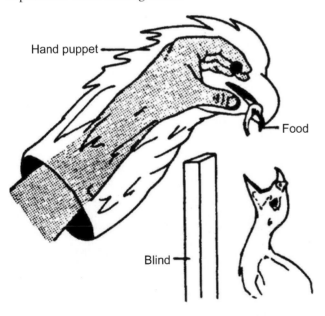

Fig. 14.4. Hand-feeding puppet used for feeding neonates. During critical imprinting periods, hand-feeding puppets should be used in conjunction with blinds to prevent a young animal from associating food with humans. (Permission for drawing use granted by the Georgia Department of Natural Resources and Branson Ritchie, DVM, MS)

Raptor Orphan Food

Young raptors eat enormous amounts of food and often three to four times the amount of an adult. Weigh the chick in the morning before feeding and then feed 8–10% of body weight. The first few meals should be less to allow the digestive tract time to adjust to the changes. The crop should be allowed to fully empty before offering the next meal. Unlike hawks, owls do not have crops but tend to turn away from food when full (Crawford 1988).

Very young chicks, 0 to 7 days old, should eat just the soft muscle organ meat of prey foods dipped into vitamin water. The parents would remove all skin, fur, and bones initially from the meals. These young raptor chicks should eat, until they are satisfied, every 3–4 hours. Feed them until the crop is half to three-quarters full but not so full that it feels hard or extended. Meals should not be skipped, and birds should be fed for a 12-hour day.

Once they are 7 to 10 days old, one can begin to introduce small amounts of moistened hair, skin, and small bones into the diet, which will serve as roughage and later be casted up.

Around days 10–20, the chicks can be fed larger moistened pieces of meat with bones, skin, and fur for three feedings a day. Starting at 3 weeks of age, the young should be able to eat the entire mouse cut into three to four pieces and will start to pick these up on their own.

One should feed the 3-week-olds to fledge twice a day and offer whole-prey items for them to tear on their own. One should then continue to hand-feed them until it is certain that they are picking up enough food on their own to sustain themselves.

Once fledged, one can feed these birds once daily (owls in the evening, hawks in the morning).

Whether the baby is staying at the veterinary hospital for one meal or many, it is the clinic's responsibility to *NOT* allow this animal (or any wild animal) the opportunity to improperly imprint on human beings. If this is allowed to occur, the raptor will be deemed unreleasable and usually will need to be euthanized.

Raptor Orphan Housing

A small cardboard box lined with cloth works well for a very young raptor. A twisted towel made into a circle with the baby placed inside the "doughnut" serves well for support. Walls may need to be covered or cleaned daily because hawks and eagles tend to shoot when they excrete feces. Use of an incubator, heat lamp, or heating pad to provide external heat for the very young (2 weeks old or younger) will be necessary.

Healthy raptors do not need as much heat as other birds, but if it seems lethargic or shivers, it may be cold. A panting chick is too warm. Housing temperatures are outlined below in the initial care section (fig. 14.5).

As the young become more active, pieces of branches can be placed on the nest bottom to provide the birds with foot-gripping exercise, which is necessary to develop coordination and strength.

When raptors fledge, they need a larger enclosure with stable perches that are larger around than the bird's grip. The enclosure should have solid sides to prevent the flight feathers from sticking out and becoming damaged. The growing chick will now need room to hop and flap its wings.

Misting these newly feathered birds daily with water will help stimulate them to preen and activate their uropygial gland for waterproofing. Once they are eating on their own, acclimated to the outside, and waterproofed, juvenile raptors are ready for outdoor flight caging. By now the bird should be transferred to a raptor rehabilitator to train on catching live food and prepare for release.

ALTRICIAL ORPHAN SONGBIRD BASIC CARE

This section is to be used as general information only. It should be kept in mind that every bird is slightly different in development and behavior. These guidelines are to be used by the veterinary technician until the bird can be transferred to a licensed rehabilitator.

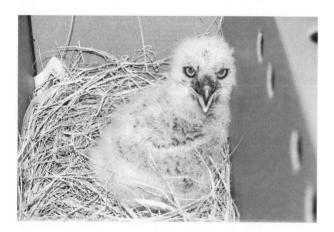

Fig. 14.5. Baby hawk. (photo courtesy of Melanie Haire)

Altricial birds are those that are hatched blind, naked, unable to control body temperature, and completely helpless (blue jays, robins, mockingbirds).

Development
The development of the altricial bird is generally five stages. All species follow these stages but at different rates depending on their natural history.

1. Hatchling—0–4 days old, newly hatched, no voice, eyes closed, naked, or sparsely downy
2. Nestling—5–10 days old, eyes open, partially feathered, feeding call
3. Fledgling—11–14 days, almost fully feathered, can perch, hop, first attempts to fly, ready to leave the nest, able to thermoregulate, frequently preening, wing stretching, short tail feathers
4. Juvenile—fully grown, defensive, independence begins, lasts until sexual maturity
5. Adult—sexually mature

Initial Care
An animal should never be fed until it is warm. Use an incubator, a brooder, heat light, or heating pad to warm up a chilled infant and keep the baby on heat until it is feathered. Altricial baby birds' temperature guidelines are:

- Hatchlings—should be kept at 80°F–90°F
- Nestlings— should be kept at 80°F–85°F
- Fledglings—should be kept at 70°F–80°F

Once the bird is warm, it should be hydrated by offering drops of Pedialyte or lactated Ringer's solution orally every 5–10 minutes until the baby passes a normal fecal sac. For most birds this should consist of a dark solid part (stool) and a milky white softer part (urates) contained within a clear sac.

The baby bird should be examined for injuries, bruises, puncture wounds, and bites, mites, and so on.

Identification of what species it is needs to be made to determine proper diet and feeding schedule.

Begin offering the infant hand-rearing formula.

Identification
To determine the type of bird, the bird rehabilitator should be called for help, and one can also refer to appendix 5.

Information should be obtained about where and how the bird was found from the person who found it. These details not only help identify what type of bird it is, but also may help determine if the bird needs further help or if it can be returned to its parents.

The following items help to identify altricial nestling species:

1. Mouth color—The inside membranes of the mouth are usually brightly colored to attract attention from the feeding parent bird.
2. Gape flanges color—The fleshy "lips" that edge the mouth may be a different color than the inside of the mouth.
3. Beak description—The length and shape of the beak helps identify a species by what it eats. Insect eaters tend to have long, slender beaks and seed eaters tend to have thick, short, and conical shaped beaks.
4. Skin color or color of down—Presence or absence of down, natal down, and skin color are also species specific.
5. Vocalizations—Many songbird species have unique feeding calls.
6. Location baby was found—Was the baby found in a tree cavity (woodpeckers, nuthatches), a fireplace (chimney swifts), hanging planters (wrens, finches)?
7. Body size—When the tail feathers emerge from their sheaths, a baby bird has reached its full body size.

Housing Nestlings

The baby bird should be placed in a homemade nest constructed out of a berry basket, small plastic bowl, or margarine tub lined with unscented toilet or facial tissues.

A cuplike cavity with the nesting material can be constructed so the baby can nestle down but still receive support from all sides. The baby could develop leg problems if not properly supported during the nesting stage. For extra support, a paper towel can be rolled (snakelike) and coiled around the inside of the nest, and then the tissue placed over the top.

If the tissue is piled high enough (within one-half inch of the nest container top), the baby can defecate over the side of the nest and help keep the inside clean.

Replace the tissue as it gets soiled.

Do not use the old natural nest because it may contain parasites and is too difficult to clean. Do not line the artificial nest with fresh grass because it is too cold and damp.

If the baby bird is very young, using an incubator with a wet sponge or other source of moisture for humidity may be necessary. A homemade incubator can be made out of a small plastic tote with air holes put in the lid. Care should be taken to provide enough ventilation that the humidity does not build up and allow moisture to collect on the inside of the container, which in turn allows rapid growth of pathogens.

Instructions for how to make a homemade incubator are available on the International Wildlife Rehabilitation Council (IWRC) web page: www.iwrc-online.org.

If an incubator is not being used, the nest should be placed inside a safe container such as a lidded box or basket to prevent any unfortunate mishaps from babies falling out or pets getting into the nest. This especially applies to the technician who has the babies at work in a busy veterinary practice.

The nest should be kept on the heating pad or under the heat lamp at all times to keep the baby from chilling.

A thermometer should *always* be used to monitor the ambient air. The warmth should circulate around the infant (fig. 14.6).

A tissue or soft wash cloth should be draped over the top of the baby to hold in the warmth and to simulate the security of a brooding parent.

Baby birds can usually come off the heat when they feather out as long as they are active and healthy.

Housing Fledglings

Once the babies are ready to leave the nest, they will require a larger cage. The nest can be placed inside a small flight cage so the youngsters can hop in and out of their nests until they no longer return to it. The cage should be large enough to allow the birds to take short

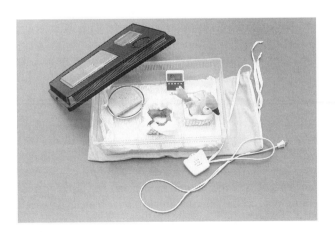

Fig. 14.6. Baby bird incubator with hygrometer, wet sponge, nest with facial tissues, and a heating pad. (photo courtesy of Melanie Haire)

flights and hop from perch to perch but small enough to be easily carried inside and out.

The sides should be constructed out of or lined with soft netting or nylon mesh to prevent injury to the bird or its feathers. Reptariums, affordable commercially available soft-sided mesh cages, can be purchased and successfully used to house fledgling and injured adult songbirds. These cages are available in different sizes and are easy to clean because the mesh zips off the plastic frame and can be machine washed.

Wire bird or mammal cages should *never* be used. If the feathers stick out from between the cage bars they will fray, break off, and possibly become too damaged to support flight. At best these birds with damaged plumage will have to be held over until they molt out a new set of flight feathers. With many songbird species this may take up to a year. Occasionally these birds develop permanent feather follicle damage and need to be euthanized.

The cage bottom can be lined with paper towels and should be changed out daily.

Several secured low branches should be included to allow for landing and perching practice.

If the weather is mild, the cage should be moved outside during the day but brought inside at night to start acclimating the birds to outdoor temperatures, sights, and sounds.

In addition to introducing the young bird to natural temperatures, the sunlight will provide vital and accurate doses of vitamin D_3. Birds require a proper balance of calcium and phosphorus in their diet for the development of normal, healthy bones. Vitamin D_3 is necessary to ensure that the body can absorb the dietary calcium. Without this proper absorption, the body cannot form normal bones, and the bones and the bill can become rubbery and soft. This deficiency, called metabolic bone disease, results in bone deformities or even stress fractures that are difficult at best to treat. Prevention is the best medicine, and a combination of 30 minutes a day of direct daylight or 30–60 minutes a day with artificial full-spectrum light plus a balanced diet will meet the requirements.

Plastic and glass filter out the necessary ultraviolet light so sunlight coming through a window or aquarium will not provide adequate light.

The entire cage should never be placed in direct sunlight. The babies can quickly overheat if a shaded area is not easily accessible. Ultraviolet rays from the sun are still available on cloudy days and in the shade.

The enclosure should never be left unprotected from possible predators. A screened porch or a fenced yard is no protection from a stray cat or hungry raccoon. Predator-proof caging can be affordably built

but will not be discussed in this chapter. All hand raised wild bird releases should be done by a licensed bird rehabilitator. Many of the rehabilitation manuals listed on the source pages have instructions for building prerelease and release caging.

Feeding Methods

There are many feeding methods in practice for feeding wild baby birds (fig. 14.7).

Blunt forceps, tweezers, pipettes, syringes, eyedroppers, small artists paint brushes, Popsicle sticks, blunted toothpicks, and fingers are just some of the tools that can be used for administering food.

A discussion of feeding techniques with a local avian rehabilitator will aid in choosing the one that works best.

Many of the above feeding implements only work with certain types of formulas, and sometimes a combination works well. Often the thickness of the formula depends on the age of the bird, so feeding several birds of different ages may require the use of more than one tool.

Many healthy nestlings and fledglings will gape readily and hungrily making feeding time for the caregiver much easier. These willing participants will continue to gape, for the most part, until their crops are full. Care should be taken to avoid over filling the crop. If the bird is slow to swallow or flings food, it might be full or too dehydrated.

If the baby is hesitant to gape, it may be dehydrated or otherwise ill, not hungry, too frightened, or nervous, or it may not recognize the gesture as a feeding attempt.

One can tap on the side of the nest and whistle softly in an attempt to imitate the parent bird's arrival to

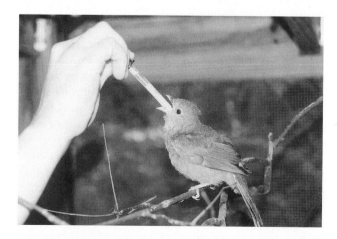

Fig. 14.7. Hand-feeding a baby cardinal. (photo courtesy of Melanie Haire)

the nest. This may require patience and several tries with different chirping sounds. Gaping nestmates often help stimulate gaping in all individuals including newcomers.

If the baby is hydrated and healthy but still will not gape, gently prying the beak open with fingers and placing a small amount of food toward the back of its mouth may be necessary. Some birds will get the picture quickly and only need one or two force-feedings to understand that they are being offered food and will not be harmed.

Once birds imprint on their parents and are old enough to have developed fear of humans in the wild, they become more difficult to hand-feed and may need to be force-fed until they become self-feeding. Introducing a bowl of food into their cage for this older fledgling group may be the answer.

Several altricial species of baby birds (i.e., some swifts, swallows, nighthawks, pigeons, and all doves) never gape, and knowing the identification of these species will save a lot of time and frustration. These individuals will need to be fed in a different manner.

The fledgling or juvenile swifts, swallows, and nighthawks are examples of birds that will probably need to be force- or tube fed until release. Hatchlings and nestlings may adjust to hand-feedings but need to be fed by holding the food up to the bird's beak.

Pigeon and dove babies do not gape but they do beg. They naturally feed by sticking their beaks inside their parent's mouth, which is the opposite position of many songbirds. So the concept of willingly opening their mouths to the sight of an eyedropper full of food has no meaning to them. These birds will need to be tube fed until they are self-feeding. Once the birds are 7 days old or older, a feeder can be made that resembles the feeding technique naturally used by this group.

Pigeon and Dove Feeder

A 12 or 20 cc syringe casing can be filled with a balanced parakeet seed mix (small seeds without a lot of hulls or shelled sunflower seeds) and tightly wrapped with Vetrap over the opened bottom of the case to keep the seeds in. A quarter- to half-inch slit is then cut in the center of the Vetrap (long enough for the bird's beak to fit through but not too big to allow seeds to spill out around beak). Next the bird's beak can be inserted into the slit in the Vetrap, and while holding the back of the bird's head to keep it from pulling out of the dispenser, the syringe can be tapped to simulate the movement of the parent bird. See figure 14.8. It will take several attempts to get the bird to quit struggling and pulling away from the feeder. Once

it swallows some seeds (probably by accident the first time), it will quickly start self-feeding right out of the dispenser. Then in addition to tube feeding into their crop with a hand-rearing formula, one can offer the baby the feeder several times a day to facilitate the self-feeding and weaning process.

A size 10 or 12 red rubber catheter cut to about 3 inches in length can be used to crop tube feed pigeons and doves. Exact, Pretty Bird, and Lefabers are examples of quality hand-rearing powdered diets commercially available at pet stores.

Food Prep

The bird formulas ideally should be made up fresh daily and refrigerated until use. Each feeding should be allowed to warm to room temperature before feeding it to the bird.

The consistency will vary depending on the diet and the age of the bird. Most diets are thick like oatmeal when hand mixed but can be blended down to a slurry that can be pushed through a syringe or dropper. Some formulas tend to thicken over the day during refrigeration, and a little water may need to be added to keep it at the proper consistency. Remember that baby birds need as many calories as possible so do not thin formulas down more than absolutely necessary. Runny or drippy formulas should never be fed because the food could drip down into the trachea and cause aspiration pneumonia.

Many diets can be made in batches and stored in the freezer for short periods of time. Making a week's worth of food at once and freezing it in ice cube trays can save a lot of time. One can thaw out as many cubes as needed for the day, and a back up supply is available if more babies are received.

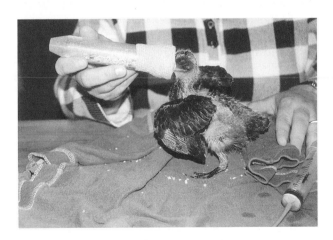

Fig. 14.8. Pigeon feeder. (photo courtesy of Melanie Haire)

One should be knowledgeable about nutrition because some ingredients lose dietary value when frozen or stored for long periods of time. One should always start with fresh, good quality ingredients.

Feeding Frequency

Feeding frequency should follow this guideline:

Hatchling—Feed every 10–20 min (6 a.m.–10 p.m.)
Nestling—Feed every 20–30 min (6 a.m.–10 p.m.)
Fledgling—Feed every 45–60 min (7 a.m.–10 p.m.)
Juveniles—Feed every 2 hours (7 a.m.–9 p.m.)

In the wild, baby birds are fed from sunup to sundown. A technician should not make the mistake of thinking that they can be fed enough calories in a 9:00–5:00 workday. Hand-raising a baby bird is not a part-time responsibility. If the bird cannot be transferred over to a rehabilitator the same day, feeding arrangements must be made for the baby for a full 12–14-hour day. The biggest single mistake made, by well-meaning people, with hand-rearing baby wild birds is to underfeed them. The caretaker cannot make up for several missed feedings by feeding larger volumes at the next couple of feedings.

The only flexibility a caretaker has is to pick when the 12–14 hours begins and ends. By covering the cage and making it dark or leaving the lights on in the nursery past sundown, one can slightly alter the "daytime" if need be. This is not recommended for the long term or with older juvenile birds because they need to develop a sense of natural time.

Diets

It is ideal to feed the same diet that the rehabilitator will be using to prevent the stress of change to the baby's gastrointestinal tract. The recipes and ingredients should be kept on hand prior to the start of baby season in order to be always prepared. All too often the babies seem to come in at 10:00 p.m. on a Sunday night just as the pet stores close.

Proper bird species identification is necessary to choose the best diet recipe. By reading as much natural history information as is available, one can learn about food preferences, feeding methods, food presentation, and normal behavior.

The following are some examples of passerine hand-rearing formulas used at rehabilitation centers:

1. 1 part soaked Hill's Science Diet Feline growth
   1 part Gerber's High Protein Cereal
   1 tsp. bone meal
   Water to proper consistency (Evans 1986)

2. 1 cup soaked puppy chow
   1 T baby food beef
   1 T hard-boiled egg yolk
   3–4 drops balanced avian vitamins (Avitron)
   ½ t ground egg shell
   (Johnson 1991)

3. 1 cup soaked Hill's Science Diet Feline growth
   ½ cup chick starter added to ½ cup boiling water
   3–4 drops balanced avian vitamins (Avitron)
   ½ t Rep-cal (calcium w/vitamin D_3, phosphorus-free)
   1 t powdered Benebac
   Mix cat food and hot chick starter together in blender. Add other ingredients after mix cools (Ivie 1999).

These sample diets can be fed to a wide variety of species with the exception of doves and pigeons. These diets are a balanced base. Depending on the bird species, food items can be added to more closely match their natural diet.

- Insectivorous birds such as woodpeckers, swifts, and wrens should have insects added to the base. Mealworms, wax worms, crickets, and freeze-dried insects are examples of such supplements that should make up to 50% of the diet.
- Frugivores such as waxwings and orioles should have chopped fruit added.
- Birds with a tendency to develop a calcium deficiency such as mockingbirds, thrashers, and kingbirds should have food items rich in calcium or a calcium supplement added to the diet.
- Doves and pigeons being strictly seed and grain feeders can be tube fed with a commercial brand of baby bird food formulated for psittacines. These powdered diets are available, ready to use after adding water, in most pet stores.
- Hummingbirds need a commercial nectar such as Nekton or Roudybush. Pet store or homemade sugar-water diets (although good for providing energy) only provide calories and will not keep a hummingbird alive long term.

Additional Information

Avoid allowing formula to dry on the baby's beak, nares, or feathers. Remove any spilled food while it is still moist and easier to remove. If food is allowed to dry on feathers, it may cause feather loss or a skin infection. One should use a damp cotton swab to clean food off of the baby; wiping should be in the direction of the feather growth.

One should always try to house single baby birds with conspecifics. The rehabilitator should be contacted to help place the baby with other same-species orphans or, even better, into a foster parent situation. Arrangements should be made to get them together as soon as possible. The benefits of orphaned animals being raised with natural or foster siblings are immeasurable. They learn critical behavioral and social skills from interacting with the correct species.

Never forget that the goal of wildlife rehabilitation is to provide temporary care with the goal of releasing the animal with its best chances to survive. Technicians must above all do no harm and never release an animal that cannot properly care for itself.

- Limit talking around wildlife.
- Avoid improper imprinting.
- Adequate notes should be kept that can be used as reference material later. Good record keeping may also prevent mishaps due to shift changes in caregivers.
- One should limit handling and activity to feeding and cleaning time only.
- Wild birds should never be housed near domestic pets, especially pet birds.
- All food containers and tools should be cleaned with hot soapy water after each use and allowed to air dry or towel dry before next use. Dip feeding instruments in 5% diluted bleach or soak in 10% diluted Nolvasan for 30 minutes once daily.

CARING FOR ADULT PASSERINE (SONG) BIRDS

Initial Care

The bird's history should be obtained on the intake form to help formulate the diagnosis of why the bird came in to the clinic. The rescuer might know for certain that it was hit by a car, flew into a window, or was caught by a cat. If no cause is known, good "investigative" questions should help find the answer. If the bird was found in the driveway, it should be asked if there is a nearby garage with windows it might have collided with. If the bird was found under a bird feeder and has had its tail feathers pulled out, the founder should be questioned about the possibilities of outdoor cats in the area.

After the history taking, a visual exam should be performed first before touching the bird. The bird should be observed for signs of disease or illness such as ruffled feathers, squinted or closed eyes, sneezing, clicking, mouth breathing, dull feathers, lethargy,

diarrhea, squatting instead of standing, and wing droops.

Next a physical examination should be performed looking for obvious wounds and fractures along with more subtle signs of shock and dehydration. (See the section on performing the physical exam under "Initial Exam" above). Body and feather condition should be checked and noted. The keel should be palpated to determine if the bird is thin or emaciated. When checking for lacerations or bruising, feathers can be blown out of the way to better visualize the skin underneath.

Restraint for adult songbirds is relatively easy. Pressure should not be placed on a bird's sternum since they breathe by expanding their chest and abdominal cavities. Use of the "bander's" hold, enables the examiner to check the bird thoroughly while keeping a secure yet gentle hold on the patient. (See figure 14.9.) This hold should be used for any handling, medicating or force-feeding procedures.

An accurate weight in grams should be obtained and monitored every 24–48 hours.

The bird should be kept warm and hydrated before attempting to feed it. If the bird feels thin, has bright green stools, sunken eyes, wrinkled skin, or is weak and lethargic, it should be offered two to four drops of rehydrating solution orally by placing the drops behind the glottis into the throat every 15 minutes for the first 1–2 hours.

Dehydrated birds can receive SQ fluids injected into their wing web or into the loose medial skin folds where the legs join to the body. Injecting fluids, although more painful than delivering oral fluids due to the needle prick, may be less stressful in the end due to the larger volume that can be given at one time,

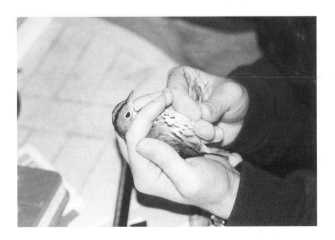

Fig. 14.9. Bird bander's hold. (photo courtesy of Melanie Haire)

which decreases the number of times needed to restrain the bird.

Immobilizing Fractures

Immobilization of any fractures should be performed as soon as possible so the bird does not further injure itself.

The wildlife veterinary technician should know how to apply all of the following bandages. The veterinarians may not be able to look at every bird that comes in with a fracture but if the proper stabilizing wrap is applied, the fracture may have all it needs to heal properly. Do not allow a bird with a fractured bone to sit in the hospital without a proper bandage. Waiting one or two days to apply the wrap could be too late.

If the bone needs more than a bandage to properly mend (long bones on larger birds such as ducks, owls, and hawks), the wrap should still be applied until the veterinarian can schedule the bone surgery procedure.

If the lower leg (tibiotarsus or tarsometatarsus) is fractured, on a small bird, a tape splint usually works well (fig. 14.10). The leg is held in a natural "perch" position and tape is placed on each side of the leg. One should seal the tape firmly up to the leg by pinching it with a pair of hemostats. The more tape applied, the more stable the splint but it should be kept in mind the weight of the apparatus versus the small size of your patient. The bird should be able to stand and perch with this type of bandage if it is properly trimmed.

The femur needs more than tape if it has been fractured. Cast padding and a splint (made of toothpicks, tongue depressors, halved syringe case, etc.) covered in Vetrap depending on the size of the bird will be

needed. The joint above and below the fracture site needs to be covered. If this is not possible, it is best not to bandage at all and arrange to have the bird transported to an experienced avian veterinarian or rehabilitator immediately.

Any leg bandage applied too tightly will prevent blood flow from leaving the foot, and the foot and toes may swell. The toes must be evaluated daily for swelling, loss of function, or discoloration.

Foot injuries can be bandaged several different ways. In small songbirds, their toes can be taped down individually onto a cardboard "snowshoe." In larger birds, a padded ball bandage can be made to keep the toes aligned and the talons from puncturing the footpads fig. 14.11). A circular piece of cardboard is cut that fits in the bottom of the bird's foot and is padded with cotton. The pad is taped in place by wrapping the cotton padding with Vetrap between the bird's toes. The toe tips should be slightly visible to be checked for bandage tightness. The bandages should be kept as

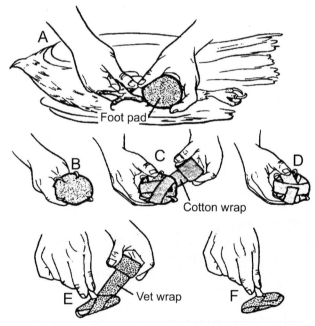

Fig. 14.11. Padded bandage used in avian foot and leg injuries. **A.** *Cardboard plate is cut to fit the foot and is padded with cotton wrap and covered with tape.* **B.** *Foot pad is placed against the bottom of the foot with the toes properly positioned and in extension.* **C&D.** *Foot pad is wrapped in place with cotton padding.* **E.** *Cotton padding is covered with Vetrap.* **F.** *Completed bandage. (Permission for drawing use granted by the Georgia Department of Natural Resources and Branson Ritchie, DVM, MS)*

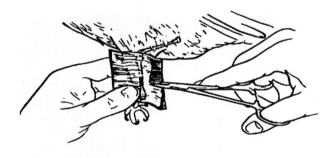

Fig. 14.10. Tape splint used for fracture immobilization in the lower leg bones of small birds. Tape is placed on each side of the leg with the sticky sides facing each other. The tape is pressed together with hemostats. (Permission for drawing use granted by the Georgia Department of Natural Resources and Branson Ritchie, DVM, MS)

clean and dry as possible because replacing the wrap before the bone is healed will delay or prevent healing.

For wing fractures, as with all fractures, the joint above and below the fracture site should be immobilized. The figure-eight bandage holds the wing closed in a natural position and is adequate to immobilize a fracture on any portion of the wing as well as to reduce the weight of the wing on the shoulder. If the fracture involves the humerus, continue the wing bandage around the body to immobilize the shoulder joint (joint above the fracture).

If using the body wrap, one must be sure to pass the tape *under* the good wing on the opposite side and across the body on the upper keel (fig. 14.12). The fit should be snug but not tight enough to interfere with respiration or circulation.

When this bandage is properly applied, the bird should be able to stand and perch while holding the wing in a normal anatomic position. All wing feathers should be in alignment as well. If the bandage pulls the wing in an abnormal position, the bandage should be removed and reapplied.

Bird bones heal much more quickly then mammal bones do so bandages usually only have to remain on for 2–3 weeks as long as the bird is confined to strict

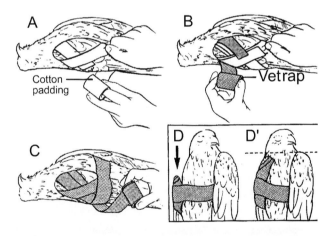

Fig. 14.12. *Figure-eight bandage used for the immobilization of the avian wing.* **A.** *Cotton padding is wrapped from the carpus to the humerus and back to the carpus.* **B.** *The same pattern is repeated with Vetrap.* **C.** *Vetrap is passed around the midbody and taped in place.* **D.** *A properly bandaged wing should be held at the same level as the normal wing.* **D'.** *If the wing drops below the level of the normal wing, the bandage should be removed and reapplied. (Permission for drawing use granted by the Georgia Department of Natural Resources and Branson Ritchie, DVM, MS.)*

cage rest for several days after the bandage is removed. After this cage-rest period, the bird should have manual limb massage and gradual limb extensions. After a good callus is formed, the bird can be placed in a flight cage.

Housing Adult Birds

Make sure the housing is as stress free as possible. Cover the fronts of all bird caging and if possible give the bird natural materials to hide in. Reptariums (under mesh cages in appendix 10) and the collapsible framed, mesh laundry hampers (available at discount stores) make excellent injured adult bird caging due to their soft-sided, feather protecting material and light weight. Reptariums are machine washable.

Perching of various heights should be provided if the bird is capable of standing.

As soon as its hospital stay is over, the patient should be transferred over to the rehabilitator in order to be housed in an appropriate aviary.

Feeding Adult Birds

Adult birds should be encouraged to eat on their own by providing natural food items that they may recognize. One can use whole berries, millet sprays, seed mixes, and live insects along with grains, cracked corn, bran, and chopped fruits. A stressed bird usually will not eat, so noise, bright lights, visual disturbances, and extreme temperatures should be reduced to allow the avian patient to settle down and eat.

If after one day the bird has not eaten, it must be force-fed at least four times a day. This can be performed by gently placing a thumb and forefinger at the corners of the mouth and either pressing it to open or by using the other hand to open the mouth and placing food carefully down the throat behind the glottis. Most birds will swallow when food is placed back far enough. Use one of the homemade diets in the nestling care section for hand-feeding or Emeraid II (powdered diet for debilitated birds) for tube feeding.

Sometimes force-feeding a bird several times is all it takes to get it to start self-feeding. One should make sure it is eating enough and maintaining a healthy weight.

Live insects (wax worms, mealworms, and crickets) should be "gut-loaded" with healthy, nutritionally rich ingredients and not fed off the shelf from a bait store. When insects are purchased, they usually have eaten much of the food that was in the container they have been living in so they will need to be provided with at least 24 hours of nutrition before feeding them to wildlife patients. Mealworms can be put into a plastic tub, with a ventilated lid, at room temperature with coarsely ground whole grains such as corn meal, rolled oats, wheat bran, or game bird starter. For moisture, a cut-up potato can be added to the top of the mixture. Crickets and wax worms can also eat this mixture.

Fresh-dug earthworms are also good to offer insectivorous or omnivorous birds especially robins, thrashers, ducks, thrushes, jays, and mockingbirds.

See appendix 6 for average weight of selected North American songbirds.

PRECOCIAL BIRD BASIC CARE

At hatching, precocial birds are covered in feather down, are self-feeding, are ready to leave the nest, and can see, hear, run, and swim. These baby birds have no flanges on the sides of the mouth and have small, developed wings. The eggs of the precocial bird contain more nutrients and require more time to hatch, but the chick hatches out fully developed.

These birds (ducks, geese, killdeer, pheasant, quail, woodcock, and other shorebirds) have different dietary and housing needs from that of altricial birds.

Initial Orphan Care

One should never feed any animal until it is warm. An incubator, brooder, or heat light should be used to warm up a chilled infant. Despite their downy covering, precocial chicks need to be kept at slightly warmer ambient air temperature than altricial ones.

Newborn chick (0–7 days): 90°F–95°F
Chicks developing quills: 85°F–90°F
Birds with quills and developing feathers: 60°F–85°F

These chicks, if healthy, will usually readily eat and drink on their own. They are social and eat better in groups of similar species and ages.

If the chick is not eating, its dehydration and temperature should be checked. Some chicks can be quite nervous, and covering the box or cage with a towel may help them to eat.

If the bird is dehydrated, it can be offered drops of Pedialyte every 15 minutes for the first several hours or until it passes a normal stool. The fluid may have to be placed into the throat beyond the glottis if the baby is weak and dehydrated.

The bird should be examined for injuries, cuts, mites, or wounds.

Species identification should be determined in order to determine its proper diet and feeding schedule. One should begin offering the infant hand-rearing formula.

Identification

A bird rehabilitator should be contacted to help identify the species. Field guides may also be helpful. Ducks and some dabbling water birds have webbed feet or toes. Hatchling wood ducks have a visible egg tooth on the tip of the bill. Most shore birds have very long legs and can run quite fast.

One should be sure to look at the beak shape. Ducks and geese have wide, flat bills while the killdeer have thinner, tapered beaks (fig. 14.13). Quails and pheasant have short, sturdy, conical beaks.

Housing

A box or plastic tote lined with newspaper covered with paper or ravel-free cloth towels will do. The container should be covered with a screen top because some ducks (wood ducks) can jump very high. These birds are messy and cardboard will become soiled and need to be replaced often.

A wild bird should never be housed in a wire pet bird or mammal cage. A ceramic brooder-heating element or a brooder heat light can be hung in one half of the cage, making sure the enclosure is large to allow the birds to move in and out of the heated area.

It is very important to provide these birds with hiding places, such as a small box on its side. One can hang a feather duster down inside the cage so babies can snuggle up under it for security, shelter, and comfort. All these cage items will get soiled and need to be cleaned and kept dry as possible.

Waterfowl will splash in the water bowl and then seek the heat lamp to dry off underneath. As the birds grow feathers and spend less time under the lamp, it can be gradually raised up until you wean the birds off of the supplemental heat.

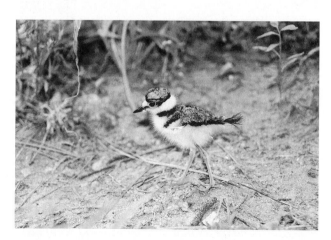

Fig. 14.13. One-week-old killdeer. (Photo courtesy of Melanie Haire)

Do not provide waterfowl with a pool unless directed to do so by an avian rehabilitator. Baby ducks and geese should never be left unattended during swimming time. If instructed to provide "swim time," a painter's roller tray can be used that will provide a ramp and shallow swimming area.

These young chicks need appropriate shelter and a quiet room to prevent stress that can oftentimes be fatal.

As they grow, so should their housing. Older juveniles and adults need to have a large outside predator-proof pen with a pool. This type of setup can not usually be provided at a veterinary clinic or at most people's homes so transferring the birds to the rehabilitator or wildlife center is recommended.

Feeding

Food and water bowls should be placed on the side away from the heat.

Caution must be used with the selection of water bowl used to prevent babies getting soaked and chilled. Using a Mason jar filled with water and inverted over a shallow lid or a commercial chicken waterer (available at most feed and farm stores) works well. A small water bowl filled three-fourths full with rocks or marbles also provides a readily available drinking source and keeps the babies from jumping into the water.

Food varies slightly between species but most do well on crumbled unmedicated chicken starter. One can sprinkle some on the cage floor as well as provide some in a food bowl.

A very young, single chick may be unsure how and what to eat. It learns these skills by watching and imitating its mother. Other bird rehabilitators should be contacted immediately to locate another chick to place it with. Sometimes these birds will need to be force-fed until placement can be found. In the meantime, one can try to teach the youngster by "pecking" at the food with a finger. Food in motion also seems to help stimulate feeding behavior so the grain can be gently rolled around and tiny live mealworms, earthworms, or crickets offered to inspire the infant to begin to peck. Also, floating chopped greens and small amounts of chick starter on water tends to stimulate unsure waterfowl.

The food should be changed twice a day, and one can begin offering small live mealworms, chopped greens and berries, cracked corn, and crickets as the babies grow. Fresh food should always be available, as the birds will eat free choice.

ADULT PRECOCIAL BIRDS (INCLUDING WATERFOWL AND WADING BIRDS)

Identification of the species and familiarity with its natural history, food preferences, and habitat is required.

An examination for injuries should be performed. Care must be taken of the water birds with long-pointed beaks. Herons, cranes, kingfishers, loons, and egrets will stab at faces and eyes when feeling threatened. Smaller birds such as grebes, coots, gulls, and rails can strike very quickly with short sturdy beaks and give quite a pinch as well. Coots will kick and use the spurs on their legs to defend themselves.

Ducks, geese, and swans can be difficult to restrain as well due to their strength and size. These birds will bite and twist with their powerful bills as well as beat at their restrainer with their very powerful wings.

One should take precautions, wear goggles, secure their heads, and work in pairs when restraining these animals. Even the small species are surprisingly strong and difficult to restrain.

Examination, body temperatures, hydration, and treatments are similar to other adult birds. See chapter 2, "The Avian Patient."

These species are particularly susceptible to lead poisoning (from ingesting fishing sinkers and lead birdshot used for duck hunting), fish hook ingestion, monofilament entanglement, and botulism due to their aquatic nature.

Diving birds (grebes, some sea ducks, loons, etc.) are built for floating, swimming, and diving but not walking, so many times these birds are presented with "broken legs" because they will not or cannot stand. The legs on these birds are positioned far back on the body for propelling through the water instead of underneath the body for walking. Many times these birds get tired during migrational movements and come down for a rest. If a loon lands on a wet pavement or parking lot thinking it looked like water, it has no way to take off again. Many times these birds just need a few meals and to be placed on a large body of water to allow for takeoff. This is a good example of why learning about a patient's natural history is so important.

Housing

If a water bird needs to be housed, a plastic pet kennel works well. Due to the large volume of liquid stool they produce, keeping the pen clean can be challenging. If the bird is too weak to hold itself upright or has a fractured leg, placing it in a box half filled with shredded newspapers makes a good body support setup and also allows the feces to drop away from the bird, which keeps the feathers and vent clean.

Water birds must keep their feathers in perfect condition and naturally do so by constant preening and bathing. If the birds are strong enough and do not have a bandage on, they can be provided with a bathwater source either in the enclosure or in a sink or tub to allow them to bathe and keep their feathers waterproof. Caution should be used with pools because even ducks can drown, especially if they are weak or not waterproof. It may be best to transfer these birds out as soon as possible and allow the rehabilitator to do this process.

Many water-type birds do not have feet designed for long-term perching. A kennel, box, or mesh cage can have a flat "shelf-type" perch or a split log available to those who feel comfortable standing up off the ground.

These adult birds, especially the herons, rails, and egrets, are quite nervous and will pace and wear themselves out trying to escape if they do not feel secure and hidden. These birds should be provided with the quietest place possible with covering on all sides of the caging.

Feeding

Although the commercial game bird grain mixes are sufficient in nutrition for short-term care of many of these species, getting them to eat it is the biggest challenge. These birds, with the possible exception of some ducks and geese, tend to be very difficult captive feeders. One problem is that many are normally used to feeding in or while on the water. Sitting on a towel in a box is too unnatural for them, and they don't understand the concept of eating with a bowl of food in front of them. Also, due to their nervous nature, they might not ever feel secure enough to eat.

Oftentimes these species will need to be tube fed or force-fed while they remain in captivity. Kingfishers, herons, and gulls must be fed fish, insects, and/or mice. To force-feed a fish, one must be sure to insert the fish headfirst into the bird's mouth and gently push the fish down the throat until the bird swallows. Holding the head in an upright position for several moments after feeding each fish may help prevent the bird from regurgitating the meal.

Several tube feeding formulas that can be used depending on the diet requirements of the species include Emeraid II, infant bird hand-rearing powdered diets, Clinicare (liquid diets made for dehabilitated dogs or cats), ground game bird pellets mixed with water, or blended fish.

All the medical procedures, cleaning, moving, and so on should be done before feeding is attempted. Feeding should always be the last procedure done on any animal and should be *immediately* followed by low stress, quiet, and privacy to aid the animal in the digestion process. Sudden loud noises or big movements may cause the animal to regurgitate the food and possibly even aspirate it.

Some fish eaters will learn to fish live minnows or gold fish out of a pan or bucket. Ducks, geese, coots, shorebirds, and similar species may eat live insects and chopped greens if provided in addition to the grain diet. Another hint is to float grain, insects, and greens on top of a dish of water. Sometimes this more natural presentation stimulates the birds to stab or dabble at the groceries.

GENERAL ORPHAN MAMMAL CARE

What to Do First

One should never feed any animal until it is warm and hydrated. A heat lamp, heating pad on low and always under cage not inside, or warm water bath to warm up a cold baby should be used. Once the baby is at normal body temperature, then one can start to rehydrate it.

Use of oral fluids such as lactated Ringer's solution (LRS) or Pedialyte is the preferred method of rehydration with infants. Subcutaneous fluids (LRS) can be used if the animal is moderately dehydrated. One should consider all animals that come into rehabilitation to be dehydrated to some extent. Fluids should always be warmed first before administering regardless of route.

The infant should be weighed and fluids provided at the rate of 40–50 ml/kg over a 12–24 period or until hydration is complete. See fluid chart in the glossary in appendix 9 under "Dehydration."

Introducing Formula

Once the baby animal is warm and properly hydrated, feeding formula can gradually begin. It should be introduced slowly to prevent digestive problems.

One should never start an animal on full-strength formula. It should take 24–72 hours to introduce a milk formula depending on the degree of initial dehydration. A severely dehydrated animal's digestive tract cannot handle full-strength or solid foods. Feeding these food items prematurely could prove to be fatal.

The following dilution procedure should be followed:

Day 1: 25% full-strength formula/75% water or Pedialyte

Day 2: 50% full-strength formula/50% water or Pedialyte

Day 3: 75% full-strength formuly/25% water or Pedialyte; or, 100% full-strength formula, if no diarrhea develops and infant remains hydrated

If diarrhea or bloating develops, at any stage, the concentration of formula should be reduced or replaced entirely with Pedialyte until the situation clears up. If problems persist for more than 24 hours, veterinary advice should be sought.

If bloating occurs, one can gently message the infant's abdomen while submerging the bottom half of the infant's body in a warm water bath. One can also consider giving oral simethicone drops for gas relief if the massaging is not completely effective.

Using a probiotic (*Lactobacillus*) product, such as Benebac, can be helpful to reduce stress to the babies' intestinal tract and help prevent or treat diarrhea.

If the neonate regurgitates formula, feeding should be discontinued and that feeding skipped altogether. At the next feeding, the formula can be thinned with water by half and the volume reduced. If the vomiting continues, veterinary advice should be sought.

Preparing Formulas
Milk formulas should be mixed by the label's instructions using warm water to help dissolve the powdered milk. Ready-to-use liquid formulas are also available, but they tend to be more expensive. Once the can is opened, unused milk must be discarded after 72 hours making this sometimes wasteful (fig. 14.14).

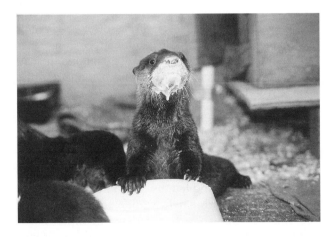

Fig. 14.14. Three-month-old river otter enjoying a bowl of Esbilac milk formula. (Photo courtesy of Melanie Haire)

Enough milk formula should be made up to last for 24 hours and kept refrigerated. When ready to feed, only enough should be heated for one feeding to 100°–102°F (warm but not hot on a wrist). One way to warm formula is to drop formula-filled syringes into a mug of warm water. Using an electric coffee mug warmer may be helpful to keep multiple syringes warm. Also, one should remember to cap syringes or milk will leak out and mug water will refill syringe resulting in diluted formula.

Do not use the microwave to heat formula. This method tends to cook the milk and leaves contents unevenly heated.

The infant should be weighed and the species care pages in the appendix used to determine quantity of food intake.

Some infants prefer to be stimulated to urinate and defecate prior to feeding. Use of a cotton ball or soft facial tissue dipped in warm water to lightly wipe babies' abdomen and genitals will suffice. This process also seems to stimulate the nursing reflex in some species.

Selecting Milk Formulas
There are many brands of milk replacers available as well as many variations of how to use them. Again, this is where contacting a local rehabilitator becomes critical. The importance of using the correct diet cannot be stressed enough. One should try not to switch formulas unless the baby is having trouble digesting the milk replacer chosen. By using the same formula that the rehabilitator will be using, the animal transfer process will be made much easier on the infant.

Of the many commercial formulas available, no one milk substitute will meet the needs of all species. Substitute domestic animal milk formulas for puppies, kittens, lambs, and foals have been successfully used. Recently a commercial line of milk replacers, formulated for wildlife, has become available. Due to space limitations this chapter will not cover detailed wildlife nutritional requirements and comparisons. One should refer to the species care sheets in appendix 7 for general diet guidelines. There are good reference articles and books available through the NWRA and IWRC on wildlife nutritional requirements.

The company Pet-Ag has been manufacturing milk replacer products since 1930 and most of the wildlife nutritional studies have been done on their products (e.g., Esbilac, KMR, Multi-Milk, Zoological Milk Matrix).

Homemade formulas are sometimes used but these rarely meet the complete nutritional requirements for wildlife. Cow's milk is not compatible with the natural milk of most wild animals and tends to cause gastrointestinal problems.

Syringe Feeding

Use the smallest size syringe that will hold the needed volume of formula. This provides the most accurate measurement of the animal's formula intake and the best flow control.

Many animals resist the first few feeding attempts due to the newness of the plastic feeder and the taste of the formula. However, after several feedings, they begin to accept their foster care.

Use of a soft rubber nipple (Catac) or silicone nipple (Mothering Kit) on the end of the syringe often helps facilitate the feedings. To help keep the nipple from slipping off the syringe tip, one needs to remember to wipe the syringe's slip tip dry and roughen the surface up slightly with a hemostat before slipping the nipple on. One needs to make sure that an overeager youngster does not pull the nipple all the way off and choke on it. Also, once rodents' incisors appear, discontinued use of the nipple may be necessary due to their ability to chew the tip off and possibly ingest it.

In the case of the tiny neonate (i.e., newborn chipmunk, flying squirrels, mice), a handmade "preemie nipple" can be made from two common veterinary supplies. A size 16 gauge intravenous indwelling catheter cut off about one-half inch from the end can be used as the base for the nipple apparatus as it fits onto any slip-tipped syringe. The nipple is made from the rubber sleeve that covers the needle of a multiple-sample blood collection needle used to draw blood. First, the rubber sleeve should be pulled down and punctured with the collection needle to make the nipple hole. Then the sleeve is pulled off of the blood collection device and slipped over the cut catheter. A size 16 gauge catheter provides a snug fit for the nipple, and the apparatus is ready to attach to the feeding syringe (fig. 14.15).

Other feeding syringe attachment examples are tomcat catheters, feeding tubes, or teat infusion cannulas.

Any slip-tip syringe will work but the o-ring type syringe is much smoother, and the rubber plunger doesn't stick and wear out as fast as the regular plungers do. (See suppliers list in appendix 10.)

Slow and steady pressure on the base of the syringe should be used to allow infants to drink small amounts at a time. Some species will nurse (i.e., squirrels, chipmunks, raccoons, and beavers) while others may lap (i.e., cottontails, opossums, and mink) at the tip of the nipple or syringe.

Use the following methods to help control the formula flow rate:

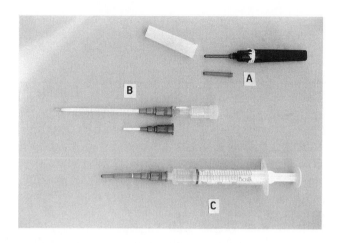

Fig. 14.15. "Preemie" feeding nipple. *A. A multiple sample collection needle. B. 16 gauge IV indwelling catheter. C. Assembled. (Photo courtesy of Melanie Haire)*

To increase flow rate

- Apply more pressure on syringe.
- Allow air into the syringe.
- Enlarge the opening of the syringe tip or nipple.
- Thin down the formula.
- Use a smaller size syringe.

To decrease flow rate

- Hold back on the syringe plunger.
- Remove air from syringe.
- Use another nipple with a smaller hole.
- Add rice baby cereal to thicken formula.
- Use a larger size syringe.

Each animal is different and one may need several different syringes and nipple combinations even when feeding littermates (fig. 14.16). Individual infants may drink too quickly regardless of what is done and the syringe will have to be moved away every few seconds to reduce the chance of the baby choking or aspirating formula.

Other Feeding Implements

Bottle-feeding can be used for some species of animals. Pet nursers and puppy and kitten bottles are sometimes used with small wildlife such as squirrels and rabbits. Human baby bottles and nipples will work for such species as large felids, canids, older raccoons, and otters. Neonatal carnivores should be started out on a human premature-infant-sized nipple. Hoofstock prefer a goat/foal-type nipple and bottle due to the size and shape of their mouths. This

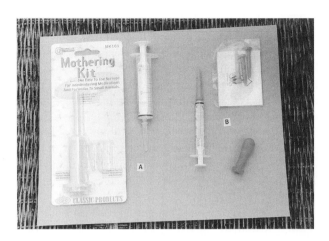

Fig. 14.16. A. Mothering Kit silicone feeding nipples. B. Catac rubber feeding nipples. C. Pet nurser nipple tip tied to a catheter tip syringe. (Photo courtesy of Melanie Haire)

method offers a faster formula delivery system but less control over milk flow speed and quantity.

One needs to remember to make the size of the nipple hole appropriate for the animal at hand. Holes can be made in the nipple by several methods. By cutting the tip off with a scissors or cutting an "x" into the tip, different flow patterns are created. To create a very small round hole, an appropriate-sized gauge needle is heated with the beveled tip in the flame. When the needle tip is hot, allow it to melt through the center of the end of the nipple. With the needle still in place, the entire apparatus should be placed in cold water until cool. Once the needle is removed, the hole remains approximately the same size as the needle gauge.

Eyedroppers can be used for hand-feeding but tend to produce air bubbles and make the milk flow difficult to control.

Gavage feeding, or stomach tubing, is another option for difficult feeders, such as armadillos, opossums, and nervous cottontails, who do not suck or drink consistently from other implements.

Stomach tubing can also be a lifesaving technique used with older juveniles and adult mammals but can also be the most difficult to do correctly and safely. When using the stomach tube method, one should never feed more then the calculated stomach capacity volume. It should be kept in mind that an emaciated animal's stomach capacity may be reduced by as much as 50%. Due to space limitation of this chapter, the gavage technique will not be covered here. This method is covered in chapter 9 under "Techniques."

Feeding Procedure

Infant mammals should be fed in an upright position on a soft, warm surface. Some babies like to feel secure and be wrapped in a cloth. They should never be fed on their backs as this could result in aspiration of the formula (fig. 14.17).

Mammals should be fed their calculated amounts until their stomachs are rounded but not tight. One should never overfeed a baby as it can lead to diarrhea, bloating, and perhaps death.

Even with every effect made, occasionally babies will aspirate formula and get milk in their nose or lungs. If this happens, feeding should immediately be discontinued, and the baby should be turned nose down and lightly tapped on its back. Any bubbles or drops should immediately be wiped off as they come out of the infant's nose or mouth to prevent reinhalation.

Once fed, all formula needs to be wiped off of the mammal. Allowing the milk to dry on the skin or hair of an infant can result in hair loss or skin infections. If the baby was not stimulated to eliminate before the feeding, it should be done afterward. One can gently stroke the belly and anal area with a warm, moist cloth until the flow stops. After about a minute, stimulation should be discontinued whether the baby has defecated or not. When the infant's eyes are open and there is evidence that it is eliminating on its own, stimulation can be discontinued. Any uneaten formula should be thrown away, as reheated milk should never be saved.

All feeding implements should be cleaned with hot soapy water after each feeding and a bottlebrush used to remove milk residue from hard to reach places inside the syringes/bottles. Syringes, bottles, and nip-

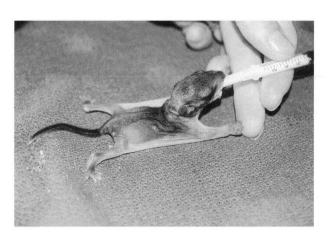

Fig. 14.17. Three-week-old flying squirrel being fed with a silicone nipple and syringe. (Photo courtesy of Melanie Haire)

ples should be disinfected once daily by soaking in an appropriate cleaning solution such as diluted 10% Nolvasan or 5% bleach for 10–15 minutes followed by a thorough rinse.

All items should be allowed to completely dry before each use to reduce the chance of bacterial overgrowth. Once they are cleaned and rinsed, feeding materials should be stored on an absorbent material such as a clean hand or paper towel or in a drying rack until the next feeding.

Orphan Mammal Housing

Most eyes-closed mammal infants can be housed in an incubator generally kept at 85°F–95°F. A set of plans to make an incubator is available on-line at the IWRC web site: www.iwrc-online.org. A homemade incubator can be made from a lidded plastic tote with ventilation holes. Some rehabilitators use glass or plastic aquariums, cardboard boxes, plastic pet carriers, or laundry baskets, of appropriate height and size, for this stage. A heating pad set on low, placed a quarter of the way to halfway under the tote, can provide the heat, and a water-soaked sponge placed in a plastic container with holes for evaporation can provide the humidity. One should make sure that moisture does not collect on the inside of the incubator by providing enough ventilation. A heat lamp can be used in place of a heating pad but both should never be used at the same time (fig. 14.18).

A soft, ravel-free cloth such as cotton T-shirt, sweatshirt, or flannel or fleece material can be considered for bedding. Terry cloth should never be used because their fingers, toes, and nails are too easily caught and twisted in the loops.

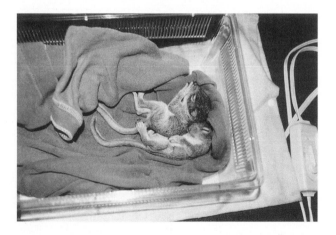

Fig. 14.18. *Two four-week-old gray squirrels on supplemental heat. (Photo courtesy of Melanie Haire)*

When the mammals become more active, they can be placed in a larger enclosure to allow for more room to exercise, dig, or climb. Once their eyes are open, baby mammals tend to become more active and they begin to explore their surroundings. One needs to be careful that the adventurous youngster cannot escape out of too large kennel door holes or unsecured cage lids. The supplemental heat and humidity can be removed when the baby is furred, able to thermoregulate, and spends most of its time away from the heat. This time varies from species to species and even from individual to individual.

Once the heat is no longer needed, one should begin to acclimate the babies by placing their cage outside for short periods of time at first and then gradually lengthening the time. Caution and common sense should be used with the placement of the cage, and one should be watchful for predators and sudden inclement weather and be sure to provide shade. The acclimation process usually can wait until the animal has been transferred to the rehabilitator's facility. Features such as nest boxes, hammocks, shelves, and natural items can be added to the cage at this stage.

The next phase usually begins once the mammals are weaned, eating natural foods, acclimated to the outside temperatures, and grown out of their cage. Preparing them for release by placing them in the large prerelease cages should be done at the rehabilitator's facility.

Recommended housing materials, sizes, and standards are also available on line at the IWRC web site, www.iwrc-online.org.

SPECIES CARE SHEETS

The species summary sheets provided in appendix 7, are meant for quick reference only. Entire books have been written on the care of each of these species and, whenever possible, one should refer to more than one source for more complete and detailed care. The charts are included to serve as a summary of age determinators and growth characteristics to provide the technician with enough general information to accurately confirm age and thus temporarily care for the most common species. Due to regional variations, standardized weights and infant developmental patterns are difficult to predict. Factors such as geographical location, subspecies, weather, season, and quantity and quality of food are just a few things that determine how fast or large an animal can grow. The species care sheets in appendix 7 should only be referred to after reading the general orphan mammal care section. See appendix 10 for a list of products mentioned in this chapter.

ACKNOWLEDGMENTS

Avian illustrations (figs. 14.2, 14.3, & 14.4): Illustrated by Linda A. Orebaugh, MS, AMI, from the *Care and Rehabilitation of Injured Native Wildlife* training manual. Permission for use granted by the Georgia Department of Natural Resources & Branson W. Richie, DVM, MS.

Raptor Tail Wrap Procedure (appendix 4): from *Raptor Rehabilitation, A Manual of Guidelines Offered by the Carolina Raptor Center*. Permission to use granted by Mathias Engelmann and Pat Marcum.

State and Federal Wildlife Permit Offices Lists (appendix 1): International Wildlife Rehabilitation Council Membership Directory 2001. Names and numbers are likely to change.

Raptor Restraint Illustration (fig. 14.1): Illustrated by George Carpenter. *Raptor Restraint, Handling, and Transport Methods* by Terry A. Schulz from the NWRA Volume 8 Symposium Proceedings. Permission for use granted by the National Wildlife Rehabilitators Association.

Photos: by Melanie Haire

Admission, Examination, and Animal Care Record Forms (appendix 2): by Janet Howard

Handling and Restraint of Wildlife Species Paper: by Florina S. Tseng, DVM, from IWRC 1991 Conference Proceedings. Permission granted for use by International Wildlife Rehabilitation Council.

Guide to Identification of Hatchling and Nestling Songbirds (appendix 5): by Marty Johnson from *NWRA Principles of Wildlife Rehabilitation, The Essential Guide for Novice and Experienced Rehabilitators*. Permission granted for use by the National Wildlife Rehabilitators Association.

Special Thanks: To Michael Haire, Veola Herron, Michael Ellis, Mike Fost, and Sue Barnard for all their help.

REFERENCES

Adams, P, Johnson, V, Goodrich, P, & Haas, R. 1991. *Wild Animal Care and Rehabilitation Manual*. Kalamazoo Nature Center. Kalamazoo: Beech Leaf Press.

Beaver, P. 1984. *Imprinting and Wildlife Rehabilitation*. Suisun, CA: International Wildlife Rehabilitation Council.

Campbell, TW. 1995. Raptor Rehabilitation in the Private Veterinary Hospital. In *Exotic Animals: A Veterinary Handbook*, pp. 121–25. Trenton: Veterinary Learning Systems Co., Inc.

Chapman, JA, & Feldhamer, GA (eds.). 1982. *Wild Mammals of North America*. Baltimore: Johns Hopkins University Press.

Crawford, WC. 1988. Hand Rearing Birds of Prey. In *IWRC Proceedings*, pp. 1–6. Suisan, CA: International Wildlife Rehabilitation Council.

Diehl, S, & Stokhaug, C. 1991. Release Criteria for Rehabilitated Wild Animals. *Symposium Proceedings*, pp. 159–81. St. Cloud: National Rehabilitators Association.

Dunning, JB. 1984. *Body Weights of 686 Species of North American Birds*. Suisun, CA: IWRC.

Ehrlich, PR, Dobkin, DS, Wheye, D. 1988. *The Birder's Handbook, A Field Guide to the Natural History of North American Birds*. Fireside: Simon & Schuster.

Engelmann, M, & Marcum, P. 1993, *Raptor Rehabilitation, A Manual of Guidelines Offered by the Carolina Raptor Center*. Charlotte: Carolina Raptor Center.

Evans, AT, & Evans, RH. 1995. Rearing Raccoons for Release: Part II: Rehabilitation and Diet. *Veterinary Technician* 6 (6):296–306.

Evans, RH. 1986. Care and feeding of orphan mammals and birds. In *Current Veterinary Therapy IX*, edited by R. B. Kirk. Philadelphia: W.B. Saunders Co.

Evans, RH. 1987. Rearing Orphaned Wild Mammals. In *Veterinary Clinics of North America: Small Animal Practice* 17(3): 755–783.

Fowler, ME. 1986. *Zoo and Wild Animal Medicine*. 2d ed. Philadelphia: W.B. Saunders Co.

Fowler, ME. 1979. Care of Orphaned Wild Animals. In *Veterinary Clinics of North America: Small Animal Practice* 9 (3): 447–70.

Fowler, ME. 1983. *Restraint and Handling of Wild and Domestic Animals*. Ames: Iowa State University Press.

Hanes, PC. 1988. Hand-Rearing Infant Tree Squirrels. *IWRC 1988 Proceedings*, 77–93. Suisan, CA: International Rehabilitation Council.

Ivie, D. 1999. Individual bird rehabilitator personal communication.

Johnson, V. 1991. *Wild Animal and Rehabilitation Manual, Kalamazoo Nature Center*. Kalamazo: Beech Leaf Press.

Klinghammer, E. 1991. Imprint and Early Experience: How to Avoid Problems with Tame Animals. *Symposium Proceedings*. St. Cloud: National Wildlife Rehabilitators Association.

Merritt, JF. 1987. *Guide to the Mammals of Pennsylvania*. Pittsburgh: University of Pittsburgh Press.

Moore, AT, Joosten, S. 1995a. Euthanasia—The three stages of euthanasia. In *NWRA—Principles of Wildlife Rehabilitation, The Essential Guide for Novice and Experienced Rehabilitators*. St. Cloud: National Wildlife Rehabilitators Association.

Moore, AT, Joosten, S. 1995b. *NWRA—Principles of Wildlife Rehabilitation, The Essential Guide for Novice and Experienced Rehabilitators*. St. Cloud: National Wildlife Rehabilitators Association.

Morzenti, A. 1998. *Captive Raptor Management*. Madison: Omnipress.

Pokras, M. 1995. *NWRA—Principles of Wildlife Rehabilitation, Introduction*. St. Cloud: National Wildlife Rehabilitators Assoc.

Raley, P. 1991. *Primer of Wildlife Care and Rehabilitation*. Troy: Brukner Nature Center.

Rue, LL. 1981. *Furbearing Animals of North America*. New York: Crown Publishers, Inc.

Schwartz, CW, and Schwartz, ER. 1974. *Mammals of Missouri.* Columbia: University of Missouri Press.

Stokes, D, Stokes, L. 1979. *Stokes Nature Guides, A Guide to Bird Behavior,* Volumes 1–3. Boston: Little Brown & Co.

Stokes, D, Stokes, L. 1986. *Stokes Nature Guides, A Guide to Animal Tracking and Behavior.* Boston: Little Brown & Co.

Wasserman, J. 1988. Raising Orphaned Flying Squirrels. *IWRC 1988 Proceedings.* Suisun, CA: International Wildlife Rehabilitation Council.

White, J. 2000. *IWRC—Basic Wildlife Rehabilitation 1AB Skills Manual.* Suisun, CA: International Wildlife Rehabilitation Council.

CHAPTER FIFTEEN

Avian and Reptile Hematology

Denise I. Bounous

INTRODUCTION

Birds and reptiles are not so different as one may suppose. Phylogenetically, these species emerge closer to each other than to mammals (Gauthier et al. 1988). Hematology of both is similar, in that they have nucleated erythrocytes that develop and mature in the bone marrow sinusoids, unlike mammalian erythrocytes, which migrate into the sinusoids and into vessels after developing into mature anucleate erythrocytes (Campbell 1967). However, these nucleated erythrocytes present problems for complete blood analysis. Automated hematology instruments do not accurately count nucleated erythrocytes. The morphology of blood cells may vary, not only between animal groups of birds and reptiles, but also between species within a group (e.g., iguanas and chameleons or boas and rat snakes). Additionally, there are variations in the white blood cell differential among the different genera of birds and reptiles. In some snakes, such as the boidae family (e.g., boa constrictors, pythons), the predominant leukocyte is the azurophil, whereas other snakes, such as rat snakes, have predominantly heterophils. Morphology of peripheral blood constituents can also vary. Thrombocytes of some birds and boid snakes are elongate and easily differentiated from small lymphocytes (see color plate 15.1), but thrombocytes of the rat snake are small and round, very similar to lymphocytes (Bounous et al. 1996) (see color plate 15.2). When performing a differential leukocyte count on birds or reptiles, it is advisable to scan the smear, examining each cell type, and identifying what characteristics can be used to classify the cell types before actually starting the count.

BLOOD COLLECTION

Avian and reptilian blood volume is approximately 10% and 5 to 8% of body weight, respectively, and approximately 10% of blood volume can be taken from a healthy bird or reptile with no ill effects (Mader 2000; Campbell 1995). Therefore, approximately 3.5 mL can be withdrawn from an Amazon parrot weighing 350 grams, but only 0.35 mL from a budgerigar weighing 35 grams. Thus, it is necessary to prioritize which assays are to be performed when only small volumes are available.

Blood for hematologic procedures must be collected in anticoagulant. Potential anticoagulants include EDTA (ethylenediaminetetracetic acid), heparin, or sodium citrate. Heparin can interfere with staining of blood cells, and using sodium citrate causes dilution of the blood resulting in incorrect cell counts. Comparison studies with the three anticoagulants show that citrate causes significant changes in PCV as well as increased cell lysis. Samples for hematology that are collected into any of these anticoagulants should be evaluated within 12 hours of collection for best results, as greater than 50% lysis can occur at 24 hours. Heparin is frequently used as the anticoagulant for avian and reptile blood samples only because it allows both hematology and biochemistry analysis to be performed on the same sample tube. Blood for biochemical analysis can be collected into lithium heparin or into "serum" tubes without anticoagulant. However, glucose, potassium, and chloride concentrations were shown to change significantly at 24 hours in python samples collected in lithium heparin (Davidson et al. 2002). When possible, EDTA is the optimal anticoagulant for hematology analysis and serum for biochemistry; however, the volume of blood that can be removed from birds and reptiles frequently limits this optimization. Blood collected for biochemistry into heparin or into tubes without anticoagulant should be separated immediately to prevent artifactual changes.

BLOOD SMEAR AND ASSESSMENT

Smears should be made as soon as possible after blood collection to avoid any deterioration of the cells. Methods for making smears include (1) using a spreader slide across the slide containing the drop of blood and (2) placing a cover slip on top of another cover slip containing a blood drop, then pulling the two cover slips apart. The cover slip method requires extra care in staining and must be fixed to a regular glass slide in order to evaluate microscopically. Blood smears are stained with classical Romanowsky-type stains, containing the dyes azure A, azure B, methylene violet, and methylene blue (e.g., Wrights stain, Giemsa stain, or rapid stains such as Diff-Quick or Accustain). A properly made smear can be used to assess the number of leukocytes and platelets, as well as evaluate erythrocyte morphology.

Leukocytes

Total Leukocyte Count

Leukocytes from birds are classified as heterophils, eosinophils, basophils, monocytes, and lymphocytes (Campbell 2000). Reptiles have an additional leukocyte, the azurophil (Hawkey & Dennett 1989; Frye 1991). In general, electronic counters cannot be used for avian and reptilian leukocyte counts. Avian and reptilian leukocytes are best enumerated using a hemocytometer. Various stains have been reported for use in differentiating and counting types of leukocytes from thrombocytes and erythrocytes. Using the Natt and Herricks staining method, all leukocytes and thrombocytes stain varying degrees of a blue-violet color. One must be able to identify thrombocytes from leukocytes in the hemocytometer in order to calculate the leukocyte count. Use of the Unopette #5877 eosinophil system containing phloxine B, which stains avian granulocytes (heterophils, eosinophils, basophils) is an indirect method for leukocyte counting. This procedure requires an accurate differential to calculate the number of leukocytes. After counting the number of cells staining an orange-red color on both sides of the hemocytometer chamber, the count is corrected for all leukocytes (to include monocytes, lymphocytes, and azurophils) based on the differential as follows:

Total WBC =

$$\frac{\text{\# of cells stained in the chamber} \times 1.1 \times 16}{\text{\% granulocytes}/100}$$

$$\text{Example: } \frac{300 \times 1.1 \times 16}{.60} = 8{,}800 \text{ cells/}\mu\text{l}$$

Estimating the leukocyte count is highly variable and not very accurate. A "guestimate" of the number of leukocytes/μl blood can be made from a well-made smear by counting the number of leukocytes per high power field (40× objective) in ten fields, taking the average of the ten, and multiplying by 1,500.

Heterophils

Heterophils are functionally similar to the mammalian neutrophil. Heterophils are usually the most numerous leukocytes in pet bird blood (see color plate 15.3). They are round cells with clear cytoplasm and prominent eosinophilic, rod-shaped to oval granules, which may partially obscure the nucleus. The nucleus of a mature heterophil usually has two to three lobes containing coarse, purple-staining chromatin. Immature heterophils are rarely present in peripheral blood of birds or reptiles, and usually are associated with inflammation (Bounous et al. 1989). The nuclei of these immature cells (toxic heterophils) have fewer lobes and may appear mononuclear with more basophilic cytoplasm and less mature granules (see color plate 15.4). Very early granulocytes may be so poorly differentiated that granules are round and exhibit staining characteristics of both eosinophilia and basophilia (see color plate 15.5).

Heterophils of reptiles are similar to birds, with some subtle differences. This cell can account for approximately 30–45% of leukocytes in reptiles. Mature heterophils of reptiles contain an oval-to-lenticular nucleus that can be eccentrically located in the cell with a chromatin pattern similar to that of birds. The nuclear color may range from more light blue in lizards to purple in other reptiles. The reddish-orange granules can be pleomorphic across the species, ranging from needlelike to oval and from large to small (see color plate 15.6). Heterophil cytoplasm of reptiles can frequently have a foamy appearance. As in birds, immature heterophils in the peripheral blood of reptiles indicates an increased demand for heterophils, such as in conditions of inflammation (Mateo et al. 1984).

Heterophilia, increase in number of circulating heterophils, is usually a response to stress or inflammation. Heteropenia may also occur with severe inflammation that exceeds or affects bone marrow production.

Eosinophils

Eosinophils are uncommon to few in the peripheral blood of birds and reptiles. They are round peroxidase positive cells, with pale basophilic cytoplasm and many spherical reddish-orange cytoplasmic granules (see color plate 15.7). Eosinophil granules from birds may appear brighter than heterophil granules. The nucleus is eccentrically located, and nuclear lobulation is less than in heterophils. Reptilian eosinophil size varies with species, with snakes having the largest

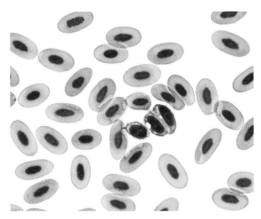

Plate 15.1. *Blood smear from owl: cluster of elongate thrombocytes. (Wright stain, EDTA, original magnification ×100)*

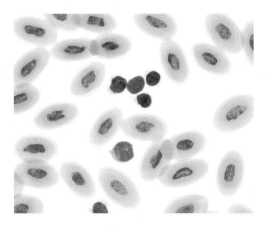

Plate 15.2. *Blood smear from rat snake: cluster of small round thrombocytes, one lymphocyte. (Wright stain, EDTA, original magnification ×100)*

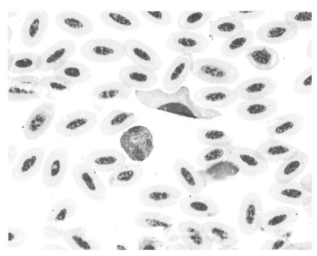

Plate 15.3. *Blood smear from hawk: heterophil, erythrocytes containing hemoparasite,* Leucocytozoon. *(Wright stain, EDTA, original magnification ×100)*

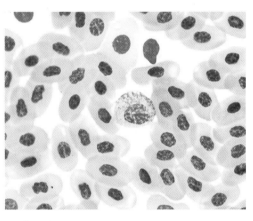

Plate 15.4. *Blood smear from tortoise: heterophil with band-shaped nucleus and area of basophilic cytoplasm. (Wright stain, EDTA, original magnification ×100)*

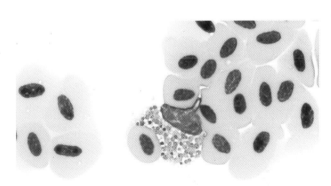

Plate 15.5. *Blood smear from owl: toxic mononuclear heterophil with eccentric nucleus and both basophilic and eosinophilic granules. (Wright stain, EDTA, original magnification ×100)*

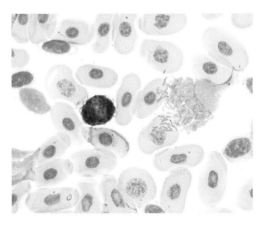

Plate 15.6. *Blood smear from a tortoise: basophil with granules obscuring the nucleus, ruptured heterophil with loose granules. (Wright stain, EDTA, original magnification ×100)*

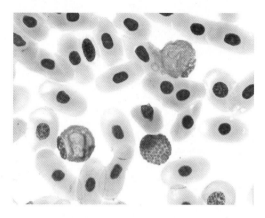

Plate 15.7. *Blood smear from a tortoise: heterophil with ill-defined rod-shaped granules, eosinophil with round distinct granules, heterophil. (Wright stain, EDTA, original magnification ×100)*

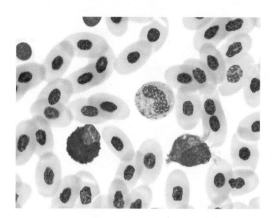

Plate 15.8. *Blood smear from a lizard: basophil, band heterophil, monocyte. (Wright stain, EDTA, original magnification ×100)*

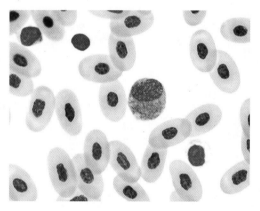

Plate 15.9. *Blood smear from a lizard: monocyte with gray-blue cytoplasm and oval nucleus. (Wright stain, EDTA, original magnification ×100)*

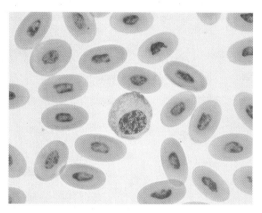

Plate 15.10. *Blood smear from a rat snake: azurophil with granules at cytoplasmic periphery instilling a pinkish-purple hue. (Wright stain, EDTA, original magnification ×100)*

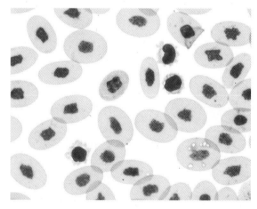

Plate 15.11. *Blood smear from a lizard: basophilic erythrocyte in center, two thrombocytes. Note irregularly shaped erythrocyte nuclei, tiny cytoplasmic vacuoles in erythrocytes. (Wright stain, EDTA, original magnification ×100)*

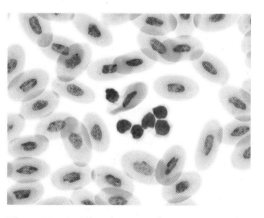

Plate 15.12. *Blood smear from a rat snake: cluster of thrombocytes. (Wright stain, EDTA, original magnification ×100)*

cells, turtles and crocodilians having intermediate-sized cells, and lizards having the smallest eosinophils. Eosinophils can make up from 7% to 20% of the leukocytes in healthy reptiles. Increased eosinophil numbers in pet birds have been associated with parasitism (Campbell 1994).

Basophils

Basophils are uncommonly seen in the peripheral blood of birds and most reptiles. Depending on the species, they may compose from 0 to 40% of the leukocytes in reptiles, turtles having the highest percentage. Basophils are easily identified because of their large, round, deeply basophilic granules. The round to oval nucleus is centrally or eccentrically located and frequently obscured by the granules (see color plates 15.6 and 15.8). Reptilian basophils, as mammalian basophils, appear to be involved in processing immunoglobulin and histamine release (Sypek & Borysenko 1988).

Lymphocytes

Lymphocytes occur in different sizes and somewhat different morphology. They are round or oval mononuclear cells with variation in the appearance of the nucleus and cytoplasm. Most are small to medium sized (5 to 10 μm) round cells with a centrally located nucleus containing densely aggregated chromatin. Nuclear shape is usually round to indented, and cytoplasm is pale blue. The nuclear to cytoplasmic ratio of small lymphocytes is high. Larger lymphocytes (15 μm) can have larger nuclei with more dispersed or reticulated chromatin and more cytoplasm, so that the N:C ratio is less. Lymphocytes may have cytoplasmic blebs and sometimes deeper blue staining cytoplasm at the periphery of the cytoplasm. Occasionally a few azurophilic granules may be present. Lymphocytes may occasionally appear to be indented by surrounding cells on the smear. In some parrots (e.g., Amazons, Electus), lymphocytes are reported to be the most common leukocytes in peripheral blood. Reptilian lymphocytes are similar, and can compose as high as 80% of the circulating leukocytes (see color plate 15.2). Reactive lymphocytes are larger cells with large nuclei containing dispersed chromatin and deeply basophilic cytoplasm. Reactive lymphocytes may result from antigenic stimulation of the immune system due to infection or inflammation. Lymphocytosis in reptiles can occur with viral diseases, inflammation, wound healing, and certain parasitic infections (Campbell 1996).

Monocytes

Monocytes are large mononuclear cells found less commonly in peripheral blood of birds and reptiles than lymphocytes. These cells are more variable than most other types of leukocytes. They can be round to oval to rhomboid shape. The nucleus may be small or large and round, indented, bilobed, or U-shaped. Monocytes may appear similar to large lymphocytes, but with finely granular cytoplasm that is blue-gray, and may also occasionally contain vacuoles. Monocyte nuclear chromatin is usually less clumped when compared to lymphocytes (see color plate 15.9). Monocytosis in birds can occur with chronic illness, such as tuberculosis, chlamydia, and aspergillosis.

Azurophils

Azurophils are unique cells identified only in reptiles. (These cells eventually may be determined to be a type of monocyte.) They are similar in size to heterophils with abundant cytoplasm that is finely to coarsely granular and may sometimes contain vacuoles. Granules may impart a purplish hue to the cytoplasm, particularly to the outer region (see color plate 15.10). Occasionally azurophils are observed with vacuolated cytoplasm (Dotson et al. 1995).

Erythrocytes

Early erythrocytes are round with round nuclei. The cells and nuclei become more oval, and the nuclear chromatin becomes increasingly condensed as the cell matures. Mature avian and reptile erythrocytes appear oval to elliptical on the blood smear with a centrally located nucleus that is also oval. It is not unusual for the erythrocyte nucleus to be irregularly shaped in some reptiles (see color plate 15.11). The cytoplasm of the early erythrocyte is basophilic, becoming polychromatic, and then pale orange to pink when the hemoglobin and cell is mature. The change in color from basophilic to eosinophilic as the erythrocyte matures parallels the maturation of hemoglobin in the cell. The mature erythrocyte varies in size, and to some degree, in shape, depending on the species of bird or reptile. A slight variation in the size of erythrocytes is normal. Polychromatophilic erythrocytes make up less than 5% of erythrocytes in the peripheral blood (see color plate 15.11). These cells can be identified and enumerated as reticulocytes by staining with a supravital stain, such as new methylene blue. Variation in size of erythrocytes and number of reticulocytes can be used to classify anemia. A greater degree of anisocytosis in the presence of increased polychromasia is indicative of responsive anemia. A large number of hypochromatic erythrocytes is associated with an erythrocyte disorder such as iron deficiency anemia. Marked poikilocytosis may indicate a maturation dysfunction. Occasionally erythrocytes of reptiles may contain small, clear cytoplasmic vacuoles that are not associated with any pathology (see color plate 15.11).

Thrombocytes

Mature thrombocytes in birds and reptiles are round to oval with a round to oval nucleus containing clumped chromatin. Their shape can vary from one species to another, but the cytoplasm is colorless to pale gray. Thrombocytes frequently contain a few small azurophilic granules. In some animals, thrombocytes are difficult to discern from small lymphocytes. Thrombocytes occasionally occur in closely associated groups in the smear, and this characteristic can be helpful in identifying thrombocytes from small lymphocytes (see color plate 15.12). Thrombocytes have been reported to have potential phagocytotic capabilities, but in general function as do mammalian platelets (Bounous et al. 1989).

REFERENCES

Bounous, DI, Dotson, TK, Brooks, RL, Jr, Ramsay, EC. 1996. Cytochemical staining and ultrastructural characteristics of peripheral blood leukocytes from the yellow rat snake (*Elaphe obsoleta quadrivitatta*). *Comp Haematol Int* 6:86–91.

Bounous, DI, Schaeffer, DO, Roy, A. 1989. Diagnosis of a coagulase negative Staphylococcus sp septicemia in a lovebird. *J Am Vet Med Assoc* 195:1120–22.

Campbell, F. 1967. Fine structure of the bone marrow of the chicken and pigeon. *J Morphol* 123:405–40.

Campbell, TW. 1994. Hematology. In *Avian Medicine: Principles and Application*. edited by Ritchie, BW, Harrison GJ, Harrison LP, pp.176–98. Lake Worth: Wingers Publishing Inc.

Campbell, TW. 1995. *Avian Hematology and Cytology*, 2d ed. Ames: Iowa State University Press.

Campbell, TW. 1996. Clinical pathology. In *Reptile Medicine and Surgery*, edited by Mader DR, pp. 248–57. Philadelphia: W.B. Saunders Co.

Campbell, TW. 2000. Hematology of Psittacines. In *Schalm's Veterinary Hematology*, edited by BF Feldman, JG Zinkl, NC Jain, 5th ed., 1155–60. Baltimore: Lippincott Williams and Wilkins.

Davidson, D, Harr, K, Raskin, R. Hematologic and biochemical changes caused by commonly used anticoagulants on Burmese python (*Python molurus bivittatus*) blood over time. *Vet Pathol*, in press.

Dotson, TK, Ramsay, EC, Bounous, DI. 1995. A color atlas of blood cells of the yellow rat snake. *Compend Contin Educ Pract Vet* 17:1013–17.

Frye, FL. 1991. Hematology as applied to clinical reptile medicine. In *Biomedical and Surgical Aspects of Captive Reptile Husbandry*, edited by FL Frye. 2d ed. Malabar: Krieger Publishing Company.

Gauthier, J, Kluge, AG, Rowe, T. 1988. The early evolution of Amniota. In *The Phylogeny and Classification of the Tetrapods*, edited by MJ Benton, Volume 1: *Amphibians, Reptiles, Birds*. Oxford: Clarendon Press.

Hawkey, CM, Dennett TB. 1989. *Color Atlas of Comparative Veterinary Hematology*. Ames: Iowa State University Press.

Mader, DR. 2000. Normal hematology of reptiles. *Schalm's Veterinary Hematology*, edited by BF Feldman, JG Zinkl, NC Jain, 5th ed., 1126–32. Baltimore: Lippincott Williams and Wilkins.

Mateo, MR, Roberts, ED, Enright, FM. 1984. Morphological, cytochemical, and functional studies of peripheral blood cells of young healthy American alligators (*Alligator mississippiensis*). *Am J Vet Res* 45: 1046–1053.

Sypek J, Borysenko M. 1988. Reptiles. In *Vetebrate Blood Cells*, edited by AF Rowley, NA Ratcliff. Cambridge: Cambridge University Press.

State/Federal Wildlife Permit Offices

STATE AND U.S. TERRITORY WILDLIFE PERMIT OFFICES

Listings are alphabetical by state or territory.

Chief of Law Enforcement, Division of Wildlife/Freshwater Fisheries, PO Box 301456, Montgomery, AL 36130-1456; 334-242-3467; ghouston@dcnr.state.al.us

Director of Wildlife Conservation, Department of Fish and Game, PO Box 25526, Juneau, AK 99802-5526; 907-465-6197

Wildlife Building Coordinator, Arizona Game and Fish Department, 2221 W. Greenway Rd., Phoenix, AZ 85023-4312; 602-789-3370, 602-256-7627 fax; azwildbd@primenet.com

Karen Rowe, Wildlife Permit Officer, AR Game and Fish Commission, 31 Hallowel Lane, Humphrey, AR 72073; 870-873-4302; krowe@agfc.state.ar.us

CA Department of Fish and Game, PO Box 944209, 1416 Ninth St., Sacramento, CA 95814-2090; 916-227-1305

Wildlife Permit Officer, CDOW/Special Licensing, PO Box 49128, Colorado Springs, CO 80919; 719-268-0143, 719-268-0144 fax; kathy.konishi@state.co.us

Wildlife Permit Officer, Department of Env. Protection, Wildlife Division, 79 Elm St., Hartford, CT 06106-5127; 860-424-3011, 860-424-4078 fax; laurie.fortin@po.state.ct.us

Kenneth Reynolds, Program Manager, Division of Fish and Wildlife, 4876 Hay Point Landing Rd., Smyrna, DE 19997; 302-739-5297, 302-653-3431 fax; mkreynolds@state.de.us

Wildlife Permit Officer, Florida Fish and Wildlife Conservation Commission, 620 S. Meridian St., Tallahassee, FL 32399-1600; 850-488-6253

Wildlife Permit Officer, Georgia DNR, Wildlife Resources Division, 2109 US Hwy 278 SE, Social Circle, GA 30025; 770-761-3044, 706-557-3060 fax; marykay_blalock@mail.dnr.state.ga.us

Administrator of Forestry and Wildlife, 1151 Punchbowl St., Honolulu, HI 96813; 808-587-0166

Wayne Melquist, Department of Fish and Game, 600 S. Walnut, Boise, ID 83707-0025; 208-334-2920

Permit Officer, Department of Natural Resources, 524 S. 2nd St., Springfield, IL 62701-1787; 217-782-6431; bclark1@dnrmail.state.il.us

Linnea Floyd, Wildlife Permit Officer, IN DNR, 402 W. Washington St. #W273, Indianapolis, IN 46204-2212; 317-233-6527, 317-232-8150 fax

Daryl Howell, IA DNR, Wallace State Office Bldg., 502 E 9th St., Des Moines, IA 50319-0034; 515-281-8524, 515-281-6794 fax; daryl.howell@dnr.state.ia.us

Wildlife Permit Officer, KS Department of Wildlife and Parks, 512 S.E. 25th Ave., Pratt, KS 67124-8174; 620-672-5911, 620-672-2972 fax; kenb@wp.state.ks.us

Wildlife Permit Officer, Department of Fish and Wildlife Resources, #1 Game Farm Rd., Frankfort, KY 40601; 502-564-3400

Nongame Biologist, LA Department of Wildlife and Fisheries, Natural Heritage Program, PO Box 98000, Baton Rouge, LA 70898-9000; 225-765-2976, 225-765-2607 fax; higginbotham_ne@wlf.state.la.us

Beth Turcotte, Department of Inland Fish and Wildlife, 284 State St, Station #41, Augusta, ME 04333-0041; 207-287-5240

Wildlife Permit Officer, DNR 580 Taylor Ave., Tawes State Office Bldg., Annapolis, MD 21401; 410-260-8540; mscanlan@dnr.state.md.us

Wildlife Permit Officer, Division of Fisheries and Wildlife, 251 Causeway St., Suite 400, Boston, MA 02114-2104; 617-727-3151, ext. 327

Jim Jansen, DNR, Box 30444, Lansing, MI 48909-7944; 517-373-9329

Nancy Huonder, WL Rehab. Program Coordinator, DNR Sect. of Wildlife, 500 Lafayette Rd., Box 25, St. Paul, MN 55155-4025; 651-297-8040, 651-297-4961 fax; nahuonde@dnr.state.mn.us

Richard G. Rummel, Department of Wildlife, Fish and Parks, MS Museum of Nat. Science, 2148 Riverside Dr., Jackson, MS 39202-1353; 601-354-7303, 601-354-7227 fax; richardr@mmns.state.ms.us

Bill Heatherly, Department of Conservation, PO Box 180, Jefferson City, MO 65102-0180; 573-751-4115, ext. 3262, 573-526-4663 fax; heathb@mail.conservation.state.mo.us

MT Fish, Wildlife and Parks, 1420 E. Sixth Ave, PO Box 200701, Helena, MT 59620-0701; 406-444-1267, 406-444-4952 fax; rcunningham@state.mt.us

Dana Miller, Wildlife Permit Officer, Game and Parks Commission, 105 W. 2nd, Suite #201, Lincoln, NE 69201; 402-376-3116; dkmiller@inebraska.com

Law Enforcement, NV Division of Wildlife, 1100 Valley Road, Reno, NV 89512; 775-688-1500

Attn: S. Wheeler, NH Fish and Game Department, 2 Hazen Dr., Concord, NH 03301; 603-271-2501

Wildlife Permit Officer, NJ Division of Fish, Game and Wildlife, PO Box 400, Trenton, NJ 08625-0400; 609-292-2965, 609-984-1414 fax; www.state.nj.us/dep/fgw

NM Department of Game and Fish, Special Use Permits Program, Law Enforcement Division, PO Box 25112, Santa Fe, NM 87507; 505-476-8064

Patrick P. Martin, NYS Department Env. Con., 625 Broadway, Albany, NY 12233-4752; 518-402-8985, 518-402-8925 fax; pxmartin@qw.dec.state.ny.us

Wildlife Permit Officer, PO Box 29613, Raleigh, NC 27626-0613; 919-661-4872

Chris Grondahl, ND Game and Fish Department, 100 N. Bismarck Expressway, Bismarck, ND 58501; 701-328-6351

Carolyn Caldwell, Asst. Administrator, Wildlife Management and Research, Division of Wildlife, 1840 Belcher Dr., Columbus, OH 43224; 614-254-6300, 614-262-1143 fax; carolyn.caldwell@dnr.state.oh.us

Law Enforcement Division, Department of Wildlife Conservation, 1801 N. Lincoln, Oklahoma City, OK 73105; 405-521-3719, 405-522-3486 fax

Dale Nelson, Department of Fish and Wildlife, 2501 S.W. 1st Ave, PO Box 59, Portland, OR 97207; 503-872-5260, x5348, 503-872-5269 fax; dale.c.nelson@state.or.us

Wildlife Permit Officer, Game Commission, 2001 Elmerton Ave., Harrisburg, PA 17110-9797; 717-783-8164

Wildlife Permit Officer, Division of Fish and Wildlife, Box 218, West Kingston, RI 02892; 401-789-0281, 401-783-7490 fax; lsuprock@mindspring.com

Wildlife Permit Coordinator, Sandhills Research and Education Center, PO Box 23205, Columbia, SC 29224-3205; 803-419-9645

Wildlife Permit Officer, Game, Fish and Parks Department, Division of Wildlife, 523 E. Capitol Ave., Pierre, SD 57501-3182; 605-773-4191

Captive Wildlife Coordinator, TWRA/Law Enforcement Division, PO Box 40747, Ellington Ag Center, Nashville, TN 37204; 615-781-6647

Wildlife Permit Officer, Parks and Wildlife Department, 4200 Smith School Rd., Austin, TX 78744-3291; 512-389-4481

DNR Division of Wildlife Resources, 1594 W. North Temple, Suite 2110, PO Box 146301, Salt Lake City, UT 84114-6301; 801-538-4701

Law Enforcement Assistant, Agency of Natural Resources, Fish and Wildlife Department, 103 S. Main St., 10 South, Waterbury, VT 05671-0501; 802-241-3727, 802-241-3295 fax; mallen@fwd.anr.state.vt.us

Judy Pierce, Wildlife Permit Officer, VA Department of Game and Inland Fisheries, PO Box 11104, Richmond, VA 23230-1104; 804-367-1076, 804-367-0488 fax

Division of Fish and Wildlife, 6291 Estate Nazareth 101, St. Thomas, VI 00802-1104; 340-775-6762, 340-775-3972 fax; sula@vitelcom.net

Peggy Crain, Department of Fish and Wildlife, 600 Capitol Way N., Olympia, WA 98501-1091; 360-902-2513, 360-902-2162 fax; crainpsc@dfw.wa.gov

Wildlife Permit Officer, Division of Natural Resources, Wildlife Resources, 1900 Kanawha Blvd., Bldg. 3, Rm. 816, Charleston, WV 25305; 304-558-2771

Wildlife Veterinarian-J. Langenberg, DNR Bureau of Wildlife Management, Box 7921, 101 S. Webster St., Madison, WI 53707-7921; 608-266-3143, 608-267-7857 fax; langej@dnr.state.wi.us

Law Enforcement Coordinator, Game and Fish Department, 5400 Bishop Blvd., Cheyenne, WY 82006; 307-777-4579

UNITED STATES MIGRATORY BIRD PERMIT OFFICES

The following list includes only the US Fish and Wildlife Service Migratory Bird Permit Offices.

Region 1: CA, HI, ID, NV, OR, WA
Tami Tate-Hall, US Fish and Wildlife Service, Migratory Bird Permit Office, 911 N.E. 11th Ave., Portland, OR 97232-4181; 503-872-2715, 503-231-2019 fax; tami_tatehall@fws.gov

Region 2: AZ, NM, OK, TX
Kamile McKeever, US Fish and Wildlife Service, Migratory Bird Permit Office, PO Box 709, Albuquerque, NM 87103-0709; 505-248-7882, 505-248-7885 fax; kamile_mckeever@fws.gov

Region 3: IL, IN, IA, MI, MN, MO, OH, WI
Marlys Bulander, US Fish and Wildlife Service, Migratory Bird Permit Office, Region 3, 1 Federal Dr., Fort Snelling, MN 55111; 612-713-5449 (direct office), 612-713-5436 (general line), 612-713-5393 fax; marlys_bulander@fws.gov

Region 4: AL, AR, FL, GA, KY, LA, MS, NC, SC, TN
Carmen Simonton, US Fish and Wildlife Service, Migratory Bird Permit Office, PO Box 49208, Atlanta, GA 30359; 404-679-4130, 404-679-7285 fax; carmensimonton@fws.gov

Region 5: CT, DE, ME, MD, MA, NH, NJ, NY, PA, RI, VT, VA, WV
David Dobias, Migratory Bird Permit Office, PO Box 779, Hadley, MA 01035-0779; 413-253-8643

Region 6: CO, KS, MT, NE, ND, SD, UT, WY
Laura Whalen, US Fish and Wildlife Service, Migratory Bird Permit Office, PO Box 25486 DFC 60154, Denver, CO 80225-0486; 303-236-8171 x630, 303-236-8017 fax; laura_whalen@fws.gov

Region 7: AK
Karen Laing, US Fish and Wildlife Service, Migratory Bird Permit Office, 1011 E. Tudor Rd., Anchorage, AK 99503; 907-786-3459, 907-786-3641 fax; karen_laing@fws.gov

Wildlife Admissions/Exam/Care Forms

Admission Form
Clinic Name • Address • Phone Number

Date Admitted: _____ / _____ / _____   Case No. _____
Time Admitted: _____ AM / PM

Rescuer Information

Name: _____
Address: _____
City: _____ State: _____ Zip _____
Phone: _____
Do you wish to be contacted via email about the animal's status?   □Yes   □No
Email Address: _____

Animal Information

Species: _____   □ Young   □ Adult
Date and time found: ____ / _____ / _____   Time: _____ AM / PM
Have you fed or medicated the animal? □No   □Yes, I gave it _____
Location Found:

_____

Describe circumstances found:

_____

Was anyone bitten or scratched by the animal ? □ Yes □No
Did you come in contact with blood/urine/feces/saliva? □ Yes □No
Other treatment/ comments:

Condition (Mark all that apply):

Cause of Admission:
(circle one)
- □ Cat / Dog Attack
- □ Hit by car
- □ Found on ground
- □ In road
- □ Abused
- □ Exposed to Chemicals
- □ Disease suspected
- □ Nest disturbed
- □ Hit window
- □ Shot
- □ Other: _____

Observations:
- □ Easy to catch
- □ Limping
- □ Can't stand
- □ Can't walk
- □ Panting
- □ Bleeding
- □ Wet
- □ Oiled
- □ Cold
- □ No apparent injury
- □ Other: _____

Describe condition: _____

_____

Disposition:

Date: _____ / _____ / _____
Circle One: R   TR   TD   TE   P   DOA   DIC   EOA   E
Location: _____
□ US F&WS Notification (Illegal activity, E/TH species, B/G eagle) Date: _____

Examination Form

Clinic Name • Address • Phone Number

Case No.: _____
Date: _____ / _____ / _____   Time: _____ AM / PM

Basic Information:

Species: _____   Age: _____
Sex: ☐ Male   ☐ Female   Weight: _____

Visual Observation:

Weight Distribution: ☐ Even ☐ Abnormal   Notes: _____
Movement/Attitude: ☐ Walks in circles ☐ Head tilt Notes: _____
Alertness: ☐ Comatose ☐ Lethargic ☐ Normal ☐ Excitable   Notes: _____
Body Condition: ☐ Emaciated   ☐ Underweight   ☐ Normal   ☐ Overweight

Temp: ☐ Hypothermic   ☐ Cool   ☐ Normal   ☐ Warm   ☐ Hyperthermic
Hydration: ☐ Severely Dehydrated   ☐ Moderate dehydration   ☐ Normal

Mouth: ☐ Normal ☐Plaque/Lesions   ☐ Cap Refill _____ seconds
       Notes:_____
Eyes: ☐ Follows movement ☐ Proper Dilation ☐ Abrasions/Cuts ☐ Consensual
                                                              Response
       Notes: _____
Ears: ☐ Normal ☐ Parasites ☐ Discharge/bleeding   Notes: _____
Nose: ☐ Normal ☐ Discharge/bleeding ☐ Cuts/Abrasions Notes: _____
Fur/Skin: ☐ Cuts/Wounds ☐ Abrasions ☐ Bald Spots ☐ Parasites Notes: _____

Gastrointestinal: ☐ Normal   ☐ Mouth odor ☐ Vomiting ☐ Blood
Urogenital: ☐ Normal   ☐ Discharge ☐ No urine/stool
Notes_____
Anal Area: ☐Normal ☐ Clogged ☐ Loose ☐ Parasites Notes: _____
Abdomen: ☐ Normal ☐ Bloated ☐ Painful ☐ Cuts/Abrasions Notes: _____

Cardio/Pulmonary: ☐ HR _____/min.   ☐ RR _____/min.
          ☐ Cough   ☐ Chest Sounds   Notes: _____
Muscular/Skeletal: ☐ Swelling ☐ Lameness ☐ Fractures/Dislocation ☐ Pain
                                                              Response

Animal Care Record
Clinic Name • Address • Phone Number

Case No.: _____

Species: _____   Description: _____

Weight Record

Date	Weight	Date	Weight	Date	Weight	Date	Weight

Feeding Chart

Date	Food Description	Amount per feeding	# Feedings Daily	Feeding Frequency	Comments

Treatment

Date	Medication/ Treatment	Comments/ Observations

Veterinary Care

Date	Description

Handling and Restraint of Wildlife Species

Florina S. Tseng, DVM
HOWL Wildlife Center
P. O. Box 1037
Lynnwood, WA 98046

INTRODUCTION

Wildlife rehabilitation involves the care of sick, injured and orphaned wildlife. These animals, while in captivity, require special husbandry practices—they must be transported, housed and fed. When they are ill, they must be examined and treated. In addition, it will sometimes be necessary to relocate "nuisance" wildlife to more appropriate locations. All of these situations will necessitate the handling and restraint of wildlife species.

CONSIDERATIONS

Restraint can be as direct as holding the animal in your hands or as indirect as restriction of an animal's movement by fencing. The responsibility for the animal's welfare is in the hands of the rehabilitator. The amount of restraint on the animal should be as minimal as possible, yet enough to accomplish the purpose of the restraint and afford the handler maximum safety.

There are four basic considerations in the selection of a restraint technique:

A. *Human safety* always comes first in the execution of any capture or restraint plan. If a person is injured during an attempt to handle the animal, all attention will be focused on the care of that person and the capture will be unsuccessful.
B. *Animal safety* if the animal is hurt or dies during the capture/handling, you will not have achieved your goal!
C. Choose the *proper technique* to accomplish the desired result. Have you chosen a technique that is likely to work given the environment and the expected behavior of the species?

D. *Can the animal be observed* during and after the procedure? Observation of the animal during and after capture/handling and transport will allow you to act in a timely manner if problems arise, e.g., breathing difficulties, hyperthermia etc.

In addition to the above basic considerations, there are also *environmental, behavioral* and *humane* factors in handling and restraint. A major environmental consideration should be the possibility of hyperthermia generated during the capture procedure. In order to restrain an animal, you usually have to chase and catch it, which means increased muscle activity for the animal. This, in turn, translates into heat generation, especially if the air temperature and humidity are high. Smaller species tend to overheat faster than larger species because they have a higher metabolic rate. So, keep these factors in mind when planning restraint, e.g. try to plan activities for cooler times of the day, if possible, and try to work quickly and efficiently if it is necessary to work during the hotter times of the day. Animals dissipate heat by a variety of methods, including excretion of moisture via urine, feces etc. and evaporation. Moisture can be evaporated from the skin (as long as the relative humidity is not too high) and the skin can become wet from sweat glands, from the animals' licking themselves, etc. Evaporation also takes place from the lungs of all breathing animals, so panting serves to increase cooling from the respiratory tract. Be aware of restraint techniques that inhibit heat dissipation—e.g. stockinette placed around a bird's body will prevent them from spreading their wings to allow convection cooling; wrapping a mammal in a heavy towel will decrease evaporative cooling, or taping a beak shut will inhibit the ability of the bird to pant.

Reprinted with permission from IWRC Proceedings 1991 "Handle with Care."

Clinical signs of hyperthermia include increased heart and respiratory rates, open-mouth breathing, and increased salivation/sweating in those species that are capable of sweating. These signs may, in turn, lead to dehydration and subsequent loss of cooling ability, weakness, depression, incoordination and, if the temperature rises above 108°F, eventually convulsions, collapse and death will occur.

The converse side is hypothermia or low body temperature. This occurs when you are working outdoors in cold temperature, or when you have animals housed in outside areas on cold concrete or other surfaces. It may also occur when you have a weak or sedated animal that has lost the ability to shiver and generate heat. Be wary of placing these animals on a cold exam table because their body temperature will quickly drop.

Be aware of the immediate surroundings you are working in. You may be able to use the physical environment to your advantage in capturing an animal—for instance, herding an animal using portable barriers (plywood) into a large pen or shed or against a fence or cliff, will make the final capture much easier. You must also be aware of physical hazards in the environment that the animal may encounter during a capture episode.

You can also use the physical environment to decrease the animal's sense perceptions. If, for instance, the animal is nocturnal, try to capture it during daylight hours. Conversely, if they are diurnal, try to work at night or dim the lights during the capture attempt.

What are some behavioral considerations in deciding on your capture technique? You must know the natural history of the species—is it nocturnal or diurnal, when is the breeding season, when are young raised, what are the food habits, what is the habitat occupied etc. These factors will aid in your decisions—e.g. if you capture an adult of the species, will you potentially be leaving young behind?

Animals have a natural fear of predators—this fear is what drives the flight or fight response. As you approach an animal, the first response will be to flee, if this is possible. If this is not possible and/or you come within a critical distance of the animal, the fight response will then be initiated. You may be able to use long handled nets, poles, or projectiles to extend the effective range of capture by staying outside of this critical distance until the animal is effectively restrained.

Know what the animal's fight response will be! Wild felid kits respond to being grabbed by the nape of the neck much as a domestic kitten does. However, this is not true of adults! Raccoons will turn and bite if you hold them in this manner. Knowing the behavior of the species helps you to determine what an animal will do next—e.g. buteo hawks will use their feet more than their beaks whereas falcons will use both feet and beaks; eagles are perfectly willing to bite, too, whereas vultures will regurgitate. Pigeons and waterfowl will beat their wings when alarmed etc. If you understand behavior, you will be able to give more complete and better care to your patients.

Never underestimate the power of confidence on your part! Your voice, eye contact and body language can all be used to psychologically restrain an animal or, conversely, will let the animal know that you are afraid. Be sure of yourself, but never let yourself become overly confident.

"Every restraint procedure should be preceded by an evaluation as to whether or not the procedure will result in the greatest good for that animal" (Fowler, *Handling and Restraint of Wild and Domestic Animals,* p. 5). Lastly, you must consider the most humane method of capture. You should try to reduce stress to the animal as much as possible during the capture. These stressors include visual, auditory, olfactory, tactile or psychological factors. Be sensitive but do your job. This means being prepared ahead of time so you can work as quickly as possible. In addition, try to minimize exacerbating any preexisting injury or condition during the capture and handling episode.

PREPARATION

Try to work in pairs whenever possible—having a backup person ensures the safety and efficacy of the plan. Next, decide on the technique you'll use beforehand—talk it through to make sure that everyone understands their role. Be prepared for all eventualities—especially the worst case scenario! Then, make sure all necessary equipment is ready and in working order before you attempt the capture. Protective clothing is helpful in most situations—long pants, long sleeved shirt, boots, gloves, and goggles.

TOOLS OF RESTRAINT

The first tool of restraint is *psychological restraint*—have confidence in your abilities. Everyone is aware that animals can sense when a person is afraid of them and react accordingly. Next, consider *diminishing sensory perceptions*. The more you can decrease or eliminate visual, auditory or other sensory stimuli during the restraint episode, the easier it will be on both humans and animals.

Physical barriers include using items such as shields made of plywood, Plexiglas, blankets etc. to herd animals from one area to another and provide a protective device between the handler and the animal. *Confinement techniques* include the use of squeeze cages, restraint bags, plastic tubes for holding snakes etc.

It is also possible to use equipment to act as *extensions of your arms*—e.g., nets, snares and tongs.

1. *Nets*—come in all sizes and shapes. By placing a net on the animal, many manipulative procedures, such as injections, examinations, or obtaining samples for blood work can be carried out. Hoop nets with long handles are commonly used. Be aware that the hoop edge can injure the animal. Better to allow the animal to enter the net than to swing the net at the animal. The net should be of sufficient depth to allow the hoop to be twisted, trapping the animal in the bottom of the net. If it is too shallow, the animal will be able to climb out. If you place the net on the ground or against the wall, it will help to restrict escape. Birds with talons or animals with claws are difficult to handle in large mesh nets. They may poke their limbs through the netting, possibly causing feather damage and fractured bones.

They may also cling to the netting with their talons, making it difficult to extract them. Try to use smooth netting for birds. If the mesh is too large, the animal may also force a head through the mesh and strangle. Know the characteristics of the materials with which the net is constructed. Nylon, cotton, and manila all withstand different degrees of stretch and wear. Inspect for flaws before use!

Rectangular nets can be placed in the path of various types of animals. As the animal runs towards it, the net is extended, then dropped over the animal. *Mist nets* are used to capture small birds and bats. *Cannon nets* are shot over the top of the animal or herd. Nets can also be suspended over feeding areas and dropped over the animal to entangle it.

2. *Snares*—used carelessly can cause unnecessary pain or strangle an animal. Commercial snares are designed with swivels for humane and effective manipulation. Quick release snares (Ketch-all TM) permit the animal to twist without being suffocated. Always try to include one front leg through the snare as well as encircling the neck to decrease any problems with twisting. Don't catch the animal around the chest or abdomen because you may cause crushing injuries to this part of the body and because this also allows too much mobility of the head. Animals with good forelimb dexterity, like raccoons, are sometimes difficult to catch with snares. Once you have the animal snared, grasp the tail and bring the animal taut to the pole, control the head and remove the snare as quickly as possible.

3. *Tongs*—vise tongs grasp an animal at the neck. They act like snares but do not completely encircle the neck—they clamp behind the back of the head. These are used for initial control.

The use of *physical force* involves using your hands to grasp the animal. You must know where and how to grasp, how much pressure to use and how this varies from species to species. The greatest protection you have is detailed knowledge of the animal. Gloves vary from thin cotton gloves to heavy, double layered coarse leather gloves. Leather welder's gloves are good for general use. The thicker and heavier the glove, the less ability you have to determine how tightly you are grasping the animal or to feel the animal's response. Try to keep the glove loose on your hand so you can slip your fingers up or out of the way if teeth penetrate the leather. Gloves do not protect from crushing injuries! Chain mail gloves alone or within leather gloves offer more protection against the tearing effects of large canine teeth. Lastly, *chemical restraint* can be administered via injection, pole syringe, blow-dart, or pistol. These techniques and the restraint drugs used are further detailed in *Restraint and Handling of Wild and Domestic Animals* by Murray E. Fowler.

SPECIFIC TECHNIQUES BY SPECIES

A. Opossums

Danger potential—sharp claws and 50 small sharp teeth! *Technique*—Fortunately, they usually move slowly during the daytime and will oftentimes "play possum" when stressed. Be careful if there are fetuses in the pouch, you may cause the fetuses to pull away from the nipples and they will need to be replaced right away. Opossums can be netted, snared, tonged or manually handled by covering the head with a towel, grasping at the base of the tail and supporting under the chest or grasping at the scruff of the neck.

B. Rabbits

Danger potential—will scratch with sharp claws and have powerful back legs. *Technique*—

be aware that rabbits can kick so strongly with their rear legs that they can fracture their spines! Grasp the loose skin over the back of the neck, lift the hindquarters with the other hand for added support and cradle the animal against your body. Rabbits can be induced into a torpid state by placing and holding them on their backs for a few seconds or blindfolding them.

C. Rodents

Danger potential—those sharp incisor teeth especially adapted for chewing and gnawing and sharp claws for burrowing. *Technique*—be aware that rodents possess no specialized thermoregulatory mechanisms—they achieve homeostasis by a high level of behavioral activity. Therefore, they are predisposed to hyperthermia when handled and hypothermia when sedated or anesthetized.

Squirrels, chipmunks—Can use fine mesh net, though claws sometimes become entangled. Can use a towel and gloves (they can bite through gloves!), and try to grasp behind the neck and one foreleg.

Beaver—do not lift them up by their tail, since they are so heavy, you can cause spinal injuries. Restrain with a snare or tongs around the neck, then lift up and hold at base of tail. Or some people feel that they don't have much in the way of a neck and prefer to wrap them up in a blanket and just pick them up manually; they do not tend to be very aggressive

Porcupine—separate porcupines that are in a group before attempting to capture one or they may bump into one another, cause quill discharge and injury to one another. Approach from the rear when the porcupine is facing into a corner, reach under the tail and grab the underhairs, pull backward and don't let the tail flip up or it will discharge quills into you. Then, slide your other hand beneath the tail and up under the body. You can also use a snare around the base of the tail and other snares on each foot to stretch the animal if you need to get a blood sample for any reason.

D. Carnivores

Danger potential—teeth designed for grasping and tearing prey with well-developed jaw muscles. Claws can rip and tear. *Technique*—in general, control the head first then the body. Wear gloves to guard against scratches, most can bite through gloves.

Fox, coyote, wolf—smaller canids can be netted or grasped by the base of the tail, and then manipulated until the scruff of the neck can be grasped. Can also use tongs around the neck for initial control, and can muzzle for further control of the mouth (though you are decreasing their ability to pant).

Bear—these animals have extremely powerful paws and limbs. Immature bears less than five months old may be hand-held or controlled with nets or snares. Mature bears can be handled only with squeeze cages and chemical restraint.

Raccoons—nets, squeeze cages, tongs, snares. Great forelimb dexterity.

Skunks—use a shield of plate glass or plastic, wear goggles or protective clothing. Use a net to capture, then sedate or anesthetize to handle further.

Mink, weasel—snares or manually grasping at base of tail, pulling up and out of cage, then grasping behind the neck you must move quickly! Sometimes it is best to simply try to pin them behind the neck then sort out where the rest of the body is.

Otters—river otters can be netted or snared. Sea otters require specialized techniques. They are trapped in the wild using basket nets from beneath while the otters float on the surface of the sea. The net is closed with a drawstring, then lifted out of the water. They are extremely susceptible to stress and have no insulating blubber layer. They are protected from hypothermia by their dense fur coats. You must prevent soiling of the coat.

Cats—infants are easily handled manually or wrapped in towels or canvas restraint bags. If the cat is under 30 lbs., they can be netted with a fine mesh net, snare or tongs, then the tail is grasped with a gloved hand. Squeeze cages can be used for the larger species. One of our secret techniques for luring them into cages is to use catnip!

E. Hoofed Stock

Danger potential—antlers, sharp hooves. *Technique*—small cervids without antlers can be handled manually. With one arm, hold under the abdomen in front of the rear legs and with the other arm, hold under the neck, lift the animal up and away from the ground and point the legs away from the handler's body. Larger cervids usually need to be chemically immobilized in order to work on individual animals. For herding or transporting, be aware that deer do not recognize chain link or wire net fences as barriers, therefore you should drape these with opaque plastic sheeting. You can also use plastic sheeting to herd them toward a certain area. Most injuries occur during herding and transport—try to arrange it so that you can funnel them via chutes into their new enclosure or a transportation crate. You must select the correct sized crate—if it is too large, they may try to turn around and injure themselves. Capture myopathy is a big problem in cervids.

F. Birds

Waterfowl—can be captured with nets or hooks or manually. Drape a towel over the wings to hold them against the body, then grasp behind the head. To carry, support the body, restrain the head and let the legs dangle.

Shorebirds—will try to bite and stab with long, sharp bills. Protect your face with goggles if necessary. Can net birds like gulls or place a towel over them. Control the wings first, then the head.

Herons, cranes, etc—their long, thin legs are easily broken by rough handling. They will aim for your eyes with their beaks and are fully capable of spearing an extremity—exercise extreme caution and always control the head first.

Raptors—beaks and talons are adapted for grasping and tearing flesh. Vultures will employ their beaks but have very weak feet. Wear heavy leather gloves, use a hood or towel on their heads to decrease visual stimuli. If a bird is on the floor of an enclosure, throw a towel or heavy cloth over the bird, wrap the bird in the fabric and then grasp the feet, then the head. Try to remove the gloves after the initial capture to facilitate handling. The feet should be grasped with one hand above the talons (but not too far above the foot or you will lose control of the talons) and with your finger between the two feet, the head should be grasped from behind without obstructing the trachea. If the bird is perched, it can be approached from in front or in back. If coming from the front, grasp the legs first, one in each hand, then transfer the legs to one hand and grasp behind the head. If coming from the back, grasp the wings, body and legs together, then separate the legs in one hand and the head with the other hand.

Galliform birds—usually docile but have claws and some males have well-developed tarsal spurs. Do NOT grab them by the feathers, especially the tail feathers, as the bird will release them into your hand. Hold the wings close to the body and try to control the legs.

Pigeons/doves—do not scratch, don't peck, have mild dispositions. Will attempt to beat their wings when alarmed. Grasp them from above and behind and press the wings close to the bird's body.

Small passeriformes—capture with a net in the aviary, hold cupped in one hand with fingers around the base of the head. Do not completely surround the sternum and interfere with respiration. Sometimes it helps to darken the room and approach from behind.

G. Reptiles and Amphibians

Chelonians—small species can be handled manually. Hold them on either side of the carapace, you may need to insert a finger between carapace and plastron to prevent the shell from completely closing. Do not rapidly turn the animal upside down then right-side up again as it is possible to cause a torsion of the bowel by this sudden movement. Snapping turtles are capable of inflicting serious bite wounds—grasp them at the base of the tail, lift off the ground then grab the carapace just behind the head. You can turn them over onto the carapace; they usually relax in this position.

Snakes

Danger potential—can bite, produce venom, or constrict. *Technique*—grasp behind the head (if nonpoisonous), then support the body. If unsupported, the snake can thrash so much that it dislocates or fractures its vertebrae. Snake hooks can be used to pin the head to the ground. Snakes can be cooled for procedures that require only mild restraint but respiratory ailments are a possibility after prolonged chilling. Handling poisonous snakes is beyond the scope of this talk—suffice it to say that you must be extremely careful, always have antivenin on hand and know what you are doing!

Amphibians

Danger potential—toothless but can bite with hard-keratinized plates in mouth. None are venomous. *Technique*—they can be netted, then surround the body with your hand—two fingers surround the neck and the rest of the hand encircles the body and back legs.

CONCLUSION

Just as there are a myriad of different animal *species* that the wildlife rehabilitator may be called upon to handle, there are similarly a wide variety of handling and restraint techniques that are available for use. Our job as knowledgeable rehabilitators should include familiarity with the proper techniques to use for each individual animal in each individual situation. In this way, we will best serve the interests of our unique patients.

REFERENCE

Fowler, ME. 1985. *Restraint and Handling of Wild and Domestic Animals*. Iowa State University Press, Ames.

Tail Wrapping

A. Standard wrap (to be used with tail feathers not in molt)
   1. Materials
      a. 1–2 tongue depressors
      b. Spray bottle with water (set on mist)
      c. Gummed paper packaging tape (sticky when wet)
      d. Used X-ray film or other plastic
      e. Scissors
      f. Stapler
      g. Adhesive tape
   2. Procedure
      a. Tear or cut off several strips of paper tape (2–3 inches long for American kestrel, 6–8 inches red-tailed hawk).
      b. Cut a strip of X-ray film about ⅓ the length of the tail and about the same width as the folded tail. Fold it in half and staple it at the fold.
      c. Gather all tail feathers fairly close together without bending them—the narrower the tail wrap, the stronger and less cumbersome it will be.
      d. Place the tongue depressor along the center of the tail so that one end is flush with the feather tips and the other end almost reaches the bird's body. You may have to trim the tongue depressor.
      e. Fit X-ray "sleeve" over the tips of the tail and tongue depressor.
      f. Wet the first strip of paper and fold it around the end section of the tail making sure no feathers are bent (see fig. A4.1).

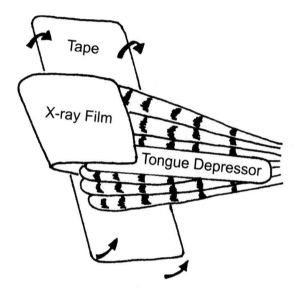

Fig. A4.1. *Wrapping the paper tape around the tail feathers.*

   g. Repeat with as many strips as necessary to cover the tail to the bare shafts making sure that each strip overlaps the previous one; do not include tail coverts (downy feathers on underside of tail). Try to conform shape of wrap to natural curvature of tail feathers.
   h. Finally, fold one long strip lengthwise around the tip of the tail wrap and press all strips firmly together, making sure they all stick well (see fig. A4.2).

Tail wrapping article reprinted with permission from the Carolina Raptor Center, www.birdsofprey.org, *Raptor Rehabilitation, A Manual of Guidelines*, pp. 30–31.

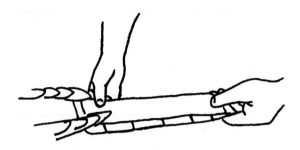

Fig. A4.2. The completed tail wrap.

3. Notes
   a. For long-tailed birds (cooper's hawk, etc.), you may have to tape two tongue depressors together.
   b. For American kestrals, you may have to cut one off a little.
   c. Make wraps as lightweight as possible.
   d. Press edges together firmly and dry the tail wrap. A wet or loose wrap will slide off as soon as the bird is returned to its cage.
   e. Tail wraps will have to be repaired or replaced periodically.
4. To remove this tail wrap
   a. Soak the whole tail in a pitcher or bucket filled with warm water. Gently begin separating the tape from feathers with your fingers. After 30–45 seconds the whole wrap will often slide off in one piece. Do not try to cut or tear the wrap off dry—it will permanently damage feathers.

B. Modified wrap (To be used with tail feathers in molt)
   1. Materials
      a. Piece of used X-ray film or similar lightweight plastic
      b. Masking tape
      c. Stapler
   2. Procedure
      a. Cut a piece of plastic as long as the tail and twice as wide as the folded tail (not fanned out).
      b. Fold this piece in half lengthwise so it now matches the shape of the folded-up tail fairly well.
      c. Place a few staples along the long edge (where two edges meet) and along one short edge. You should now have an "envelope" with one short side still open.
      d. Carefully slide this sleeve over the folded-up tail.
      e. Attach the sleeve to some of the downy coverts on the underside and backside with some strips of masking tape. Be sure not to cover up the oil gland or the feathers covering the vent area.
   3. Notes
      a. Depending on the material used this wrap may be stiff enough without the addition of tongue depressors.
      b. If the bird is active or when the masking tape wears out, this wrap will have to be repaired/replaced.
      c. Standard-size sleeves can be prepared and kept on hand for quick applications.

Guide to Identification of Hatchling and Nestling Songbirds

Table A5.1. Yellow to Orange Mouth Birds*

Species	Mouth color	Gape flanges	Beak contour	Down	Legs/feet	Approximate weight in grams			Feeding call	Feathers	Special features
						Hatchling	Nestling	Adult (F)			
Starling	bright yellow	bright yellow, very prominent, lower larger than upper	very wide	grayish-white, long and plentiful on head, back, and wings	long legs	5.5–30	40–60	80	hatchling—single squeaky note	gray-black	
Mockingbird	yellow	yellow	wide	dark gray, plentiful	long legs	5–18	20–32	43	hatchling—single, clear, piping note; then throaty bark	gray and white striped wings and tail	gray, irides, crescent marking on roof of mouth
Robin	yellow to yellow-orange	pale yellow	wide	sparse, cream on head, back, legs	long legs	5–35	40–60	77	hatchling—staccato trill	rust-tipped speckly chest	skin often yellowish
Black phoebe	bright yellow-orange	bright yellow	wide, flat, tapering to a point	gray and sparse	long, thin legs	2–5	7–15	18	peep-peep	brown-tipped black feathers	insect eater
Pacific slope flycatcher	bright yellow-orange	yellow	flat, wide, pointy tip, "arrowhead" look	white on head, back and wings in a "star" cluster	long, thin, delicate, dark blue-gray, white toenails	2–6	7–8	11	insistent—crowlike squawk, frog-like when older	buff abdomen, buf and white striped wings	insect eater
Cliff swallow	orange-yellow	flesh	very wide, flat, pointy beak	light gray head and back	short legs, small chubby feet	2–13	13–15	22	barking type chirp	nestlings—light tan on back by tail, otherwise adult	insect eater, cavity nest
Violet-green swallow	orange-yellow	cream	very wide, pointy beak	cream on head, shoulders and back	short legs	1.5–8	8–10	14		white eyebrows	insect eater, cavity nest

Species	Mouth color	Gape flanges	Beak contour	Down	Legs/feet	Approximate weight in grams			Feeding call	Feathers	Special features
						Hatchling	Nestling	Adult (F)			
California thrasher	orange-yellow	cream	curves down as nestling grows	dark gray on head, back, wings, thighs, plentiful	long legs	6–35	40–60	84		medium gray	
Chestnut-backed chickadee	orange-yellow	very yellow, prominent	flat, wide	gray on head and back	long, pale bluish-purple	1–4	6–8	10	squeaky cheep	buff abdomen, black head, buff—white circles on side of head	insect eater
Bewick's wren	orange	yellow	flat, wide, pointy	long, gray on head only	long, delicate	1–4	6–8	10		circles	
Bushtit	deep orange-yellow	yellow	short	none	long, delicate	1–3	3.5–4	5	3 syllable "locator" call, "mohawk" look	gray, first feathers on crown of head	females have blue eyes, cavity nesters
Wrentit	deep orange	yellow	pointy	none		1.5–6	7–11	14		gray-brown	yellow irides.

Source: Marty Johnson, Wildlife Rescue, Inc., Palo Alto, CA 94303, 1995.

*Bushtits, chickadees, creepers, dippers, flycatchers, mockingbirds, robins, shrikes, starlings, swallows, thrashers, thrushes, titmice, wrens, and vireos.

Table A5.2. Pink to Red Mouth Birds*

Species	Mouth color	Gape flanges	Beak contour	Down	Legs/feet	Approximate weight in grams			Feeding call	Feathers	Special features
						Hatchling	Nestling	Adult (F)			
House sparrow	pink	med. yellow, prominent	short-cone-shaped	none	short, chunky	2–13	14–20	27	melodic, single chirp	smooth, gray-white chest	
Rufous sided towhee	pink	pale yellow	conical and pointed	dark gray	long legs, big feet	3–18	20–29	39		dark back, white spots on wings and tail	
California towhee	pink to red	pale yellow not prominent	conical and pointed	long, brown-gray on head, back and wings	long legs, big feet	4–20	25–39	52	high-pitched repeated, like crickets, changes to single peep	brown	
Brown-headed cowbird	deep pink	white to cream not prominent	heavy, to a point narrower than a towee's	long, snow-white	long legs, big feet, blk. tipped nails	2–20	25–30	39	continuous, high-pitched vibrating sound	breast yellowish when coming in	bald face, parasitic, often found in nests of towhees
Northern oriole	deep pink	pale yellow	long, pointed, narrow	long, white-lt. gray on bk, wngs, 2 rows on head	long, slate-gray legs	2.5–18	20–25	33	high, staccato, repeated notes, similar to blackbird	yellow breast, gray back, white wing bars	insect eater
Lesser goldfinch	red	pale yellow	similar to finch	grayish	short, pink, stubby	1–6	7–8	10	green to rust back, yellow abdomen	red dot at corner of gape flanges	
Red-winged blackbird	red	yellow, not prominent	long, pointed	scant, white on back, lower wings, and thighs	long legs	3–15	20–30	42		bald face, similar to cowbirds	
Brewer's blackbird	red	white, not prominent	long, pointed	blackish-gray fairly plentiful	long legs, white toenails	3–15	20–30	42	raucous, repeated call, sounds like a rusty hinge	black	

Species	Mouth color	Gape flanges	Beak contour	Down	Legs/feet	Approximate weight in grams			Feeding call	Feathers	Special features
						Hatchling	Nestling	Adult (F)			
Scrub jay	red	white, not prom inent	long and wide	none	long legs, grabby feet, white toenails	6–30	35–70	87	hatchling-short repeated peeping, later a single squawk	furry gray head, blue wings and tail	ruddy skin
House finch	red	white to yellowish	short, conical	white, long and plentiful. 4 rows on head	short, stocky	1.5–8	10–15	21	none when newly	stripey, gray/ hatched, then high-pitched peeping	white chest
Crow	red	white	very long, large, heavy	sparse, gray-brown on head, underparts	long, heavy	18–70	70–328	438		black	ruddy skin

Source: Marty Johnson, Wildlife Rescue, Inc., Palo Alto, CA 94303, 1995.
*Blackbirds, cowbirds, crows, finches, goldfinches, grosbeaks, jays, orioles, sparrows, tanagers, towhees, and waxwings.

APPENDIX SIX

Average Body Weights of Selected North American Songbirds

Bird species	Weight range (g)	Avg. weight (g)
American robin		77
Bluebird, eastern		31
Cardinal	33.6–64.0	45
Carolina wren		21
Chickadee, black-capped	8.2–13.6	10.8
Crow, American		448
Dove, mourning		126
Duck, mallard	720–1580	1,082
Finch, house	19–25.5	21
Flicker, yellow-shafted	130	106–164
Goldfinch, American	8.6–20.7	12.6
Grackle, common		115
Hummingbird, ruby-throated	2.4–4.1	3.0
Jay, blue	64.1–109	85
Mockingbird	36.2–55.7	49
Oriole, orchard	16.0–25.1	19.6
Pigeon		270
Purple martin		49.4
Sparrow, house	20.1–34.5	27.4
Swallow, barn	13.4–23.4	19
Thrasher, brown	57.6–89.0	69
Titmouse, tufted	17.5–26.1	21.6
Warbler, pine	9.4–15.1	11.9
Woodpecker, pileated		290
Woodpecker, red-headed	56.1–90.5	72

Species Care Sheets

Table A7.1. *Raccoon Care Sheet*

Age (weeks)	Weights (g)	Age determinates	Diet	Amount	Frequency
0–1	50–100	Faint tail rings and mask, very lightly furred, ears pressed against head	KMR	Volume by B.W.	q 3 hr, 1 PM feeding
1–2	100–150	Face mask furred, eye slit visible, crawling on belly	KMR		q 3.5 hr, 1 PM feeding
2–3	100–200	Ear canals open, 18–24 d eyes open	KMR		q 3.5 hr, no PM feeding
3–4	200–300	Fully furred tail rings, responds to sight and sound	KMR, add cereal		q 4 hr
4–5	175–300	Able to walk, eyes open but cloudy blue, deciduous teeth erupting	KMR, add soaked kibble		q 4 hr
5–6	300–400	Able to run and climb, eyes darken			QID
6–7	400–600	Adult pelage begins (ends 12–14 weeks)			TID
7–8	600–650	2nd & 3rd premolars erupt, full sight & hearing	Start weaning		TID
8–9	650–675	1st permanent incisors erupt	Start dish feeding		BID
9–10	675–700	1st premolars erupt	No bottle feedings		SID
10–11	700–775	Wean 10–12 weeks	Weaned		
11–12	775–825				
12–13	825–875	3rd permanent incisors erupt			
13–14	875–900				
14–15	900–1,100				

RACCOONS

Raccoon Diet and Feeding
Formula: 1 part powdered KMR : 2 parts water.

- Stomach capacity is 50–66 ml/kg (5%–7%) Use 50 ml/kg to reduce chances of diarrhea. (.05 × B.W. in g =_____ml.) There are 30 ml / fluid ounce.
- Do not allow free choice formula feeding because some raccoons will overeat and develop diarrhea or bloat.
- Very young raccoons can be fed with a dropper, pet nurser bottle or nipple attached to a syringe. The pet nurser has the least amount of flow control so use them with caution.
- Older juveniles are often fed with preemie baby bottles and nipples. After bottle feeding always remember to burp the baby by patting firmly between the shoulder blades and down the infant's back.
- New incoming infants may take several days to become accustomed to the new diet and feeding instrument.
- Scratching the back of a raccoon's neck, while holding the nurser in its mouth, usually stimulates a suckling reflex.
- Once baby raccoons get the idea of bottle nursing, the rest of the feeding times are spent trying to slow them down. They tend to drink very fast and you must pull the bottle away after they have received the measured formula amount or they will swallow air.
- Stimulate before feeding until eyes open and self-elimination is evident (4–5 weeks).
- Add baby rice cereal to formula as a thickener to slow down overzealous nursers.
- Gradually begin introducing solid foods (applesauce, yogurt, baby foods, softened puppy food), either in with the formula or separate, once raccoons have their eyes open and are beginning to get teeth (4 weeks).
- Once they have a taste for the puppy food in the formula, start offering it dry.
- Gradually decrease the bottle feeding until weaned (7–12 weeks).
- Begin to offer drinking water when raccoons begin to eat solid foods but plan to refill water bowl several times a day because they love to climb in and also dunk their food items in bowl.
- Some rehabilitators prefer to teach the babies how to lap formula out of a bowl. This method takes patience and a lot of wash cloths to clean up afterward.
- Raccoons may resist weaning and lose weight at first.
- Dry puppy food (Science Diet Canine Growth) should constitute 90% of the post-weaning diet.
- Remaining 10% of diet should be apples, grapes, berries, eggs, vegetables, sweet potatoes, fish, worms, clams, small rodents, chicks, and crayfish.
- By 12 weeks old raccoons should be able to kill crayfish.
- By 14 weeks old raccoons should be able to kill young rats.
- Some individuals need to be fasted for 24 hours before they will try new foods.
- Use caution and protective clothing when handling raccoons since they are a rabies vector species.

Raccoon Housing
- From 0–5 weeks old, a cardboard box or pet carrier works best because it can be thrown out after it becomes soiled. Due to the zoonotic concern with the internal parasite *Baylisascaris procyonis*, any fecal contaminated materials should be burned or thrown out. Never reuse any cages or caging materials used with raccoons with any other species since disinfectants are ineffective in killing the raccoon roundworm. Fresh feces are not infective, but becomes so in 3 to 4 weeks. Intake procedure for raccoons should include weekly dewormings of pyrantel pamoate suspension 4.5 mg/ml at 0.5–1 cc/lb.
- Use soft, ravel-free cloth as bedding. No terry cloth because their fingernails get caught in the loops too easily.
- Provide supplemental heat until they are 4 weeks old.
- At 6 weeks provide animal with a wire cage with logs, natural substrate, tree limbs for climbing, and a hammock made from canvas or tight-weave netting should be hung near the top of the enclosure. The hammocks are a good substitute for wooden nest boxes because they can be changed and washed.
- By 8 weeks, raccoons are very active and need a large cage with lots of natural items to help keep them from getting bored (i.e., hollow logs, rocks, live plants, dirt for digging, water bowls for dunking food, pine cones, small pool).
- Outdoor acclimation usually starts at 6 weeks and finishes by 12 weeks.

Raccoon Release
- Release age is 4–5 months when they are self-feeding and acclimated to the outdoors.

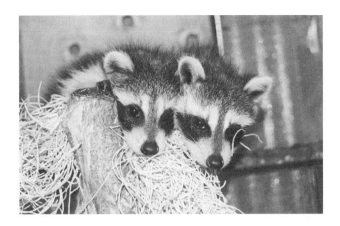

Fig. A7.1. Racoon babies.

- This page will not cover raccoon release due to the regulations on possessing rabies vector species in many states and the numerous difficulties one can face with this procedure. Turning all raccoons over to a licensed rehabilitator, vaccinated against rabies, is recommended.

FLYING SQUIRRELS

Flying Squirrel Diet and Feeding
Formula: 1 part powdered Esbilac: 2 parts water.

- Feed with a 1 or 3 cc O-ring syringe with silicone nipple.
- Flying squirrels have a good suckling reflex and the formula may need to be thickened to prevent aspiration.
- Gradually thicken formula with rice baby cereal starting at 3 weeks.
- Stimulate after each meal until the eyes are open and there is evidence of self-elimination in cage.
- Once eyes are open begin to introduce solid food items.
- Start decreasing number of formula feedings as solid food is being consumed (4–5 weeks).
- Wait at least 4 days between feeding reductions.
- A useful weaning tool is to add powdered rodent or primate chow to the formula starting at 5 weeks.

Table A7.2. Flying Squirrel Care Sheet

Age (weeks)	Weights (g)	Age determinates	Diet	Amounts	Frequency
0–1	3–6	Pink, no fur, eyes closed, few whiskers	Esbilac	0.2–0.3 ml	q 2 hr, 2 PM feedings
1–2	6–10	Short hairs appear, toes separate	Esbilac	0.3–0.6 ml	q 2 hr, 1 PM feeding
2–3	10–15	Downy hair darkens, able to right themselves, ear canals open, lower incisors erupt	Esbilac	0.6–1.0 ml	q 3 hr, no PM feeding
3–4	17–23	Lateral tail hairs develop, responds to loud noises	Esbilac, add cereal	1.0–1.5 ml	q 3 hr
4–5	25–30	Fur covers body, upper incisors erupt, days 28–32 eyes open	Esbilac, cereal, add solid food	1.5–2.0 ml	q 4 hr
5–6	30–38	Miniature version of adult	Weaning begins	2.0–2.5 ml	TID
6–7	38–43		Add rodent pellets	2.5–3.0 ml	BID
7–8	40–47		Add natural foods	3.0–5.0 ml	SID-BID
8–10	47–53		Wk 8–9 weaned		
12–14	60	Ready for release			

- Examples of weaning foods include dog chow, raw nuts, fresh corn on the cob, apple, grapes, rodent blocks, primate chow, seed mix, vegetables, sweet potatoes, carrots, broccoli, wheat germ, etc.
- Natural food items to offer include mushrooms, lichens, bark, buds, insects, acorns, hickory nuts, pine cones, beech nuts, berries, green buds, etc.
- Diet ratio of food groups should be: 80% rodent mix (dog, primate, rodent chow); 20% fruit and vegetable matter; 1 nut/squirrel/day; 2–3 insects/squirrel/day.
- Offering squirrel "nutri-bites" (recipe under grey squirrel diet) until release will help assure proper nutrition.
- Provide drinking water in a bowl or water bottle when babies are weaned down to twice a day formula.
- Once weaned, feed the squirrels at night (since they are nocturnal) and scatter food around the cage.

Flying Squirrel Housing

- Supplemental heat is needed until they are 5–6 weeks old. Using a heating pad under half of the enclosure is recommended.
- Masters of escape, flying squirrels need to be housed in a secure enclosure with a tight lid.
- 1–4 weeks in aquarium or small box.
- 4–6 weeks in a larger wire portable cage (begin to acclimate to the outdoors).
- Provide a nesting box since these squirrels live in tree cavities in the wild.
- 6–14 weeks in outdoor prerelease pen (once acclimated). This pen needs to be large enough for the young flying squirrels to practice jumping and gliding. Minimum size of 6′ H × 6′ W × 8′ L.
- The pen needs both horizontal and vertical branches to assimilate the trees.
- Flying squirrels move from tree to tree and rarely go to the ground.

Flying Squirrel Release

- Release age is 14–16 weeks.
- Release criteria: Fully acclimated to outdoors, nocturnal behaviors, running from humans, opening shelled nuts, and eating natural food items.
- Whenever possible, raise and release flyers with a group since these animals live in colonies. Also release in a well-wooded area where other flyers have been seen or heard.

- Release by closing animals up inside their nest box 1 hr before dark outside (tape hole shut). Tie box to tree trunk (6 ft or higher up) and remove tape from nest box entrance at dusk. Flyers will exit box and explore the tree tops then sometimes return to the nest box until they find another cavity to sleep in.
- Supply back-up food by having a nearby feeding station or putting bowl on top of nest box.

Flying Squirrel Miscellaneous Information

- When startled, flying squirrels flip on their backs and box at the invader with all four feet. Wake the sleeping baby up slowly and gently to prevent this aggressive display.
- Do not worry if the infant does not eliminate each time it is stimulated. Discontinue stimulation after about a minute. As long as the squirrel has at least one bowel movement a day bloating should not occur.

OPOSSUMS

Opossum Diet and Feeding
Formula: 1 part powdered Esbilac : 2 parts water

- Stomach capacity is 50–66 ml/kg or 5%–7% of BW. (.05 × BW in g =_____ml)
- Opossums have a poorly developed suckling reflex, which makes gavage feeding the most effective method to feed young animals under 45 grams.
- Gavage tube size ranges from size 3½–5 French feeding tube.
- Pinkies should be started on very dilute formula (1:5 w/water) and gradually built up to full strength formula over 3–5 days. Until infant is on full strength, feed more often.
- 0–75 days: tube feed q 2 hr at 5% BW. Belly should be rounded but not tight after a feeding and a milk line in the stomach should be visible through the skin.
- By the time they weigh 50 g, they do not tolerate tube feedings. Even before their eyes open a jar lid of warm formula can be placed in with baby opossums. By dipping their noses in the milk and allowing them to walk through the formula they will clean the milk off of themselves (and their littermates) and learn to self-feed faster.
- When able to lap up formula out of bowl, start thickening with rice baby cereal.

Table A7.3. Opossum Care Sheet

Age (Weeks)	Weights (g)	Age determinates	Diet	Amounts	Frequency
2		Whiskers start, blond nose hairs, pink skin	Tube—Esbilac	.50 ml	q 2 hrs, 24 hr
4	20	Blond belly hairs, pink skin	Same	1 ml	q 2–3 hr, 1 PM feeding
5–6	25–35	Slight bluish coloration, ears open	Same	1–2 ml	q 2–3 hr, 1 PM feeding
6–8	35–50	Furred, eye slits developed, mouth fully open	Same	2–3 ml	q 3–4 hr, 1 PM feeding
9	45–52	Eyes open, running around, lapping formula, teeth present, white tipped guard hairs, ears erect	Bowl—Esbilac, add cereal	2.5–3 ml	QID
10–11	50–75	Self-defecating/urinating; 3–6″ excluding tail	Bowl—Esbilac, cereal, add cat or puppy chow	2.5–4 ml	QID
12	75–100	Thermoregulating; 4.5–6.5″	Start weaning	4 ml	TID
13–15	100–500	Actively climbing; 6–10″	Weaned, dry chow	5 ml	BID-TID
15–20	500–1,000	20 weeks—ready for release	Natural foods		BID

- Foods to help facilitate the weaning process: fruit yogurt, meat baby foods, bananas, grapes, cooked sweet potatoes, and apple sauce. These items can be mixed with milk formula in the bowl to encourage self-feeding.
- By 10–12 weeks gradually start adding puppy or cat chow to formula.
- By 16 weeks opossums should be weaned and eating solid food items such as fresh carrion, live crickets, mealworms and earthworms, fruit and vegetables native to area, raw eggs, dead minnows, and crayfish. Lightly sprinkle diet with a calcium supplement. Offer food in the evenings.
- Make sure there is always fresh drinking water available during and after weaning. Opossums have a habit of defecating in their food and water bowls so offer a water bottle to guarantee a clean water source.

Opossum Housing
- Housing: Small box or pet carrier with soft, ravel-free cloth, heating pad set on low, and a source of humidity until 8 weeks old. Careful to use cage lids and small (less than ½ in.) ventilation holes due to opossum's ability to easily escape.

- Maintain nest humidity at 70%.
- Move to ¼″–½″ mesh hardware cloth 2′ × 2′ × 4′ cage at 8–10 weeks.
- Use heating pad until 10 weeks or 80–90 g at external temperatures of 95°F.
- At 12 weeks begin outdoor acclimation. Opossums need exercise and a daily dose of vitamin D_3, naturally provided by sunlight, to help prevent metabolic bone disease (MBD). Opossums are very prone to MBD and must receive daily dietary calcium in addition to 30–60 minutes of unfiltered U/V light.
- Use caution when putting animals in sunlight. Opossums are prone to overheating and can die quickly if not provided with some shade and proper ventilation. They do not need to be in direct sunlight to benefit from natural U/V, just placed outside during daylight hours. Beneficial U/V rays are blocked out by glass windows.
- Move to release cage at 4 months.
- Becoming nocturnal and sleeping during the day by 4 mos.
- Small groups of same age preweanlings can be housed together. Cannibalism can result when housing together older juveniles.

Opossum Release

- Consider release when the opossums are 5 mos. old and 8–10 in. in body length, 1.5 lb., self-feeding, acclimated to weather and outside temperatures and baring teeth at caretaker.
- If the cage is on a suitable release site, open cage door 1 hour before dark and allow opossum to come and go. Provide back-up food until the animals move on.
- Some opossums will leave the cage and explore at night but come back to the nest box by morning and sleep until the next dusk.
- If the cage is not on a suitable site, be certain the animals are ready and release them near cover and trees right before dark.

Opossum Miscellaneous Information

- Opossums are sensitive to corticosteroids and Levamisole is dewormer of choice.
- Opossums tolerate sutures, bandages, and splints well.
- Orphans have immature immune systems so wash hands before/after feeding.

GREY SQUIRRELS

Grey Squirrel Diet and Feeding

Formula: 1 part powdered Esbilac : 2 parts water

- Stomach capacity is 50 ml/kg (.05 ml × BW in g =_____ml)
- Use O-ring syringe with a silicone or Catac nipple to feed orphan squirrels.
- Stimulate after each feeding until 5 weeks.
- A healthy squirrel should gain 4–7 g/day once established on Esbilac formula.
- Squirrels should be fed lying on their stomachs with heads slightly raised.
- Add rice baby cereal to thicken formula at about 3 weeks.
- Add powdered rodent blocks to further thicken formula at about 5 weeks.
- When eyes open and the squirrel is eating rodent blocks or monkey chow, start offering self-feeding diet items such as: cracked nuts, small pieces of fresh corn on the cob, apple, grapes, broccoli stems, cauliflower, and rodent seed mixes.
- Start to wean at 8 weeks and finish by 10–11 weeks.
- Diet offered ratio should be: 80% rodent/primate chow : 20% other items. Do not allow the animal "to choose" a balanced diet for itself; stick with ratio.

- Limit nuts to 1 nut/squirrel/day or they will not eat enough more nutritious foods.
- Make sure squirrel is off milk and eating solid and natural food items for at least 2 weeks prior to release.
- Post-weaning foods: rodent blocks, high quality dog chow (i.e.; Purina One, Proplan, Eukanuba), uncracked acorns, hickory nuts, pecans, buds, bark, pine cones, fungi, sun flower seeds, insects, fresh vegetables; and rodent seed mixes.
- Healthy weaning tool: "squirrel nutri-bites" recipe:

  1½ cups powdered rodent or primate chow
  ⅓ cup powdered Esbilac
  ⅔ cup warm water
  ⅓ cup chopped pecans
  ⅓ cup crushed cuttlebone, if needed.

  Mix together and roll into small meatball-size balls.
  Keep refrigerated up to 3 days or freeze for up to 6 months.

- These "squirrel nutri-bites" can be offered in place of a milk feeding and once the squirrels start eating them they can be offered free choice. Due to the milk content, do not leave them in cages long enough to spoil.

Grey Squirrel Housing

- From 0–4 weeks: lidded box, cardboard pet carrier, plastic or glass aquarium with heating pad on low under ½ of cage.
- Use soft, ravel-free cloth for bedding such as cotton T-shirt, flannel, sweat shirts, fleece.
- At 5–6 weeks discontinue heating pad use.
- Around 6–8 weeks move to a small wire flush bottom cage (½" × 1" mesh or smaller) with tree limbs for climbing and provide a nest box inside cage.
- Start acclimating to outdoor temperatures by placing cage outside during warm days and bringing back in at night. Gradually leave out for longer periods of time until squirrels can comfortably be left out overnight. Baby squirrels do not have to be brought inside if a heat lamp can be provided near one of the nest boxes.
- At 8–12 weeks move squirrel to large outdoor wire release cage (minimum size 4′ × 4′ × 6′), the larger the better. Covered waterproof roof, back, and 1 side. Hang water bottle on cage. Attach nest box to the top of cage. Natural substrate on cage bottom and inside nest box.
- House animals with similarly aged conspecifics.

Table A7.4. Grey Squirrel Care Sheet

Age (weeks)	Weights (g)	Age determinates	Diet	Amounts	Frequency
0–1	15–25	Pink, no fur, eyes closed tight—bulgy	Esbilac	0.5–1.0 ml	q 2 hr, 1pm feeding
1–2	25–35	Scant gray color to head, shoulder & back Day 10—lose umbilical cord	Esbilac	1–2 ml	q 2 hr, 1pm
2–3	35–60	Scant grayish fur, ears unglued, eyes less bulgy; Day 21—lower incisors emerge	Esbilac	2–4 ml	q 2–3 hr, no PM
3–4	60–90	Slick, shiny fur except under tail; ears open, eye slits relaxed and ready to open	Esbilac, add cereal	3–6 ml	q 3–4 hr
4–5	90–115	Downy white hair on belly, slight bush to tail, eyes open, may begin to walk	Esbilac, cereal, add rodent block	5–9 ml	QID
5–6	115–175	Thicker hair, tail curling over back, upper incisors emerge, sitting up	Same; keep thickening	5–12 ml	TID-QID
6–7	175–250	Furry all over, sleeping less, can sit up	Add small pieces fruit	9–15 ml	TID-QID
7–8		Bushy tail, back molars come in	Rodent blocks	15–20 ml	BID-TID
8–9		Looks like miniature squirrel	Begin to wean	20–25 ml	SID-BID
9–10		Furred on underside except for 1″ at base tail, tail bushy	Wean	20–30 ml	SID
10–11	300–425		Wean		
11–12		Tail completely furred	Weaned		
12–14		Ready for release			

Grey Squirrel Release

Release Criteria:
- At least 12–14 weeks of age and acclimated to the outdoors for at least 2 weeks.
- Squirrels should hide at the sight or sound of approaching people and not allow any handling even from the hand raiser.
- Squirrels should be weaned for a minimum of 2 weeks, nest building, eating natural food items, and able to crack open whole shelled raw nuts.
- If so, open cage door and allow animal to come and go. Continue to supply food until squirrels move on or at least for 3–4 weeks.

Table A7.5. Cottontail Care Sheet

Age (weeks)	Weights (g)	Age determinates	Diet	Amounts (ml)	Frequency
0–1	30–40	Pink, thin fur all over, eyes closed, ears flat and closed	KMR	0.5–1.5 ml	3–4 × /day
1–2	35–55	Fully furred, 7–10 days eyes open, ears erect	KMR, offer greens	2–6 ml	2–3 × /day
2–3	50–90	Ear length growth, 3 weeks self-defecating	Same	3–9 ml	1–2 × /day
3–4	60–120	Hopping, running, ears fully erect	Natural food; weaned		0–1 × /day
4–5	150–190	Release			

COTTONTAIL RABBITS

Cottontail Rabbit Diet and Feeding

Formula: 1 part powdered KMR : 2 parts water

- Feed with O-ring syringe and nipple or tube feed rabbits.
- Stomach capacity = 100–125 ml/kg (10%–12.5%) of BW. Safer to use 100 ml/kg or $.1 \times BW$ in gm = _____ ml
- Cottontails benefit by receiving daily Benebac to aid with digestion and diarrhea prevention.
- Rabbits can be fed with a syringe but they seldom suckle. Some will lick formula from the tip of syringe drop by drop or swallow milk as it is dripped onto their lips.
- If your new cottontail refuses to eat, try a drop of Karo syrup on the end of the nipple or adding a bit of baby food (no sugar added) applesauce to the formula. Another trick used is to add orange flavored Pedialyte to the formula to enhance the flavor.
- Allow cottontails to drink as much formula as they want per feeding. Better to feed these babies in as few feedings as possible. Twice a day is the goal as long as they get enough calories and are gaining weight.
- Gavage feeding is a faster method and ideal if there are many babies to feed or if the babies are frightened of handling and refuse to nurse. Be sure to watch a veterinarian or an experienced rehabilitator do this method before first trying it yourself. Although faster, tube feeding can be potentially lethal if done incorrectly. The rabbit's pallet skin is

very fragile and can be punctured by the soft end of the feeding tube resulting in SQ delivery of formula followed by death.

- Stimulate baby rabbits before feeding until its eyes open.
- Keep a secure hold on baby rabbits when handling. Rabbits have a habit of suddenly jumping out of your hands or off the table.
- When eyes are open, start offering diced (easily done with scissors), fresh natural greens (clover greens and flowers, grass, dandelion leaves, alfalfa, privet) twice daily. No stems of plants should be given until rabbits are approximately 3 weeks old. Offer only a small amount at first and be sure greens are clean and chemical free.
- Once they have adjusted to the new food items (3–4 days after they begin to sample it), offer larger amounts. There should always be some left over. After a week of eating solid foods, discontinue dicing the greens and offer them whole.
- Remove uneaten greens as new greens are added. Greens and grasses wilt quickly becoming undesirable to the rabbits and can mold in just a day or two.
- Provide drinking water in a shallow lid or a water bottle when young rabbits start to nibble on solid foods.
- Other solid food items include rabbit chow, rolled oats, wheat germ, corn, apple and carrot slivers, dry hay, or alfalfa fed free choice until released.
- Introduce new food items slowly and one at a time to allow their gut to adjust to the changes.
- Wean rabbits by 3–4 weeks.

Cottontail Rabbit Housing

- From 0–2 weeks use a small cardboard box or aquarium with secure lid.
- Use a heating pad on low under one half of cage or heat light on one half of cage.
- Supply soft, ravel free cloth for bedding. Rabbits like layers to burrow into and prefer to be covered up.
- Once weaned remove heating pad and cloth bedding. Instead, bed with natural substrates such as hay, grasses, leaves, or pine straw.
- At 3 weeks move to a large plastic pet carrier or enclosed rabbit hutch. Rabbits need solid sided cages and a quiet area to reduce stress.
- Do not overcrowd the cages.
- Littermates can be housed together but be careful mixing unrelated animals and do not mix different ages as they tend to fight and become stressed.
- Fatal enteritis can develop from environmental stress.
- Albon at 25–50 mg/kg PO SID × 5–14 days given to all rabbits initially may help prevent enteritis caused by stress-induced coccidiosis flare ups.
- Be sure there are no holes in the cage or cage door larger than ½ inch square because infant rabbits can squeeze out of a 1 by 1 in. hole. Cover securely any questionable holes with burlap, netting, or screen.
- Acclimate to outside temperatures once rabbits are weaned.
- Provide hiding spots such as hay to burrow into, a cardboard or wooden nest box.

Cottontail Rabbit Release

- Ready for release by the end of 4 weeks.
- Many rabbits do not do well in captivity past 5–6 weeks old and should not be kept this long unless there is a medical reason.
- Rabbits ready for release should run and hide from all humans, pets, and noise.
- Release weight is between 100–200 g, ideally about 150 g.
- Find a site with open fields or pasture with nearby cover for a release site. Open cage door and allow rabbits to hop out by themselves or place them under cover and quietly leave the area.
- Cottontails do not need back-up food if released in a proper habitat and they rarely return to release site.
- Release at dusk or dawn in mild weather.

Biological Data of Selected North American Wild Mammals

Appendix 8. Biological Data

Animal	°F body temp	Pulse rate/min	Respiration. rate/min	Weight at birth (g)	Adult weight (kg)	Weaning age (weeks)	Feeding formula	Eyes open (days)	Release age (weeks)
Armadillo	84–92			51–150.3	5–6	8	Esbilac	birth	
Badger	99–102			95	6–11	8–10	Esbilac	28–36	9–12
Bat (big brown)	95–102.2			3.3–4.0	11–16 g	6–8	Mother's Helper k-9	hrs after birth	6–8
Bat (red)	97–98.6			1.5–2.0	10–12 g	3–6		10	6–8
Bear (black)	100–102	60–90	15–30	170–227	90–214	22–26	Esbilac	35–42	1 yr.
Beaver	98–101	100	16	400–500	13–27	6–8	Esbilac	birth	10–12
Bobcat	99–102	110–140	26	283–340	6–15	8–9	KMR	3–11	16–20
Cottontail	100–103	130–325	32–60	35–45	0.9–2	2–3	KMR	6–8	3–4
Coyote	100–103	100–170		200–275	8.1–18	5–7	Esbilac	10–11	6 mo.
Deer (white tail)	101–102	70–80	16–20	2.5–4.0kg	M 34–180 F 22–112	8–12	lamb, doe, goat milk	birth	6–8 mo.
Fox (gray)	100–103			86	3–6	7–8	Esbilac	10–12	20
Fox (red)	100–103			71–119	5–7	8–10	Esbilac	8–9	24
E. Chipmunk	99–102	660–702		2.5–5.0	65–127 g	5–6	Esbilac	30–33	8
Hare (black tailed jack rabbit)	99–102			60–180	1.8–3.6	3–4	KMR	birth	
Mink	99–103	250–300	18–20	6–10	0.5–1.4	5–8	Esbilac	21–30	8–10
Muskrat	98–101	148–306*	45	21	1–2	3–4	Esbilac	14–16	8–10
Opossum (Virginia)	90–99	120–140		.2	4–6	13–15	Esbilac	58–72	15
Otter (river)	99–102	130–178	20–60	132	5–11	12–16	Esbilac	21–35	9 mo.
Porcupine	99–100	280–320	100	400–500	5–12	3–5	Esbilac	birth	10–12
Raccoon	100–103	128–180	15–30	60–75	5–16	10–16	KMR	18–24	20
Skunk (spotted)	101–102			28	.340–1.2	6–8	Esbilac	28–32	
Skunk (striped)	101–102			33	3–6	6–8	Esbilac	14–28	9–12
Squirrel (S. flying)	98–102			3–6	50–79 g	8–9	Esbilac	29–40	12
Squirrels (fox)	98–102			14–18	0.5–1.4	8–9	Esbilac	28–35	12
Squirrel (grey)	98–102	390*		14–18	0.038–0.069	8–9	Esbilac	28–35	12
Weasel (least)	100–103	172–192		1.0–1.5	38–69 g	2–3		26–29	6–8
Wolf	100–102			454	23.5	6–8	Esbilac	11–15	
Woodchuck	99–100	180–264*		28.4–42.5	1.8–6.3	8–12	Esbilac	30	12

Source: Information in part from Evans (1987), Fowler (1979), Stokes (1986), and Schwartz (1974).
* Pulse rate under anesthesia.

Glossary of Medical Conditions and Treatments

Bloat: Causes of bloat include a change in diet, internal parasites, improper diet, feeding a cold infant, overfeeding, or constipation. If an infant bloats, hold its belly down on a heating pad and gently but firmly massage its side from top to bottom of abdomen. Also use gas relief medications such as Di-gel, simethicone, activated charcoal, or powdered calcium carbonate dissolved in water orally in addition to warmth and massage. Long-term treatment is to eliminate the cause of the bloat.

Broken Blood Feathers: Feathers that are actively growing (pin feathers) contain a blood supply and when damaged may bleed. These feathers need to be removed by grasping the quill at the skin surface with hemostats, supporting the bone with the other hand and pulling straight out. The entire feather must be cleanly removed from the follicle for the bleeding to stop.

Bumblefoot: A generalized inflammation of the foot that is most commonly seen in raptors but could occur in any bird. The condition usually starts out as a cut, puncture, swelling, bruising, crack, or abrasion on the bottom of the foot. Bacteria then enter the break in the skin and cause a generalized infection. The problem is often caused by improper or unclean perches and cages. Therapy must include topical cleaning and flushing of the wounds, proper bandaging, and often systemic antibiotics.

Constipation: In infant mammals constipation may be due to over feeding, change in diet, internal parasites, dehydration, intestinal obstruction or too long since stimulation. If increasing the fluid intake and stimulating for a longer than normal time does not work, remove impacted feces in the colon by a warm water or mineral oil enema. A couple of drops of mineral oil or Laxatone orally may help alleviate constipation.

Crop Stasis: "Sour crop" or crop stasis occurs when the contents of the crop fails to empty out. This sometimes occurs when the food was fed too cold, the crop was overfilled, foreign bodies are present or food was sour when fed. Crop infections such as trichomoniasis and systemic illness are other causes. Since the contents must be removed, administer a small amount of sterile water and gently massaging the crop. If the crop does not empty on its own within a few hours, the contents must be removed by drawing the material out with the tube and syringe used to feed the bird. Flush the crop with warm sterile water. Possible treatments consist of antimicrobial therapy and correction of dehydration and nutrition.

Dehydration: The excessive loss of fluid from the body. Dehydration is life threatening and prevents every system in the body from functioning properly. The body cannot digest food, maintain body temperature, deliver proper oxygen or blood flow or excrete toxins in a dehydrated state. The condition must be

Table A9.1. Method to Determine Degree of Dehydration

% Dehydration	Skin turgor in seconds	Clinical signs
6%	1–2	Tented skin; slight loss of skin elasticity
8%	2–3	Eyes slightly depressed; slow CRT; dry tacky mucous membranes
10%	3–5	Sunken eyes and cere; dry, tented, scaly skin; very slow CRT; wrinkling of foot, cere, and eyelid skin; pale oral membranes; feces dry
12%	>5	Early signs of hypovolemic shock; easily collapsible peripheral veins

quickly assessed by determining the level of dehydration and the fluid treatment should be started immediately. Neonates need 2–3 times the fluid requirement of adults.

Maintenance: 50 ml/kg/day (OR) BW in g × .05 = daily mls fluids

Replacement: decimal value of % dehydration × BW in g = daily mls needed 0.10 = 10% (replaces fluid loss volume for volume e.g. diarrhea, hemorrhage)

Dehydration: 100 ml/kg/day (OR) BW in g × .10 = daily mls fluids (give ½ volume over 2–6 hrs; then ½ volume + maintenance over next 24 hours OR 50 ml/kg BID until rehydrated)

The daily volume must be divided by the number of times you wish to administer fluids. Use the least evasive method to resolve the dehydration. Oral is preferred for birds provided the animal is conscious and its bowels are functional. IV therapy is mandatory in cases of dehydration and shock, comatose animals, and starvation.

Emaciation: Body weights and degree of muscle wasting are diagnostic. These animals should slowly be weaned onto solid food depending on category stage. First offer a rehydrating solution such as LRS or LRS with 2.5% Dextrose orally. Then start with a diet such as Ultracal, Ensure, or Isocal. These liquid diets are high calorie, low volume, isotonic (requiring minimum energy for digestion) food sources that can be fed to birds or mammals. Probiotics should be offered to help reestablish normal healthy gut flora. When the animal is hydrated and passing normal looking stools, begin to offer diets for dehabilitated animals such as Clinicare, Hill's A/D, or Emeraid II.

The progression time period from fluids to solid foods will vary from category to category as well as from patient to patient. Always slowly mix new foods in with old diet to make the changes gradual (over several days) and easier on the animal. Meals should be small and as often as possible (weighed against frequent handling stress). These animals should be on vitamin supplementation to promote appetite. Supportive care should include heat and a stress free environment.

Fleas, Ticks: Use VIP flea powder, 5% pyrethrin dust or powder safe for kittens and puppies. Manually remove ticks.

Glue Traps: Use a light sprinkle of cornstarch to neutralize the glue and prevent the animal from becoming more entangled. Cut away as much of the trap as possible. Warm Canola oil to 102–104°F and apply oil to stuck feathers or fur by gently working it in with your fingers. The warmed oil will soften the adhesive bond and after several minutes allow you to remove the animal from the trap. Work the soft gummy substance that forms up and off of the animal without pulling on the feathers or fur directly. After several more minutes most of the glue should be soft enough to be removed or washed out. If the Canola oil leaves a residue you may need to do a Dawn bath and rinse as described under "soiled feathers."

Hyperthermia: Abnormally high body temperature. Factors which predispose animals to hyperthermia are fever, infection, excessive muscular exertion, exposure to high ambient temperatures or high humidity. These patients need to be cooled down quickly. Submerge animals in a cold water bath and perform cold water enemas. Utilizing a circulating air fan will help provide evaporation cooling. The danger here is taking the body temperature down below normal levels so be sure to discontinue cooling methods once temperature nears normal.

Hypothermia: Abnormally low body temperature. Hypothermic animals must be warmed slowly. With temperatures 10–15° below normal, the animal is likely to become comatose and unable to respond or even

Table A9.2. Method to Determine Degree of Emaciation

Category I	Category II	Category III
90–100% BW	75–90% BW	50–70% BW
Not eaten in 1 day	Not eaten in several days	Not eaten in 1 week
Hypoglycemic	Seizures	Near comatose
Mild muscle atrophy	Moderate muscle atrophy	Severe atrophy
Generally salvageable	Difficult to save	Few recoveries

shiver. At this point it is critical that you understand why a heating pad will NOT be effective. Circulation is decreased to the peripheral parts of the body due to the body's attempt to conserve blood for the vital organs so contact heat from a heating pad is wasted. The body is not capable of carrying heat from the skin touching the warm pad into the rest of the body. The best sources of heat are from heat lamps, incubators or a warm water bath that supplies radiant heat evenly over the entire body at one time. Warm water enemas are helpful as well. Gradually increase the temperature and make sure the animal does not burn or get heated up too fast which is equally damaging.

Maggots: In small numbers, best removed manually. Heavy infestations may require flushing with peroxide to kill them. Applying cornstarch to the maggots dries them out and they often fall off. A dose of Ivermectin will kill any remaining maggots and any eggs that may hatch. If the infestation is advanced and they have entered the body cavities, euthanasia is recommended.

Malocclusion: Improper tooth alignment is most critical with rodents and lagomorphs. These animals have two upper and two lower incisors that continue to grow throughout the animal's life. They normally wear down from chewing on hard objects and grinding teeth. Maligned incisors may continue to grow and overgrow resulting in starvation (from not being able to chew food) or self-induced puncture wounds (from the lower teeth puncturing the roof of the mouth). The prognosis is poor with this condition but manually trimming the teeth biweekly or so may allow the teeth time to grow back normally after the animal has healed from the fractured jaw or other facial injury that caused the trauma.

Mites: Dust baby and adult birds with an avian mite powder. Ivermectin applied to the back of the neck will treat birds for mites but be sure to accurately measure dose by body weight not just by applying "a

drop." Ivermectin is effective against mites in mammals by injecting one dose SQ.

Ruptured Air Sac: Appears like an air bubble under the bird's skin often caused by impact trauma such as falling from nest. Small SQ pockets that do no interfere with the bird's mobility or breathing can be left to heal on their own. Otherwise clean the skin over the bubble and make a small incision about ⅛"–¼" long with a sterile scissors to let the air out. Be sure to avoid the cutaneous blood vessels that can usually be seen through the skin.

Shock: The definition of shock is an acute failure of the heart to provide adequate blood flow to the tissues. Signs of shock include glassy eyes, a fixed stare, unresponsive pupils, rigidity of the limbs, paleness of gums, listlessness, decrease in blood pressure, increase in pulse, lower body temperature, or unresponsiveness to stimuli. Treatment is a combination of heat, fluids, medications, oxygen, and stress removal. Seek veterinary care for animals that come into the clinic in this condition.

Soiled Feathers (oil, tar, dirt): Feathers need to remain clean and waterproof to provide insulation and flight. If a bird comes in with soiled feathers or becomes soiled during rehabilitation, a warm water bath (103–104°F) using Dawn dishwashing detergent followed by a clean warm water rinse will remove caked on food, feces, oil, and glue. It is very important to keep the bird warm at all times until completely dry. Wash and dry under a heat lamp if possible. Fill a container with warm soapy water and dip the bird into the solution carefully wiping with the grain of the feathers. Agitate the bird's body around in the solution being careful to keep the animal's head dry. Then dip bird into warm clean rinse water until all soap and residue are gone. Repeat if necessary until water beads on feathers. This procedure is very stressful and should only be done on stable animals.

Wildlife Product Sources

Product Sources

Products	Manufacturer/Supplier	Products	Manufacturer/Supplier
Aviary netting	J.A. Cissel Cutler's Pheasant Supply 3805 Washington Rd. Carsonville, MI 48419 www.cutlersupply.com Memphis Net & Twine Co., Inc. 2481 Matthews Ave. P.O. Box 80331 Memphis, Tennessee 38108-0331 Phone: 800-238-6380 E-mail: memnet@memphisnet.net Sterling Net Co., Inc. 18 Label St., Montclair, NJ 07042 Phone: 800-342-0316 www.sterlingnets.com	Dried insects	www.sirius.com/~monterey/dry_ fish_food.htm Skipios Tillamook, OR Phone: 503-842-5988 www.skipio.com Any good fish, reptile, or pet store
Nipples "Catac" (Latex rubber nursing nipples, 3 sizes,) fits on slip tip or catheter tip syringes	Summit Pet Products 400 Quaint Acres Drive Sliver Springs, MD 20904 Phone: 800-882-9410	Live insects: mealworms, crickets	Grubo, Inc. P.O. Box 15001 Hamilton, OH 45015-0001 Phone: 800-222-3563 www.herp.com/grubco Rainbow Mealworms Inc. Phone: 800-777-9676 www.herp.com/rainbow/ rainbow.htm
Nipples "Mothering Kit" (Silicone small tapered nipples fits on slip tip syringes) Catac nipples, Esbilac, KMR, Multi-Milk, Bene-Bac, plastic feeding cannula	Upco 3705 Pear Street P.O. Box 969 St. Joseph, MO 64502 Phone: 800-254-8726 www.upco.com discounts to licensed rehabilitators Feed stores, pet stores		Nature's Way Phone: 800-318-2611 www.herp.com/nature discount to rehabilitators
Feeding tubes, catheters, Tom Cat catheters	Sovereign Monoject Division of Sherwood Davis & Geck 1915 Olive Street St. Louis, MO 63103 Phone: 800-428-4400	Avimin (avian minerals) Avitron (avian vitamins) Syringes (O-Ring), Esbilac, KMR, Mulit-Milk, Benebac, Catac nipples, Snuggle Safe (microwavable disks that stay warm for 12 hours), Nekton nectars, Zupreem Primate Diet, scales, feeding tubes, homeopathy remedies,cannula tips, reference books, pipettes	Lambert Kay Division of Cater-Wallace, Inc. Half Acre Road P.O. Box 1418 Cranbury, NJ 08512 Phone: 609-655-6293 www.lambertkay.com The Squirrel Store Phone: 877-717-7748 www.thesquirrelstore.com
Rubber feeding catheters, flexible white syringe tip, pipettes, O-ring syringes	Coconut Creek Publishing Co. Phone: 888-WRT-1020 www.wildliferehabtoday.com		

Products	Manufacturer/Supplier	Products	Manufacturer/Supplier
Syringes (O-Ring)	Feeding Tech P.O. Box 246 Nineveh, IN 46164 Phone: 800-688-0850		Krieger Publishing Co. Natural Science & Veterinary Topics Catalog Phone: 800-724-0025 www.web4u.com/krieger- publishing/
	Medcare 246E. 131st Street Cleveland, OH 44108 Phone: 800-433-4550		Coconut Creek Publishing Co. 2300 W. Sample Rd., Suite 314 Pompano Beach, FL 33073-3046 Phone: 888-WRT-1020
Animals for food: Rats & Mice Coturnix Quail, eggs, chicks; Frozen: rats, mice, chicks, and live crickets	The Gourmet Rodent Bill & Marcia Brant 6115 SW 137th Ave. Archer, FL 32618 Phone: 352-495-9024 grmtrodent@aol.com	Monkey Biscuits/Chow	Jeffers West Plains, MO phone: 1-800-533-3377 JeffersPet.com Zupreem-primate chow
	Northwest Gamebirds 228812 E. Game Farm Rd. Kennewick, WA 99337 Phone: 509-586-0150 www.northwest-gamebirds.com	Hummingbird nectars	Guenter Enderle Enterprises, Inc. Nekton Tarpon Springs, Florida Phone: 727-938-1544 www.nekton.de
	Perfect Pets, Inc. Dept. WRT 23180 Sherwood Belleville, MI 48111 Phone: 800-366-8794 www.perfectpet.net		Roudybush Nectar Hummingbird nectars 1-800-326-1726
Zoologic Milk Matrix products, Esbilac, KMR, Multi-Milk	Pet- Ag, Inc. Phone: 800-323-0877	CliniCare	Abbott Laboratories- Animal Health Feline and Canine Liquid Diet 1-847-935-4849
Mesh cages (reptariums)	That Pet Place 237 Centerville Road Lancaster, PA 17603 Phone: 717-299-5691 www.thatpetplace.com	Isocal	Mead Johnson & Company Evansville, Indiana 47721
		Human Tube-Feeding Formula	Order from local pharmacy
Wildlife related book sources—Mail-order catalogues specializing in: Natural history books, field guides, veterinary topics, rehabilitation manuals	Zoo Book Sales 403 Parkway Ave. N Mail To: P.O. Box 405 Lanesboro, MN 55949-0405 Phone: 507-467-8733 www.zoobooksales.com	Emeraid I & II	Lafeber Company Cornell, IL Phone: 800-842-6445 ext. 888 www.lafeber.com
	Wild Ones Animal Books P.O. Box 275 Half Moon Bay, CA 94019 Phone: 800-539-0210 wildonesbooks@compuserve.com	Rodent blocks	Kaytee Products, Inc., Chilton, WI phone: 1-800-KAYTEE-1 www.Kaytee.com
			Pet stores that sell Kaytee products
	Wildlife Publications PMB 293 897 Oak Park Blvd., Pismo Beach, CA 93449 Phone: 805-489-0411 www.wildcare.com	Animal-related catalogues: Animal handling & restraint Nets, Traps, Punch Poles, Animal Handling Gloves, Blowpipes, Darting Equipment, Ketch-All Poles, Snake Hooks	Aces Animal Care Equipment & Services, Inc. P.O. Box 3275 340 Highway 138 Crestline, CA 92325 Phone: 800-338-ACES www.animal-care.com

Products	Manufacturer/Supplier	Products	Manufacturer/Supplier
	Tomahawk Live Trap P.O. Box 323 Tomahawk, WI 54487 Phone: 800-272-8727 www.livetrap.com		R.C. Steele 1989 Transit Way P.O. Box 910 Brockport, NY 14420-0910 Phone: 800-872-3773
	Ketch All Company Phone: 877-538-2425 www.ketch-all.com	Animal Caging Products Cages, wire, netting, latches, watering systems, cage building supplies, incubators, brooders, heat lights, etc.	Valentine Inc. 4259 S. Western Blvd Chicago, IL 60609 Phone: 800-GET-STUFF
ThermoCare Intensive Care Units	Thermocare Inc. P.O. Box 6069 Incline Village, NV 89450 Phone: 800-262-4020		Stromberg's P.O. Box 400 Pine River, MN 56474 Phone: 800-720-1134
Banding & tagging supplies	National Band & Tag Company 721 York Street P.O. Box 72430 Newport, KY 41072-0430 Phone: 859-261-2035	Chicken / Duck starter Crumbled balanced diet for growing ducks, chicken, geese	Feed stores and some larger pet stores
			Usually sold by 10 lb. or 25 lb. bags
Pet Store Products: Bowls, vitamins, foods, milk formulas, cages, water bottles, vaccines, Nutri-cal, books, etc.	Upco Phone: 800-254-UPCO www.upco.com	Falconry equipment, raptor books, raptor handling gloves	Northwoods Limited P.O. Box 874 Rainier, WA 98576 Phone: 800-446-5080 www.northwoodsfalconry.com
	That Pet Place Phone: 888-THAT-PET www.thatpetplace.com	Reptile Equipment Tongs, hooks, transport bags, heat lamps, U/V light bulbs, light stands, etc.	Mid-West Products 14505 S. Harris Rd. Greenwood, MO 64034 Phone: 816-537-4444 www.tongs.com
	Pet Warehouse P.O. Box 310 Xenia, OH 45385-0310 Phone: 800-443-1160		

Additional Reading

NATURAL HISTORY

Eastman, J. 1997. *Birds of Forest, Yard and Thicket.* Mechanicsburg, PA: Stackpole Books.

Eastman, J. 1999. *Birds of Lake, Pond and Marsh.* Mechanicsburg, PA: Stackpole Books.

Eastman, J. 2000. *Birds of Field and Shore.* Mechanicsburg, PA: Stackpole Books.

Ehrlich PR, Dobkin DS, and Wheye, D. 1988. *The Birder's Handbook, A Field Guide to the Natural History of North American Birds.* Fireside, Simon & Schuster.

Fox, N. 1995. *Understanding the Birds of Prey.* Blaine, WA: Hancock House Publishers.

Johnsgard, P. 1988. *North American Owls, Biology and Natural History.* Smithsonian Institution.

Peterson, RT. 1980. *Peterson Field Guides.* Boston: Houghton Mifflin Company.

Rue, LL, III. 1981. *Furbearing Animals of North America.* New York: Crown Publishers, Inc.

Stokes, D, and Stokes, L. 1986. *Stokes Nature Guides, A Guide to Animal Tracking and Behavior.* Boston: Little Brown & Co.

Stokes, D, and Stokes, L. 1979. *Stokes Nature Guides, A Guide to Bird Behavior.* Volumes 1–3. Boston: Little Brown & Co.

Terres JK. 1980. *The Audubon Encyclopedia of North America Birds.* New York: Alfred A. Knopf, Inc.

Tyrrell, EQ. 1985. *Hummingbirds, Their Life and Behavior.* New York: Crown Publishers, Inc.

RODENTS

Allen, EG. 1938. The Habits and Life History of the Eastern Chipmunk (Tamias striatus lysteri*). NY State Museum Bulletin.*

Barkalow, F, and Shorten, M. 1973. *The World of the Gray Squirrel.* New York: J.B. Lippincott Co.

Booth, ES. 1946. Notes on the Life History of the Flying Squirrel. *Journal of Mammalogy* 27 (1): 28–30.

Costello, DF. 1966. *The World of the Porcupine.* New York: Lippincott Co.

Nichols, JT. 1958. Food Habits and Behavior of the Grey Squirrel. *Journal of Mammalogy* 39 (3): 376–80.

Rue, LL, III. 1964. *The World of the Beaver.* Philadelphia: J.B. Lippincott.

LAGOMORPHS

Lockley, RM. 1964. *The Private Life of the Rabbit.* New York: Macmillan Publishing Co., Inc.

OPOSSUM

Keefe, JF, & Wooldridge, D. 1967. *The World of the Opossum.* Philadelphia: J.B. Lippincott.

McManus, J. 1974. *Didelphis virginian.* Mammalian Species, No. 40: 1–6.

Nave, P, and Lacy, J. 1983. Rehabilitation notes: Opossum (*Didelphis marsupialis*). WRC J, Winter, 7–10.

CANIDS

Fox, MW. 1971. *Behavior of Wolves, Dogs and Related Canids.* New York: Harper & Row.

Rue, LL, III. 1969. *The World of the Red Fox.* Philadelphia: J.B. Lippincott.

Van Wormer, J. 1964. *The World of the Coyote.* Philadelphia: J.B. Lippincott.

MUSTELIDS

Caine-Stage, M. 1990. American River Otter, *Lutra canadensis.* Wildlife Journal 13(1): 7–10.

Hall, RR. 1951. *American Weasels.* Lawrence: University of Kansas Press.

357

Park, E. 1971. *The World of the Otter.* New York: J.B. Lippincott.

Verts, BJ. 1967. *Biology of the Striped Skunk.* Urbana, IL: University of Illinois Press.

PROCYONS

Goldman, EA. 1950. *Raccoons of North and Middle America.* U.S. Department of Interior, U.S. Fish and Wildlife Services, North American Fauna 60. Washington, DC.

Rue, LL, III. 1964. *The World of the Raccoon.* Philadelphia: J.B. Lippincott.

Stuewer, FW. 1943. *Raccoons: Their Habits and Management in Michigan.* Michigan Ecol Monograph, 13:203–57.

WILDLIFE REHABILITATION ORGANIZATIONS

Basically Bats Wildlife Conservation Society, Inc.
6146 Fieldcrest Dr., Morrow, GA 30260

BCI—Bat Conservation International
P.O. Box 162603, Austin, TX 78716
phone: (512) 327-9721
www.batcon.org

IWRC—International Wildlife Rehabilitation Council
4437 Central Place, Suite B-4 Suisun, CA 94585-1633
phone: (707) 864-1761
fax: (707) 864-3106
iwrc@inreach.com
www.iwrc-online.org. This site offers wildlife care, literature catalogues, non-releasable animal placement, jobline, symposium information, standards, rehabilitation links.

NOS—National Opossum Society, Inc.
Anita M. Henness, DVM
P.O. Box 3091, Orange, CA 92857-0091
phone: (714) 539-3896
Yearly Subscription

NWRA—National Wildlife Rehabilitation Association
14 North 7th Ave, St. Cloud, MN 56303
phone: (320) 259-4086
nwra@cloudnet.com

www.nwrawildlife.org. This site offers NWRA/IWRC Minimum Standards, state and federal permit agency listings, career page, baby animal care, publications, literature order reprints, upcoming events, and symposium.

Wildlife Rehabilitation Today
semiannual magazine
Coconut Creek Publishing Company
2300 West Sample Road, Suite 314
Pompano Beach, FL 33073-3046
home (954) 977-5058
fax (954) 977-5158
www.wildliferehabtoday.com

REHABILITATION BOOKS

These books can be purchased from the IWRC or NWRA web sites or the other book companies listed on the product source pages.

Bats in Captivity. 1995. By Susan M. Barnard. Now available free of charge on line at www.basically-bats.org/onlinebook.htm.

Care and Management of Captive Raptors. 1996. By Lori Arent and Mark Martelli; The Raptor Center of The University of Minnesota; www.raptor.cvm.umn.edu.

Care and Rehabilitation of Injured Owls, 4th ed., 1987. By Katherine Mckeever. The Owl Rehabilitation Research Foundation, Vineland, Ontario, Canada.

Complete Rehabilitation Guide for North American Bats. By Amanda Lollar, Barbara French, and Patricia Winters.

IWRC—Basic Wildlife Rehabilitation 1AB Skills Seminar, 5th ed. rev. By Jan White, DVM. An interpretation of existing biological and veterinary literature for the wildlife rehabilitator. Includes anatomy, physiology, calculating drug dosages, nutrition, housing, release, euthanasia, and more.

Medical Management of Birds of Prey: A Collection of Notes on Selected Topics. 1993. By Patrick Redig, D.V.M., Ph.D. University of Minnesota.

North American River Otter, Lontra canadensis, *Husbandry Notebook,* 2nd ed. 2001. By Janice Reed-Smith. John Ball Zoological Gardens, Grand Rapids, MI.

NWRA Quick Reference. Includes a glossary, abbreviations, tables, calculations, and anatomy pertaining to wildlife.

NWRA—Principles of Wildlife Rehabilitation, The Essential Guide for Novice and Experienced Rehabilitators. By Adele T. Moore and Sally Joosten. Printed by Burgess International Group Inc., Edina, MN.

NWRA/IWRC Minimum Standards for Wildlife Rehabilitation. Includes basic housing requirements for mammals and birds, euthanasia standards, and disease transmission (available free on IWRC/NWRA web site).

Raptor Rehabilitation: A Manual of Guidelines. By Mathias Engelmann, Pat Marcum. The Carolina Raptor Center (1993); www.birdsofprey.org.

Wild Animal Care and Rehabilitation Manual, 4th ed. 1991. Kalamazoo Nature Center, 7000 North Westedge Ave. Kalamazoo, MI 49007; phone (616) 381-1574; fax (616) 381-2557.

Wildlife Neighbors: The Humane Approach to Living with Wildlife. 1997. Edited by John Hadidian, Guy R. Hodge, and John W. Grandy. The Humane Society of the United States.

WEB SITES AND MAILING LISTS USEFUL TO REHABILITATORS

- Centers for Disease Control and Prevention: www.cdc.gov
- Diseases and zoonotics: www.cdc.gov/ncidod/diseases/diseases/htm
- Links to hundreds of veterinary related sites: www.netvet.wustl.edu
- Merck Veterinary Manual: www.merck.com
  This site includes rehabilitation laws, publications, online bulletin board, locating a rehabilitator, information on nuisance wildlife, helping wildlife, and other wildlife web site links.
- Tips on dealing with urban wildlife: www.ianr.unl.edu/wildlife
- Tri-State Bird Rescue and Research: www.tristatebird.org
- USF&W home page: www.fws.gov
- Wildlife health: www.emtc.nbs.gov/http_data/whip/
- Wildlife Rehabilitation Information Directory: www.tc.umn.edu/~devo0028/index.htm
- WLREHAB—Internet mailing list for wildlife rehabilitators: To Subscribe, send an e-mail to: listserve@listserv.nodak.edu with a blank subject line and text that reads: subscribe WLREHAB.

TECHNICAL PERIODICALS

Available at local, university, or state libraries.

American Naturalist
American Zoology
Ecology
International Zoo Yearbook
Journal of American Veterinary Association
Journal of Herpetology
Journal of Mammalogy
Journal of Wildlife Diseases
Journal of Wildlife Management
Journal of Zoo Animal Medicine
Journal of Zoology
Natural History
Natural Magazine

Supplies Necessary for an Exotic Practice

3.5–5 red French rubber catheters
Drinking water bottles
Electrocautery unit
Avian feeding formulas
2–3.5mm Endotracheal tubes
Feeding tubes
Gavage needles of various sizes
Gram scale
Gram stain kit
Heat lamps
Heated cages
Heating pads
Incubators
Induction chamber/Oxygen cage
Instrument pack with small hemostats, scissors, forceps, and needle holders

Isoflurane or sevoflurane precision vaporizer
Microdrip IV sets and pumps
Microtainer blood collection tubes
Mouth speculum (stainless steel and rubber)
Nasolacrimal cannulas
Nolvasan solution and scrub
Perches of different sizes
Rigid endoscope
Small anesthesia masks (cones)
Small hand towels
Small nonrebreathing circuit
Small rebreathing bag for an anesthesia machine
Sterile cotton tip applicators
Uncuffed endotracheal tubes
Wing trimming scissors

Index

Note: Page numbers in *italics* refer to illustrations and those followed by "t" refer to tables.